# Introductory Head and Neck Imaging

# Introductory Head and Neck Imaging

**Eugene Yu** MD FRCPC
University of Toronto
Canada

**Lalitha Shankar** MD FRCPC
University of Toronto
Canada

*Foreword*
**Suresh K Mukherji**

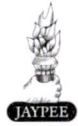

**JAYPEE BROTHERS MEDICAL PUBLISHERS**
*The Health Sciences Publisher*
New Delhi | London

## Jaypee Brothers Medical Publishers (P) Ltd.

**Headquarter**
EMCA House
23/23-B, Ansari Road, Daryaganj
New Delhi 110 002, India
Landline: +91-11-23272143, +91-11-23272703
+91-11-23282021, +91-11-23245672
E-mail: jaypee@jaypeebrothers.com

**Corporate Office**
4838/24, Ansari Road, Daryaganj
New Delhi 110 002, India
Phone: +91-11-43574357
Fax: +91-11-43574314
E-mail: jaypee@jaypeebrothers.com

**Overseas Office**
J.P. Medical Ltd.
83, Victoria Street, London
SW1H 0HW (UK)
Phone: +44-2031708910
E-mail: info@jpmedpub.com

**EU GPSR** Authorised Representative
Logos Europe, 9 rue Nicolas Poussin
17000, La Rochelle, France
Phone: +33 (0) 6 67 93 73 78
E-mail: contact@logoseurope.eu

Website: www.jaypeebrothers.com
Website: www.jaypeedigital.com

© 2014, Jaypee Brothers Medical Publishers

The views and opinions expressed in this book are solely those of the original contributor(s)/author(s) and do not necessarily represent those of editor(s) of the book.

All rights reserved. No part of this publication may be reproduced, stored or transmitted in any form or by any means, electronic, mechanical, photo copying, recording or otherwise, without the prior permission in writing of the publishers.

All brand names and product names used in this book are trade names, service marks, trademarks or registered trademarks of their respective owners. The publisher is not associated with any product or vendor mentioned in this book.

Medical knowledge and practice change constantly. This book is designed to provide accurate, authoritative information about the subject matter in question. However, readers are advised to check the most current information available on procedures included and check information from the manufacturer of each product to be administered, to verify the recommended dose, formula, method and duration of administration, adverse effects and contra indications. It is the responsibility of the practitioner to take all appropriate safety precautions. Neither the publisher nor the author(s)/editor(s) assume any liability for any injury and/or damage to persons or property arising from or related to use of material in this book.

This book is sold on the understanding that the publisher is not engaged in providing professional medical services. If such advice or services are required, the services of a competent medical professional should be sought.

Every effort has been made where necessary to contact holders of copyright to obtain permission to reproduce copy-right material. If any have been inadvertently overlooked, the publisher will be pleased to make the necessary arrange-ments at the first opportunity.

**Inquiries for bulk sales may be solicited at:** jaypee@jaypeebrothers.com

### *Introductory Head and Neck Imaging*

*First Edition*: 2014
*Reprint*: **2026**

ISBN 978-93-5152-207-2

*Printed in India*

**Dedicated to**

My wife Grace, for her continual support and understanding,
and for entertaining our two children
Ryan and Charlotte during this venture.

*Eugene Yu*


My husband Shanky, a pillar of support and lets my dreams
come true and my two children Samantha and Meghana
who have read through many of these chapters and
have assisted me throughout this project.

*Lalitha Shankar*

# Contributors

**Aditya Bharatha** MD
Division of Neuroradiology
Department of Medical Imaging
Victoria Hospital, London
Health Sciences Center
University of Western Ontario
London, Ontario, Canada

**Alan Johnson** MD
Assistant Professor
Department of Neuroradiology
Division Chief of
Neuroradiology
Long Island Jewish Medical
Center
Long Island, New York, USA

**Andrew Law** MBBS
Neurological Intervention and
Imaging Service of
Western Australia (NIISWA)
Sir Charles Gairdner Hospital
and Royal Perth Hospital
Perth, Western Australia
Australia

**Andrew Thompson** MBBS
Neurological Intervention and
Imaging Service of
Western Australia (NIISWA)
Sir Charles Gairdner Hospital
and Royal Perth Hospital
Perth, Western Australia
Australia

**Annie Hsu** MD PhD
Department of
Radiation Oncology
Stanford University Medical
Center
Stanford, California, USA

**Arjun Sahgal** MD
Department of
Radiation Oncology
Princess Margaret Hospital
and the Sunnybrook Health
Sciences Center
University of Toronto
Toronto, Ontario, Canada

**Claudia Kirsch** MD
Associate Professor
Department of Neuroradiology
and Head and Neck Radiology
Section Chief
Head and Neck Radiology
Director
Radiology Medical Student
Teaching
Associate Radiology Resident
Director
The Ohio State University
College of Medicine, USA

**Colin S Poon** MD PhD FRCPC
University of Chicago
Chicago, USA

**Daniel M Mandell** MD
University of Toronto
Ontario, Canada

**David Ashton** MBBS
Radiology Consultant
Sydney, Australia

**Dorothy Lazinski** MD
Division of Neuroradiology
University of Toronto
Ontario, Canada

**Dzung Vu** MBBS
Radiology Consultant
Sydney, Australia

**Edward Kassel** MD DDS FRCPC
Division of Neuroradiology
University of Toronto
Ontario, Canada

**Eric Bartlett** MD FRCPC
Assistant Professor
Department of Neuroradiology
Head and Neck Division
Joint Department of Medical
Imaging
Otolaryngology, Head and Neck
Surgery
Princess Margaret Hospital
University of Toronto
Toronto, Ontario, Canada

**Eugene Yu** MD
Department of
Medical Imaging and
Otolaryngology
Head and Neck Surgery
University Health Network
Mount Sinai Hospital and
Women's College Hospital
University of Toronto
Toronto, Ontario, Canada

**Hugh D Curtin** MD FACR
Chief of Radiology
Massachusetts Eye and Ear
Infirmary, Boston
Professor of Radiology
Harvard Medical School
Boston, MA, USA

# Contributors

**Jessie Aw** MD FRCR
University of Chicago
Chicago, USA

**Juan Pablo Cruz** MD
Division of Neuroradiology
St. Michael's Hospital
University of Toronto
Toronto, Ontario, Canada

**Karen P Chu** MD
Department of Radiation Oncology
Princess Margaret Hospital
University of Toronto
Toronto, Ontario, Canada

**Keng-Yeow Tay** MBBS
Division of Neuroradiology
Department of Medical Imaging
Victoria Hospital, London Health Sciences Center
University of Western Ontario
London, Ontario, Canada

**Kristin McNamara** DDS
Assistant Professor
Department of Oral and Maxillofacial Surgery
Anesthesiology and Pathology
The Ohio State University College of Dentistry
Columbus, OH, USA

**Lalitha Shankar** MD
University of Toronto
Toronto, Ontario, Canada

**Laurent Létourneau-Guillon** MD
Department of Medical Imaging
University Health Network
University of Toronto
Toronto, Ontario, Canada

**Makki Almuntashri** FRCPC
University of Toronto
Toronto, Ontario, Canada

**Manas Sharma** MBBS
Department of Medical Imaging
University Health Network
University of Toronto
Toronto, Ontario, Canada

**Peter Yang**
Medical Student Trainee
University of Toronto
Toronto, Ontario, Canada

**Reza Forghani** MD PhD FRCPC DABR
Associate Chief
Department of Radiology
Sir Mortimer B. Davis Jewish General Hospital
Assistant Professor of Radiology
McGill University
Montreal, Quebec, Canada

**Samantha Shankar** MD
PGY-5 Radiology Resident
Long Island Jewish Medical Center
Long Island, New York, USA

**Timo Krings** MD
Division of Neuroradiology
Toronto Western Hospital
Toronto, Ontario, Canada

**Tom Marotta** MD
Division of Neuroradiology
St. Michael's Hospital
University of Toronto
Toronto, Ontario, Canada

**Vinh Nguyen** MD
Assistant Professor
Department of Neuroradiology
Section Chief of Head and Neck Radiology
Long Island Jewish Medical Center
Long Island, New York, USA

# Foreword

I was extremely honored when I was invited to write this foreword for *Introductory Head and Neck Imaging*. I think this is a very important textbook that meets an essential educational need. Our subspecialty is complex enough and my job as an educator is made even harder by each new "comprehensive" head and neck textbook that is published. I think the hardest part about head and neck imaging is to have the will to first open the study! If a teacher can get his audience to have the desire to first look at a head and neck study, then it is very likely they will enjoy our subspecialty.

*Introductory Head and Neck Imaging* achieves this goal and is written for radiology residents, neuroradiology fellows and general radiologists with its goal to introduce the reader to our terrific subspecialty. The name of the textbook underscores the intent which is to provide a basic core of knowledge in head and neck imaging. The work is not meant to be an exhaustive treatise in head and neck imaging but instead to provide the readers with a digestible introduction to the field. Those interested could then supplement their knowledge through targeted review articles or a more comprehensive textbook.

I can speak from experience when I say that such a textbook is long overdue. I remember my first introduction to head and neck imaging which was reading a small introductory textbook by June Unger. That textbook introduced me to the field that eventually became my career. I am convinced that Lalitha Shankar and Eugene Yu have created a textbook that will be an important asset to any individual who cares for patients with head and neck disorders. I would recommend this textbook to radiologists, regardless of training level or subspecialty and I am sure this interesting and readable textbook will help achieve my ultimate goal…which is to make every radiologist a head and neck radiologist!

**Suresh K Mukherji** MD FACR
Professor of Radiology
Otolaryngology, Head and Neck Surgery and Radiation Oncology
Division Director of Neuroradiology
University of Michigan Health System

Professor of Periodontics and Oral Medicine
University of Michigan School of Dentistry
Ann Arbor, MI, USA

# Preface

"Observation is more than seeing; it is knowing what you see and comprehending its significance."
                                                         –*Anonymous*

Our textbook is an introduction to the field of head and neck imaging. This work is intended primarily for radiology residents and neuroradiology fellows and its goal is to provide a solid foundation upon which the reader can build and develop their knowledge and comprehension of this fascinating subspecialty.

We chose to name this textbook *Introductory Head and Neck Imaging* in order to emphasize our intention of providing the readers with a basic core of information and knowledge that adequately covers the various components of head and neck imaging in a manner that is easily readable and comprehendible. The work is not meant to be an exhaustive reference text of head and neck imaging but instead provides the readers with an approachable introduction to the field.

We are fortunate to have been able to assemble together a group of talented educators that have devoted a significant amount of their time and energy to present and introduce the readers to the imaging of some of the most complex anatomical regions and pathological entities in radiology. The contributors are confident that the results of their dedication and efforts have produced a textbook that will be an asset to radiologists-in-training, fellows, general radiologists and also physicians in affiliated specialties such as otolaryngology, and radiation oncology.

Each of the chapters focuses on a particular anatomic region of the extracranial head and neck. Chapters begin by introducing the reader to the imaging anatomy of that particular area. This is followed by a discussion and review of some of the more common pathologic entities that affect that particular region of anatomy. The textbook also includes an introductory chapter on the Introduction of Radiation Oncology. The contributors feel strongly that this will provide valuable insight for the non-radiation oncologist readers and help enhance their knowledge of a field with whom the contemporary head and neck image works in partnership with very closely.

Finally, we would like to thank all of the talented contributors and teachers who have contributed their valuable time, dedication and unique skills in the preparation of the textbook. We also note the help and continued support of the dedicated editorial team of M/s Jaypee Brothers Medical Publishers (P) Ltd, New Delhi, India, without all of them, the textbook would not have been possible.

**Eugene Yu**
**Lalitha Shankar**

# Contents

## 1. Imaging techniques in head and neck — 1
*Colin S Poon, Jessie Aw*

- Computed tomography  *2*
- Magnetic resonance imaging  *4*
- Positron emission tomography  *9*
- Ultrasound  *10*
- X-ray esophagram  *12*

## 2. Radiographic anatomy and pathology of the temporal bone — 15
*Samantha Shankar, Alan Johnson, Vinh Nguyen*

- Embryology  *15*

### Normal CT and MRI anatomy of the temporal bone  *16*
- The external ear  *16*
- The middle ear  *18*
- The facial nerve  *25*
- The inner ear  *25*
- Imaging of the temporal bone with CT and MRI  *36*

### Temporal bone pathology  *37*
- The external ear  *37*
- The middle ear  *48*
- Facial nerve  *63*
- The inner ear  *68*
- Trauma  *79*

## 3. Imaging of the orbit — 86
*Makki Almuntashri, Edward Kassel*

- Anatomy of the orbit  *86*
- Congenital anomalies  *92*

- Orbital infections  98
- Orbital neoplasms  105
- Inflammatory diseases of the orbit  122
- Trauma of the orbit  129
- Intraocular detachments  133
- Some overall thoughts about the orbit  134

## 4. Imaging of the paranasal sinuses  142
*David Ashton, Dzung Vu, Lalitha Shankar, Eugene Yu*

- Normal anatomy  142
- Paranasal sinus imaging anatomy  146
- Benign lesions  215

## 5. Diseases of the nasopharynx  229
*Manas Sharma, Eugene Yu, Peter Yang*

- Anatomy  229
- Imaging of the nasopharynx  230
- Diseases of the nasopharynx  231
- Nasopharyngeal cysts  231
- Lymphoid hyperplasia/hyperplastic adenoid  233
- Juvenile angiofibroma  234
- Nasopharyngeal tuberculosis  237
- Nasopharyngeal carcinoma  240
- Lymphoma  247
- Other rare nasopharyngeal disorders  251

## 6. Imaging of the masticator and parapharyngeal spaces  257
*Dorothy Lazinski*

### Part I: The masticator space  257
- Anatomy  257
- Imaging anatomy  259
- Muscles of mastication  262

- Mandible  *267*
- Odontogenic tumor  *269*
- Neurogenic lesions  *273*

**Part II: The parapharyngeal space**  *279*
- Anatomy  *279*
- Pathology  *283*
- Patterns of parapharyngeal fat displacement  *284*
- Infection  *286*
- Tumors  *287*
- Retrostyloid parapharyngeal space  *294*

## 7. Radiographic anatomy and pathology of the oral cavity  302
*Claudia Kirsch, Kristin McNamara*

- Cross-sectional anatomy of the oral cavity  *303*
- Imaging of the oral cavity with CT and MRI  *309*
- Pathology  *310*

## 8. Oropharynx  333
*Aditya Bharatha, Keng-Yeow Tay*

- Radiologic anatomy  *333*

## 9. Diseases of the parotid gland  355
*Andrew Law, Andrew Thompson*

- Embryology  *355*
- Anatomy  *355*
- Imaging overview  *357*
- Normal variants  *360*
- Pathology  *360*
- Autoimmune/inflammatory/infiltrative  *364*
- Trauma  *369*
- Benign neoplasms  *369*
- Malignant neoplasms  *382*

## 10. Perineural disease in the head and neck — 394
*Manas Sharma, Laurent Létourneau-Guillon*

- Anatomy  *398*
- Imaging considerations: techniques and features  *409*
- Normal variants and differential diagnosis  *419*

## 11. Imaging evaluation of cervical lymph nodes — 421
*Reza Forghani, Hugh D Curtin*

- Physiology and radiologic anatomy of cervical nodes  *422*
- Pathology  *447*

## 12. The larynx and the hypopharynx — 505
*Eric S Bartlett*

- The role of imaging  *507*
- Imaging anatomy—larynx  *509*
- Imaging anatomy—hypopharynx  *516*
- Anatomic details  *518*
- Pathology  *519*

## 13. Carotid, prevertebral, and perivertebral spaces — 531
*Daniel M Mandell*

### Carotid space  *531*
- Anatomy  *531*
- Pseudolesions  *532*
- Vascular diseases  *533*
- Neoplastic  *539*
- Nerve sheath neoplasms  *543*

### Retropharyngeal space  *548*
- Anatomy  *548*
- Infectious or inflammatory  *549*
- Neoplastic  *552*

### Perivertebral space  *555*
- Anatomy  *555*
- Infectious or inflammatory  *555*
- Neoplastic  *557*

## 14. Vascular lesions of the head and neck  560
*Juan Pablo Cruz, Timo Krings, Tom Marotta*

- Vascular malformations  *560*
- Traumatic vascular lesions  *572*
- Other vascular diseases  *579*
- Vascular tumors  *584*
- Hypervascular lymphadenopathies  *603*

## 15. Diseases of the thyroid gland  610
*Andrew Law, Andrew Thompson*

- Embryology  *610*
- Anatomy  *610*
- Imaging overview  *612*
- Pathology  *617*
- Inflammatory  *618*

## 16. Introduction to radiation oncology  634
*Karen P Chu, Annie Hsu, Arjun Sahgal*

- Clinical radiation oncology  *643*
- Clinical radiotherapy planning  *646*

*Index*  659

## Plate 1

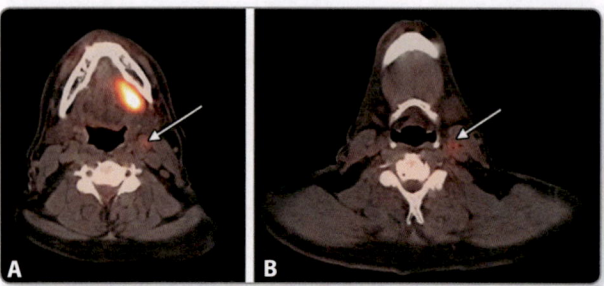

**Figures 1.7A and B** Squamous cell carcinoma of oral tongue with metastatic lymphadenopathy. (A, B) Axial fused PET-CT images demonstrate avid uptake in the left oral tongue squamous cell carcinoma. Abnormal uptake in left level 2 nodes is seen (arrows); subsequently proven to be pathological although not enlarged

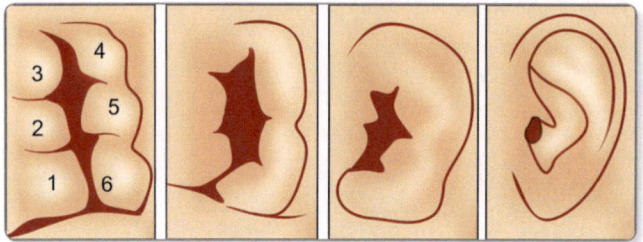

**Figure 2.1** Embryology of the auricle. Six hillocks form around the dorsal extremity of the embryo from the first branchial groove which fuses to form the external pinna

Plate 2

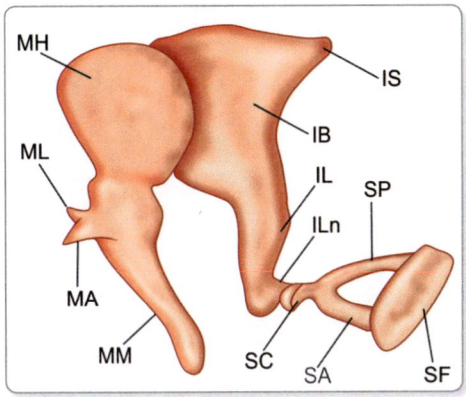

**Figure 2.3A** Diagram of the middle ear ossicles. Malleolar head (MH), malleus anterior process (MA), malleus lateral process (ML), manubrium of malleus (MM), incus body (IB), incus long process (IL), incus short process (IS), lenticular process of incus (ILn), stapes capitellum (SC), anterior stapes anterior crura (SA), posterior stapes crura (SP) and stapes footplate (SF)

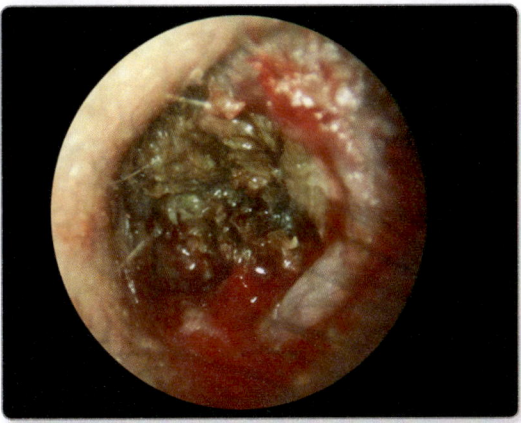

**Figure 2.7A** 30-year-old patient with otalgia and conductive hearing loss. Otoscopic image of the EAC demonstrating a large, bleeding, keratinous mass obstructing the EAC with erosion and widening of the EAC

## Plate 3

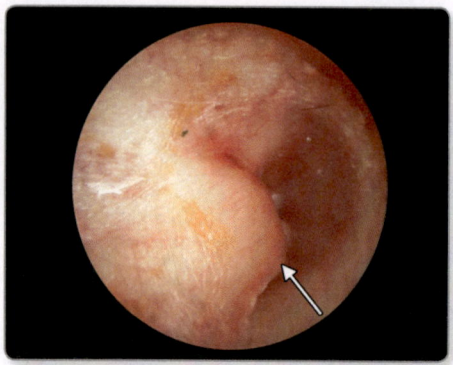

**Figure 2.9A** Otoscopic image of the EAC demonstrating the presence of large masses (white arrow) in the EAC

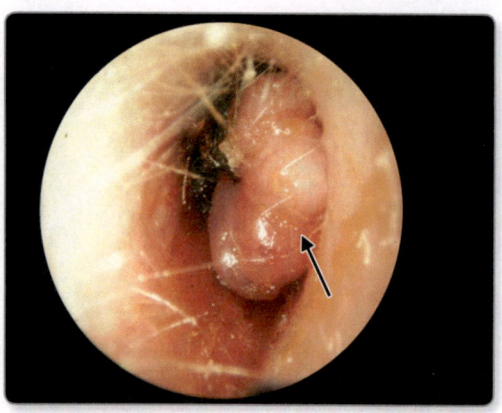

**Figure 2.10A** Otoscopic image of the EAC demonstrates an incidental mass (black arrow) seen on otoscopy with normal skin covering the neoplasm

## Plate 4

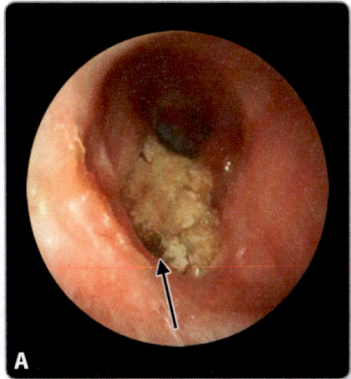

**Figures 2.12A and B** The patient had radiation treatment for a basal cell carcinoma of the head and neck four years prior. Otoscopic image of the EAC demonstrates non viable bone in the floor of the EAC (black arrow). Axial CT image of the right temporal bone demonstrates bony erosion of the posterior wall of the EAC (white arrow) with opacification of the underlying mastoid air cells. This patient required debridement of the EAC and removal of the nonviable or bony sequestrum from the EAC

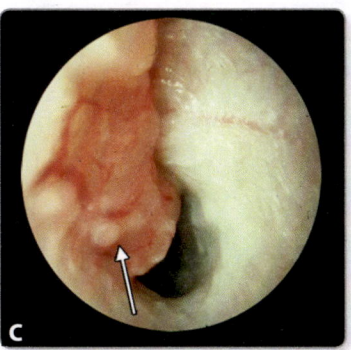

**Figures 2.13C and D** Otoscopic and axial CT image demonstrating parotid tumor invading the EAC. On otoscopy, a pinkish white tumor is seen invading the EAC (white arrow). CT imaging demonstrates a lobulated mass protruding into the canal (black arrow)

## Plate 5

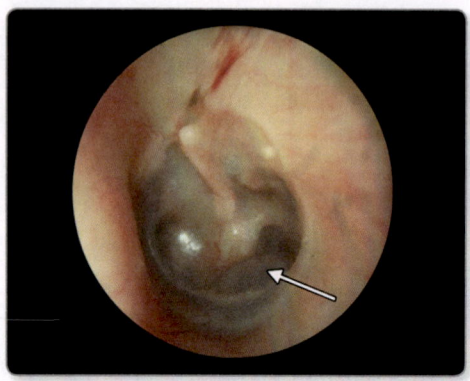

**Figure 2.15A** Otoscopic image demonstrating a bluish retrotympanic mass (white arrow) below the ossicles found to represent a high-riding dehiscent jugular bulb

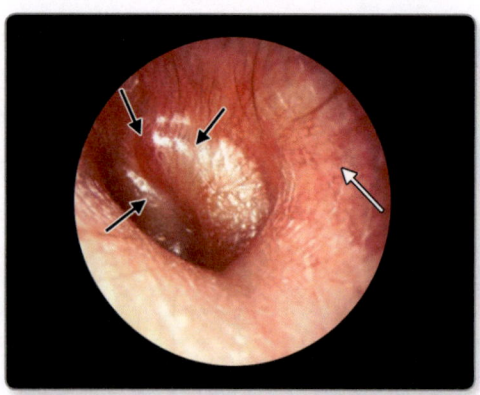

**Figure 2.17A** Otoscopic image of the tympanic membrane demonstrates reddish inflammation of the tympanic membrane (black arrows) with an erythematous EAC (white arrow)

## Plate 6

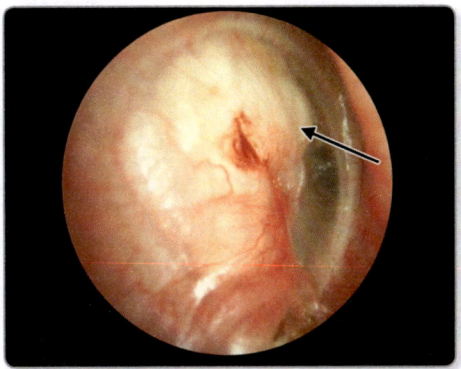

**Figure 2.19A** Otoscopic image of the tympanic membrane demonstrating a large ivory-yellow retrotympanic mass

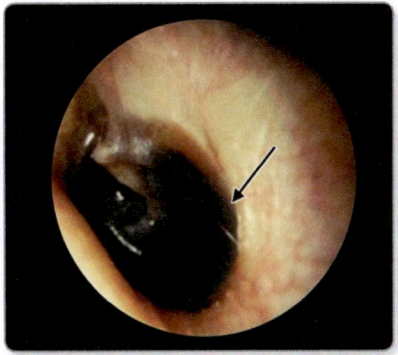

**Figure 2.20A** Otoscopic image of a tympanic membrane demonstrates a bluish-black retrotympanic mass (black arrow) protruding from the middle ear corresponding to a cholesterol granuloma

## Plate 7

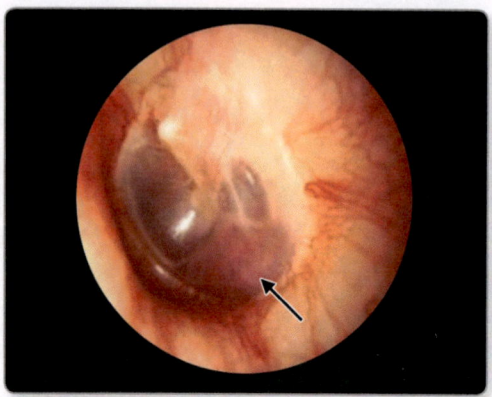

**Figure 2.21A** Otoscopic image of the tympanic membrane demonstrates a purplish-bluish retrotympanic mass (black arrow) in the hypotympanum found to be a glomus jugulotympanicum

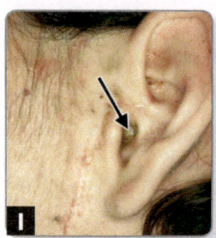

**Figures 2.34I to K** Otoscopic image of the left ear and axial and coronal CT images of the left temporal bone in a patient status post remote trauma to the left ear. On external exam, a false fundus (black arrow) is present with shortening of the EAC length. CT imaging demonstrates soft tissue filling the EAC (white arrows) secondary to scarring consistent with post-traumatic EAC stenosis

**Figures 2.34L and M** Otoscopic image of the right tympanic membrane and axial CT image of the right temporal bone in a patient status post blunt trauma to the right ear. On otoscopic exam, bluish material (B) is present filling the middle ear cavity. CT imaging demonstrates opacification of the middle ear in the same patient consistent with middle ear hemorrhage (H)

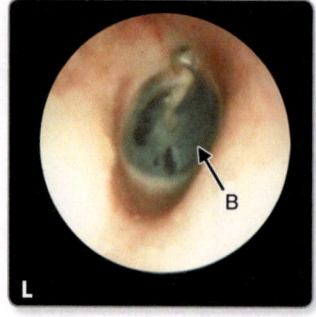

## Plate 8

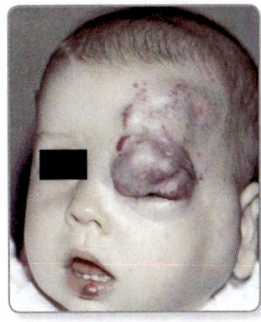

**Figure 3.27** Infant with left orbital capillary hemangioma. Digital subtracted angiogram (DSA) was done for management planning and shows high vascularity of the lesion (*Courtesy*: Dr Karl Terbrugge, Professor and Chairman of Neuroradiology, University Health Network, University of Toronto)

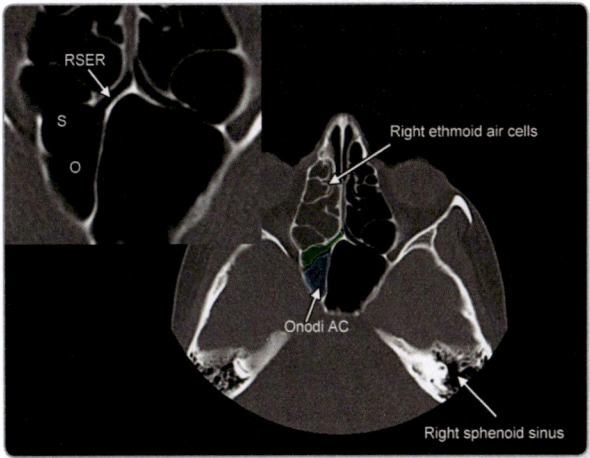

**Figure 4.8** Magnified view now shows communications between right sphenoethmoid recess (RSER) with the aire cell (S) which is the right sphenoid sinus. The larger air cell (O) located behind it is an Onodi air cell. Shaded green: Communication between RSER and right sphenoid sinus; Shaded blue: Right Onodi air cell

## Plate 9

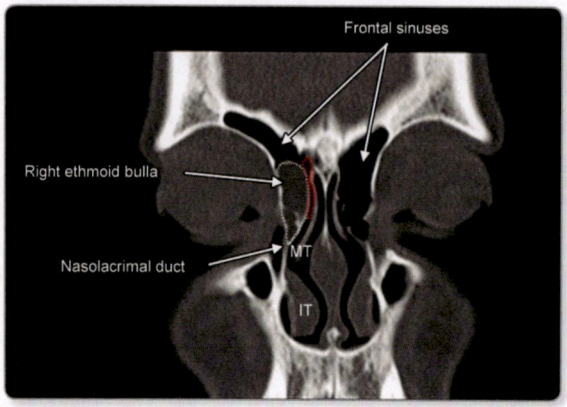

**Figure 4.15** MT: middle turbinate; IT: inferior turbinate; Red shaded: frontal recess

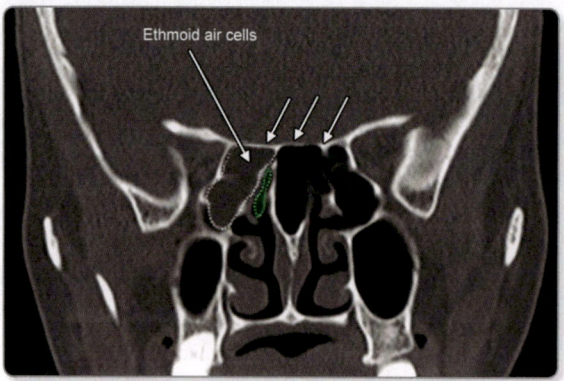

**Figure 4.20** Green shaded: Sphenoethmoid recess; Three short arrows: Planum sphenoidale

**Plate 10**

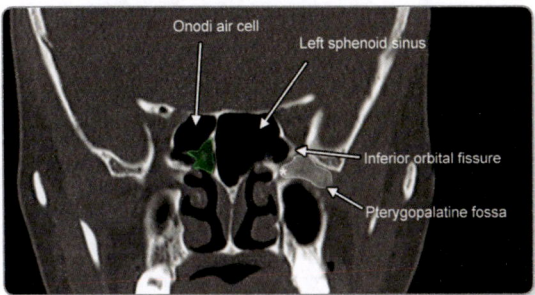

**Figure 4.21** Green shaded: Sphenoethmoid recess

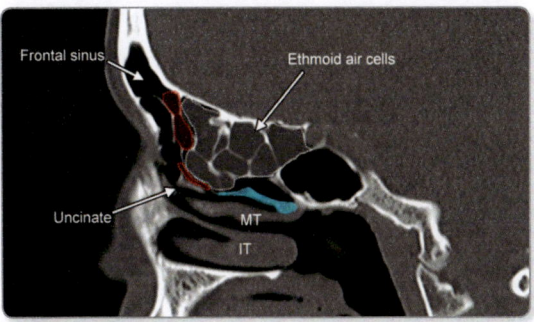

**Figure 4.29** Red shaded: Frontal recess; Blue shaded: Basal lamina of middle turbinate

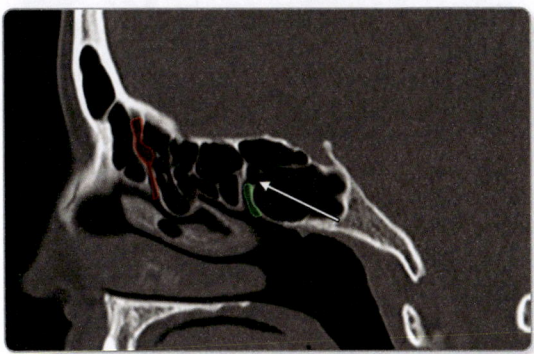

**Figure 4.30** Red shaded: Frontal recess; Green shaded: Sphenoethmoid recess; Arrow: Sphenoid ostium

## Plate 11

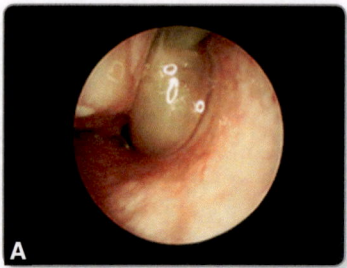

**Figures 4.64A to D** Antrochoanal polyps. This polyp is extending through a widened accessory maxillary sinus ostium to protrude into the right nasal cavity

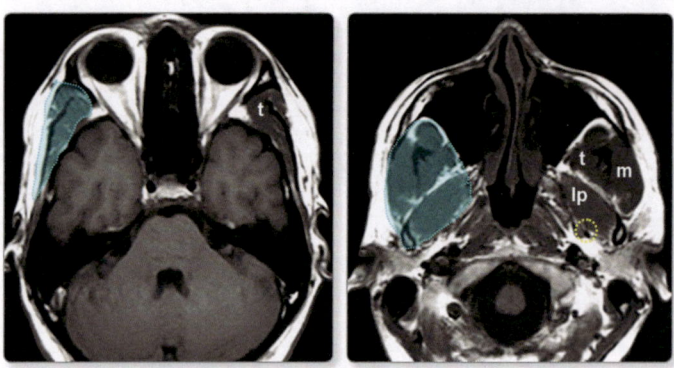

Figure 6.I.1                    Figure 6.I.2

**Figures 6.I.1 and 6.I.2** Infrazygomatic masticator space (shaded) includes the inferior temporalis (t), lateral pterygoid (lp) and masseter (m) muscles. The muscles, temporomandibular joint and the mandibular division of the trigeminal nerve, V3, (yellow circle) are invested in the superficial layer of the deep cervical fascia

## Plate 12

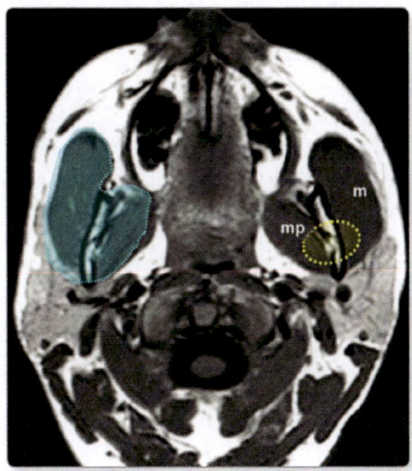

**Figure 6.I.3** Infrazygomatic mastication (lower section): medial pterygoid (mp) and masseter (m) muscles, intervening mandible and mandibular division of V3 (yellow oval) are invested in the superficial layer of the deep cervical fascia

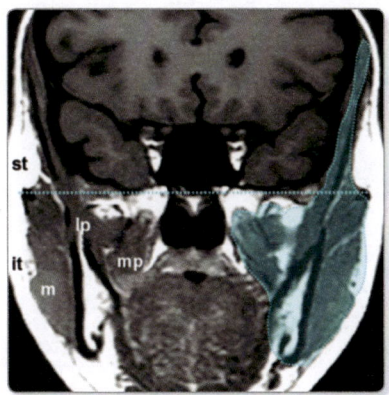

**Figure 6.I.4** Supra-(st) and infra-zygomatic temporalis (it) muscles (zygomatic boundary-dotted line), medial (mp) and lateral (lp) pterygoid and masseter (m) muscles as well as mandible and mandibular division of V3 are invested in the superficial layer of the deep cervical fascia

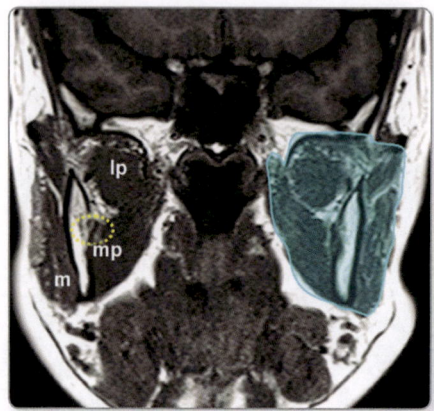

**Figure 6.I.5** Masseter (m), medial (mp) and lateral pterygoid (lp) muscles with intervening mandible and mandibular division of V3 (yellow oval) invested in the superficial layer of the deep cervical fascia

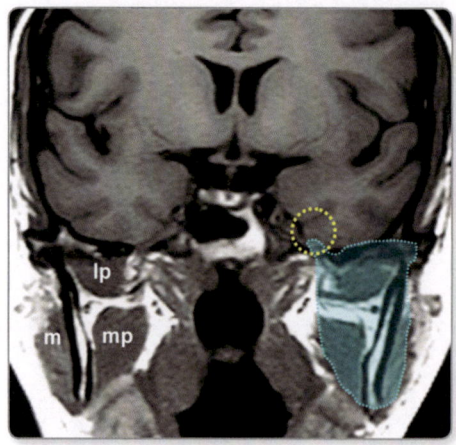

**Figure 6.I.6** Medial (mp) and lateral (lp) pterygoid and masseter (m) muscles as well as V3 at level of foramen ovale (yellow circle) invested in fascia

## Plate 14

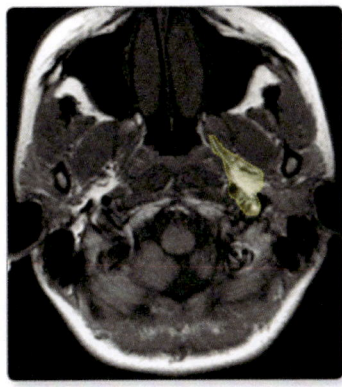

**Figure 6.II.2** Shaded region corresponds to the parapharyngeal space on axial imaging (outlined by yellow dotted line). It can be further subdivided into the prestyloid space (anterolateral to white dashed line) and retrostyloid space (posteromedial to white dashed line). White dashed line corresponds to the tensor vascular styloid fascia

**Figures 6.II.3A and B** Triangular shaped area of fat (outlined in yellow) bordered by the masticator space laterally, visceral space medially and parotid space posterolaterally. This corresponds to the prestyloid portion of the PPS. The red shaded area corresponds to the retrostyloid component which some refer to as the carotid space

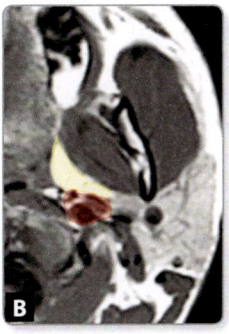

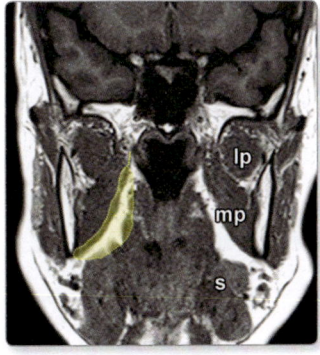

**Figure 6.II.4** Fat-filled space (yellow shaded area) medial to the muscles of mastication, [medial pterygoid (mp) and lateral pterygoid (lp) muscles]

## Plate 15

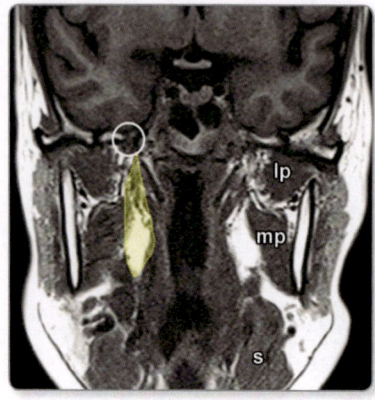

**Figure 6.II.5** Fat-filled space (yellow shaded area) tapering superiorly at skull base medial to foramen ovale (circle); [lateral pterygoid (lp) and medial pterygoid (mp) muscles]

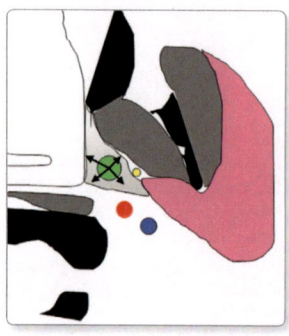

**Figure 6.II.7** A lesion centered within the parapharyngeal space is surrounded by fat. An uninterrupted rim of fat will confirm its parapharyngeal origin. As the lesion enlarges, it will efface the fat according to its direction of growth

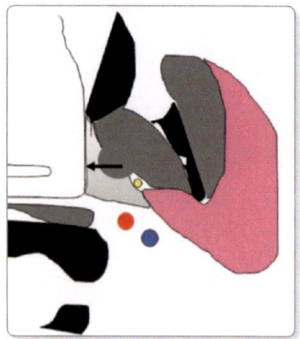

**Figure 6.II.8** A lesion centered within the masticator space will displace and compress the parapharyngeal fat predominantly medially

## Plate 16

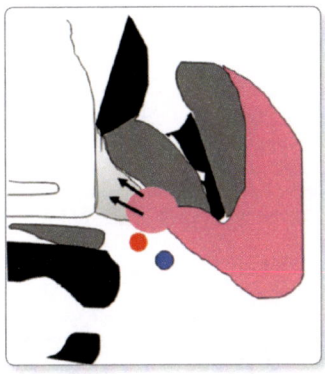

**Figure 6.II.9** A lesion centered within the parotid space widens the stylomandibular tunnel and will displace and compress the parapharyngeal fat anteriorly as well as medially

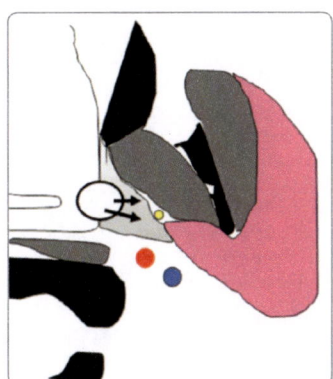

**Figure 6.II.10** A lesion centered within the visceral space will displace and compress the parapharyngeal fat predominantly laterally

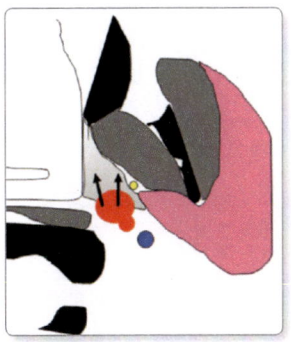

**Figure 6.II.11** A lesion centered within the retrostyloid parapharyngeal space will displace and compress the parapharyngeal fat anteriorly

## Plate 17

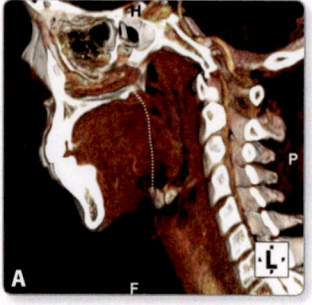

**Figures 7.1A and B** Sagittal CT of the normal oral cavity anatomy in 3D reconstruction and sagittal plane. The dotted line shows the posterior margin of the oral cavity. It marks the posterior margin of the hard palate and the circumvallate papillae. The oral tongue is anterior to the line and the tongue base is posterior

**Figures 11.21A and B** Metastatic node on PET. (A) Conventional axial contrast enhanced CT demonstrates an infiltrative lesion of the lateral right oral tongue and right floor of the mouth corresponding to a pathologically confirmed squamous cell carcinoma (black *). (B) PET component of a PET-CT performed subsequently demonstrates a highly FDG avid lesion corresponding to the invasive right tongue and floor of the mouth lesion. There is also increased asymmetric FDG uptake (short black arrow) that corresponded to a 6 mm, size-insignificant node on the nonenhanced fusion CT (*Adapted from Forghani, Smoker, and Curtin in Som and Curtin, Head and Neck Imaging, 5th Edition, Elsevier, 2011*)

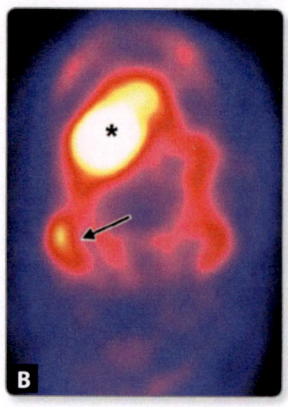

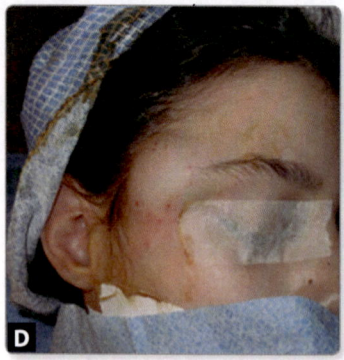

**Figures 14.3A to D** VVM. (A) Axial T1WI, (B) Axial T2WI, (C) Gadolinium enhanced T1WI and (D) Intraoperative picture. Superficial intramuscular VVM located in the temporalis muscle, with intermediate T1 signal, markedly hyperintense T2 signal and internal delayed enhancement after gadolinium administration. Intraoperative picture shows the corresponding local volume increase

Plate 18

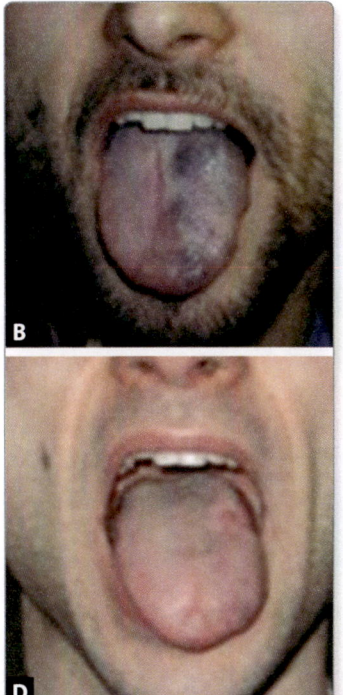

**Figures 14.5A to D** VVM (A, B) Pre- and (C, D) Postembolization axial T2WI and picture of a lingual VVM. High T2 signal multicystic lesion involving the left side of the tongue and sublingual space. Note the interval decrease in size after the embolization procedure and the almost complete resolution of the clinical mass effect and bluish discoloration of the tongue

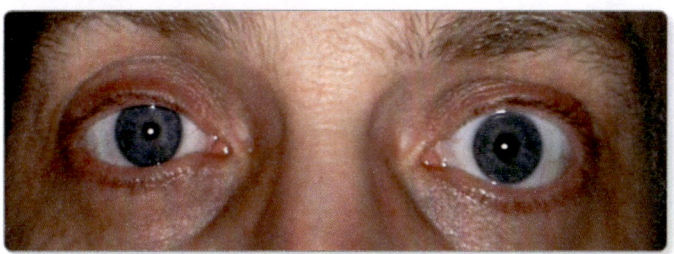

**Figure 14.7** Horner's syndrome. Patient with a right ICA dissection and Horner's syndrome characterized by right ptosis, miosis and anhydrosis

## Plate 19

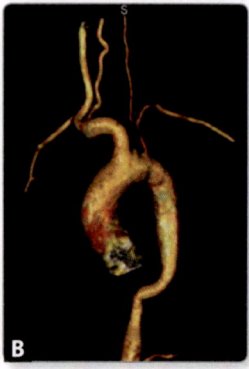

**Figures 14.16A and B** Takayasu's arteritis. (A) Contrast enhanced MRA and (B) VR images from an aortic CTA. There is occlusion of the left common carotid artery and severe diffuse circumferential narrowing of the left subclavian artery secondary to long standing arteritis. The distribution of the disease is more in keeping with a Takayasu's arteritis

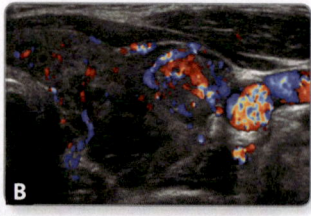

**Figures 15.11A and B** Sagittal sonographic image (A) through the right thyroid and axial Doppler image through the left thyroid and a patient with Hashimoto's thyroiditis

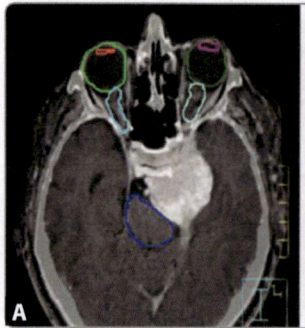 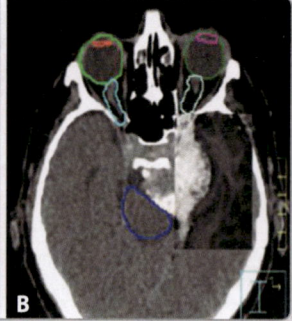

**Figures 16.9A and B** Fusion of MRI and CT data to plan radiotherapy for a cavernous sinus meningioma case. In this example, (A) demonstrates an MRI fused to the planning CT. (B) The CT simulation alone but with an overlying clipbox that allows visualization of the MRI data set for the purpose of illustrating the fusion. As can be seen on the (A), the advantage of CT to identify the bony anatomy is combined with the superior soft tissue delineation of MRI

**Plate 20**

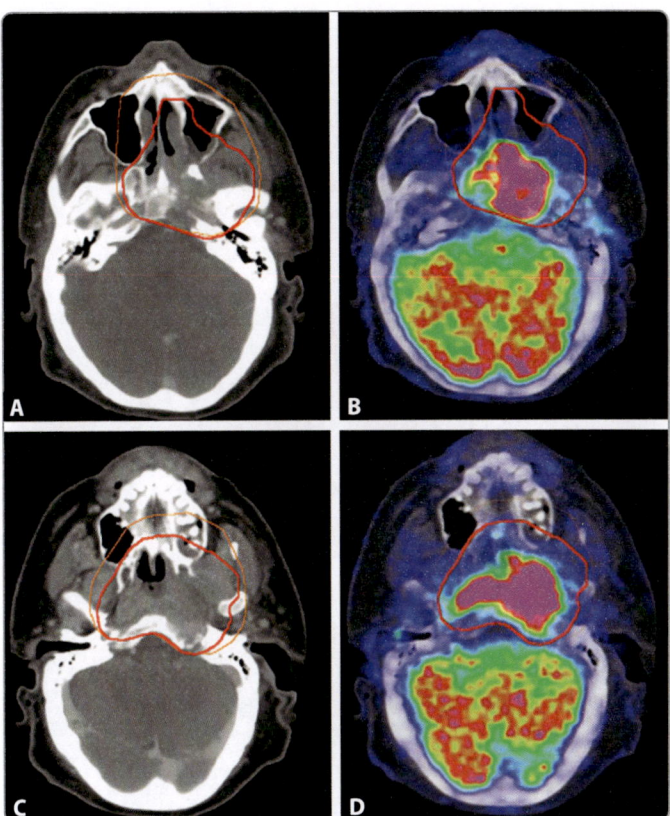

**Figures 16.10A to D** Tumor volumes. The patient had a PETCT simulation to design his therapy. The red outline illustrates the planning target volume (PTV) that encompasses the gross tumor volume (GTV) with a margin to include the areas of potential microscopic spread clinical target volume (CTV) and a margin to account for potential daily errors in set up or from patient motion. This volume was treated to 70 Gy. The orange line represents the PTV that included all potential areas of disease spread based on the known disease progression and potential pathways of spread in nasopharyngeal cancer. The volume was treated to 56 Gy

**Plate 21**

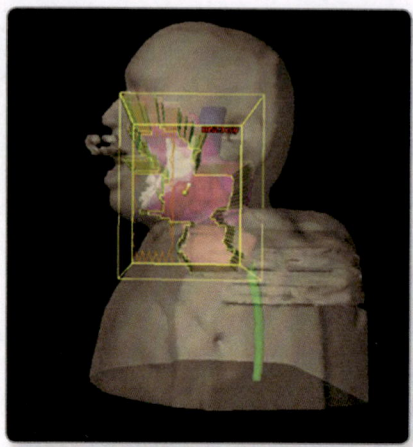

**Figure 16.11** Three-dimensional conformal radiotherapy (3DCRT). The tumor and target volumes are outlined along with the organs at risk. Using computer based programming, the structures can be reconstructed in three-dimensional imaging and overlaid on a surface rendering of the patient based on the CT simulation

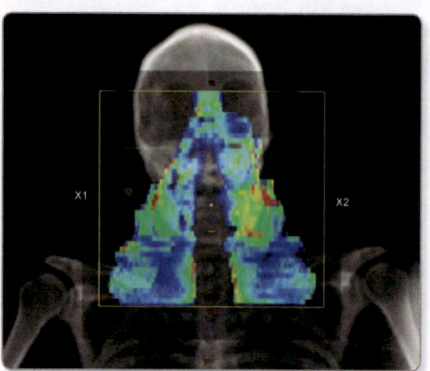

**Figure 16.12** Radiation dose distribution. Using computer software, the doses to the tumor and target volumes can be constructed and illustrated on the bony anatomy of the patient. The hotter (red/orange/yellow) colors indicate areas of higher dose while the cooler (green/blue) colors demonstrate areas receiving a lower dose. One can appreciate the large volumes of tissue that will be radiated in treating a head and neck cancer for cure as this is a typical volume treated in a nasopharyngeal cancer patient

**Plate 22**

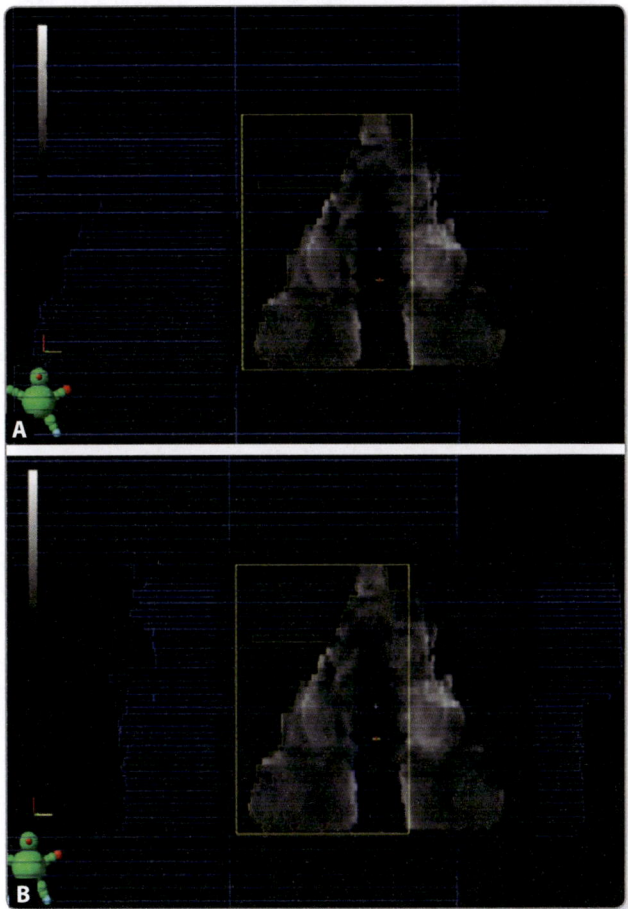

**Figures 16.13A and B** Sequencing of multileaf collimators (MLCs). In intensity modulated radiotherapy (IMRT), the dose is modulated by the MLCs within the head of the machine. The MLCs can vary their position and the time held in a single position. In this way, the beam is shaped to the tumor and target volumes. Using multiple beams with the MLCs allows for sculpting of the dose to match the tumor shape and minimize toxicities to normal structures

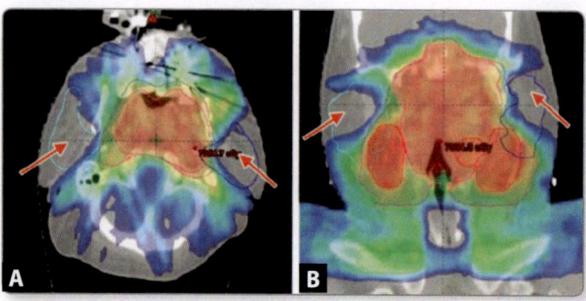

**Figures 16.14A and B** Dose sparing with intensity modulated radiotherapy. A common side effect of radiation therapy to the head and neck region is xerostomia due to the dose received by the parotids (arrows). IMRT allows the radiation oncologist to spare the parotid to a dose below the mean tolerance of 26 Gy. In the figure above, the dose distributed on the transverse and coronal slices represents a minimum of 26 Gy (dark blue) and progressively increases to 70 Gy that is focused on the actual tumor (red). The majority of the parotids is not within this dose distribution and therefore, receives less than 26 Gy

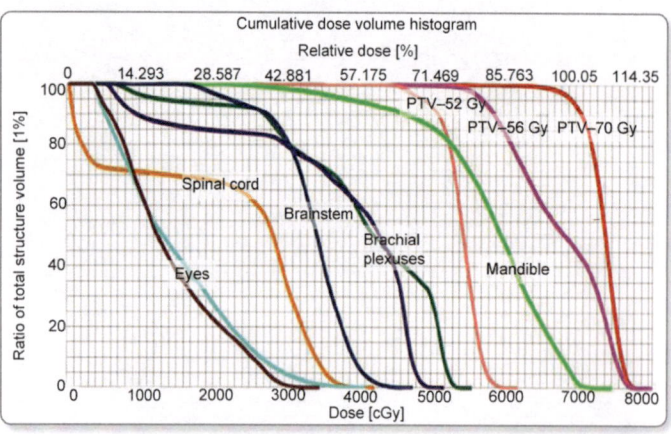

**Figure 16.15** Dose volume histogram (DVH). A DVH is a graphical representation of the dose received by all structures outlined by the radiation oncologist. The target volumes should receive the prescribed dose within approximately 5 to 10 percent. The tolerances of normal structures are known and therefore, can be used to help guide the evaluation of dose to these structures. The goal is to maximize the tumor coverage while minimizing the dose received by normal tissues. In this case the target volumes included the 70 Gy volume to cover the visible tumor, 56 Gy volume to cover high-risk areas, and a 52 Gy volume to much lower risk areas such as the low neck and supraclavicular region

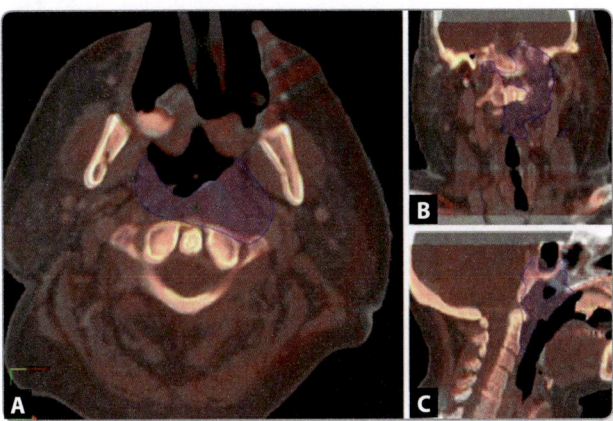

**Figures 16.16A to C** Cone-beam computed tomography (CBCT). With the proximity of critical structures such as the brainstem and the spinal cord, the room for error is minimal. Using a CBCT when the patient is set-up for daily radiation treatments allows the radiation oncologist to match the patient's soft tissue and bony anatomy with the CT simulation. The CBCT and the CT simulation images are superimposed. In addition to ensure proper patient set-up, the tumor response to radiotherapy can also be monitored

# Imaging techniques in head and neck

chapter 1

Colin S Poon, Jessie Aw

**Abstract**
This chapter reviews the major imaging modalities available – CT, MRI, PET CT, and ultrasound and examines their advantages and disadvantages in the imaging of various head and neck diseases.

**Keywords**
Imaging modalities, CT, MRI, PET, ultrasound

## Introduction

Radiological diagnosis in the head and neck requires appropriate use of imaging techniques to demonstrate optimally the complex anatomy and disease processes that affect the region. While X-ray plain films were often used historically to assess the neck soft tissues and paranasal sinuses, they lack sensitivity and specificity. In this era of wide availability of cross-sectional imaging technology, X-ray plain films no longer have much value in head and neck imaging.

One of the principles of head and neck cross-sectional imaging is to take advantage of the presence of normal fat planes that outline the normal anatomy. Disease processes in the head and neck will distort or efface the surrounding fat planes. Careful scrutiny of the head and neck fat planes helps facilitate lesion detection, localization, and the generation of a differential diagnosis.

When performing and interpreting radiological studies of the head and neck, it is important to understand that an abnormal finding can be caused by a primary cause remote from the finding. For example, vocal cord paralysis can be caused by diseases affecting the vagus nerve and its recurrent laryngeal nerve branch. A lesion therefore can be at any level from the brainstem to the superior mediastinum at the level of the aortic arch. A CT study obtained to evaluate for vocal cord paralysis should therefore cover the superior mediastinum and brainstem.

# Introductory head and neck imaging

## Computed tomography

For most diseases in the head and neck, CT is the modality of choice for initial imaging (**Figure 1.1**). CT is widely available and offers high spatial resolution, superior bone details and adequate soft tissue contrast for the head and neck. In addition, CT requires a short scan time, minimizing the problems of physiological and non-physiological motion that can be difficult to control.

Computed tomography is excellent in revealing calcifications in a lesion, which can be very helpful for lesion characterization. Diseases involving the bony structures are also well evaluated by CT.

Computed tomography scans of the neck should be performed following intravenous administration of iodinated contrast agent

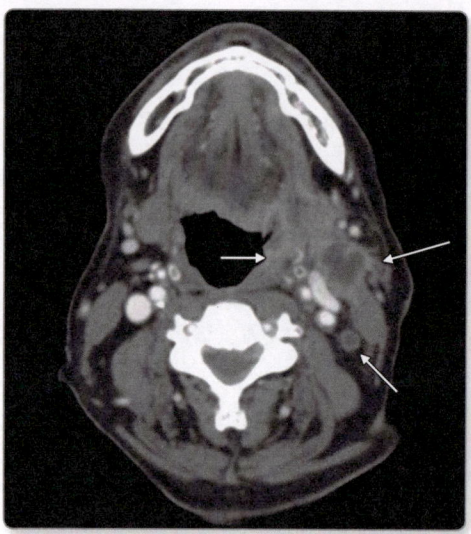

**Figure 1.1** CT of hypopharyngeal carcinoma with metastatic lymphadenopathy. Note the irregular thickening of the left lateral hypopharyngeal wall (short arrow) indicating the primary tumor. Multiple necrotic lymph nodes are noted (long arrows), indicating metastatic nodal disease. A subtle small necrotic node is present posterior to the larger node, highlighting the importance of image features in addition to size for the diagnosis of lymphadenopathy

injection. Contrast agent improves conspicuity of a lesion from normal structures and facilitates the differentiation of lymph nodes from neck vessels. The enhancement pattern may also provide additional information about the vascularity of a lesion, such as in paraganglioma. Use of contrast agent is particularly important for imaging of thin patients with little body fat. In patients with a contraindication to iodinated contrast, such as renal function impairment and history of severe contrast reaction, CT can be performed without contrast, although the accuracy of the study may be hampered.

For evaluation of mucosal lesions in the oral cavity, a "puffed cheek" technique (**Figure 1.2**) can be used.[1] The patients are asked to "puff" their cheek during CT scanning to distend the oral vestibules with air. This technique improves the visualization of subtle lesions involving the oral cavity mucosa.

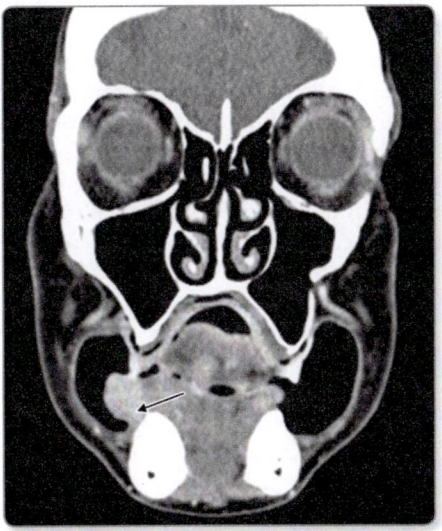

**Figure 1.2** Coronal CT image with a puffed cheek technique. This nicely demonstrates the presence of an exophytic mass along the right lateral aspect of the mandibular alveolus

When a vascular abnormality (such as carotid dissection) or hypervascular mass (such as a paraganglioma) is suspected, CT angiography (CTA) can be useful for more detailed depiction of the vascular structures. Head and neck cancer can invade vascular structures of the head and neck. Occasionally, CTA is required for further evaluation.

## Magnetic resonance imaging

Magnetic resonance imaging (MRI) is often used as a problem-solving tool in head and neck imaging. It is often requested after initial imaging has been performed with CT, but specific clinical questions still remain to be answered by radiological studies. Compared to CT, the disadvantages of MRI include its higher cost, and longer scan time making it prone to image artifacts from patient and physiological motion. MRI requires more patient cooperation, as patients are required to remain still during the examination. MRI may be contraindicated in patients with cardiac pacemakers and some other implanted electronic devices such as a cochlear implant.

MR imaging sequences used in head and neck imaging include T1-weighted imaging prior to and after intravenous injection of contrast agent, and T2-weighted imaging. Prior to intravenous injection of gadolinium contrast material, T1-weighted imaging should be performed without fat suppression to maximize the soft tissue contrast provided by the natural fat planes in the head and neck. T2-weighted and post-contrast T1-weighted imaging will benefit from fat suppression, which often increases the conspicuity of lesions. An alternative to fat suppressed T2-weighted sequence is the STIR (Short Tau Inversion Recovery) which provides reliable fat suppression at the cost of increased noise and longer scan time. The use of fat suppression in post-contrast T1-weighted imaging is a subject of debate because of the concern of inhomogeneous fat suppression due to magnetic field inhomogeneity. The resultant image artifacts, with residual high signal from failure of fat suppression, can make image interpretation difficult. However, with the introduction of more reliable fat suppression techniques such as IDEAL,[2] the concern of imperfect fat suppression should be relieved.

Because of its superior soft tissue contrast, MRI can offer an advantage over CT for a number of clinical problems. It has improved accuracy for evaluation of subtle soft tissue lesions arising from regions with paucity of natural body fat, muscular organs such as the tongue (**Figures 1.3A to D**), and lesions of the pharyngeal

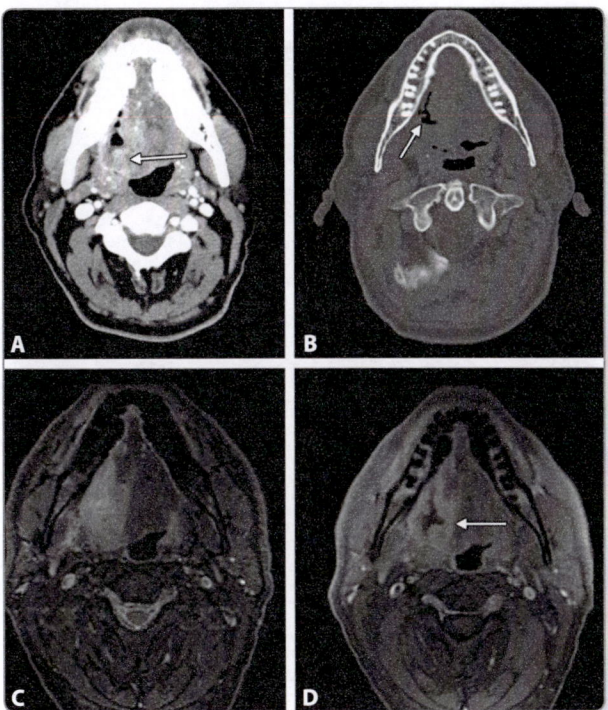

**Figures 1.3A to D** (A, B) Axial CT of the neck with soft tissue and bone windows shows an ulcerated lesion along the posterolateral aspect of the right tongue (arrows). There is subtle enhancement adjacent to the ulcerated area. The bony margin of the mandible is intact. (C) MRI STIR image shows excellent fat saturation, and provides clear depiction of the right posterior lateral tongue squamous cell carcinoma. There is also tumor involvement of the buccal mucosa immediately adjacent to the tumor. (D) MRI axial fat saturated T1 post contrast image demonstrates the tumor with central non-enhancing necrotic component (arrow). Note that the tumor is well delineated even in the absence of contrast agent, due to the intrinsic high soft tissue contrast of MRI

mucosal space (**Figures 1.4A to D**). MRI may provide a more accurate definition of the extent of head and neck lesions. For example, in laryngeal carcinoma, extralaryngeal extension of tumor and cartilage involvement can be more readily appreciated on MRI. Although CT is excellent for depiction of bony structures, MRI may demonstrate bone

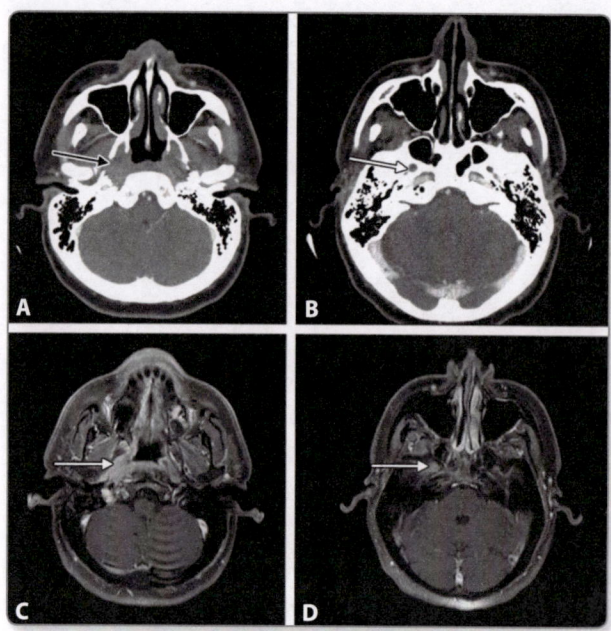

**Figures 1.4A to D** Nasopharyngeal carcinoma with perineural spread along the V3 division of trigeminal nerve. (A) CT demonstrates a soft tissue mass with minimal contrast enhancement centered in the right fossa of Rosenmueller (arrow). (B) More superiorly, there is subtle asymmetric enlargement of the right foramen of ovale (arrow). The appearance is nonspecific and may be developmental, but the diagnosis of nasopharyngeal carcinoma makes this suspicious for perineural spread. (C, D) MRI fat-saturated postcontrast T1 weighted images at the same anatomical levels demonstrates the nasopharyngeal mass with avid enhancement (arrows). There is enlargement and enhancement of right V3 nerve at the level of the foramen of ovale (arrow, Figure 1.4D), confirming the suspicion of perineural spread

involvement earlier by revealing abnormal bone marrow infiltration (**Figures 1.5A to D**).

MRI is an important adjunct evaluation of sinonasal lesions. On CT, It can be very difficult to differentiate soft tissue lesions from trapped secretion and mucosal inflammatory changes. This distinction can be more easily made on MRI (**Figures 1.6A to D**).

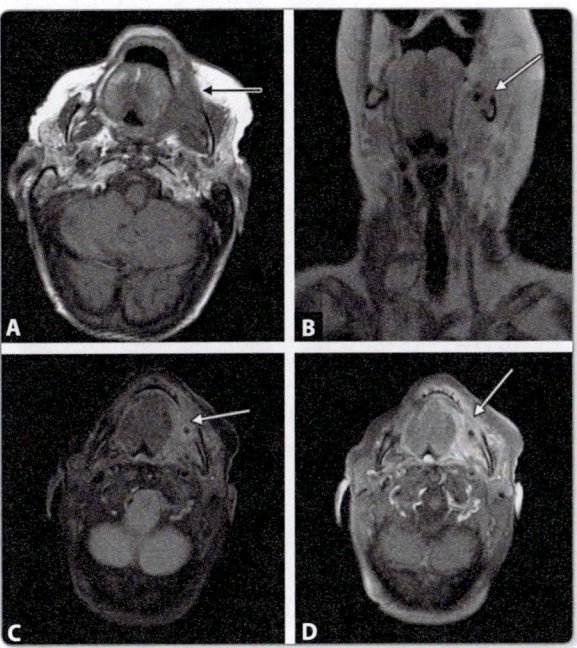

**Figures 1.5A to D** Squamous cell carcinoma of the oral cavity with mandibular invasion. MRI (A) axial and (B) coronal precontrast T1 weighted images, (C) axial T2 weighted image with fat saturation, and (D) axial post contrast fat-saturated T1 weighted image depict (arrows) a left oral cavity squamous cell carcinoma with left hemi-mandibular tumor invasion (arrows). On precontrast T1 weighted images, the tumor is hypointense, replacing the normal fat signal in soft tissues and bone marrow of the mandible. There is clear disruption of the hypointense mandibular cortex. Postcontrast images demonstrate avid enhancement of the mass

# 8 Introductory head and neck imaging

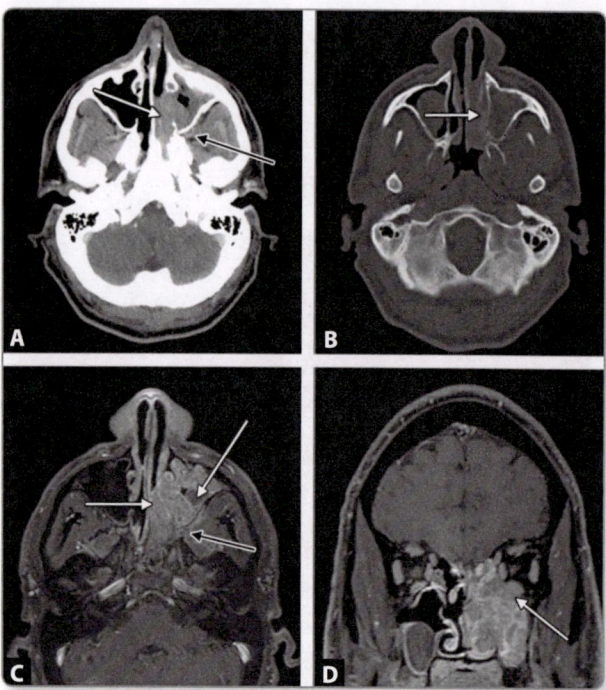

**Figures 1.6A to D** Squamous cell carcinoma of sinonasal cavity. (A) CT in soft tissue window demonstrates a soft tissue mass (white arrow) at the left maxillary sinus ostium, extending into the left maxillary sinus and nasal cavity. Very subtle soft tissue density at the left pterygopalatine fossa (black arrow) suggests its involvement by tumor. (B) CT in bone window at a more inferior level demonstrates bone erosion. (C) MRI axial enhanced T1-weighted image with fat saturation demonstrates the enhancing mass (short white arrow) similar to CT, but the involvement of the pterygopalatine fossa (black arrow) is more clearly demonstrated. In addition, trapped secretion and inflammatory sinus disease can be differentiated from enhancing tumor (long white arrow) (short white arrow), a clear advantage of MRI. (D) Coronal enhanced T1-weighted image with fat saturation demonstrates the enhancing tumor has extended into the inferior aspect of the left orbit (arrow). Note the lack of enhancement of the mucosal thickening at the floor of the right maxillary sinus from chronic sinus disease

MRI is indispensable for evaluation of diseases affecting the cranial nerves, skull base, or when intracranial extension of disease is suspected (**Figures 1.4A to D**). For this reason, MR is often requested for staging of malignancies involving the sinonasal cavity, nasopharynx, and skull base even when CT has been done.

## Positron emission tomography

Positron emission tomography (PET) is an important adjunct to cancer imaging in the head and neck. PET is often performed with PET/CT. In older units of PET/CT scanners, the CT component may not be of optimal diagnostic quality, but is used primarily for attenuation correction and anatomical localization of abnormal uptake. The technology is newer PET/CT scanners incorporate multidetector CT technology and allow diagnostic quality CT to be acquired simultaneously.

Potential benefits of PET include improved accuracy of pre-treatment staging (**Figures 1.7A and B**), detection of synchronous primary malignancies, identification of primary tumors in cases of metastatic lymphadenopathy with unknown primary, and detection of post-treatment recurrence.[3]

As in with any radiological studies, false negatives and false positives can occur with PET. False negative PET may be seen in small lesions less than 1 cm that are cystic or necrotic. Some primary

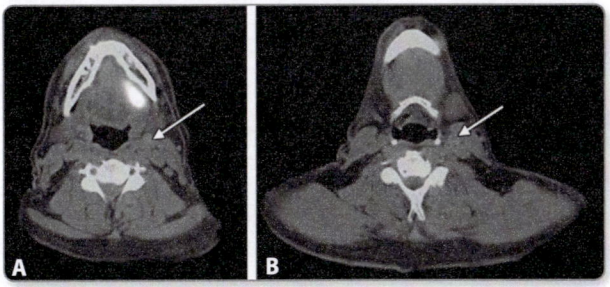

**Figures 1.7A and B** Squamous cell carcinoma of oral tongue with metastatic lymphadenopathy. (A, B) Axial fused PET-CT images demonstrate avid uptake in the left oral tongue squamous cell carcinoma. Abnormal uptake in left level 2 nodes is seen (arrows); subsequently proven to be pathological although not enlarged (*for color version see Plate 1*)

neoplasms including well-differentiated thyroid carcinoma and adenoid cystic carcinoma may not be PET-avid.

False positives of PET include physiological uptakes such as brown fat, as well as by inflammatory and infectious processes. Because false positives are commonly seen immediately after treatment, surveillance PET is not advised until 2 to 3 months post treatment.

## Ultrasound

Because of the absence of radiation, ultrasound can be used as the initial imaging choice for neck masses in pediatric patients.

Ultrasound can be used as an alternative for imaging of lymphadenopathy in adults (**Figure 1.8**). However, accurate comparison of serial images may be more difficult with ultrasound compared to CT due to variation in imaging techniques and sampling.

Ultrasound is the imaging modality of choice for characterization of thyroid nodules. It is recommended for the initial imaging of thyroid nodules, and for further workup of thyroid nodules detected incidentally on other imaging modalities.[4] Ultrasound provides an accurate assessment of the size and internal features of thyroid nodules. Features that have been shown to be associated with thyroid cancer include microcalcifications, hypoechogenicity, irregular

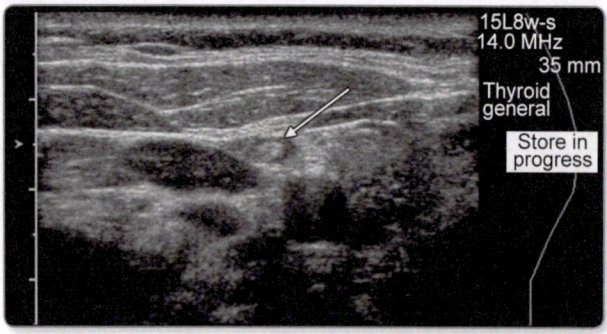

**Figure 1.8** Neck ultrasound shows a normal lymph node (arrow) with a fatty hilum

margins or absence of halo around the nodule, solid nodule, intranodular vascularity, and a "taller than wide" configuration. However, there is a significant overlap of these features between malignant and benign nodules. For this reason, fine needle aspiration is often necessary for a more definitive diagnosis. Imaging features that are highly suggestive of benign nodules include a predominantly cystic lesion, echogenic foci with "comet tail" ring down artifacts associated with inspissated colloid (**Figure 1.9**).

Sonographic features of thyroid nodules that have been recommended for fine needle aspiration include microcalcifications in nodules greater than 1 cm, nodules greater than 1.5 cm that are mostly solid or contains coarse calcifications, mixed solid – cystic nodules that are greater than 2 cm, and nodules showing substantial interval growth.[5] Slightly different criteria have also been proposed in consensus guidelines from other groups.[4]

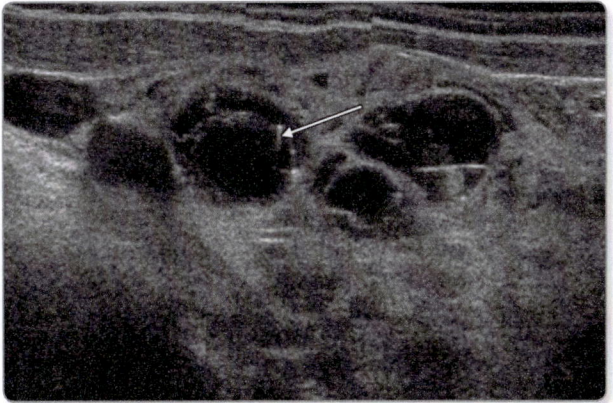

**Figure 1.9** Transverse thyroid ultrasound image shows ring down a "comet tail" artifact in a cystic nodule (arrow). The "comet tail" appearance distinguishes this echogenic focus from microcalcification which has a strong association with papillary thyroid carcinoma. The presence of "comet tail" artifact suggests the presence of colloid crystals of hyperplastic nodule

## X-ray esophagram

Application of X-ray barium studies is limited to the evaluation of esophagus. Mucosal diseases of the esophagus are best demonstrated on X-ray barium esophagram (**Figures 1.10A and B**). Although CT and even MRI may demonstrate larger esophageal lesions, their sensitivity and specificity for detection of the smaller mucosal lesions are limited.

## Summary

The ideal imaging modality for evaluation of diseases in the head and neck depends on the specific clinical scenario. Very often correlation between multiple imaging modalities is required for accurate staging of diseases.

In general, most head and neck diseases are well evaluated by CT, and therefore CT is often used as the initial imaging tool for the workup of diseases. In the head and neck pediatric patients, ultrasound can be used as the initial imaging modality of choice for neck mass. Ultrasound is also the imaging modality of choice for the initial evaluation of the thyroid glands. MRI is often used for problem solving

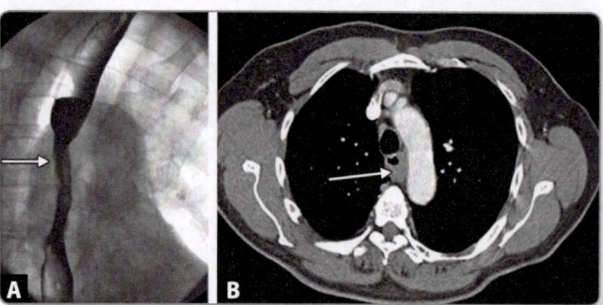

**Figures 1.10A and B** Esophageal carcinoma. (A) Double contrast barium swallow study shows lack of distension and narrowing (arrow) of the mid segment of the thoracic esophagus. The luminal margins are irregular with shouldered borders. These are typical features of an esophageal carcinoma. (B) Postcontrast staging CT confirms annular thickening and luminal narrowing of the mid esophagus (arrow). Mild esophageal thickening on CT is often a nonspecific finding, and can be due to lack of distention of the esophagus

| Clinical problems | Primary imaging modality | Secondary or alternative imaging modality |
|---|---|---|
| General screening/initial imaging | CT<br>Ultrasound for pediatric neck mass | MRI |
| Orbits | CT<br>MRI if involvement of optic nerve is suspected | |
| Infection/inflammation | CT | |
| Sinonasal cavities | CT | MRI for accurate depiction of tumor extent and perineural spread |
| Superficial and subcutaneous soft tissues of the head and neck | CT<br>Ultrasound | |
| Tongue/oral cavity | CT | MRI |
| Nasopharynx, oropharynx, hypopharynx | CT | MRI |
| Larynx | CT | MRI |
| Salivary glands and ducts | CT | MRI |
| Lymphadenopathy | CT | Ultrasound |
| Temporal bone | CT | MRI for evaluation of cranial nerve CN8, membranous labyrinths, neoplasm. |
| Trauma | CT | |
| Perineural spread of diseases | MRI | |
| Intracranial extension of diseases | MRI | |
| Thyroid nodules | Ultrasound | CT or MRI for evaluation of extent of large thyroid mass and complications such as airway compression. |
| Esophagus | Barium esophagram | |
| Head and neck cancer staging/restaging | CT | MRI<br>PET |

**Table 1.1** Indications for imaging techniques

in head and neck imaging. Its excellent soft tissue contrast resolution, makes it indispensable evaluation of malignancies involving the skull base, for which there is a high-risk of perineural spread and intracranial extension of disease. PET is often used for staging and post-treatment restaging of head and neck cancer. X-ray has limited value in head and neck imaging, except for X-ray barium esophagram which remains the best radiological study for the evaluation of esophageal mucosal diseases.

The general indications of various imaging techniques for head and neck imaging are summarized in **Table 1.1**. The optimal utilization of the different imaging techniques can be modified depending on the clinical problems.

## References

1. Weissman JL, Carrau RL. "Puffed-cheek" CT improves evaluation of the oral cavity. AJNR Am J Neuroradiol 2001; 22:741-4.
2. Barger AV, DeLone DR, Bernstein MA, Welker KM. Fat signal suppression in head and neck imaging using fast spin-echo-IDEAL technique. AJNR Am J Neuroradiol 2006;27:1292-4.
3. Agarwal V, Branstetter BF IV, Johnson JT. Indications for PET/CT in the head and neck. Otolaryngol Clin N Am 2008;41:23-49.
4. Cooper DS, Doherty GM, Haugen BR, et al. Revised American Thyroid Association management guidelines for patients with thyroid nodules and differentiated thyroid cancer. Thyroid 2009;19:1-48.
5. Frates MC, Benson CB, Charboneau JW, et al. Management of thyroid nodules detected at US: Society of Radiologists in Ultrasound consensus conference statement. Radiology 2005;237:794-800.

# Radiographic anatomy and pathology of the temporal bone

chapter 2

Samantha Shankar, Alan Johnson, Vinh Nguyen

### Abstract
The imaging anatomy of the temporal bone is discussed. A systematic review of the common congenital, infectious, inflammatory and neoplastic disease processes affecting the external, middle and inner ear are covered. A section on temporal bone trauma is also included.

### Keywords
Temporal bone, anatomy, external, middle and inner ear.

## Introduction

Temporal bone imaging can be considered one of the more challenging areas for interpretation in radiology. The complex anatomy can be difficult to conceptualize due to its multispatial orientation. High resolution CT is the modality of choice and demonstrates many of the pathologies localized to the temporal bone well. MR imaging serves as an important companion in delineating and confirming temporal bone disease. The multiplanar construction and post processing capabilities with the advent of the modern multidetector CT scanners have significantly enhanced temporal bone imaging. The exquisite bony detail with CT and the soft tissue resolution with MRI assure more accurate diagnosis and management of the myriad of disease processes in the temporal bone.

## Embryology

The auricle develops from six ectodermal hillocks which project from the first branchial groove. The auricular hillocks enlarge and fuse to form the external pinna (**Figure 2.1**). The external auditory canal develops from the first branchial groove and is ectodermal in origin.

# Introductory head and neck imaging

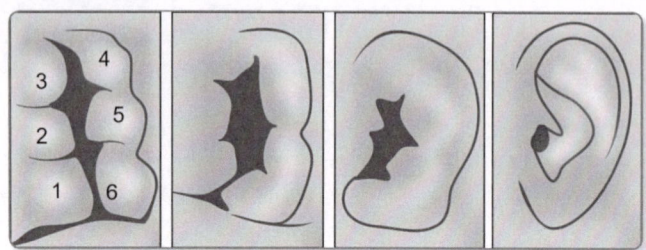

**Figure 2.1** Embryology of the auricle. Six hillocks form around the dorsal extremity of the embryo from the first branchial groove which fuses to form the external pinna (*for color version see Plate 1*)

Simultaneously, the entodermal-lined middle ear cavity is developing from the pharyngeal pouch and expanding towards the external auditory canal (EAC). A thin mesodermal plate separates the evolving EAC and middle ear cavity, which together with the outer ectoderm of the EAC and inner entoderm of the middle ear cavity forms the tympanic membrane. The middle ear structures develop from the first and second branchial arches. Meckel's cartilage, the cartilage of the first arch, gives rise to the head of the malleus and the body and short process of the incus. The tensor tympani muscle has its origin from the mesoderm of the first arch. Reichert's cartilage, the cartilage of the second arch, gives rise to the manubrium of the malleus, long process of the incus and the head and crura of the stapes. The mesoderm of the second arch forms the stapedius muscle.

Ectodermal thickening or olfactory placodes form along the side of the developing embryo and invaginate into the surrounding mesoderm to form the otic capsule. The otic capsule gives rise to the cochlea, semicircular canals and the foot plate of the stapes.

# Normal CT and MRI anatomy of the temporal bone

## The external ear (Figures 2.2A and B)

The external ear consists of the pinna and the EAC. The EAC is S-shaped and has two components, the cartilaginous component laterally and

Radiographic anatomy and pathology of the temporal bone 17

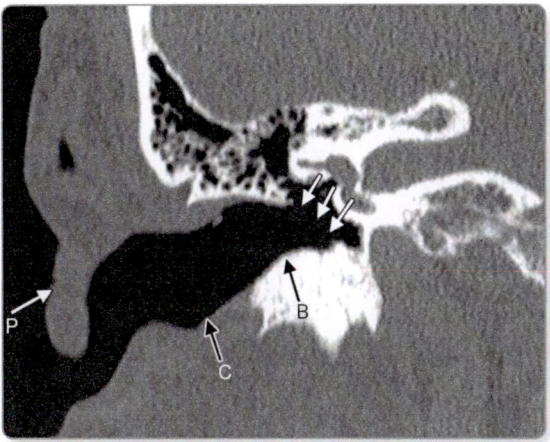

**Figure 2.2A** Coronal CT image of the right temporal bone. Pinna (P), cartilaginous EAC (C), bony EAC (B) and tympanic membrane (white arrows)

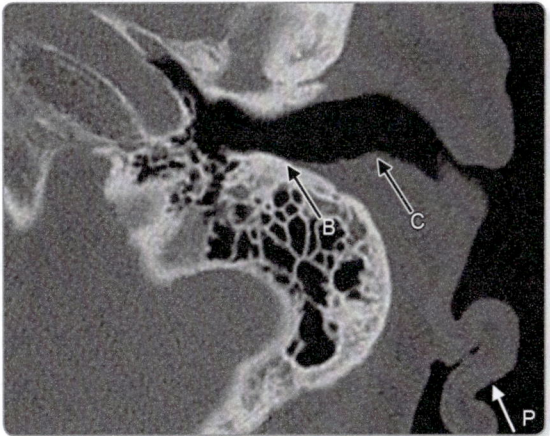

**Figure 2.2B** Axial CT image of the left temporal bone. Pinna (P), cartilaginous EAC (C) and bony EAC (B)

the bony component medially. The osseous EAC is slightly narrow as compared to its cartilaginous constituent and is bounded medially by the tympanic membrane. The posterior wall of the EAC is shorter than the anterior wall due to the angulated positioning of the tympanic membrane.

## The middle ear (Figures 2.3A to L)

The middle ear is an air-filled cavity within the temporal bone housing three mobile ossicles which bridge the gap between the tympanic drum and the oval window on the medial wall. The tympanic cavity is bordered laterally by the tympanic membrane, superiorly by the tegmen tympani, medially by the otic capsule and inferiorly by the hypotympanic floor. The cavity is arbitrarily subdivided into the mesotympanum, across from the tympanic membrane, the epitympanum, above the level of the tympanic membrane, and the hypotympanum, below the level of the tympanic membrane. The ossicular chain is composed of the malleus, incus and stapes. The tympanic membrane has two parts: the pars flaccida, denoting the lax component and the pars tensa, which denotes the taut component. The tympanic membrane sits within the tympanic sulcus, which is referred to as the scutum along its superior margin. Medial to the scutum lies an important space known as Prussak's space. This space is formed laterally by the pars flaccida, medially by the malleolar neck, superiorly by the lateral malleolar ligament and inferiorly by the short process of the malleus. The tegmen tympani forms the roof of the middle ear cavity and separates the middle ear from the middle cranial fossa. The bony floor of the middle ear cavity is separated from the petrous portion of internal carotid artery anteriorly and the posterior portion of the jugular bulb posteriorly. The internal carotid artery is separated from the jugular bulb by a bony plate termed the carotid spine. The posterior wall has a prominent process called the pyramidal eminence from which the stapedius tendon emanates. Medial to this process lies a recess called the sinus tympani and laterally lies the facial recess, which covers the upper portion of the mastoid segment of the facial nerve. The Aditus ad antrum, along the posterior wall, is a narrow conduit to the mastoid antrum, the largest of the mastoid air cells.

Radiographic anatomy and pathology of the temporal bone

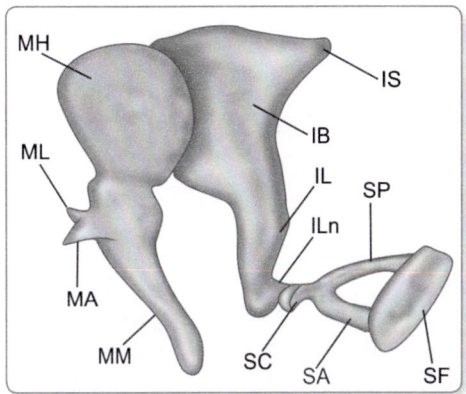

**Figure 2.3A** Diagram of the middle ear ossicles. Malleolar head (MH), malleus anterior process (MA), malleus lateral process (ML), manubrium of malleus (MM), incus body (IB), incus long process (IL), incus short process (IS), lenticular process of incus (ILn), stapes capitellum (SC), anterior stapes anterior crura (SA), posterior stapes crura (SP) and stapes footplate (SF) (*for color version see Plate 2*)

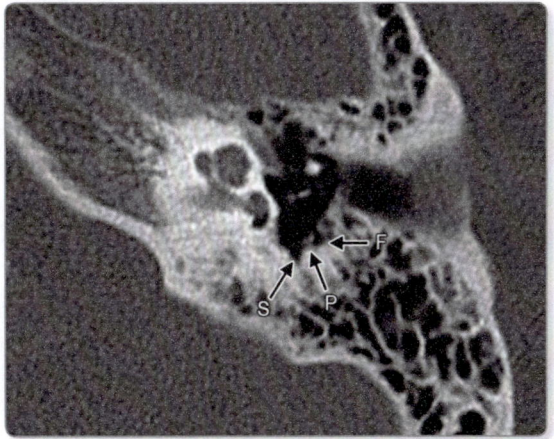

**Figure 2.3B** Axial CT image of left temporal bone. Sinus tympani (S), pyramidal eminence (P) and facial recess (F)

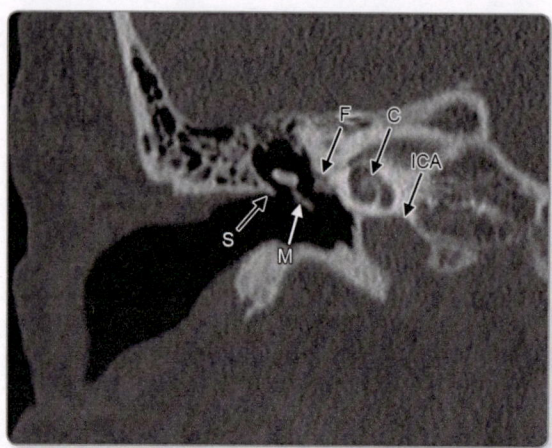

**Figure 2.3C** Coronal CT image of right temporal bone. Scutum (S), manubrium of the malleus (M), cochlea (C) and internal carotid artery (ICA). Anterior tympanic segment of facial nerve (F) with cochleariform process and tendon of tensor tympani muscle below

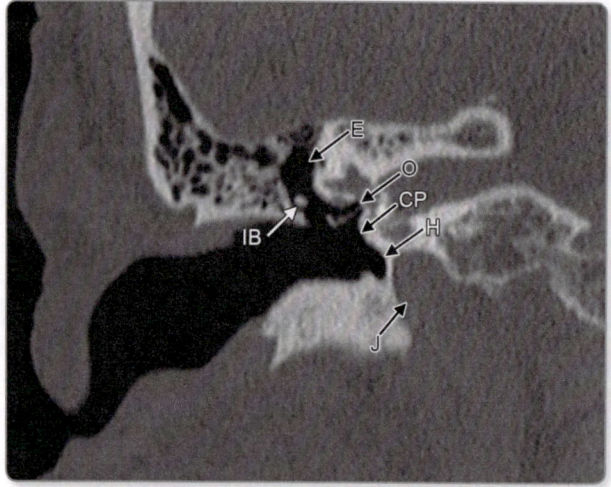

**Figure 2.3D** Coronal CT image of right temporal bone. Incus body (IB), epitympanum (E), cochlear promontory (CP), hypotympanum (H), oval window (O), and jugular bulb (J)

Radiographic anatomy and pathology of the temporal bone 21

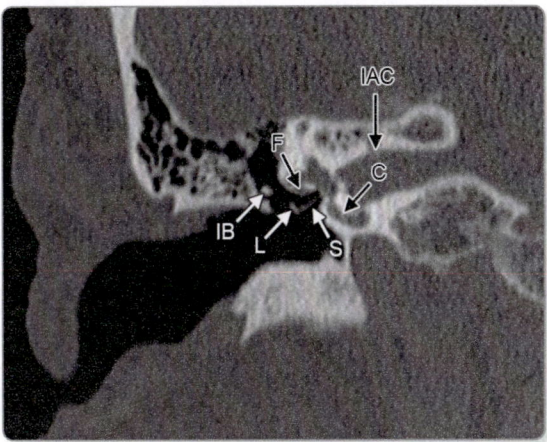

**Figure 2.3E** Coronal CT image of right temporal bone. Incus body (IB), incus lenticular process (L), stapes anterior crura (S), basal turn of the cochlea (C), tympanic segment of facial nerve (F) and internal auditory canal (IAC)

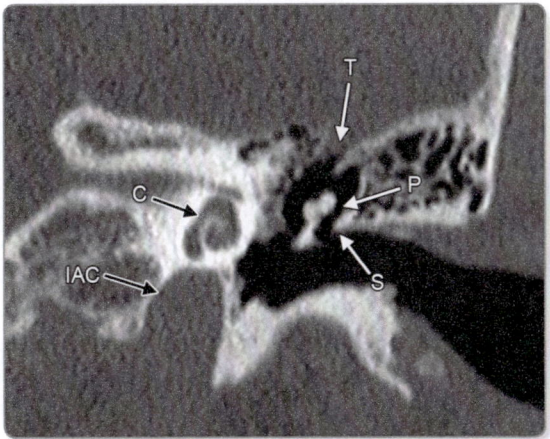

**Figure 2.3F** Coronal CT image of left temporal bone. Tegmen tympani (T), Prussak's space (P), scutum (S), cochlea (C) and internal auditory canal (IAC)

## 22 Introductory head and neck imaging

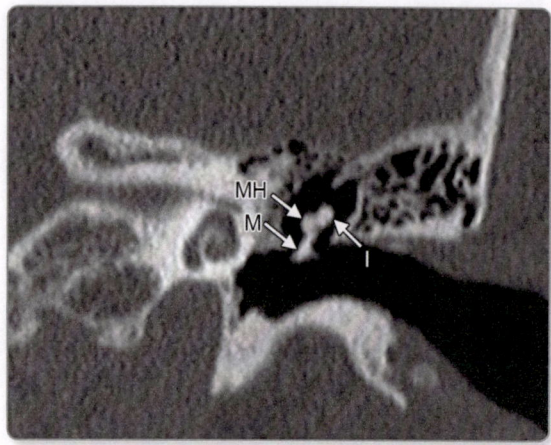

**Figure 2.3G** Coronal CT image of left temporal bone. Malleolar head (MH), manubrium of malleus (M) and incus body (I)

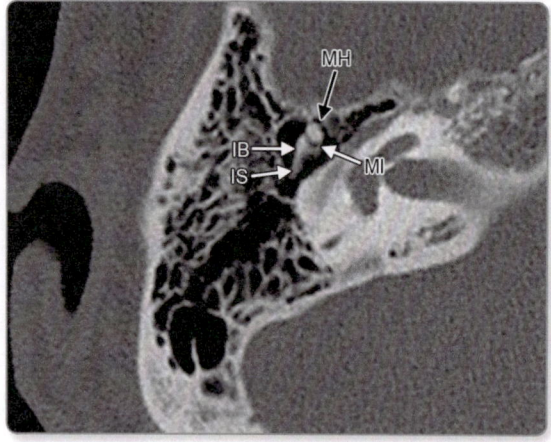

**Figure 2.3H** Axial CT image of right temporal bone. Malleolar head (MH), malleoincudal articulation (MI), incus body (IB) and incus short (IS) process

Radiographic anatomy and pathology of the temporal bone 23

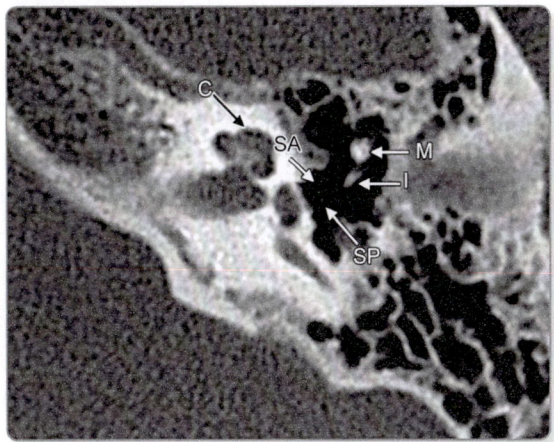

**Figure 2.3I** Axial CT image of left temporal bone. Malleus (M), long process of incus (I), stapes anterior crus (SA), stapes posterior crus (SP) and cochlea (C)

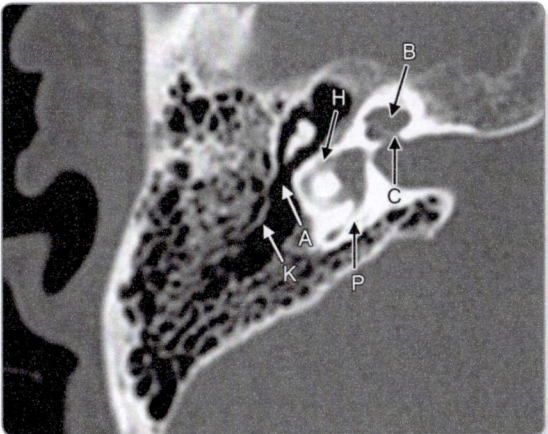

**Figure 2.3J** Axial CT image of right temporal bone. Aditus ad Antrum (A), Koerner's septum (K), horizontal semicircular canal (H), posterior semicircular canal (P), bony modiolus of the cochlea (B) and cochlear aperture (C)

## Introductory head and neck imaging

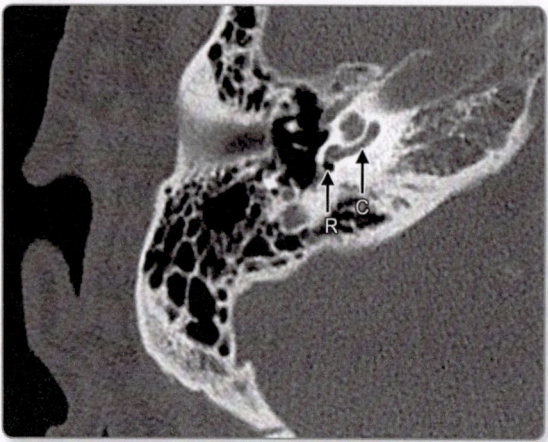

**Figure 2.3K** Axial CT image of the right temporal bone. Round window (R) and basal turn of the cochlea (C)

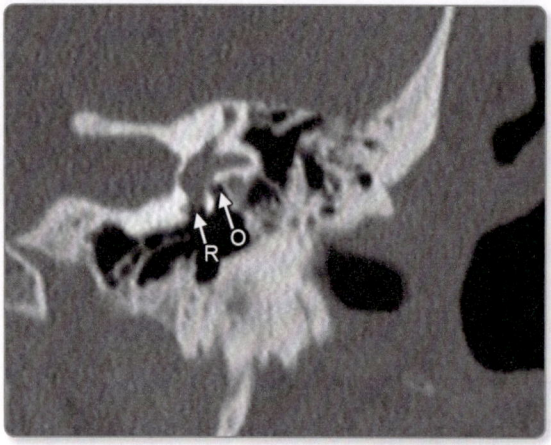

**Figure 2.3L** Coronal CT image of the right temporal bone. Round window (R) and oval window (O)

The medial wall of the tympanic cavity contains two openings, the oval and the round windows. The stapes footplate inserts on the oval window. There is a bony eminence called the cochlear promontory upon which the tensor tympani tendon travels to ultimately insert upon the malleus. Deep to the cochlear promontory lies the basal turn of the cochlea. Abutting the promontory surface is a rich plexus of sympathetic nerves. The anterior wall contains the opening of the Eustachian canal and the canal for the tensor tympani tendon.

## The facial nerve (Figures 2.4A to L)

Special attention is given to the course of the facial nerve as it has an intimate association with the structures in the temporal bone and should be evaluated on every study. The facial nerve exits the medulla anterior to the eighth cranial nerve. It crosses the cerebellopontine cistern to enter the internal auditory canal (IAC) (**Figures 2.4A and B**). The first segment of the facial nerve courses within the IAC and travels anterosuperior to the acoustic nerve (**Figures 2.4C to E**).

The facial nerve enters the fallopian or facial canal and travels superolaterally to the cochlea towards the geniculate ganglion as the second or labyrinthine segment. At the geniculate ganglion, the nerve takes a sharp hairpin turn to form the first or anterior genu of the facial nerve and redirects posteriorly (**Figures 2.4F to G**). The facial nerve continues posterolaterally along the medial wall of the middle ear, above the oval window as the third segment or tympanic segment (**Figure 2.4H**). The nerve takes an additional turn at the level of the pyramidal eminence and sinus tympani as the second genu. From the second genu, as the fourth or mastoid segment, the facial nerve travels vertically downward within the posterior wall of the middle ear cavity towards the stylomastoid foramen where it exits the temporal bone (**Figures 2.4I to L**).

## The inner ear (Figures 2.5A to I)

The inner ear labyrinth is formed by bony and membranous compartments. The membranous labyrinth is filled with endolymph and is suspended within the bony labyrinth while surrounded by perilymph. The perilymphatic space directly communicates with the subarachnoid

# Introductory head and neck imaging

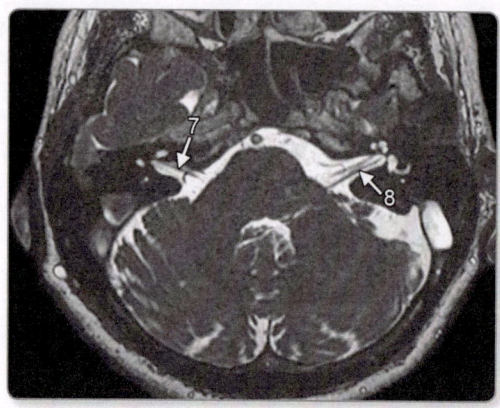

**Figure 2.4A** Axial steady state free precession gradient echo MR sequence of bilateral IAC. Facial nerve (7) and vestibulocochlear nerve (8)

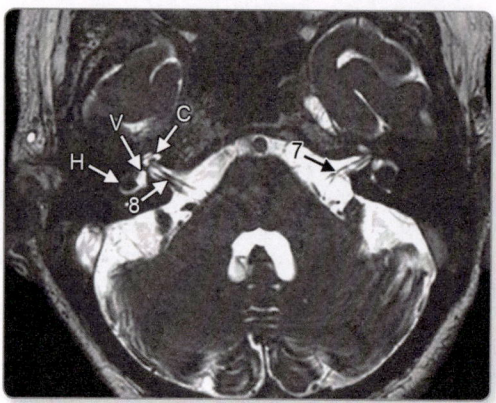

**Figure 2.4B** Axial steady state free precession gradient echo MR sequence of bilateral IAC. Facial nerve (7), vestibulocochlear nerve (8), cochlea (C), horizontal semicircular canal (H) and vestibule (V)

# Radiographic anatomy and pathology of the temporal bone

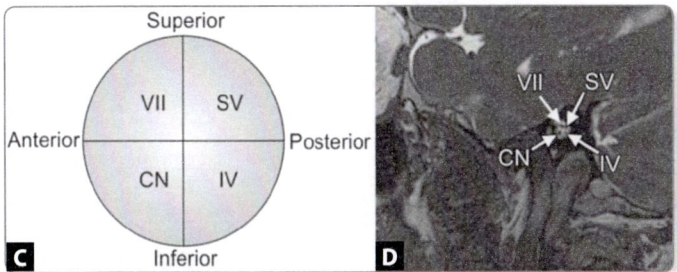

**Figures 2.4C and D** Cross-section diagrammatic view of IAC demonstrating the relationship of the cranial nerves. Within the IAC, the vestibulocochlear nerve subdivides anteriorly into the cochlear nerve (CN), which lies inferior to the facial nerve (VII) and posteriorly into the superior and inferior vestibular nerves (SV and IV respectively). Sagittal steady state free precession gradient echo sequence of the left IAC demonstrating the relation of the facial and vestibulocochlear nerves

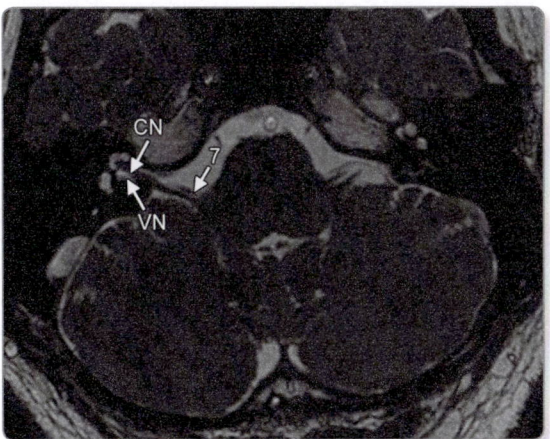

**Figure 2.4E** Axial steady state free precession MR image of bilateral IAC. Cochlear division of the vestibulocochlear nerve (CN), vestibular division of the vestibulocochlear nerve (VN) and facial nerve (7)

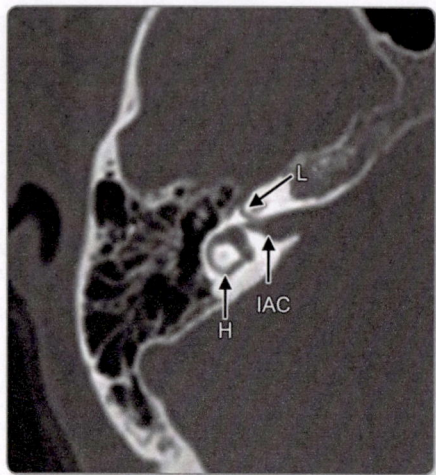

**Figure 2.4F** Axial CT image of right temporal bone. Labyrinthine segment of facial nerve (L), internal auditory canal (IAC) and horizontal semicircular canal (H)

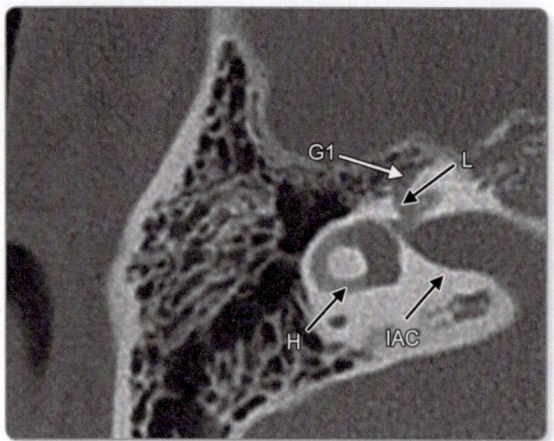

**Figure 2.4G** Axial CT image of right temporal bone. Labyrinthine segment of facial nerve (L), hairpin turn of facial nerve at 1st genu (G1), internal auditory canal (IAC) and horizontal semicircular canal (H)

# Radiographic anatomy and pathology of the temporal bone

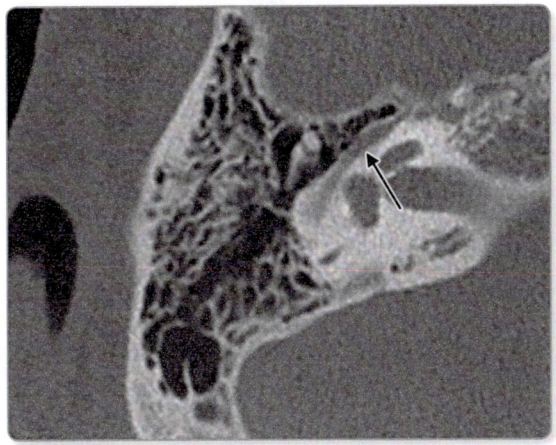

**Figure 2.4H** Axial CT image of right temporal bone. Horizontal or tympanic segment of facial nerve (black arrow)

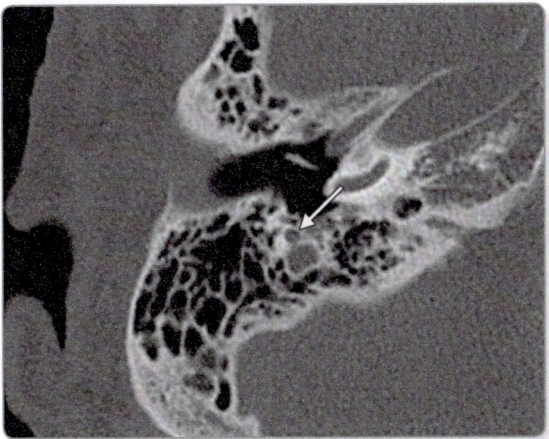

**Figure 2.4I** Axial CT image of right temporal bone. Descending or mastoid segment of facial nerve (white arrow)

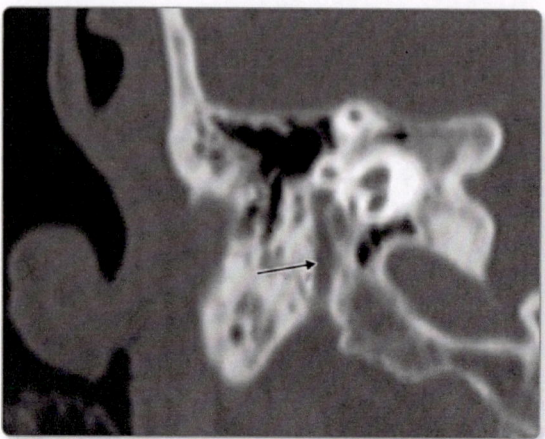

**Figure 2.4J** Coronal CT image of right temporal bone. Descending or mastoid segment of facial nerve (black arrow)

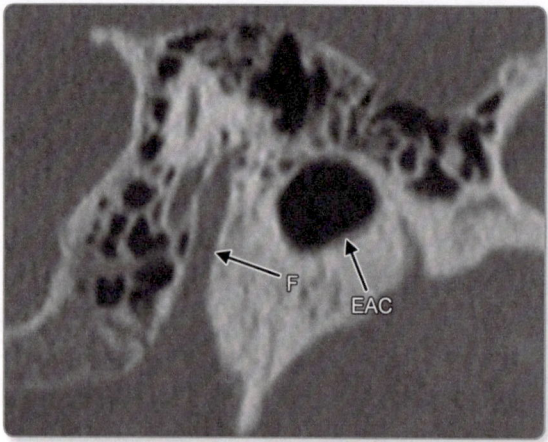

**Figure 2.4K** Sagittal CT image of right temporal bone. Descending or mastoid segment of facial nerve (F) and external auditory canal (EAC)

Radiographic anatomy and pathology of the temporal bone 31

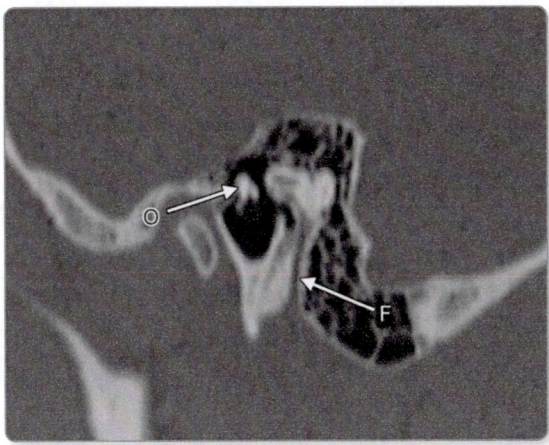

**Figure 2.4L** Sagittal CT image of right temporal bone. Descending or mastoid segment of facial nerve (F). The second genu is the angle formed between the tympanic and the mastoid segments. The typical molar tooth appearance of the Incus and malleus (O)

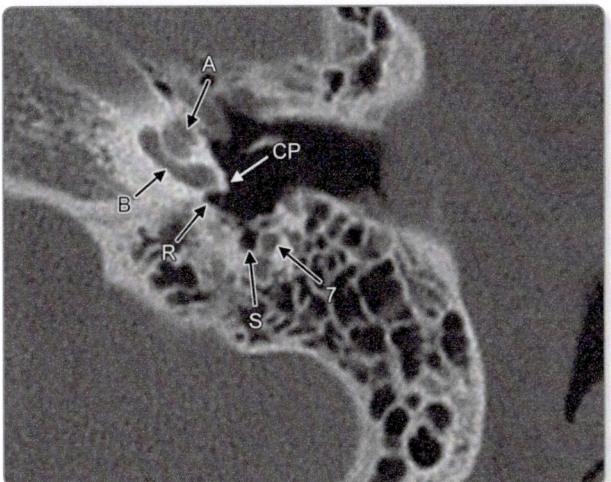

**Figure 2.5A** Axial CT image of left temporal bone. Cochlear promontory (CP), basal turn of cochlea (B), apical turn of cochlea (A), round window niche (R), sinus tympani (S) and mastoid segment of facial nerve (7)

## 32  Introductory head and neck imaging

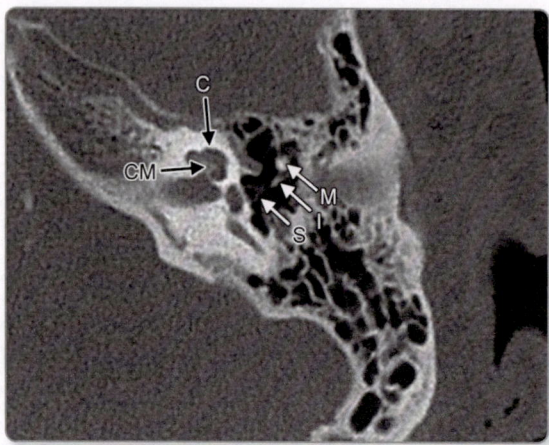

**Figure 2.5B** Axial CT image of left temporal bone. Cochlea (C), cochlear modiolus (CM), stapes at oval window (S), incus long process (I) and malleolar head (M)

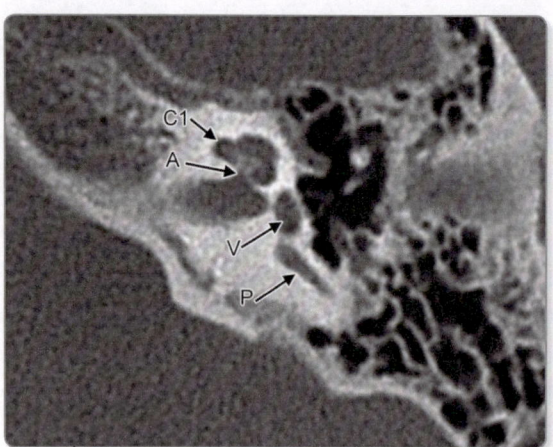

**Figure 2.5C** Axial CT image of left temporal bone. Cochlear aperture (A), first turn of cochlea (C1), vestibule (V) and posterior semicircular canal (P)

# Radiographic anatomy and pathology of the temporal bone

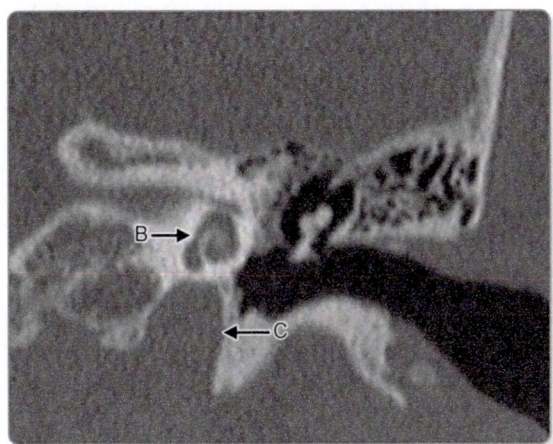

**Figure 2.5D** Coronal CT image of left temporal bone. Basal turn of cochlea (B) and carotid canal (C)

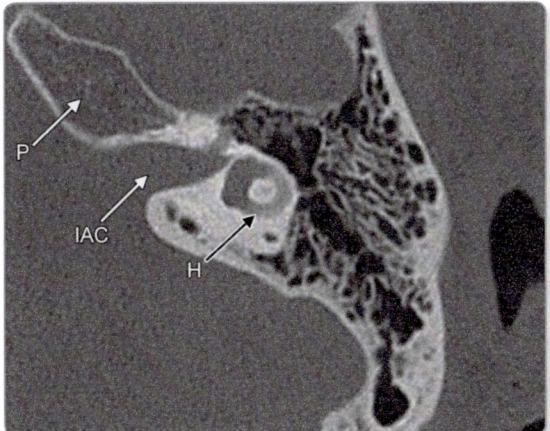

**Figure 2.5E** Axial CT image of left temporal bone. Petrous apex (P), internal auditory canal (IAC) and horizontal semicircular canal (H)

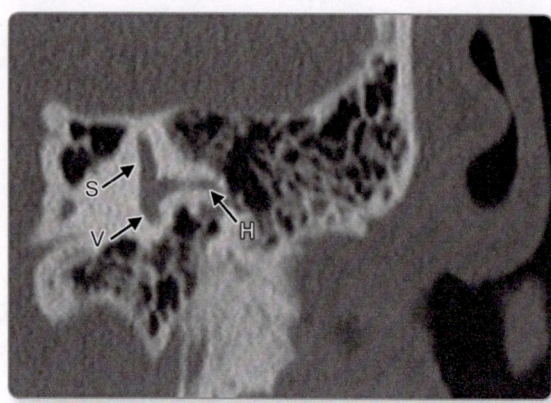

**Figure 2.5F** Coronal CT image of left temporal bone. Superior semicircular canal (S), horizontal semicircular canal (H) and vestibule (V)

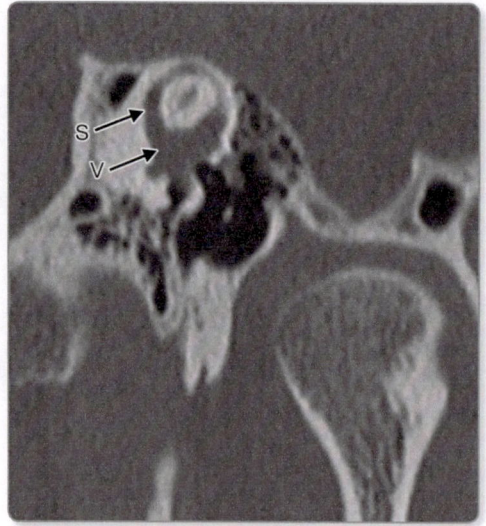

**Figure 2.5G** Coronal oblique (Poschl view) CT image of temporal bone. Superior semicircular canal (S) and vestibule (V)

# Radiographic anatomy and pathology of the temporal bone

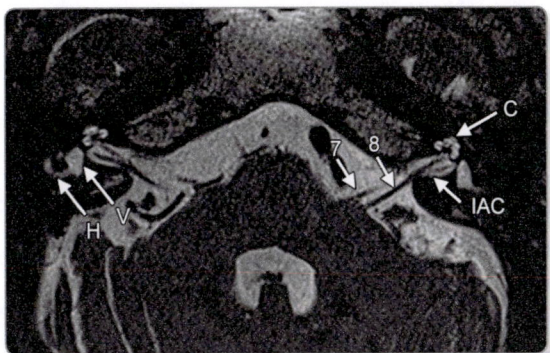

**Figure 2.5H** Axial steady state free precession gradient echo MR sequence of bilateral IAC. Cochlea (C), internal auditory canal (IAC), facial nerve (7), vestibulocochlear nerve (8), vestibule (V) and horizontal semicircular canal (H)

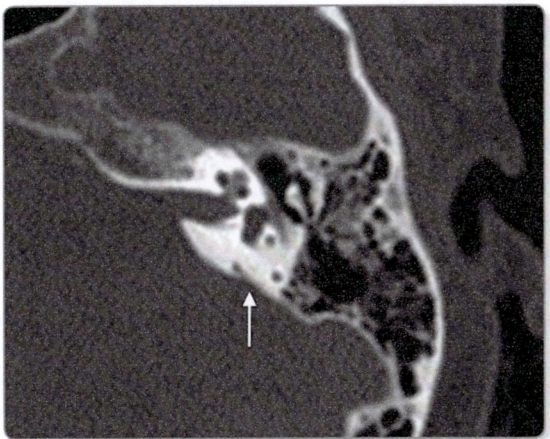

**Figure 2.5I** Axial CT image of left temporal bone. Vestibular aqueduct (white arrow)

space by way of the cochlear aqueduct. The bony labyrinth can be subdivided into the cochlea, vestibule and semicircular canals. The cochlea is a coiled structure with approximately 2.5 turns. The bony central axis of the cochlea is called the modiolus through which the cochlear nerve travels. The vestibule is continuous with the cochlea anteriorly and with the semicircular canals posteriorly. The oval and the round window open into the vestibule. The utricle and saccule are contained within the vestibule. There are three semicircular canals, superior, horizontal and posterior, which are orthogonal to each other. The vestibular aqueduct is the bony canal containing the endolymphatic duct. The vestibular aqueduct originates from the posterosuperior vestibule and courses posterior, lateral and inferiorly to open at the cisternal face of the petrous apex.

## Imaging of the temporal bone with CT and MRI

CT and MRI are routinely used to image the temporal bone. Standard technique in the imaging of the temporal bone includes 0.625 mm axial images through the temporal bone with a large field of view. These are provided in bone and soft tissue algorithm. Coned down axial and coronal bone reformations are made. Magnetic resonance imaging is a sensitive modality for evaluating the contents and pathology of the membranous labyrinth and the internal auditory canal. The standard protocol for imaging of the IAC on a 1.5 Tesla magnet includes thin section high resolution images which include the superior margin of the petrous bone, the brainstem and parotid gland. Axial and coronal precontrast T1-weighted, postcontrast fat saturated T1-weighted, coronal T2 and axial steady state free precession gradient echo sequences are obtained. Cranial nerve anatomy is best demonstrated on the steady state free precession gradient echo sequence. The T1-weighted precontrast images are helpful in the evaluation of abnormal signal in the inner ear labyrinth which may represent inner ear hemorrhage, labyrinthitis or infection. Postcontrast imaging helps to evaluate for infectious and inflammatory processes, complications of otomastoiditis and neoplasms. Fat saturation postcontrast imaging is good for the evaluation of labyrinthitis and small mass lesions such as schwannomas.

# Temporal bone pathology

## The external ear

### Congenital anomalies

*External auditory canal atresia (**Figures 2.6A and B**):* EAC atresia has a spectrum of findings and may involve the cartilaginous and/or the bony portions of the external canal. Associated deformities of the

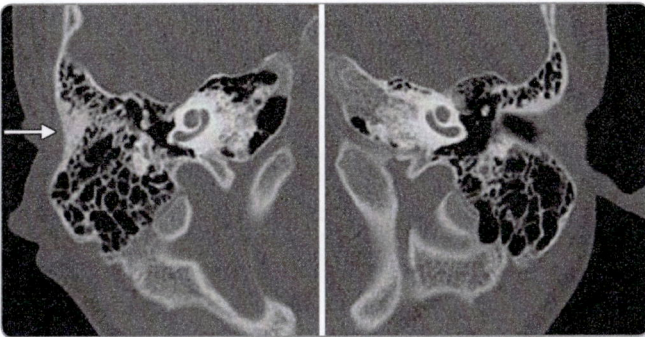

**Figure 2.6A** Axial CT images of bilateral temporal bone demonstrating absence of a normal right EAC (white arrow) as compared to the normal EAC on the left consistent with bony atresia

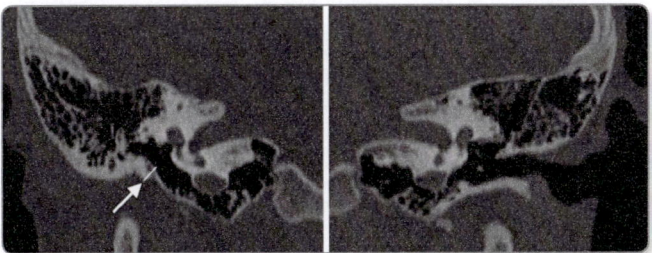

**Figure 2.6B** Coronal CT images of bilateral temporal bone demonstrating absence of a normal right EAC as compared to the normal left EAC with a right bony atretic plate (white arrow)

pinna are commonly seen. The orientation of the EAC may be altered such that it is more vertical and almost parallel to the descending segment of the facial nerve. Thus, imaging is crucial in the preoperative setting. The radiologist must provide the clinician with the type and measurement of the width of the atresia plate, as well as delineate its relationship with the facial nerve. Comment should also be made on middle ear and ossicular chain morphology, and patency of the middle ear fenestrae. The middle ear cavity can be hypoplastic resulting in a high-riding temporomandibular joint and jugular bulb. Abnormalities of the malleus and incus, including fusion, are also common.

## Acquired diseases

*Keratosis obturans (**Figures 2.7A and B**):* This condition is characterized by an abnormal accumulation of desquamated keratin within the bony EAC. The mechanism is unknown and it is important to differentiate this entity from an EAC cholesteatoma which may demonstrate local invasion and bony erosion. Imaging typically demonstrates a soft tissue plug within the EAC without bony destruction, sometimes resulting in widening and smooth bony remodeling of the canal. These patients are generally young in age, and may have a history of sinusitis and bronchiectasis. Pain and conductive hearing loss may occur due to the keratin plug which causes pressure on the EAC lining and eventual ulceration. Without treatment, this ulcer can accumulate granulation tissue and the process proceeds to erode the underlying bone in extreme cases. The process of self cleansing of the keratin where the keratin matures and migrates laterally in normal individuals is lacking in patients with keratosis obturans. The increased rate of desquamation and poor clearance results in layering of compact keratin. Resultant pressure on the bony wall can cause expansion and bony remodeling. It is often a systemic process.

*EAC cholesteatoma (**Figures 2.8A to C**):* These patients are usually elderly and may have stenosis of the external auditory canal from prior trauma or surgery. The stenosis is usually along the junction of the cartilaginous and bony portions of the EAC. With age, the normal epithelial migration in the EAC is lost and the canal is obliterated with

Radiographic anatomy and pathology of the temporal bone 39

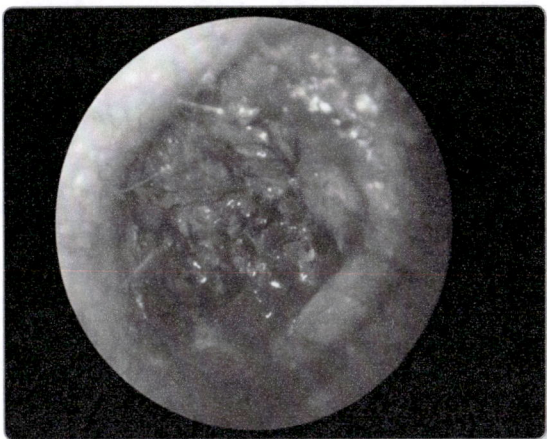

**Figure 2.7A** 30-year-old patient with otalgia and conductive hearing loss. Otoscopic image of the EAC demonstrating a large, bleeding, keratinous mass obstructing the EAC with erosion and widening of the EAC (*for color version see Plate 2*)

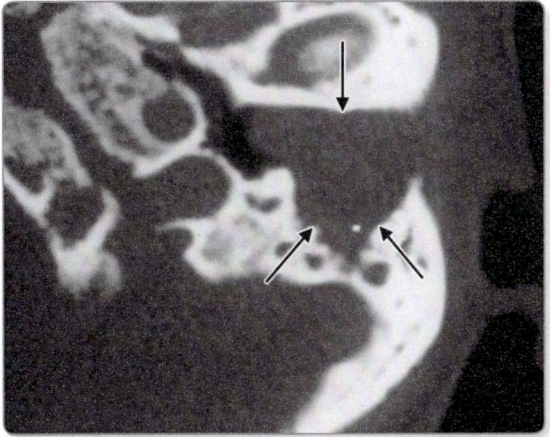

**Figure 2.7B** 30-year-old patient with otalgia and conductive hearing loss. Axial CT of the left temporal bone demonstrating a mass obliterating the EAC and eroding the mastoid bone posteriorly, which was found to represent keratosis obturans

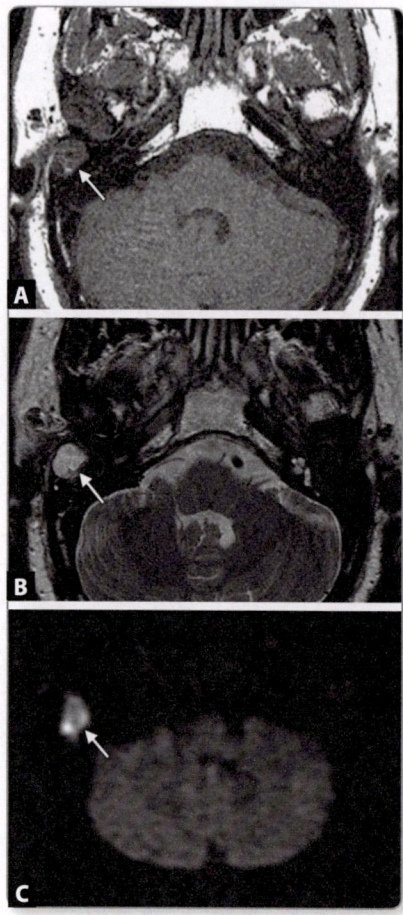

**Figures 2.8A to C** Axial T1-weighted, T2-weighted and diffusion-weighted MR images of bilateral IAC. There is a T1 hypointense, T2 hyperintense mass (white arrow) involving the right EAC which demonstrates restricted diffusion on diffusion-weighted imaging consistent with EAC cholesteatoma

a thick epithelialized membrane and fibrous tissue. Loosely packed keratin accumulates lateral to the tympanic membrane. The appearance on otoscopy is the apparent shortening of the canal and with a false fundus. The true tympanic membrane is hidden behind the fibrous epithelial matrix. There is no history of sinusitis or bronchiectasis. There are no keratin plugs and the tympanic drum is normal. These patients present with dull aching pain, with or without hearing loss and otorrhea. There may be erosive changes and periostitis localized to the posterior and inferior walls of the EAC. MR imaging will demonstrate T1 isointense, T2 hyperintense mass within the EAC which demonstrates abnormal signal on the diffusion-weighted sequence.

*EAC exostosis* (**Figures 2.9A to C**): Bony exostosis is a benign condition whereby there is focal or multifocal osseous hypertrophy of the deep bony external auditory canal. Benign bony hypertrophic reaction occur secondary to repetitive insults from exposure to cold water. The reactive vasoconstriction hyperemia results in periosteal reaction and over time new bone formation. This may result in a single or several bony masses narrowing the EAC. Typically, these masses arise along the tympanomastoid or tympanosquamous suture line and are limited medially by the tympanic membrane. Exostosis are often seen in swimmers hence the name swimmers ears. Often asymptomatic, they may cause symptoms when the exostosis is covered by wax and cerumen which may cause reactive otitis from blockage.

*Osteoma* (**Figures 2.10A and B**): Osteomas are benign bony neoplasms which are typically incidentally seen on CT imaging. These are usually attached near the petrosquamous suture and may be sessile or have a bony stalk. These are true bony neoplasm composed of cancellous or trabeculated bone as opposed to exostosis which have dense lamellar cortical bone. Patients are generally asymptomatic.

*Otitis externa* (**Figures 2.11A to F**): Otitis externa is a common infection involving the external ear in all age groups, which is usually bacterial in etiology and less commonly fungal. Evaluation with CT is usually not performed for cases of uncomplicated otits externa, however, is useful when there is suspected necrotizing otitis *eternal*. Malignant

## 42 Introductory head and neck imaging

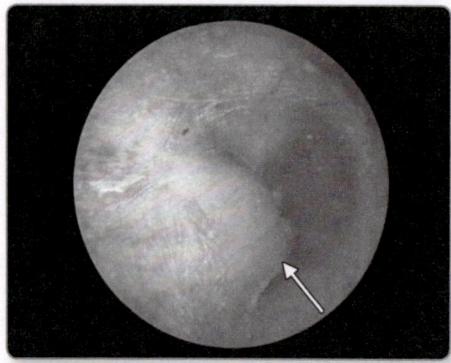

**Figure 2.9A** Otoscopic image of the EAC demonstrating the presence of large masses (white arrow) in the EAC (*for color version see Plate 3*)

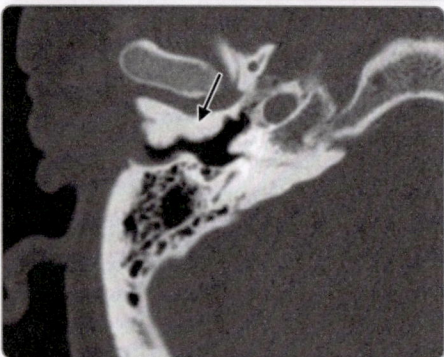

**Figure 2.9B** Axial CT of right temporal bone demonstrating lobulated bony narrowing of bony EAC (black arrow)

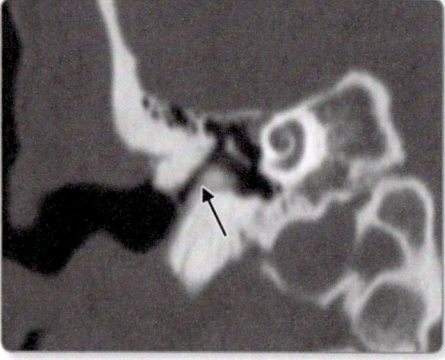

**Figure 2.9C** Coronal CT of right temporal bone demonstrating lobulated bony narrowing of bony EAC (black arrow)

Radiographic anatomy and pathology of the temporal bone 43

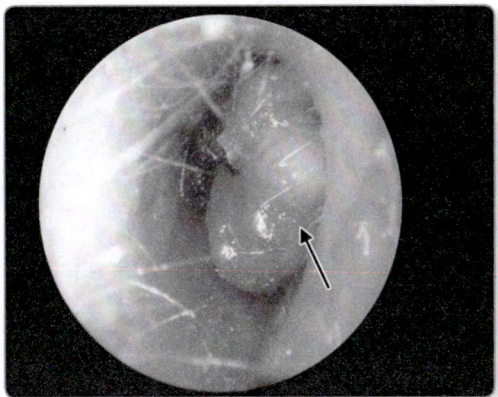

**Figure 2.10A** Otoscopic image of the EAC demonstrates an incidental mass (black arrow) seen on otoscopy with normal skin covering the neoplasm (*for color version see Plate 3*)

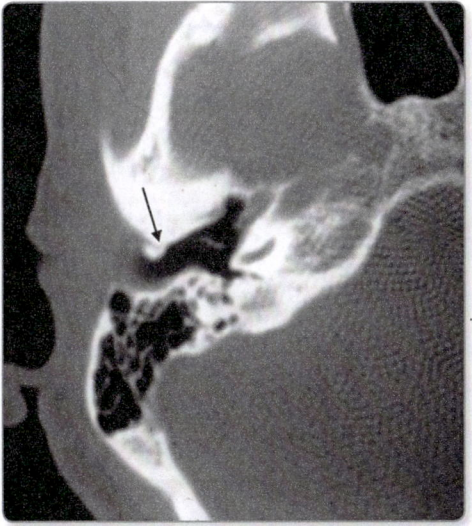

**Figure 2.10B** Axial CT image of the right temporal bone demonstrates a flat bony tumor mass on a thin bony stalk consistent with an osteoma

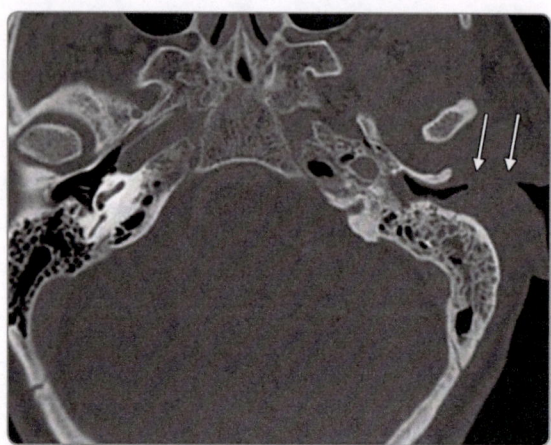

**Figure 2.11A** Axial CT of temporal bones demonstrating soft tissue swelling with narrowing of the EAC and thickening of the pinna consistent with otitis externa (white arrows). Note the absence of bony destruction or scalp abscess to suggest malignant otitis externa

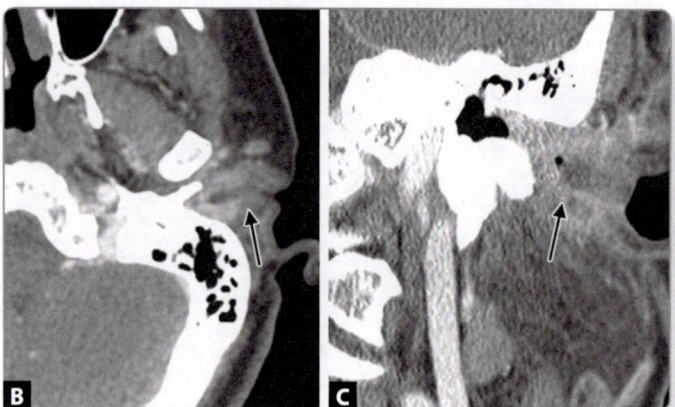

**Figures 2.11B and C** Axial and coronal contrast-enhanced CT images of the left temporal bone demonstrating soft tissue thickening with enhancement and obliteration of the EAC suggestive of otitis externa (black arrows)

Radiographic anatomy and pathology of the temporal bone 45

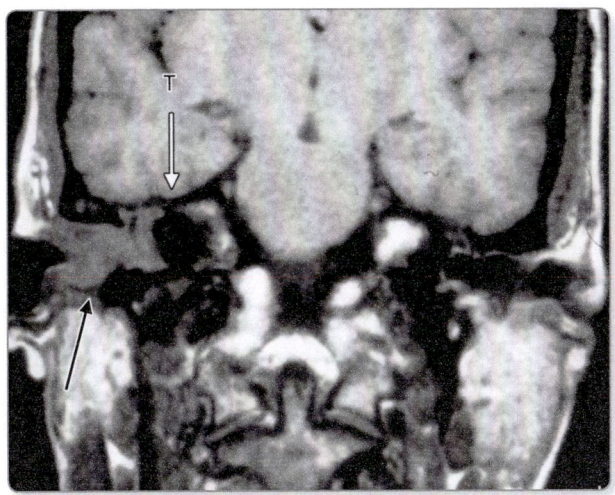

**Figure 2.11D** Coronal precontrast T1-weighted MR image of bilateral internal auditory canal (IAC)

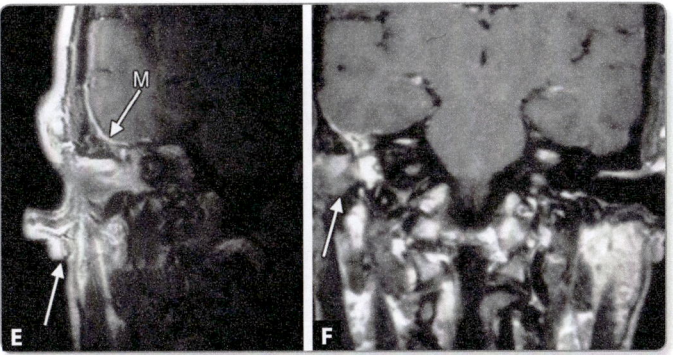

**Figures 2.11E and F** Coronal postcontrast T1-weighted MR images of bilateral internal auditory canal (IAC)

otitis externa describes an aggressive form of infection seen in the diabetic and immunosuppressed population caused by *Pseudomonas aeruginosa*. CT and MR Imaging may reveal aggressive osseous destruction with intracranial extension and cranial nerve involvement.

Coronal pre- and post-contrast MR images demonstrating soft tissue thickening along the bony and cartilaginous EAC with occlusion of EAC lumen (black arrow) and erosion of the tegmen tympani (T) (**Figures 2.11D to F**). Post-contrast imaging demonstrates enhancement along the EAC with intracranial extension of disease and enhancement of the basal meninges (M) consistent with pachymeningitis.

*Radiation osteitis (**Figures 2.12A and B**):* Patients who undergo radiation treatment for any head and neck tumors are predisposed to radiation necrosis and osteitis from radiation induced vascular injury. The inability to revascularize leads to necrosis of the external ear lining. Patients will complain of painful drainage from the EAC with a history of repetitive super-infection. On CT, there is osteolytic changes with inflammation involving the EAC lining. On CT, findings may appear

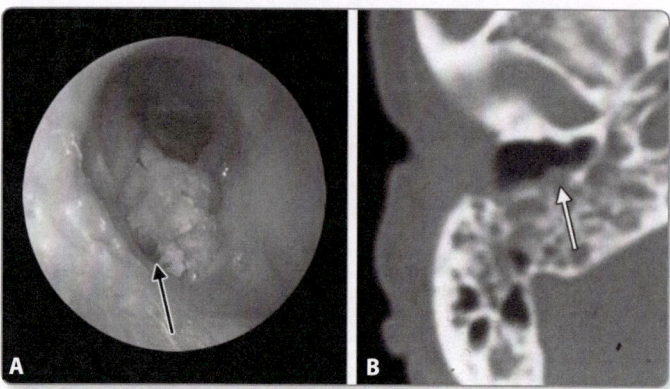

**Figures 2.12A and B** The patient had radiation treatment for a basal cell carcinoma of the head and neck four years prior. Otoscopic image of the EAC demonstrates non viable bone in the floor of the EAC (black arrow). Axial CT image of the right temporal bone demonstrates bony erosion of the posterior wall of the EAC (white arrow) with opacification of the underlying mastoid air cells. This patient required debridement of the EAC and removal of the nonviable or bony sequestrum from the EAC (*for color version of Figure 2.12A see Plate 4*)

Radiographic anatomy and pathology of the temporal bone

identical to osteomyelitis and if left untreated complications similar to osteomyelitis may ensue.

*Tumors of the external auditory canal (**Figures 2.13A to D**):* EAC tumors usually arise from the skin and are either squamous cell or basal cell carcinoma. Malignant lesions from the parotid gland can extend directly into the anterior aspect of the EAC. The ceruminous glands in the EAC can result in ceruminoma which can be a benign adenoma

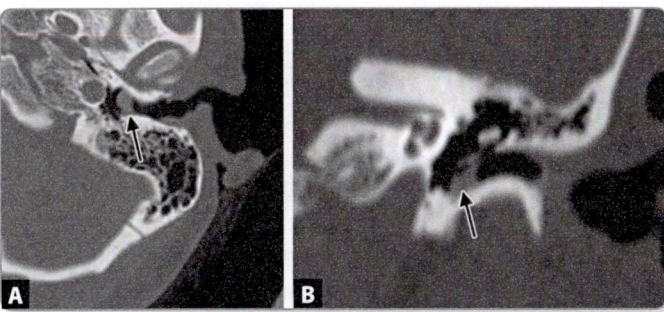

**Figures 2.13A and B** Ceruminoma of the EAC seen on the axial and coronal CT images as a soft tissue lesion without any erosion or destruction of the wall of the EAC (black arrows)

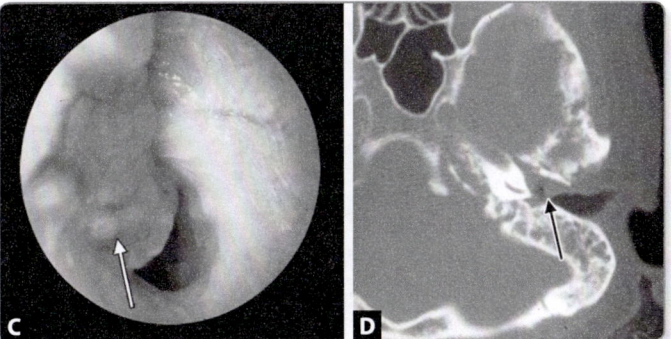

**Figures 2.13C and D** Otoscopic and axial CT image demonstrating parotid tumor invading the EAC. On otoscopy, a pinkish white tumor is seen invading the EAC (white arrow). CT imaging demonstrates a lobulated mass protruding into the canal (black arrow) (*for color version of Figure 2.13C see Plate 4*)

or an adenocarcinoma. The ceruminous glands are mainly distributed along the cartilaginous canal and are sparsely seen through out the bony canal. These tumors are locally invasive and require wide dissection to prevent recurrence.

Squamous cell carcinomas are more frequent than ceruminomas and occur more medially to invade the tympanic membrane and middle ear. These patients have a long standing history of otitis externa and often delay the diagnosis of underlying neoplasm. The change from chronic infection to more ominous symptoms such as facial nerve paralysis or bleeding should motivate reinvestigation.

# The middle ear

## Congenital anomalies

*Aberrant internal carotid artery (**Figures 2.14A and B**):* The bony course of the internal carotid artery and its relationship to the middle ear

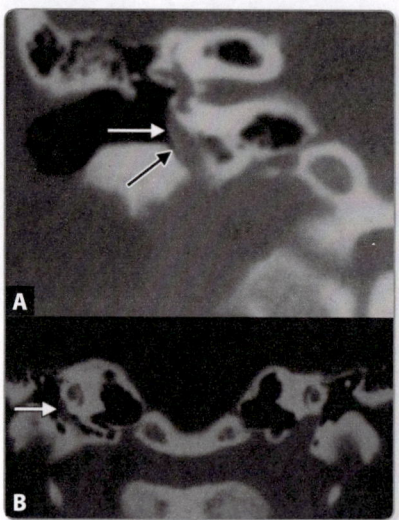

**Figures 2.14A and B** Coronal CT images of the temporal bone demonstrating a tubular structure traversing the medial tympanic cavity corresponding to an anomalous segment of ICA (white arrow) with dehiscence of bony canal (black arrow) on right

Radiographic anatomy and pathology of the temporal bone 49

cavity is well evaluated on CT. The internal carotid artery may have course to enter the middle ear cavity posteriorly via an enlarged inferior tympanic canaliculus. The internal carotid artery presents posterior and lateral to the expected site of the vertical segment of the internal carotid artery. These findings are thought to occur secondary to regression of the cervical segment of the ICA. These patients often present with pulsatile tinnitus and otoscopic examination can be nearly indistinguishable from paragangliomas. On imaging, a tubular structure can be seen traversing the medial tympanic cavity, crossing horizontally across the cochlear promontory and into the horizontal carotid canal via a dehiscent carotid plate.

*Jugular bulb dehiscence (**Figures 2.15A to C**):* Dehiscence of the jugular bulb is a congenital variant that creates a pseudomass in the middle ear. Focal absence of the sigmoid plate leads to superolateral extension of the jugular bulb into the tympanic cavity. Clinically, patients are asymptomatic. On otoscopy, a vascular retrotympanic mass is seen in the posteroinferior quadrant of the tympanic membrane. Variations of the jugular bulb can be seen with asymmetric enlargement of the jugular bulb or high-riding jugular bulb with or without bony dehiscence.

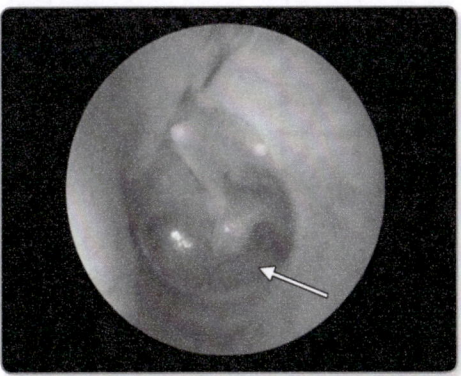

**Figure 2.15A** Otoscopic image demonstrating a bluish retrotympanic mass (white arrow) below the ossicles found to represent a high-riding dehiscent jugular bulb (*for color version see Plate 5*)

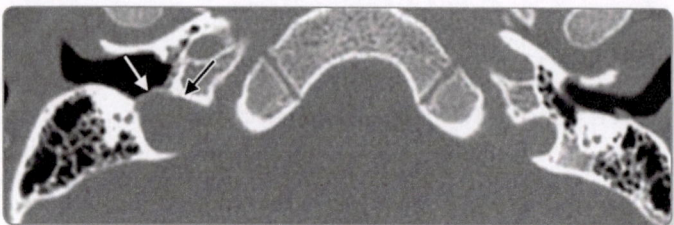

**Figure 2.15B** Axial CT of right temporal bone demonstrating a large high-riding jugular bulb (black arrow) which appears to bulge into the middle ear cavity. Note the thinned overlying bone as compared to the normal left jugular bulb (white arrow)

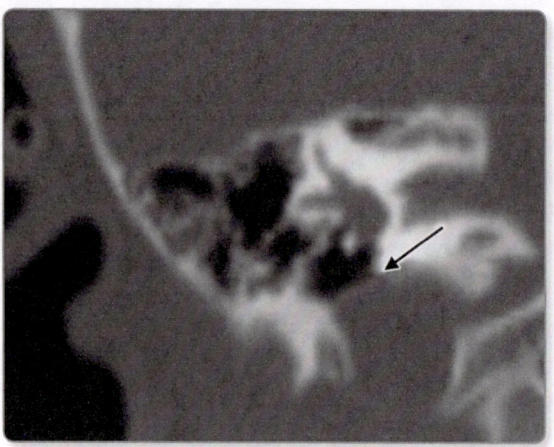

**Figure 2.15C** Coronal CT of right temporal bone demonstrating a large high-riding jugular bulb with thinning of overlying bone (black arrow)

*Congenital cholesteatoma (**Figures 2.16A and B**):* Congenital cholesteatoma is secondary to abnormal ectodermal rest migration resulting in mass-like accumulation of stratified epithelial squamous cells in the middle ear. On otology, a rounded well defined whitish retrotympanic mass is usually present. Clinically, the tympanic membrane will be intact. CT is the imaging modality of choice. Imaging will demonstrate a well circumscribed soft tissue lesion with smooth margins

Radiographic anatomy and pathology of the temporal bone 51

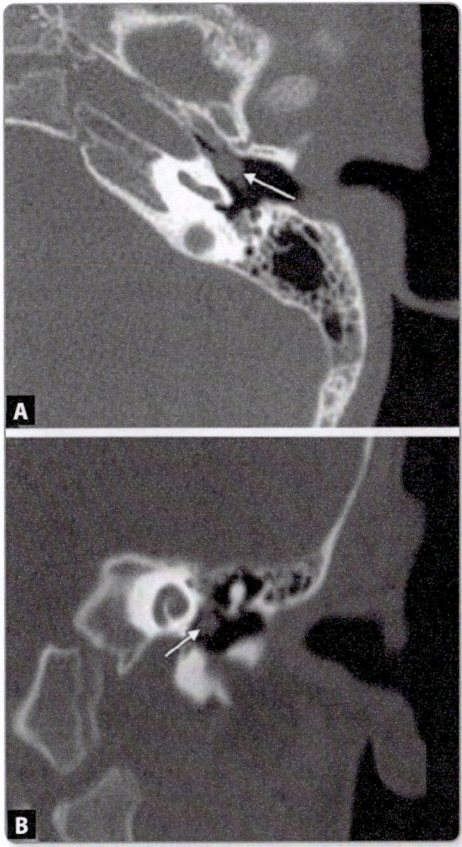

**Figures 2.16A and B** Axial and coronal CT images of left temporal bone demonstrating a soft tissue mass medial to the malleus and incus (white arrow). In the setting of an intact tympanic membrane, this mass is most consistent with a congenital cholesteatoma. Note the potential for lateral displacement of the ossicles with lesion enlargement

in the anterior aspect of the middle ear cavity. Typically, congenital cholesteatomas occur medial to the ossicles and can result in lateral displacement of the ossicular chain. Ossicular erosions can be present.

## Acquired diseases

*Acute otomastoiditis (**Figures 2.17A to L**):* The middle ear and mastoid air cells are susceptible to upper respiratory infection via direct

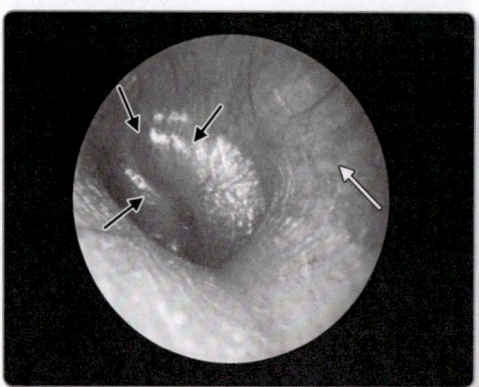

**Figure 2.17A** Otoscopic image of the tympanic membrane demonstrates reddish inflammation of the tympanic membrane (black arrows) with an erythematous EAC (white arrow) (*for color version see Plate 5*)

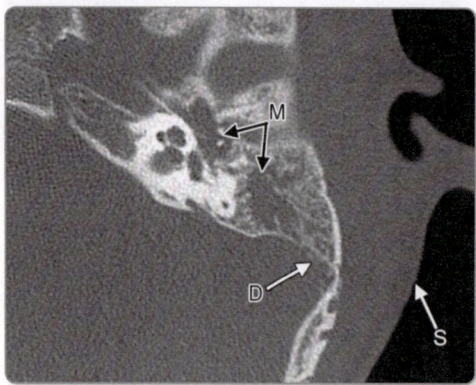

**Figure 2.17B** Axial CT image of the left temporal bone in bone window demonstrates significant swelling of the periauricular soft tissue with lateralization of the left pinna (S). There is extensive opacification of the mastoid air cells and middle ear cavity (M) consistent with acute otomastoiditis. Note the bony dehiscence of the sigmoid plate along the posterior wall of the mastoid (D)

Radiographic anatomy and pathology of the temporal bone 53

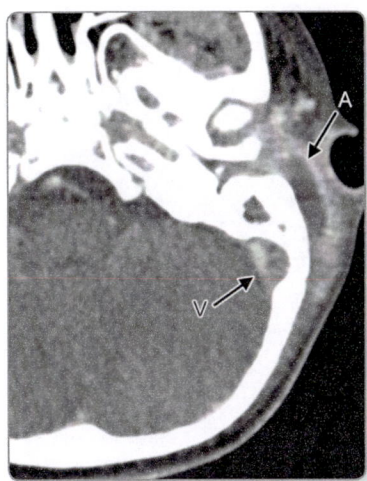

**Figure 2.17C** Contrast-enhanced axial CT image of the left temporal bone in soft tissue window of the same patient as in Figure 2.17B, demonstrating a subperiosteal abscess (A). There is partial thrombosis of the left sigmoid dural venous sinus (V)

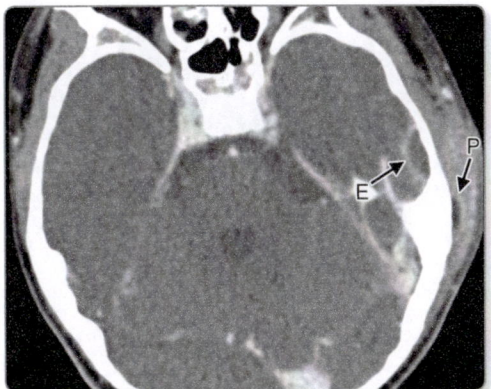

**Figure 2.17D** Contrast-enhanced axial CT image of the brain in soft tissue window of the same patient as in Figures 2.17B and C. demonstrating an additional subperiosteal abscess (P) and an epidural abscess (E) along the left temporal convexity

## 54 Introductory head and neck imaging

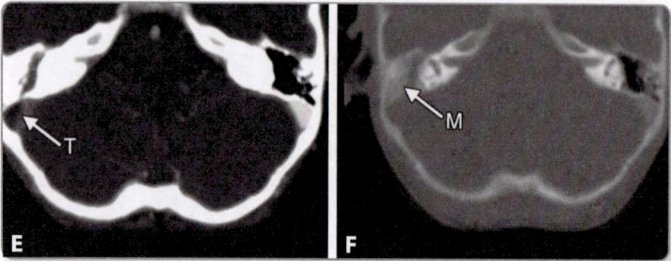

**Figures 2.17E and F** Axial CT venogram images of bilateral temporal bones demonstrating acute right sigmoid dural venous sinus thrombosis (T). In bone window, there is complete opacification of the mastoid air cells (M) consistent with mastoiditis

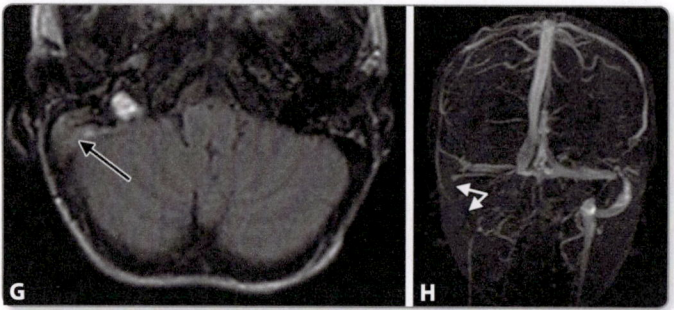

**Figures 2.17G and H** Axial FLAIR brain MR image and coronal 2D time-of-flight brain MR venogram image of the same patient as in Figures 2.17E and F. demonstrating abnormal high flair signal in the right sigmoid dural venous sinus (black arrow) which extends into the jugular fossa consistent with thrombosis. Note the normal flow void in the region of the left sigmoid dural venous sinus. On the 2D time-of-flight, there is absence of enhancement in the right sigmoid dural venous sinus (white arrows) consistent with the findings seen on the CT venogram

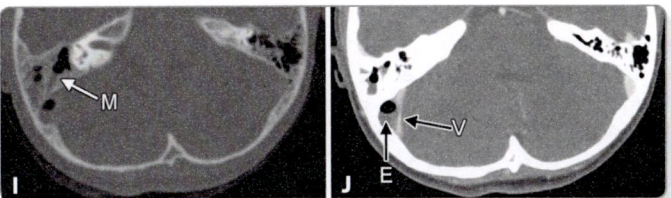

**Figures 2.17I and J** Axial CT images of bilateral temporal bones in bone and soft tissue windows demonstrating extensive opacification of the right mastoid with air-fluid levels (M) consistent with mastoiditis. There is an epidural abscess (E) in the right posterior fossa causing compression and narrowing of the right sigmoid sinus (V)

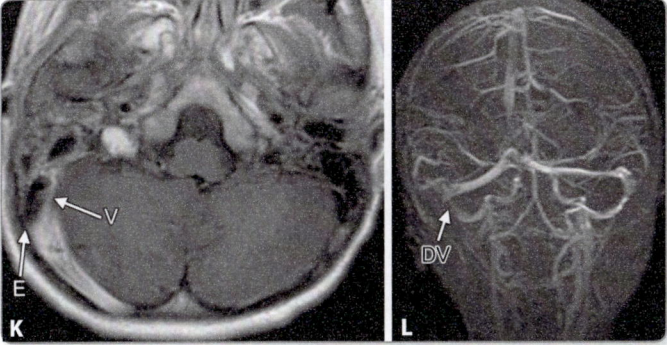

**Figures 2.17K and L** Axial T1-weighted postcontrast MR image and coronal 2D time-of-flight MR venogram image of the same patient as in Figures 2.17I and J. There is marked narrowing of the right sigmoid dural venous sinus (V) secondary to compression by an epidural abscess (E). On the coronal 2D time-of-flight MR image confirms a patent by markedly narrowed right sigmoid dural venous sinus (DV)

extension. Combined inflammation and infection of the middle ear cavity and mastoid denotes acute otomastoiditis. Both CT and MR imaging are ideal in the evaluation of acute otomastoiditis and the complications. CT findings include opacification of the otomastoid with or without air-fluid levels in an appropriate clinical picture. On

MR imaging, T2 hyperintense debris is present within the middle ear and mastoid air cells which enhance with contrast. Coalescent otomastoiditis describes acute otomastoiditis with mastoid cortical dehiscence and rarefaction of Koerner's septum and the mastoid trabeculae. Erosion of the mastoid cortex can lead to formation of a subperiosteal abscess and intracranial extension. Resultant intracranial complications include epidural abscess, subdural empyema, meningitis and dural venous thrombosis. A Bezold's abscess describes extension of infection beyond the mastoid tip into the neck deep to or within the sternocleidomastoid muscle. An important complication of acute otomastoiditis is formation of an acquired cholesteatoma.

*Chronic otomastoiditis (**Figures 2.18A and B**):* Chronic otomastoiditis is a chronic unremitting inflammation of the middle ear and mastoid air cells. CT is the mainstay imaging modality and it is important to differentiate chronic otomastoiditis from acquired cholesteatoma. MRI has little role in the evaluation of chronic otomastoiditis. CT findings include under pneumatization of the mastoid air cells with bony sclerosis and opacification. This is typically seen in the absence of acute symptoms. The degree of sinus sclerosis needs to be elucidated and characterized as being mild, moderate or severe. Soft tissue can be seen within the tympanic cavity without mass effect on the ossicular chain, unlike acquired cholesteatomas. Ossicular erosions are less common than with acquired cholesteatomas. Ossicular fixation with tympanosclerosis can be seen with increased calcific density within the tympanic membrane and middle ear cavity as a complication of chronic otitis media.

*Acquired cholesteatoma (**Figures 2.19A to I**):* An acquired cholesteatoma is an expansile soft tissue mass in the middle ear cavity which is associated with tympanic membrane retraction or perforation. This lesion can arise from the pars flaccida or pars tensa and forms as a result of abnormal accumulation of stratified squamous epithelial cells. On otoscopy, a pearly white mass can be seen with a perforated tympanic membrane. Classically, the pars flaccida cholesteatoma is seen as a soft tissue mass within Prussak's space lateral to the malleus head with or without blunting of the scutum. Medial displacement

Radiographic anatomy and pathology of the temporal bone

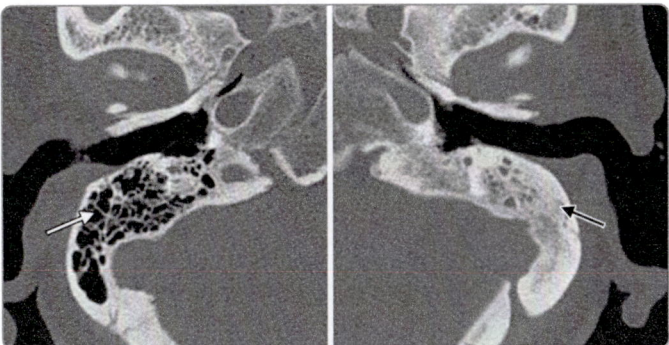

**Figure 2.18A** Axial CT images of bilateral temporal bones demonstrating under pneumatization and opacification of the left mastoid air cells (black arrow) as compared to the normal right mastoid bone (white arrow) with severe bony sclerosis

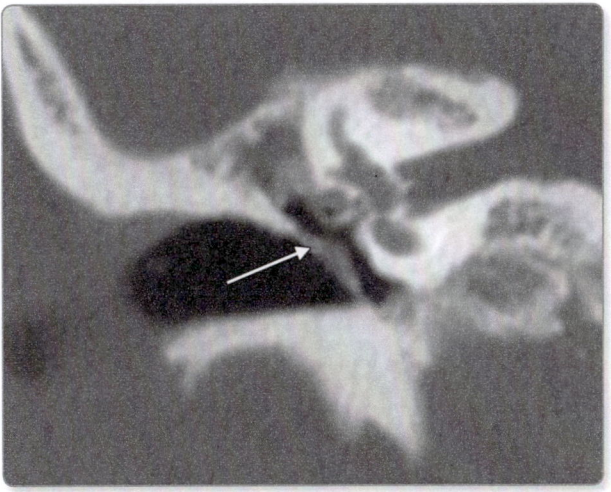

**Figure 2.18B** Coronal CT image of the right temporal bone demonstrates a thickened and partially calcified tympanic membrane (white arrow) in a patient with a history of chronic otomastoiditis consistent with tympanosclerosis

## 58 Introductory head and neck imaging

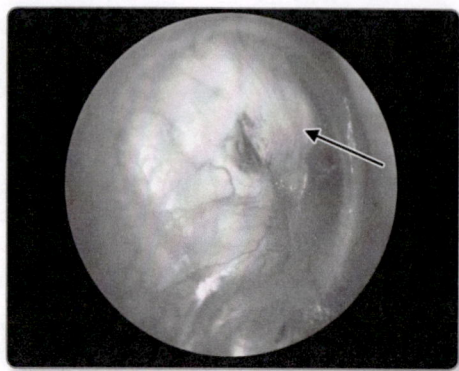

**Figure 2.19A** Otoscopic image of the tympanic membrane demonstrating a large ivory-yellow retrotympanic mass (*for color version see Plate 6*)

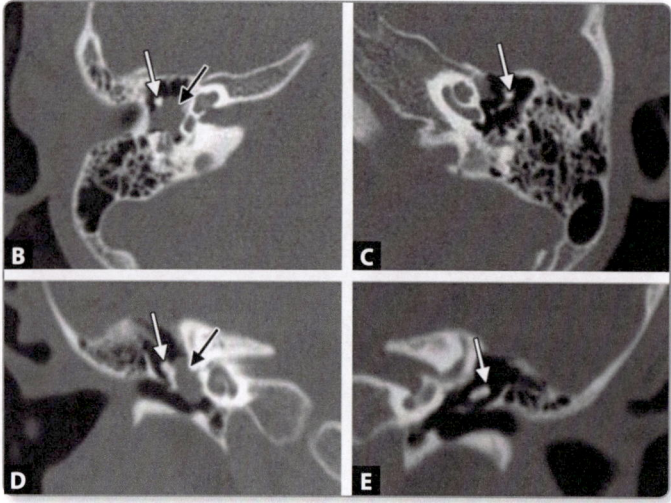

**Figures 2.19B to E** Axial and coronal CT images of bilateral temporal bones demonstrating a soft tissue mass (black arrows) in the right tympanic cavity medial to the ossicles (white arrows) in the setting of a perforated membrane consistent with a pars tensa cholesteatoma. The normal left temporal bone is provided for comparison. Note the lateral displacement of the ossicular chain by this mass

Radiographic anatomy and pathology of the temporal bone

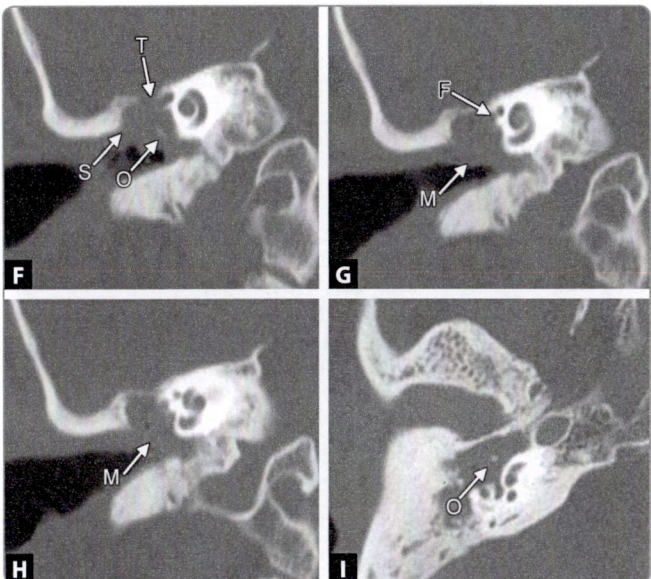

**Figures 2.19F to I** Coronal and axial CT images of the right temporal bone demonstrating the complications of acquired cholesteatoma. A soft tissue mass (M) fills the tympanic membrane causing erosion of the ossicles (O), blunting of the scutum (S), dehiscence of the tegmen tympani (T) and erosion of the bone around the horizontal segment of the facial nerve (F). Note the absence of normal ossicles

of the ossicular chain can be seen with those arising from the pars flaccida. The pars tensa cholesteatoma is commonly seen within the posterior tympanic cavity, medial to the ossicles, and may involve the sinus tympani, facial recess or aditus ad antrum. These nonenhancing lesions can continue to enlarge and erode adjacent bone. Ossicular erosions are more commonly seen in with pars tensa cholesteatomas versus pars flaccida cholesteatomas and usually depend on size.

*Cholesterol granuloma (**Figures 2.20A to E**):* Cholesterol granuloma is an acquired lesion secondary to foreign body reaction and giant cell reaction to cholesterol crystals. This is typically seen in the setting

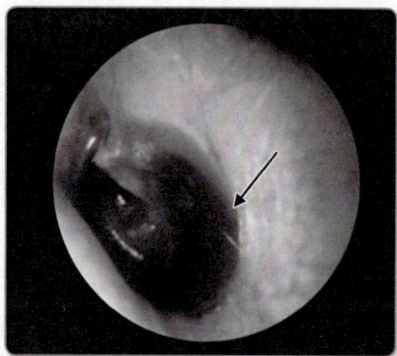

**Figure 2.20A** Otoscopic image of a tympanic membrane demonstrates a bluish-black retrotympanic mass (black arrow) protruding from the middle ear corresponding to a cholesterol granuloma (*for color version see Plate 6*)

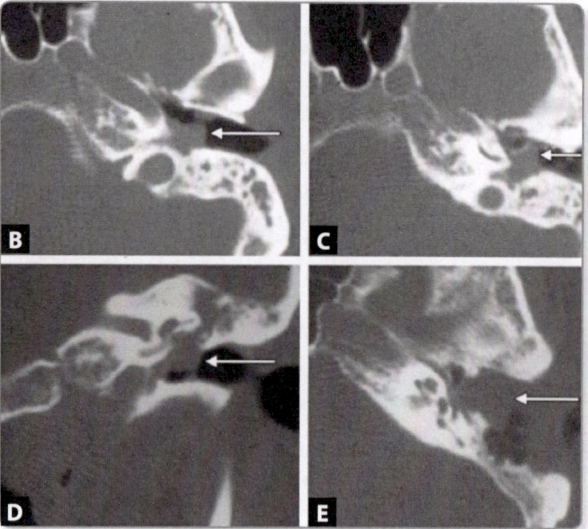

**Figures 2.20B to E** Axial and coronal CT images of the left temporal bone demonstrating a soft tissue mass (white arrows) in the tympanic cavity in a postoperative patient which appeared as a bluish retrotympanic mass on otoscopy and found to correspond to a cholesterol granuloma

of recurrent middle ear hemorrhage and chronic infection. Chronic inflammation results in the formation of mass-like granulation tissue. On otoscopy, a dark, bluish retrotympanic mass is often described and must be distinguished from vascular lesions such as dehiscence of the jugular bulb, an aberrant internal carotid artery and a paraganglioma. CT findings include a mass involving the tympanic cavity with smooth expansion of the surrounding bone. The expansile quality of this lesion is useful in distinguishing these lesions from hemorrhagic otitis media. Cholesterol granulomas appear T1 hyperintense and T2 hyperintense on MRI secondary to the cholesterol crystals. Contrast-enhanced CT imaging can be helpful in distinguishing the cholesterol granuloma from the other aforementioned vascular lesions.

## Neoplasm

*Glomus tumors (**Figures 2.21A to E**):* Paragangliomas are the most common primary tumors of the middle ear. Occurring within the temporal bone, these tumors are usually along the course of cranial nerves XI and X. When present on the cochlear promontory or within the hypotympanum, they are called glomus tympanicum tumors. Those within the jugular foramen region are known as glomus jugulare

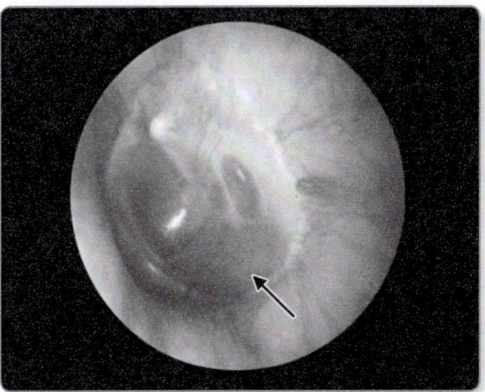

**Figure 2.21A** Otoscopic image of the tympanic membrane demonstrates a purplish-bluish retrotympanic mass (black arrow) in the hypotympanum found to be a glomus jugulotympanicum *(for color version see Plate 7)*

**62 Introductory head and neck imaging**

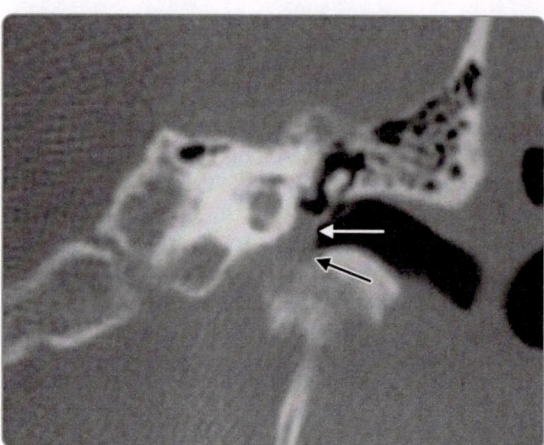

**Figure 2.21B** Coronal CT image of left temporal bone demonstrating a soft tissue mass (white arrow) within the hypotympanum with adjacent erosion of the jugular bulb bony wall (black arrow) found to be a glomus jugulotympanicum

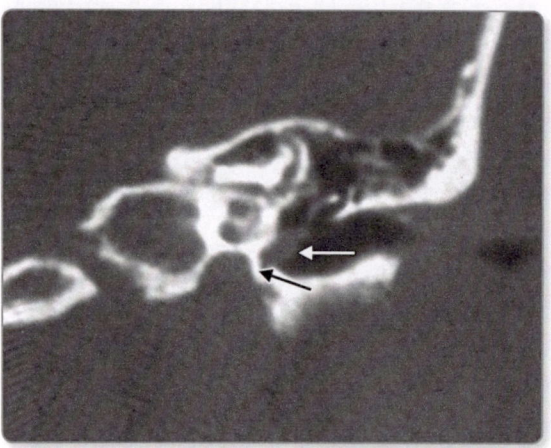

**Figure 2.21C** Coronal CT image of left temporal bone demonstrating a soft tissue mass (white arrow) in the hypotympanum adjacent to the cochlear promontory found to be a glomus tympanicum. Note the intact jugular bulb bony wall (black arrow)

Radiographic anatomy and pathology of the temporal bone    63

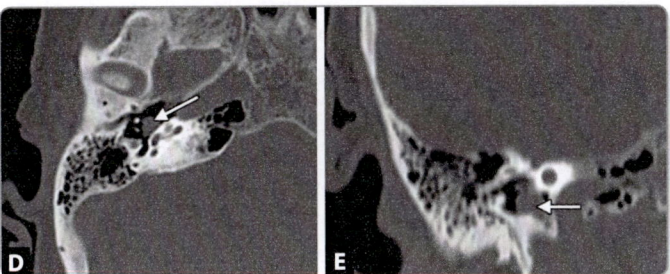

**Figures 2.21D and E** Axial and coronal CT images of the right temporal bone which demonstrates a soft tissue mass (white arrows) over the right cochlear promontory proven to be a glomus tympanicum

tumors and those along the extracranial skull base are called glomus vagale tumors. When these tumors expand from the jugular foramen to violate and occupy the tympanic cavity, they are known as glomus jugulotympanicum. Clinically, patients often present with pulsatile tinnitus, conductive hearing loss or otalgia. On otoscopy, a vascular retrotympanic mass can be seen and should be differentiated from an aberrant internal carotid artery. Both CT and MRI are relevant in evaluation of these tumors. On CT, a soft tissue mass with associated moth-eaten permeative destruction of adjacent bone. These lesions are vascular and enhance avidly on postcontrast imaging. On MRI, typically large paragangliomas have a "salt and pepper" appearance where the "pepper" corresponds to flow voids.

# Facial nerve

The facial nerve is well evaluated with a combination of MR and CT imaging. The intratemporal facial nerve can demonstrate normal variable postcontrast enhancement on MR imaging due to the surrounding rich perineural venous plexus. Normally, varying degrees of postcontrast enhancement may be seen most commonly in the geniculate ganglion, followed by the tympanic and mastoid segments, and slightly less commonly in the labyrinthine segment. Asymmetric enhancement may make differentiation from pathology challenging.

Enhancement of the cisternal, intracanalicular and extracranial segments should be considered pathologic.

## Congenital anomalies

*Abnormal course of facial nerve (**Figures 2.22A and B**):* The facial nerve may be anomalous in its course, often secondary to malformations of the adjacent structures. In EAC atresia, an associated aberrant course of the facial nerve must be elucidated to the referring clinician. Here, the tympanic and mastoid segments will appear anteriorly displaced. In the setting of a cochlear malformation, the labyrinthine segment can migrate anteromedially. Facial nerve prolapsed occurs when there is dehiscence of the bone overlying the tympanic segment allowing facial nerve protrude downwards over the oval window. This is best seen on CT in the coronal plane as a soft tissue mass overlying the oval window niche beneath the lateral semicircular canal. The surgeon should be cautioned of this finding preoperatively. A prolapsing facial nerve can be mistaken for a facial nerve schwannoma or cholesteatoma.

## Acquired diseases

*Bell's palsy (**Figures 2.23A to D**):* Bell's palsy is an idiopathic paralysis of the facial nerve and should be distinguished from facial nerve palsy secondary to trauma, tumor, infection or perineural spread of

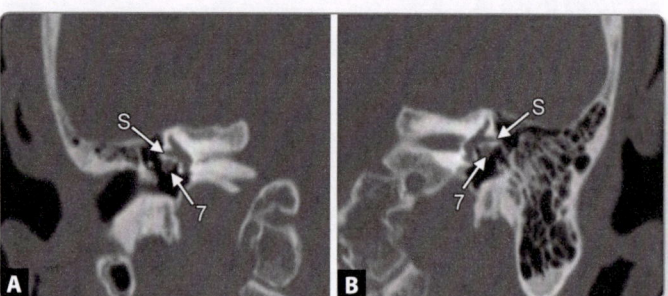

**Figures 2.22A and B** Coronal CT images of bilateral temporal bones demonstrates bilateral inferior protrusion of the facial nerves (7) over the oval windows with absence of the overlying bone. These are identified as the facial nerves, as they course beneath the lateral semicircular canals (S)

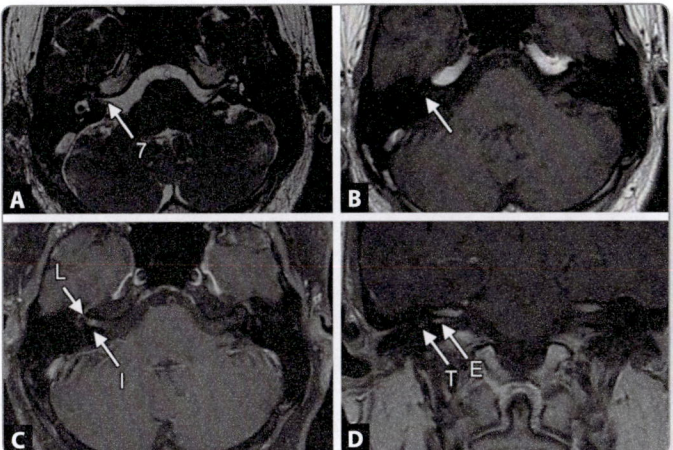

**Figures 2.23A to D** Axial steady state free precession gradient echo, axial T1-weighted pre- and postcontrast and coronal T1 postcontrast MR images in a patient with Bell's palsy. On the axial steady state free precession gradient echo sequence, the facial nerve (7) is normal in morphology without nodularity or thickening. Abnormal enhancement can be seen along the intracanalicular (I) and labyrinthine (L) segments of the facial nerve corresponding to the patient's history of Bell's palsy. Note the abnormal enhancement along the tympanic segment of the facial nerve (T) on the coronal reformat

tumor. Clinically, the patient presents with an acute onset of symptoms related to ipsilateral peripheral facial nerve paralysis which was preceded by a viral prodrome. Bell's palsy is known to spontaneously resolve, with limited or no residual deficit. CT imaging has a limited role demonstration of a normal facial nerve course without abnormal enlargement of its canal. Mainstay investigative imaging is with MR modality, MR imaging demonstrate asymmetric smooth postcontrast enhancement of the distal intracanalicular and labyrinthine segments without nodularity or enlargement of the nerve itself. Enhancement may be seen along the entire nerve. Any facial nerve nodularity or enlargement, however suggests an alternate diagnosis.

*Perineural spread of tumor (**Figures 2.24A to C**):* An important means of tumor spread, particularly in the head and neck cancer population,

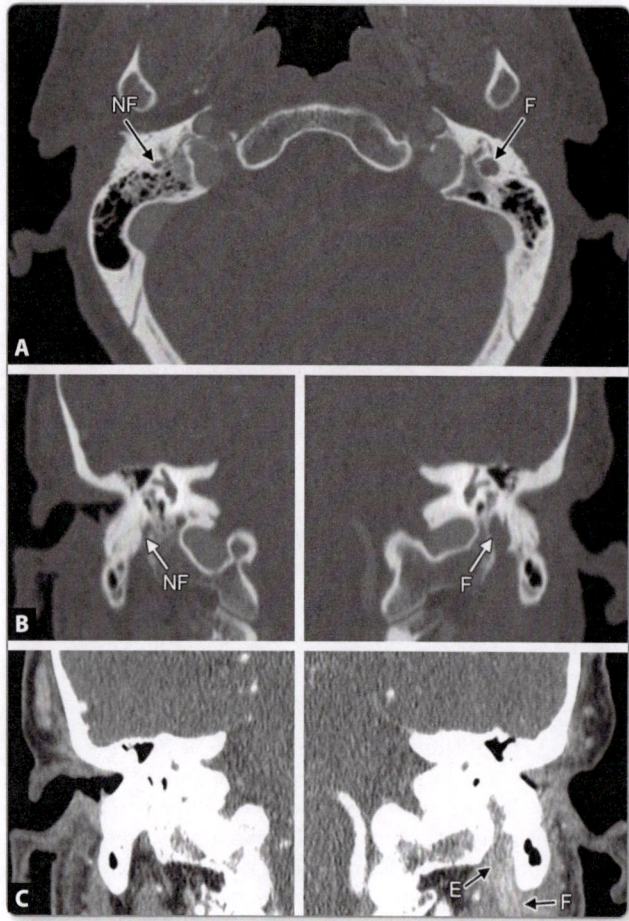

**Figures 2.24A to C** Axial and coronal contrast-enhanced CT images of bilateral temporal bones in bone and soft tissue windows in a patient with a left parotid tumor. There is soft tissue replacement of fat against the stylomastoid foramen (E) contiguously spreading asymmetric enhancing irregular enlargement of the mastoid segment of the facial nerve canal (F) secondary to perineural spread from the parotid tumor. Note the normal facial nerve canal (NF) on the right

is by direct tumor infiltration and extension along the nerves. Identification of the presence of perineural involvement may dramatically impact surgical and or nonsurgical management. There are a number of tumors implicated in perineural spread along the facial nerve, most notable of which are the parotid tumors. Both CT and MR imaging play an important role in the assessment of tumor spread along the facial nerve. CT imaging will demonstrate asymmetric enlargement of the facial nerve canal. In the setting of parotid tumors, enlargement of the stylomastoid foramen and mastoid segment is seen. Fatty replacement and soft tissue enhancement leading into an enlarged facial nerve canal on postcontrast CT imaging corresponds to tumor spread. Perineural spread is not limited to any single segment of the facial nerve and can extend to the root of the nerve. MR imaging is particularly useful in identifying the extent of disease along the intratemporal and intracranial portions of the facial nerve. On postcontrast MR sequences, the facial nerve will abnormally enhance and appear thickened along the corresponding areas of abnormal facial canal enlargement seen on CT. With parotid tumors, subtle infiltration of the stylomastoid fat can be detected on T1-weighted sequences.

## Neoplasm

*Facial nerve hemangioma:* Facial nerve hemangioma is a benign congenital vascular tumor arising from the perineural capillaries surrounding the facial nerve. Although they can occur anywhere along the course of the facial nerve, these tumors most commonly arise in the region of the geniculate ganglion and can be difficult to differentiate from facial nerve schwannomas. They are also reported in the distal IAC and mastoid segment. Because of its intimate relationship with the facial nerve, patients often present with peripheral facial nerve palsy. Both CT and MR imaging are useful in the diagnosis. On CT, a "honeycomb" bony appearance is often described in those lesions involving the region of the geniculate ganglion. Lesions arising within the IAC are better demonstrated on MR imaging. MR imaging characteristics include a lesion with T1 hypointense, T2 hyperintense signal which avidly enhances on postcontrast imaging.

*Facial nerve schwannoma (**Figures 2.25A to E**):* Facial nerve schwannomas are rare nerve sheath tumors that can occur anywhere along

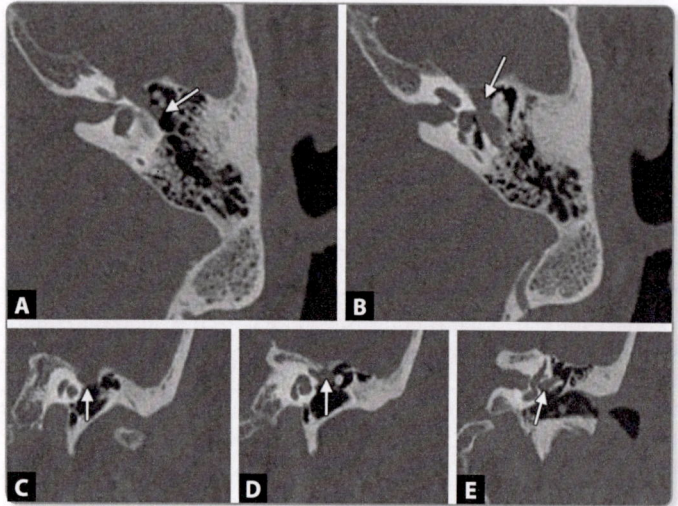

**Figures 2.25A to E** Axial and coronal CT images of the left temporal bone demonstrating a tubular soft tissue mass (white arrows) involving the first genu and tympanic segment of the left facial nerve consistent with a facial nerve schwannoma. Note the absence of the bony wall of the facial canal

the course of the facial nerve. Patients can present with hearing loss, progressive facial nerve paralysis, otalgia or facial pain. On CT imaging, smooth expansion of the intratemporal facial nerve bony canal is present. MR imaging is the mainstay modality and will demonstrate a T1 hypointense, T2 hyperintense enhancing mass which is ovoid if in the region of the geniculate ganglion, tubular in the tympanic segment or more globular if involving the mastoid segment. Facial nerve schwannomas can mimic vestibular schwannomas in the cerebellopontine angle in the absence of labyrinthine extension.

# The inner ear

## Congenital anomalies

*Mondini's malformation (**Figure 2.26**):* Mondini malformation is a congenital deformity of the cochlea resulting from arrested development

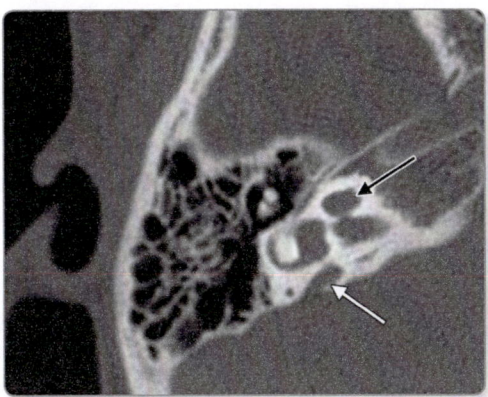

**Figure 2.26** Axial CT of right temporal bone demonstrating a coalescent cochlea (black arrow) without a bony modiolus consistent with a Mondini malformation. Note the dilated vestibular aqueduct (white arrow) which appears disproportionately enlarged relative to the horizontal semicircular canal

*in utero*. Patient's present with varying degrees of hearing loss. The abnormal cochlea will demonstrate underpartitioning of the apical and mid turns with a normal basal turn. Characteristic findings on CT include a cystic, featureless cochlea consisting of 1 ½ to 1 ¾ turns with absence of a normal bony modiolus. Abnormalities of the vestibule and semicircular canals can be seen to varying degrees. A dilated vestibular aqueduct may be an associated finding in approximately 20 percent of cases.

*Otosclerosis (**Figures 2.27A to F**):* Otosclerosis is an inherited disease of abnormal bone growth isolated to the otic capsule. Two thirds have a strong family history. It is often seen bilaterally (80%) and patients present with progressive unexplained conductive or mixed hearing loss. There is a 2:1 female predominance which presents clinically around the third decade. Otosclerosis can be subdivided into fenestral, otosclerosis or retrofenestral, also known as cochlear otosclerosis.

Fenestral otosclerosis is the more common subtype and describes disease localized to the *fissula* ante fenestram, lateral wall of the labyrinth which includes the cochlear promontory, the facial nerve and

## 70 Introductory head and neck imaging

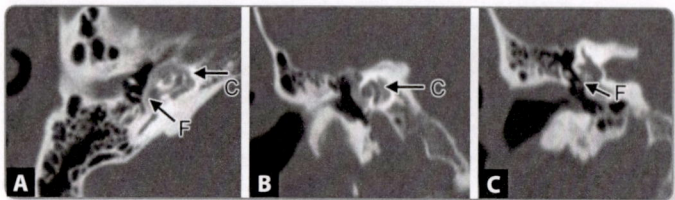

**Figures 2.27A to C** Axial and coronal images of right temporal bone demonstrating deossification surrounding the fenestral (F) and retrofenestral or cochlear (C) regions consistent with otosclerosis

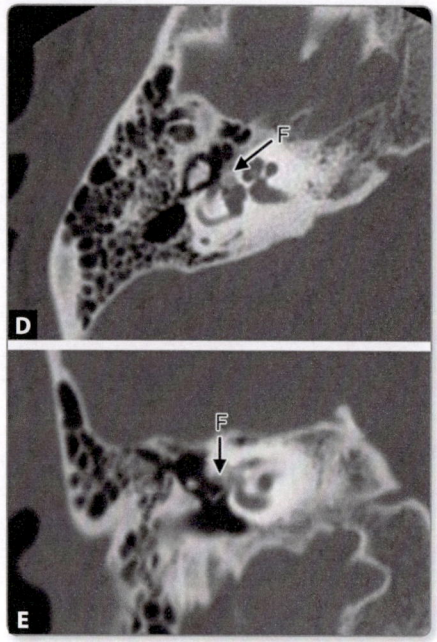

**Figures 2.27D and E** Axial and coronal CT images of right temporal bone demonstrating focal deossification in the fissula ante fenestrum (F) consistent with fenestral otosclerosis

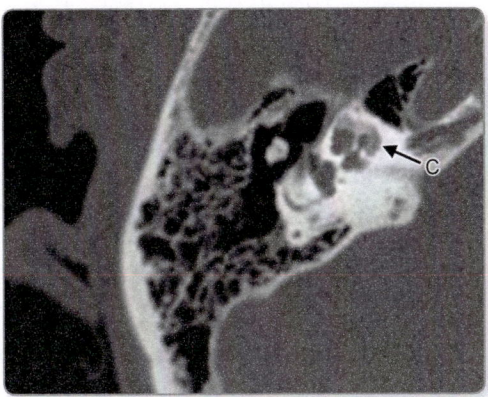

**Figure 2.27F** Axial CT of right temporal bone demonstrating focal deossification surrounding the cochlea (C) consistent with retrofenestral or cochlear otosclerosis

both oval and round windows. The less common retrofenestral type is often seen in conjunction with the fenestral subtype and describes disease involving the pericochlear otic capsule. The red hue from vascular dilatation seen over the promontory is referred to as the 'Schwartze's sign'. CT is the mainstay for diagnosis as it characterizes the extent of disease. Imaging is also used to assess failed surgery for otosclerosis. The presence of granuloma and fixation or medial migration of prosthesis or reocclusion of the oval window needs imaging if repeat surgery is contemplated. Imaging findings include abnormal lucency involving any bone of the medial tympanic cavity wall which may appear punctate initially and more confluent as the disease progresses. The stapes foot plate may be fixed to the oval window by fibrous tissue or bone. The round window may be involved in 30 to 50 percent of otosclerosis.

Histologically, in the early phase with fenestral otosclerosis, the normal endochondral bone of the otic capsule is replaced by the disorganized spongy vascular Haversian bone seen as lytic focus in the fissula ante fenestrum. In the late phase as the disease progresses from the initial deossification of the otic capsule, calcification and sclerosis and heaped up new bone formation can be seen.

Magnetic resonance imaging (MRI) is not helpful in the diagnosis or monitoring the progression of the disease. Osteogenesis imperfecta can be indistinguishable on imaging and should remain in the differential diagnosis when clinically relevant.

*Large vestibular aqueduct syndrome (**Figure 2.28**):* The vestibular aqueduct is a bony canal nestled in the posterior temporal bone which contains an endolymphatic sac. The endolymphatic sac anomaly, or enlarged vestibular aqueduct syndrome describes enlargement of the bony vestibular aqueduct and dilatation of the endolymphatic sac. Patients present with progressive congenital sensorineural hearing loss. This abnormality is considered a congenital malformation resulting from arrested development of the inner ear during the 7th week of gestation. Cochlear dysplasia is a common associated finding. CT is considered mainstay for diagnosis. If the mid portion of the vestibular aqueduct is greater than 1mm it is considered to be enlarged. A quick reference is made by comparison to the adjacent posterior semicircular canal, which should be equal to or larger in caliber to the vestibular aqueduct. MR imaging will demonstrate high T2 signal in the region of the vestibular aqueduct corresponding to the enlarged endolymphatic sac.

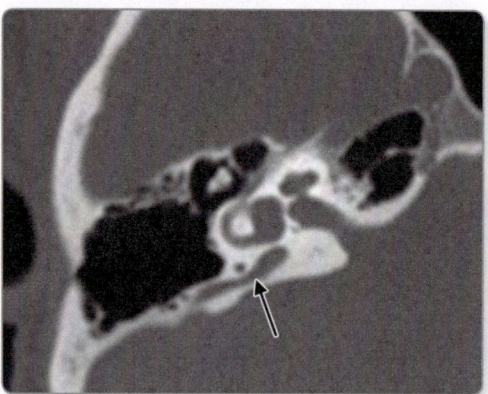

**Figure 2.28** Axial CT of right temporal bone demonstrating dilatation of the vestibular aqueduct (black arrow). Note the enlargement of the vestibular aqueduct relative to the horizontal semicircular canal

## Acquired diseases

*Labyrinthitis (**Figures 2.29A to H**):* Inflammation of the membranous labyrinth by viral, drug or immune related etiologies constitutes labyrinthitis, usually bilateral in nature. Unilateral labyrinthitis may be seen in the postsurgical or post-traumatic setting. Imaging is not typically indicated in the setting of classic symptoms such as sensorineural hearing loss, tinnitus and vertigo. The diagnosis is made with

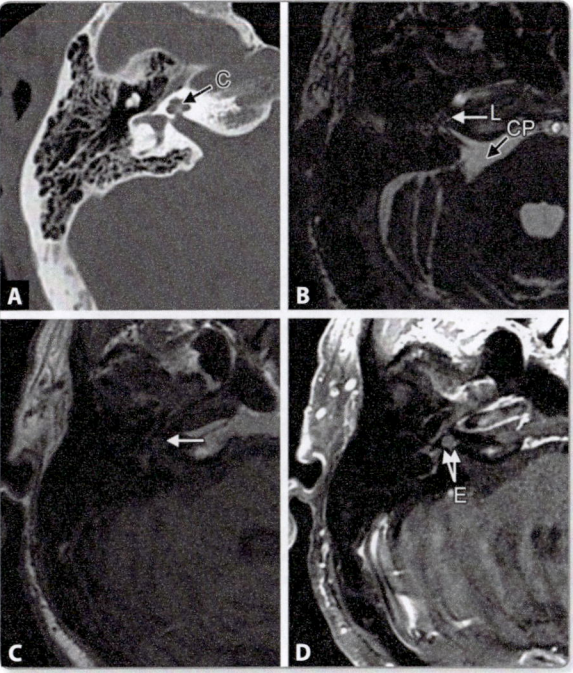

**Figures 2.29A to D** Axial CT image of the right temporal bone, axial steady state free precession gradient echo, axial pre- and postcontrast T1-weighted MR images of the right IAC demonstrates normal fluid density within the cochlea (C) on CT imaging. On the axial steady state free precession gradient echo sequence, there is decreased fluid signal within the membranous labyrinth (L) relative to the cerebellopontine cistern (CP). The membranous labyrinth demonstrates patchy abnormal postcontrast enhancement (E) consistent with acute labyrinthitis

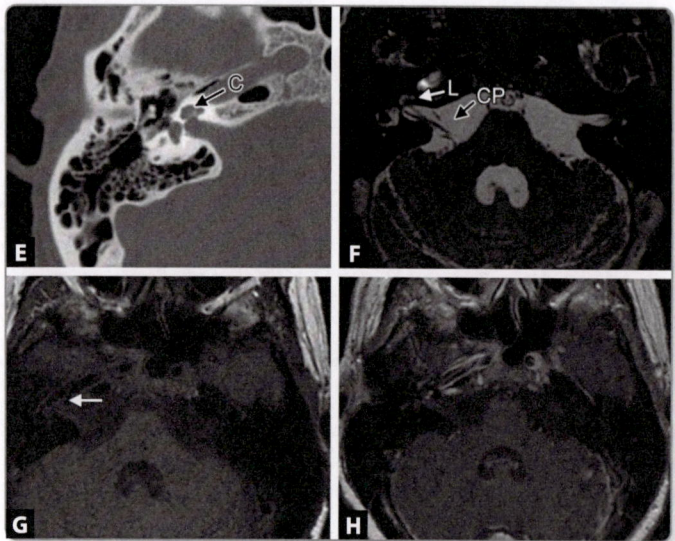

**Figures 2.29E to H** Axial CT image of the right temporal bone and axial steady state free precession gradient echo, axial pre- and postcontrast T1-weighted MR images of bilateral IAC in a patient with hearing loss status post meningitis. On CT, there is normal fluid density within the cochlea (C). There is decreased fluid signal within the membranous labyrinth (L) relative to the adjacent cistern (CP) with foci of abnormal post-contrast enhancement on MR imaging consistent with labyrinthitis

MR imaging. Abnormal T2-weighted labyrinthine filling defects and postcontrast T1-weighted enhancement is seen along the membranous labyrinth. Infection can spread to involve the facial nerve and abnormal enhancement of the nerve can be seen on postcontrast imaging in such instances.

*Labyrinthine ossificans (Figures 2.30A to E):* Labyrinthine ossificans is the healing stage of labyrinthitis typically seen in the pediatric population. Clinical presentation includes progressive sensorineural hearing loss following history of ear infection, meningitis, infection and trauma. CT imaging will demonstrate bony deposition within the membranous labyrinth and can be isolated to the cochlea or semicir-

# Radiographic anatomy and pathology of the temporal bone

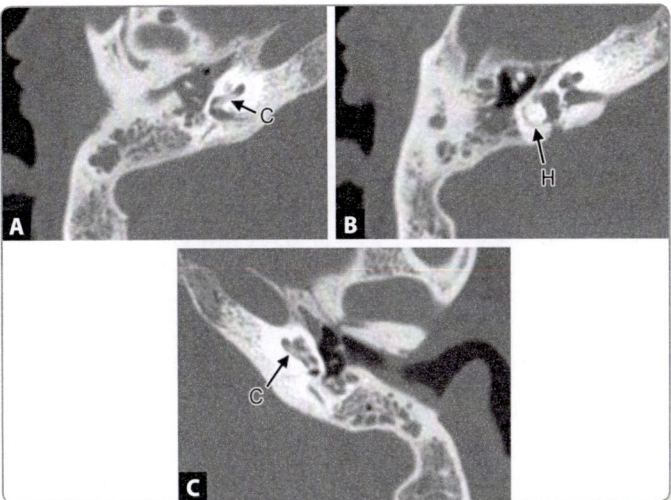

**Figures 2.30A to C** Axial CT images of bilateral temporal bones and postcontrast T1-weighted MR image of bilateral IAC demonstrating abnormal bone density in the basal turn of bilateral cochlea (C) and partial bony obliteration of the horizontal semicircular canal (H) which represents labyrinthine ossificans, the healing stage of labyrinthitis

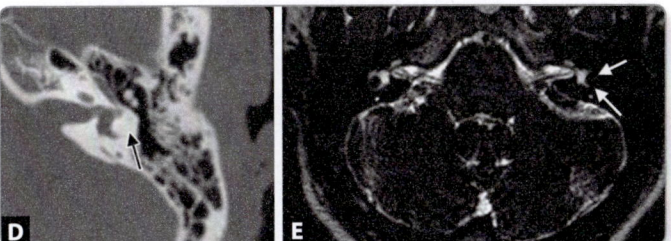

**Figures 2.30D and E** Axial CT image of the left temporal bone and axial steady state free precession MR image demonstrating abnormal bony density filling the lateral aspect of the horizontal semicircular canal (black arrow). On MR imaging, there is loss of fluid signal in the peripheral aspect of the horizontal semicircular canal (white arrows)

cular canals. On MR imaging, a loss of T2-weighted fluid signal can be seen within the affected regions of the bony labyrinth.

*Semicircular canal dehiscence (**Figures 2.31A and B**):* Semicircular canal dehiscence is diagnosed by the absence of the overlying shell of bone surrounding the superior or posterior semicircular canals. The pathophysiology is unknown and is believed by some to be a developmental anomaly. Patients present with Tullio phenomenon which constitutes sound-induced vertigo with or without nystagmus. CT imaging is the mainstay modality and thin sections are often helpful to demonstrate a bony defect overlying the superior semicircular canal. The diagnosis is excluded even if the overlying bone is thinned but present. Associated thinning of the tegmen tympani can be seen.

## Neoplasm

*Vestibular schwannoma (**Figures 2.32A to D**):* Also known as acoustic schwannoma or neuroma, vestibular schwannoma is the most common benign tumor of the Schwann cells involving the vestibulocochlear nerve. All cranial nerves except for the first and the second cranial nerve sheaths are composed of Schwann cells. In order of frequency the cranial nerve schwannomas occur in the vestibular division of cranial nerve VIII, followed by the trigeminal, facial, IX, X,

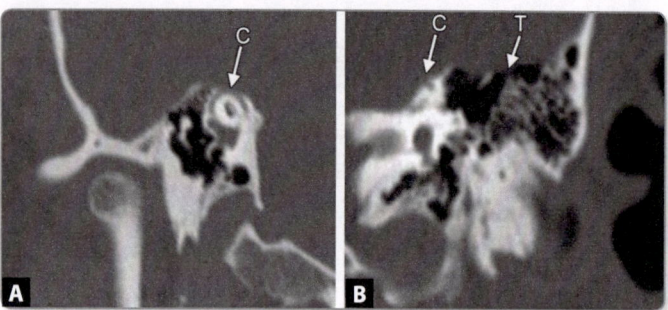

**Figures 2.31A and B** Coronal oblique and coronal CT images of the left temporal bone demonstrating bony dehiscence of the superior semicircular canal (S), which is best seen on the coronal oblique or Poschl view. Note the associated thinning of the tegmen tympani (T)

Radiographic anatomy and pathology of the temporal bone 77

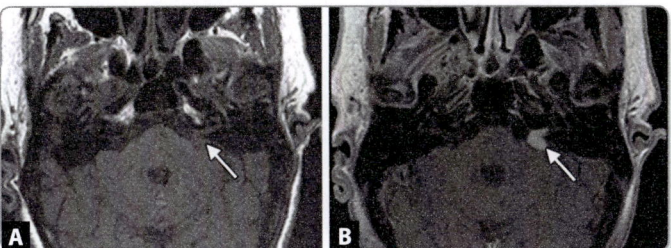

**Figures 2.32A and B** Axial T1-weighted pre- and postcontrast images of bilateral IACs demonstrate an enhancing lesion at the left cerebellopontine angle with involvement of the left IAC consistent with an acoustic schwannoma

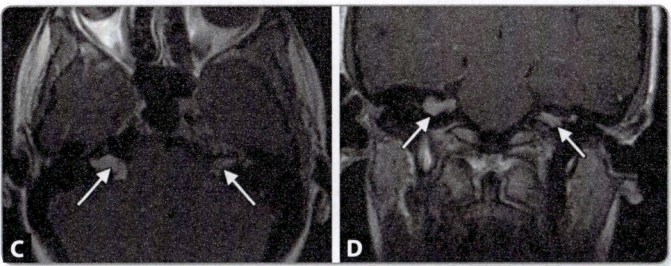

**Figures 2.32C and D** Axial and coronal postcontrast T1-weighted MR images of bilateral IAC demonstrate dumbbell-shaped, enhancing lesions (white arrows) in bilateral IAC consistent with bilateral acoustic schwannomas, diagnostic of neurofibromatosis Type 2

XI cranial nerves. Typically, patients present with gradual or sudden onset unilateral sensorineural hearing loss. The presence of bilateral vestibular schwannomas is virtually diagnostic of the genetic disorder, Neurofibromatosis type II. These lesions typically originate in the IAC as a rounded mass and expand to fill the cerebellopontine angle. Diagnosis is best made on MR imaging, however CT will demonstrate a well-circumscribed mass at the cerebellopontine angle and involving the IAC with widening of the porous acousticus. MR imaging will reveal an avidly enhancing mass in the IAC with or without extension into the Cerebellopontine angle cistern. It can be difficult to differentiate vestibular schwannomas from meningiomas, however, intracanalicular meningiomas are exceedingly rare in comparison. The presence of a dural tail and underlying bony hyperostosis on CT imaging favors meningioma.

*IAC meningioma (**Figures 2.33A to D**):* Meningiomas are benign neoplasms arising originating from arachnoid villi and account for approximately 10 to 15 percent of all cerebellopontine angle masses. Meningiomas that are intracanalicular can be difficult to differentiate from acoustic schwannomas. These tumors are typically discovered incidentally. CT and MR imaging can be helpful with the diagnosis. CT imaging often demonstrates a hyperdense mass, which in about 25 percent can have coarse calcifications. On MR imaging, meningiomas appear T1 isointense to gray matter, T2 hyperintense and may contain areas of low signal due to internal calcifications. These lesions avidly enhance on postcontrast imaging and can demonstrate a dural thickening often referred to as a "dural tail," which favors the diagnosis of meningioma over an acoustic schwannoma.

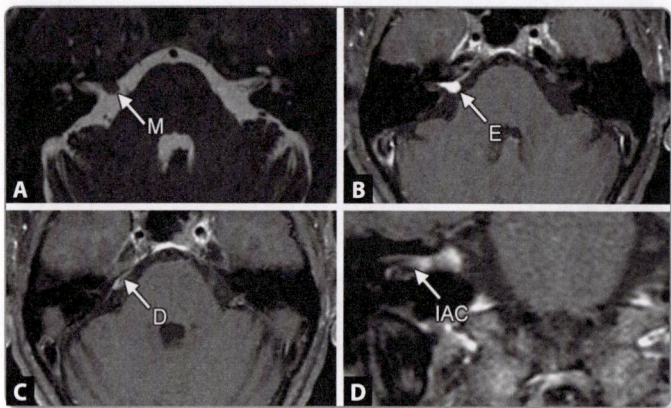

**Figures 2.33A to D** Axial T1-weighted pre- and postcontrast images of bilateral IAC and coronal T1-weighted postcontrast image fo the right IAC demonstrates a dural based mass (M) at the cerebellopontine angle which appears T1 isointense to gray matter and partially extends intracanalicularly (IAC). On postcontrast imaging, the mass avidly enhances (E) and reveals a dural tail (D) that favors the diagnosis of a meningioma

# Trauma (Figures 2.34A to S)

Temporal bone fractures are usually from blunt injury to the head. Depending upon the orientation of the fracture line in relation to the petrous bone, the force of the injury can result in longitudinal (parallel to the long axis of the petrous bone due to blunt force directed in the temporal and parietal plane), or transverse (perpendicular to the long axis from force in the frontal-occipital plane) or a combination of the two. There may be associated hemorrhage, vascular and nerve injury with or without ossicular chain disruption and intracranial injury. The potential complications include CSF leak and meningitis, facial nerve injury, hearing loss and perilymphatic fistula. Pneumolabyrinth is a rare post-traumatic finding typically seen with transverse fractures which suggests the presence of a labyrinthine fistula and requires surgical intervention. It is imperative to assess for violation of the tegmen tympani and inner ear as the patient will be at increased risk of meningitis. Facial nerve injury may be temporary and delayed in onset in the longitudinal fractures. In transverse fractures where the facial nerve is more frequently injured, deficits may be permanent. Noncontrast CT imaging is the modality of choice in the setting of temporal bone trauma. Ossicular injury varies between the individual ossicles due to their respect supportive ligaments and tendons. The incus, the most commonly injured and displaced as a result of its poor support network. With the advent of 64-slice MDCT scanners and improved spatial resolution, there are increasing reports of the more rare post-traumatic injuries such as stapes fractures being documented.

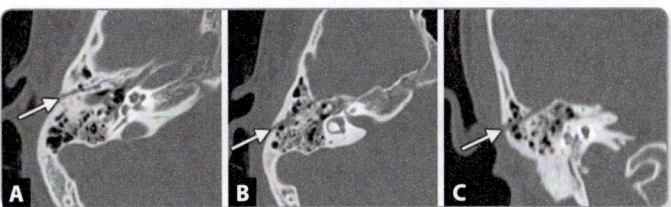

**Figures 2.34A to C** Axial and coronal CT images of the right temporal bone demonstrating a longitudinal component (white arrows) of a complex temporal bone fracture

**80** Introductory head and neck imaging

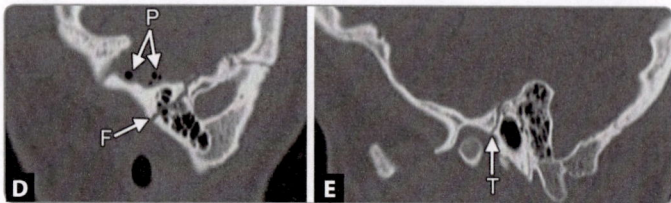

**Figures 2.34D and E** Sagittal CT images of the right temporal bone in the same patient of Figures 2.34B to D demonstrating the transverse component (F) of the complex fracture through the squamous temporal bone with pneumocephalus (P) and extension into temporomandibular joint (T)

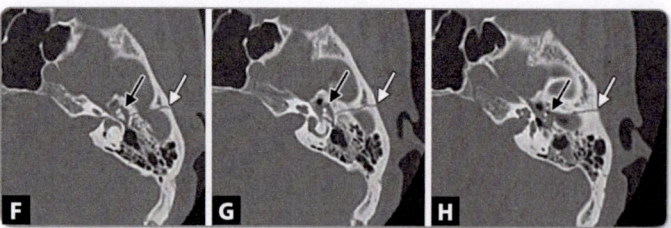

**Figures 2.34F to H** Axial CT images of the left temporal bone in a patient status post trauma to the left mastoid. There is longitudinal fracture (white arrows) through the left temporal bone with extension into the tympanic cavity. Note the middle ear effusion (black arrows)

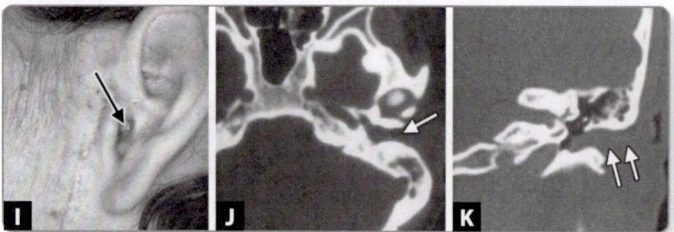

**Figures 2.34I to K** Otoscopic image of the left ear and axial and coronal CT images of the left temporal bone in a patient status post remote trauma to the left ear. On external exam, a false fundus (black arrow) is present with shortening of the EAC length. CT imaging demonstrates soft tissue filling the EAC (white arrows) secondary to scarring consistent with post-traumatic EAC stenosis (*for color version of Figure 2.34I see Plate 7*)

Radiographic anatomy and pathology of the temporal bone 81

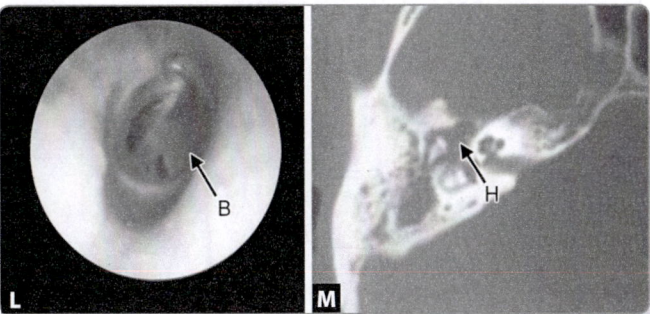

**Figures 2.34L and M** Otoscopic image of the right tympanic membrane and axial CT image of the right temporal bone in a patient status post blunt trauma to the right ear. On otoscopic exam, bluish material (B) is present filling the middle ear cavity. CT imaging demonstrates opacification of the middle ear in the same patient consistent with middle ear hemorrhage (H) (*for color version of Figure 2.34L see Plate 7*)

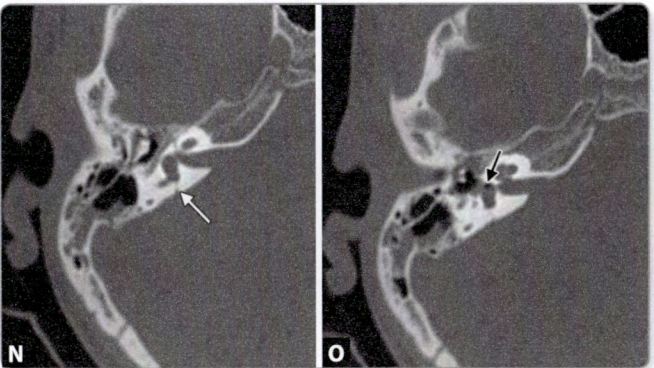

**Figures 2.34N and O** Axial CT images of the right temporal bone demonstrates a subtle transverse fracture through the posterior otic capsule (white arrow) resulting in a focus of air within the vestibule consistent with pneumolabyrinth (black arrow)

## 82  Introductory head and neck imaging

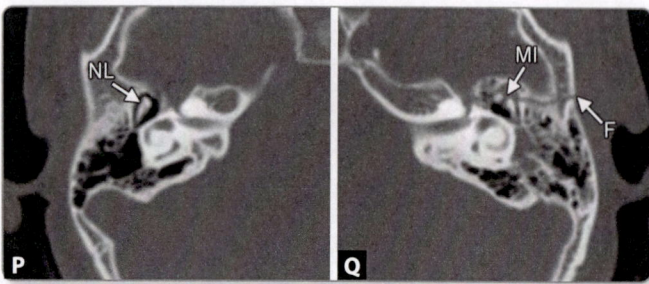

**Figures 2.34P and Q** Axial CT images of bilateral temporal bones demonstrating a longitudinal fracture (F) through the left temporal bone which extends into the tympanic cavity. There is abnormal widening of the malleoincudal joint (MI) relative to the normal right malleoincudal joint (NL) consistent with malleoincudal dislocation

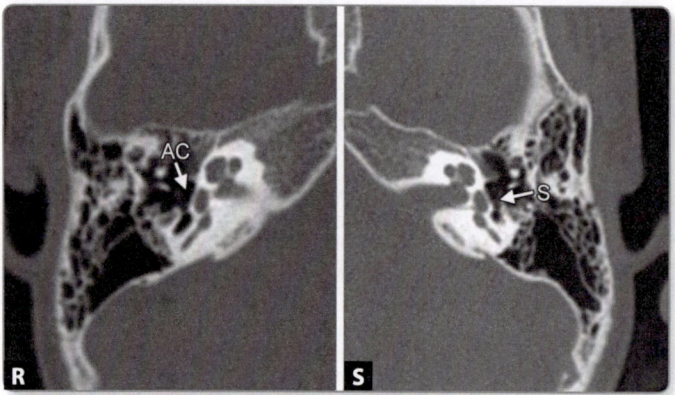

**Figures 2.34R and S** Axial CT images of bilateral temporal bones demonstrates absence of a normal anterior crura (AC) in the right stapes suggestive of a stapes fracture. The fracture was confirmed in the operating room. Note the normal appearance of the left stapes (S)

# Conclusion

The exquisite bony detail given by high resolution CT and the improved evaluation of the inner ear and IAC with MR imaging makes both modalities the standard for temporal bone imaging. Despite the advances in temporal bone imaging, correlation with clinical and otoscopic findings is an invaluable adjunct in formulating an accurate diagnosis.

# Acknowledgments

The chapter would not have been possible without the contributions of Dr Lalitha Shankar and Dr Michael Hawke of University of Toronto and Dr Loraine Wu of Long Island Jewish Medical Center.

# Bibliography

1. Aho TR, Daspit CP, Dean BL, Wallace RC. Intralabyrinthine meningioma. AJNR Am J Neuroradiol 2003;24:1642-5.
2. Becelli R, Perugini M, Carboni A, Renzi G. Diagnosis of Bell palsy with gadolinium magnetic resonance imaging. J Craniofacial Surg 2003;14(1):51-4.
3. Curtin HD. Superior semicircular canal dehiscence syndrome and multidetector row CT. Radiology 2003;226:312-4.
4. Dahlen RT, Harnsberger HR, Gray SD, Shelton C, Allen R, Parkin JL, Scalzo D. Overlapping thin-section fast spin-echo MR of the large vestibular aqueduct syndrome. AJNR Am J Neuroradiol 1997;18:67-75.
5. Daniels DL, Czervionke LF, Pojunas KW, Meyer GA, Millen SJ, Williams AL, Haughton VM. Facial nerve enhancement in MR imaging. AJNR AM J Neuroradiol 1987;8:605-7.
6. Haught K, Hogg JP, Killeffer JA, Voelker JL, Schochet Jr SS. Entirely Intracanalicular Meningioma Contrast-Enhanced MR Findings in a Rare Entity. AJNR Am J Neuroradiol 1998;19:1831–3.
7. Heilbrun ME, Salzman KL, Glastonbury CM, Harnsberger HR, Kennedy RJ, Shelton C. External auditory canal cholesteatoma: clinical and imaging spectrum. AJNR Am J Neuroradiol 2003;24:751-6.
8. Krishnan A, Mattox DE, Fountain AJ, Hudgins PA. CT arteriography and venography in pulsatile tinnitus: preliminary results. AJNR Am J Neuroradiol 2006;27:1635-8.
9. Lipkin AF, Bryan RN, Jenkins HA. Pneumolabyrinth after temporal bone fracture: documentation by high- resolution CT. AJNR Am J Neuroradiol 1985;6:294-5.
10. Lo WW, Solti-Bohman LG, McElveen Jr JT. Aberrant carotid artery: radiologic diagnosis with emphasis on high-resolution computed tomography. Radiographics 1985;5: 985-93.

11. Lowe LH, Vézina LG. Sensorineural hearing loss in children. Radiographics 1997; 17:1079-93.
12. Magliulo G, Zardo F, Bertin S, D'Amico R, Savastano V. Meningiomas of the Internal Auditory Canal: Two Case Reports. Skull base. 2002;12(1):19-26.
13. Maroldi R, Farina D, Palvarini L, Marconi A, Gadola E, Menni K, Battaglia G. Computed tomography and magnetic resonance imaging of pathologic conditions of the middle ear. Eur J Radiol 2001;40:78-93.
14. Mayer TE, Brueckmann H, Siegert R, Witt A, Weerda H. High-resolution CT of the temporal bone in dysplasia of the auricle and external auditory canal. AJNR Am J Neuroradiol 1997;18:53-65.
15. Meriot P, Veillon F, Garcia JF, Nonent M, Jezequel J, Bourjat P, Bellet M. CT appearances of ossicular injuries. Radiographics 1997;17:1445-54.
16. Parker GD, Harnsberger HR. Clinical-radiologic issues in perineural tumor spread of malignant diseases of the extracranial head and neck. Radiographics 1991;11:383-99.
17. Petrus LV, Lo WW. The anterior epitympanic recess: CT anatomy and pathology. AJNR Am J Neuroradiol 1997;18:1109-14.
18. Reis C, Lopes JM, Carneiro E, Vilarinho A, Portugal R, Duarte F, Fonseca J. Temporal Giant Cell Reparative Granuloma: A Reappraisal of Pathology and Imaging Features. AJNR Am J Neuroradiol 2006;27:1660-2.
19. Robert Y, Carcasset S, Rocourt N, Hennequin C, Dubrulle F, Lemaitre L. Congenital cholesteatoma of the temporal bone: MR findings and comparison with CT. AJNR Am J Neuroradiol 1995;16:755-61.
20. Romo LV, Curtin HD. Anomalous facial nerve canal with cochlear malformations. AJNR Am J Neuroradiol 2001;22:838-44.
21. Rubinstein D, Sandberg EJ, Cajade-law AG. Anatomy of the facial and vestibulocochlear nerves in the internal auditory canal. AJNR Am J Neuroradiol 1996;17:1099-1105.
22. Saliba I, Fayad JN. Facial nerve hemangioma of the middle ear. Ear Nose Throat J. 2009;88(9):822-3.
23. Salib RJ, Tziambazis E, McDermott AL, Chavda SV, Irving RM. The crucial role of imaging in detection of facial nerve haemangiomas. J Laryngol Otol 2001;115(6): 510-13.
24. Shelton C, Brackmann DE, Lo WW, Carberr JN. Intratemporal facial nerve hemangiomas. Otolaryngol Head Neck Surg 1991;14(1):116-21.
25. Swartz JD. Sensorineural hearing deficit; a systematic approach based on imaging findings. Radiographics 1996;16:561-74.
26. Tien R, Dillon WP, Jackler RK. Contrast-enhanced MR imaging of the facial nerve in 11 patients with Bell's palsy. AJNR Am J Neuroradiology 1990;11:735-41.
27. Turetsky DB, Vines FS, Clayman DA. Surfer's ear: exostoses of the external auditory canal. AJNR Am J Neuroradiol 1990;11:1217-8.
28. Urman SM, Talbot JM. Otic capsule dysplasia: clinical and CT findings. Radiographics 1990;10:823-38.
29. Vattoth S, Shah R, Curé JK. A Compartment-based approach for the imaging evaluation of tinnitus. AJNR Am J Neuroradiol 2010;31:211-8.

30. Vijayasekaran S, Halsted MJ, Boston M, Meinzen-Derr J, Bardo DME, Greinwald J, Benton C. When is the vestibular aqueduct enlarged? A statistical analysis of the normative distribution of vestibular aqueduct size. AJNR Am J Neuroradiol 2007; 28(6):1133.
31. Weissman L, Hirsch BE. Beyond the promontory: the multifocal origin of glomus tympanicum tumors. AJNR Am J Neuroradiol 1998;19:119-22.
32. Wiggins III RH, Harnsberger HR, Salzman KL, Shelton C, Kertesz TR, Glastonbury CM. The many faces of facial nerve schwannoma. AJNR Am J Neuroradiol 2006;27:694-9.

# Imaging of the orbit

chapter 3

Makki Almuntashri, Edward Kassel

**ABSTRACT**

A comprehensive review of the imaging anatomy of the orbit, followed by a discussion of various congenital, infectious, neoplastic, inflammatory and traumatic conditions that can affect the orbital contents.

**KEYWORDS**

Orbit, globe, eye, anatomy, infection, neoplasm

## Anatomy of the orbit

The orbit is a conical shaped cavity that contains the eye (globe), extraocular muscles, vascular supply, cranial nerves (CN) and the surrounding fat. It has four bony walls which are lateral, medial, superior and inferior. The lateral wall is formed by frontal process of zygomatic bone anteriorly and greater wing of sphenoid posteriorly. The medial wall is formed by four bones from anterior to posterior; frontal process of maxillary bone, lacrimal bone, lamina papyracea of ethmoid and lesser wing of sphenoid bone. The roof is formed by orbital process of frontal bone, complemented by the lesser wing of the sphenoid bone more posteriorly while the floor is formed by maxillary process of zygomatic bone laterally and orbital plate of maxillary bone medially which contain the infraorbital foramen (**Figures 3.1A and B**).

The orbital cavity is pyramidal shaped, narrows posteriorly forming the orbital apex which has three openings; optic canal, superior and inferior orbital fissures (**Figures 3.2A to C**). The optic canal is located superomedially within the lesser wing of sphenoid. It transmits the optic nerve (CN2) and ophthalmic artery. The superior orbital fissure, lateral to the optic canal and formed by the lesser wing of sphenoid medially and greater wing of sphenoid laterally, transmits the superior ophthalmic vein, oculomotor (CN3), trochlear (CN4),

Imaging of the orbit 87

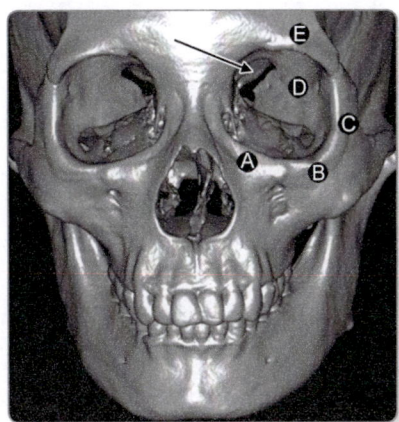

**Figure 3.1A** Orbital walls: (A) Orbital plate of maxillary bone forming medial aspect of orbital floor. (B) maxillary process of zygomatic bone forming lateral aspect of orbital floor. (C) Frontal process of zygomatic bone forming anterior aspect of lateral wall. (D) Greater wing of sphenoid forming posterior aspect of lateral wall. (E) Orbital process of frontal bone forming the roof of orbit

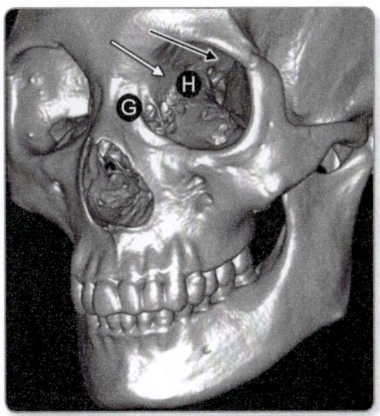

**Figure 3.1B** Medial wall from posterior to anterior: Black arrows in Figures A and B represent lesser wing of sphenoid. (H) Ethmoidal bone (lamina papyracea). White arrow: Lacrimal bone. (G) Frontal process of maxillary

## Introductory head and neck imaging

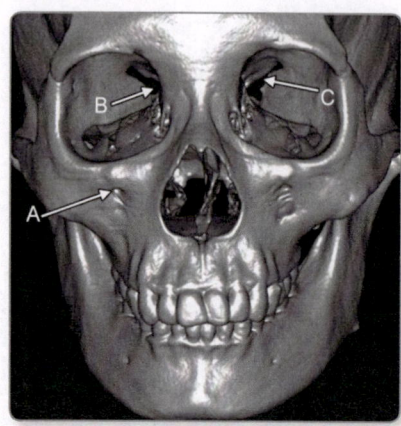

**Figure 3.2A** Foramina: Arrow (A) Infraorbital foramen. Arrow (B) Optic canal. Arrow (C) Superior orbital fissure

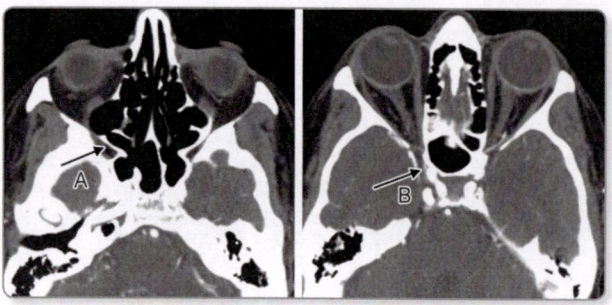

**Figure 3.2B** Foramina: Arrow (A) Right inferior orbital foramen. Arrow (B) Right superior orbital foramen

ophthalmic division of trigeminal (CN V1) and abducent nerves (CN 6). The inferior orbital fissure inferolaterally, bordered by the maxillary bone medially and greater wing of sphenoid laterally, communicates with the pterygopalatine fossa and transmits the maxillary division of trigeminal nerve (CN V2) intracranially by its communication with foramen rotundum.

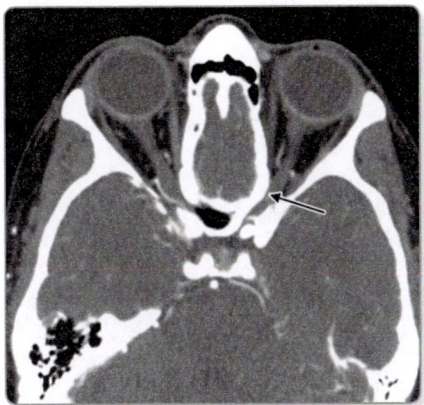

**Figure 3.2C** Optic canal

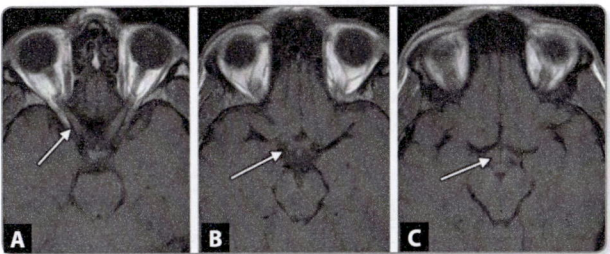

**Figures 3.3A to C** Optic pathway: (A) Optic nerve extending from the intraorbital portion to prechiasmatic portion (arrow). (B) Optic chiasma. (C) Optic tract extends from the optic chiasm to optic radiations in the occipital lobe

The optic nerve is formed from brain tissue (oligodendrocyte) without surrounding Schwann cells in contrast to peripheral nerves. It is surrounded by cerebrospinal fluid (CSF) and covered by three meningeal layers in a fashion similar to the brain, i.e. an outer dura, middle arachnoid and inner pia layers and called the optic nerve sheath, and courses from the optic disc at the retina to the optic chiasm at the suprasellar region carrying sensation to the visual cortex in the occipital lobes via optic tracts and radiations (**Figures 3.3A to C**).

CN V1, a sensory division of the trigeminal nerve, supplies the skin about the upper eyelid and superior aspect of the orbit.

CN 3, 4 and 6 are motor nerves that supply the extraocular muscles, which include four recti muscles (superior rectus, inferior rectus, medial rectus and lateral rectus muscles), two oblique muscles (superior and inferior oblique) and the levator palpebrae superioris (**Figures 3.4A and B**).

The superior oblique muscle is supplied by the trochlear nerve (CN4) and the lateral rectus muscle is supplied by the abducent nerve (CN6), with the remaining extraocular muscles supplied by the oculomotor nerve (CN3). A helpful mnemonic to remember the nerve supply to the extraocular muscles is SO4 LR6 (SO4 = superior oblique is supplied by CN4, LR6 = lateral rectus is supplied by CN6).

The eyeball (eye or globe) is protected by the bony orbit and covered anteriorly by the eyelid. With the exception of the cornea and conjunctiva at the anterior aspect of the globe, the wall of the globe is formed from three layers: outer sclera, middle uvea and inner retina. Clinically the eyeball refers to just the sclera and choroid layers, with the retina offering no appreciable thickness. The outer layer of the globe is covered by Tenon's capsule, a fibroelastic membrane that forms a socket enclosing the posterior 4/5 of the globe, separating

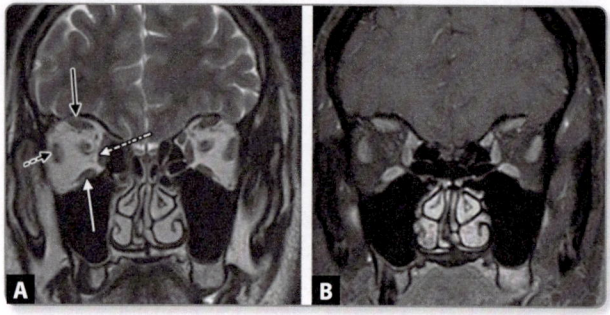

**Figures 3.4A and B** Extraocular muscles: (A) Coronal T2 of orbit shows superior rectus muscle (black arrow), lateral rectus muscle (black dotted arrow), inferior rectus muscle (white arrow), and medial rectus muscle (white dotted arrow). (B) Coronal T1 fat sat after gadolinium: Note normal enhancement of the muscles

the globe from the surrounding orbital fat, to allow free movement of the globe. Tenon's space is that space between the capsule and the sclera.

The sclera represents the large posterior opaque globe covering, formed from collagen-elastic tissue that extends from the optic nerve attachment posteriorly to the corneoscleral junction anteriorly. The cornea will cover the small transparent anterior segment of the eye. The uvea, a pigmented richly vascular layer, consists of three components; the choroid posteriorly, iris anteriorly and ciliary body connecting the choroid to iris. The iris is a thin pigmented membrane behind the cornea and anterior to the lens, surrounding a central opening called the pupil. The thin inner retinal layer is the neural sensory layer.

The lens, formed from epithelium, fibers and surrounding capsule, is located behind the iris and held in position by the suspensory ligament of the lens (Zonule) that is attached to the ciliary body on each side.

The globe is divided into anterior and posterior segments by the ciliary body. The anterior segment is divided by the iris into anterior and posterior chambers. These chambers are filled by the aqueous humor secreted by the ciliary bodies and communicate with

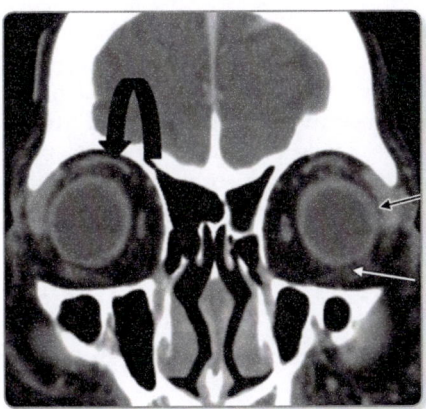

**Figure 3.4C** Coronal CT orbit shows superior oblique muscle (large circular black arrow), inferior oblique muscle (straight white arrow) and lacrimal gland (straight black arrow)

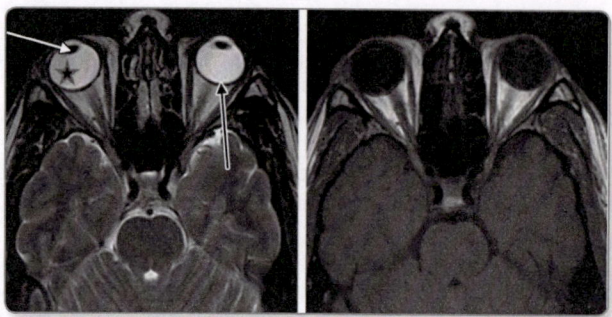

**Figure 3.5** MR of the eye (T2WI and corresponding T1WI) show the lens (white arrow), vitreous (5-points star) and eye wall (black arrow) formed by sclera, uvea and retina from outer to inner

each other through the pupil. The posterior segment is filled by the vitreous humor which contains mostly water with small amount of protein (**Figure 3.5**).

The lacrimal gland, located in the superolateral portion of the orbit (**Figure 3.4C**), secretes clear fluid which flows across the anterior orbit to drain into the lacrimal sac, at the medial inferior aspect of the orbit, and nasolacrimal duct to reach the inferior meatus of the nasal cavity.

The orbit receives its blood supply by the ophthalmic artery, which is the first branch of the internal carotid artery, and drains via the superior and inferior ophthalmic veins. The superior ophthalmic vein drains into the cavernous sinus and the inferior vein anastomoses with the pterygoid plexus (**Figures 3.6A and B**).

# Congenital anomalies

## Anophthalmia

Anophthalmia or absence of the eye is an extremely rare congenital defect.

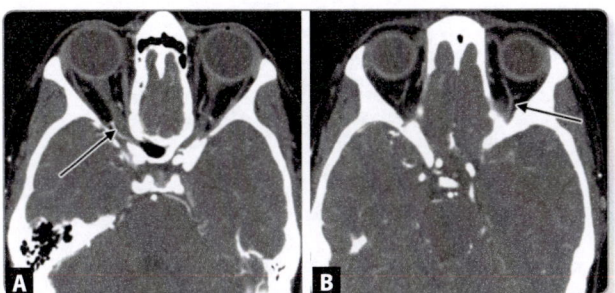

**Figures 3.6A and B** Axial CT angiogram shows ophthalmic artery running from the ICA to orbit (A) and superior ophthalmic vein (B)

## Microphthalmia

Microphthalmia denotes a small globe and can be either congenital or acquired. Congenital microphthalmia may be isolated, syndromic, or associated with other entities such as congenital infections or persistent hyperplastic primary vitreous. When the globe is congenitally small, the orbit is underdeveloped as opposed to acquired diminution of the eye.

Acquired microphthalmia, seen as a result of trauma, surgery or inflammation, is termed phthisis bulbi. In Phthisis bulbi, the eye is small, frequently irregular in configuration, and calcification may be present (**Figure 3.7**).

## Persistent hyperplastic primary vitreous

Persistent hyperplastic primary vitreous (PHPV) is a congenital ocular abnormality due to incomplete regression of embryonic ocular blood supply. It is characterized by presence of a central hyaloid artery remnant in a small globe. CT imaging shows a dense vitreous due to the presence of hemorrhage, debris and rarely calcifications. MR imaging (**Figure 3.8**) typically shows abnormally high signal on T1 and T2-weighted images of the vitreous that varies based on age of the blood contents. Common clinical presenting symptoms/signs are leukokoria, poor vision and retinal detachment.

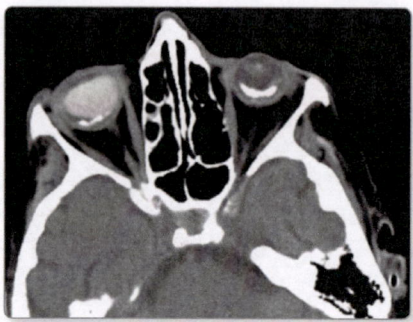

**Figure 3.7** CT head of 54-year-old male with bilateral phthisis bulbi. Both globes are small with irregular outline. There is calcification at posterior aspect of both eyes. Note dense vitreous on the right

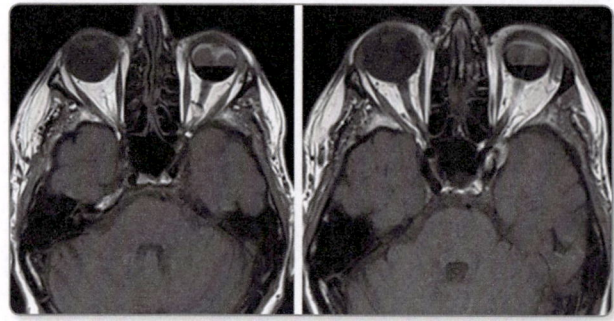

**Figure 3.8** Axial T1 MRI of orbit: 57-year-old patient with left eye blindness. Images show small left eye with persistent hyaloid artery in mid vitreous in keeping with persistent hyperplastic primary vitreous. Note dark signal in the dependent portion of eye in keeping with hemosiderin related to old hemorrhage

## Macrophthalmia

Macrophthalmia represents enlargement of the globe that may be related to various etiologies as mentioned below. The most common cause is axial myopia (**Figure 3.9**).

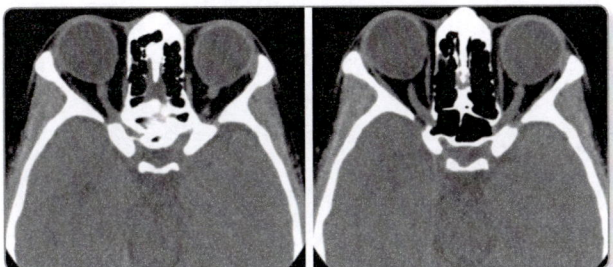

**Figure 3.9** CT images of orbits of 29-year-old female with elongation of both eyes related to myopia

## Buphthalmos (Ox eye)

Buphthalmos represents enlargement of the globe, seen in infants and children with glaucoma due to elevated intraocular pressure, characterized by increased axial diameter, with sclera thickening. Approximately 50 percent of patients with neurofibromatosis type 1 who have orbital involvement have glaucoma.

## Staphyloma

Staphyloma represents a nonspecific enlargement of the globe related to thinning of the sclera-uveal wall and has an association with myopia. Staphyloma (**Figure 3.10**) tends to be a more focal enlargement or bulge, usually posterotemporal and may also be caused by radiation or previous infection.

## Coloboma

Coloboma is a focal congenital gap or defect of the ocular tissue with outpouching of the vitreous, typically located at the optic nerve head insertion or the posterior globe and is commonly bilateral. If confined to the optic disc, it is termed an optic disc coloboma and if separated or extending beyond the optic disc, it is a chorioretinal coloboma. Clinical presentations in colobomas are variable based on extent of involvement and ranges from a decrease in visual acuity

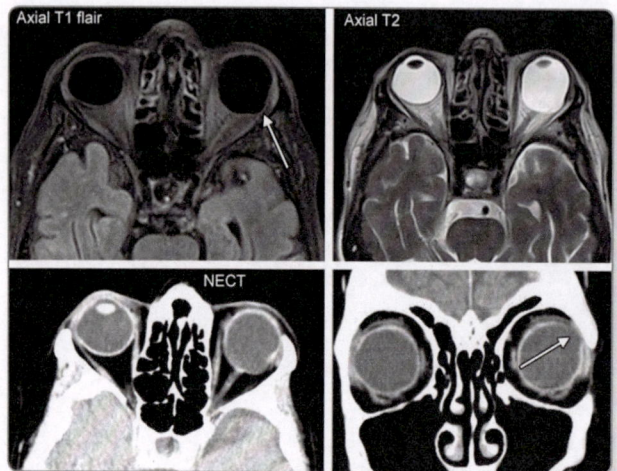

**Figure 3.10** MR and CT orbits of 81-year-old female with focal bulge posterotemporal aspect left globe seen on axial T1 FLAIR, axial T2 and axial/coronal unenhanced CT. Note focal decreased thickness of the eyewall (arrows) at the posterior bulge (Staphyloma) and adjacent posterior aspect of the globe

which is the most common to visual loss when retinal detachment is present (**Figures 3.11A to C**). Coloboma may be sporadic, autosomal dominant when nonsyndromic, or syndromic and usually autosomal recessive.

### Dermoid and epidermoid cysts

Dermoid and epidermoid cysts are developmental, non-neoplastic cysts caused by congenital failure of ectoderm to separate from the underlying structures, and sequestration of surface ectoderm or inclusion of dermal elements at site of suture closure. They represent 5 percent of orbital masses, with the majority (about 65–75%) being extraconal in the superolateral aspect of anterior orbit at the fronto-zygomatic suture. The remainder mostly occurs in the superonasal aspect of the frontolacrimal suture with other sites infrequent.

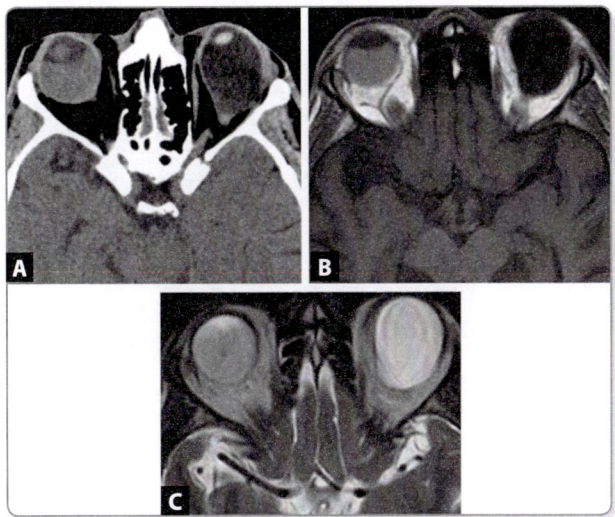

**Figures 3.11A to C** A 43-year-old female with bilateral coloboma and hemorrhage in right vitreous. (A) (Non enhanced CT orbit) shows dense hemorrhage in the vitreous of right eye. (B) and (C) (T1WI and T2WI MR) show bilateral coloboma. The hemorrhage is hyperintense on T1 and intermediate/slightly hypointense on T2

These cysts tend to be non-tender painless masses, fixed to the underlying bone (in opposition to sebaceous cysts), but may present as an enlarged painful mass if inflamed by associated infection or rupture, whether spontaneously or following trauma.

Imaging of dermoid and epidermoid demonstrates well demarcated cysts with thin rim. Presence of fat (HU -30 to -80 on CT) and/or high signal on T1WI on MR is characteristic of dermoid (**Figure 3.12**), while high signal (restricted diffusion) on DWI (MR diffusion weighted images) is indicative of epidermoid cyst. Scalloping and thinning of adjacent bone are common due to pressure erosion by the longstanding, slow growth of these lesions. Surgical resection is curative.

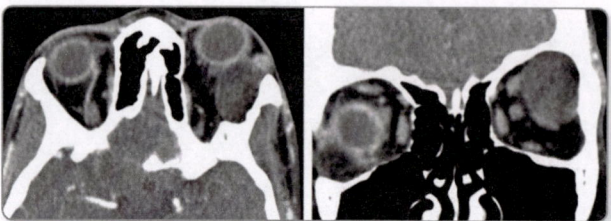

**Figure 3.12** CT orbit of 22-year-old female with left eye proptosis. Images show low attenuated mass with smooth thin capsule in the superior lateral left orbit, displacing lacrimal gland anteriorly, lateral rectus muscle inferiorly and causing bone erosions of lateral and superior orbital walls. The low attenuation content, especially of fat tissue range, and the well-defined capsule suggest the diagnosis of dermoid. This is the most common location of dermoid

# Orbital infections

## Preseptal cellulitis

Preseptal cellulitis represents a form of infection limited to the preseptal orbital soft tissues characterized by varying degrees of pain, swelling, erythema, and mild edema of eyelid and subcutaneous soft tissues. Imaging (CT or MRI), while showing soft tissue thickening or phlegmon (**Figures 3.13 and 3.14**), is more important to rule out preseptal abscess or more urgent intervention of postseptal extension of cellulitis, abscess formation or bone destruction. Early medical treatment with antimicrobial agent is usually sufficient. This preseptal infectious process should not be mistaken for an allergic soft tissue reaction.

## Postseptal cellulitis

When infection involves the orbital tissues posterior to the orbital septum the involvement is called postseptal cellulitis. Postseptal orbital cellulitis has significantly more severe implications requiring urgent treatment to save vision and prevent extension leading to orbital abscess, ophthalmic vein or cavernous sinus thrombosis. Postseptal cellulitis is suggested by increasing pain, proptosis and limitation of extraocular eye movement. Such clinical signs, in a

Imaging of the orbit 99

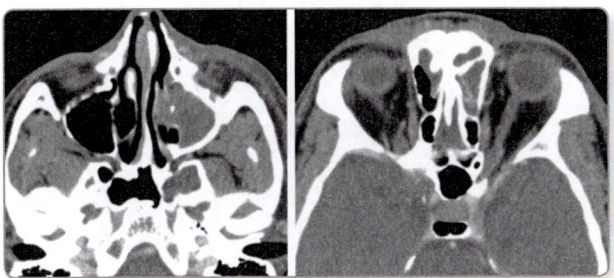

**Figure 3.13** CT of orbit of 30-year-old male with acute swelling over left orbit. It shows soft tissue swelling over left eye in keeping with preseptal cellulitis. Note right maxillary and ethmoidal opacification related to sinusitis

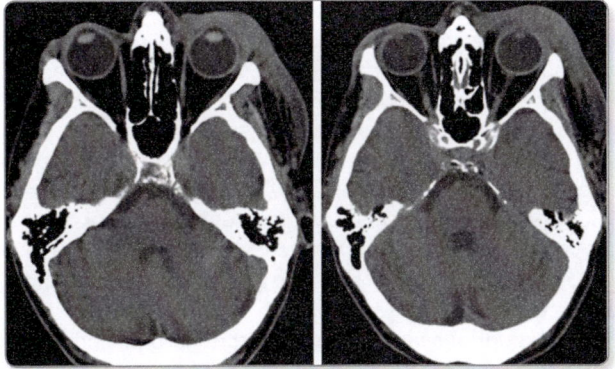

**Figure 3.14** CT orbit of 54-year-old male with fever and swelling over the left eye. Images show preseptal soft tissue thickening, swelling and fat stranding in keeping with preseptal cellulitis

patient who presented with preseptal soft tissue swelling, with limited symptoms, suggest the progression to postseptal cellulitis and its potential associated complications (**Figure 3.15**). The changes within the postseptal orbit tend to be intraconal and ill-defined and spread rapidly toward the orbit apex, with a lack of intraconal tissue

## Introductory head and neck imaging

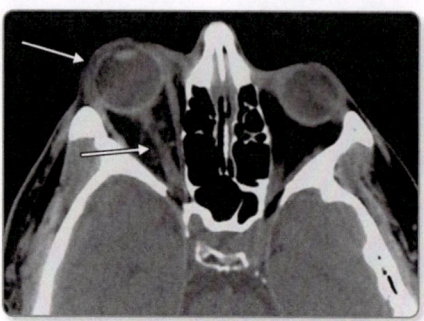

**Figure 3.15** Axial CT orbit of a patient presented with acute onset of right orbit pain and proptosis. There is a retrobulbar subtle infiltrate that can be emphasized by assessment with wider window, mild preseptal cellulitis and significant mass effect from postseptal cellulitis (see arrows)

barriers. On imaging, this postseptal infiltrate may be subtle initially and should not be underestimated. It is a key to rule out an orbital abscess or cavernous sinus involvement.

In a patient, who presents with symptoms and signs of postseptal orbital inflammation, and no preseptal inflammatory stage or signs, suggests the inflammatory etiology may be sinonasal in etiology. A contained periorbital (subperiosteal) abscess may have unappreciated symptoms of the underlying sinonasal inflammation. The sudden onset of orbital signs suggests rupture of the subperiosteal abscess intraorbitally, with a large infectious "load" that quickly extends through and overwhelms the intraconal orbit and cavernous sinus structures. Urgent imaging is required, assessing the presence of sinonasal disease, subperiosteal abscess, postseptal cellulitis and/or orbital abscess formation and cavernous sinus involvement. The degree of proptosis, stretching of the optic nerve and alteration of the configuration of the posterior globe (tenting) suggest the urgency of surgical intervention of the postseptal inflammatory disease, whether such inflammatory process arose from preseptal, sinonasal or penetrating trauma etiology.

## Orbital abscesses

Orbital abscess represents a purulent fluid collection that may be a primary process or following cellulitis and represents approximately 20 percent of orbital infections. Purulent fluid accumulating within the orbit, but contained by the orbital periosteum, is called a subperiosteal abscess and is most frequently located deep to the medial wall (lamina papyracea) of the orbit. The subperiosteal abscess may be intact or ruptured into the postseptal orbit with the inflammatory changes within the adjacent paranasal sinuses readily apparent.

## Etiology

Infections can spread to orbits via direct extension, preseptal or sinonasal infections, particularly ethmoid air cells through lamina papyracea, or by transmission of bacteria through the ophthalmic venous system in bacteremia. Other causes to be considered would include trauma, especially if penetrating, or from skin infections such as impetigo. A frontal sinus origin has higher risk of intracranial spread of infection.

## Clinical presentations

The most common symptoms/signs are eye swelling, proptosis, limitation of extraocular eye movement and fever. Complications include visual disturbances that may be due to acute optic nerve inflammation (neuritis), retinal artery ischemia resulting from retinal artery occlusion or thrombophlebitis. Other complications include cavernous sinus thrombosis and resultant cranial neuropathies. Intracranial extension can occur due to spread of infection through diploic vessels causing meningitis, cerebritis, subdural empyema or brain abscess.

## Imaging findings

Imaging can distinguish between preseptal cellulitis, postseptal cellulitis, subperiosteal abscess and orbital abscess and evaluate the cavernous sinus for thrombophlebitis, or the intracranial structures for associated subdural empyema, ventriculitis/ependymitis, meningitis, cerebritis or brain abscesses. Enhanced CT of the orbit is the modality of choice in evaluating orbital or sinonasal infections

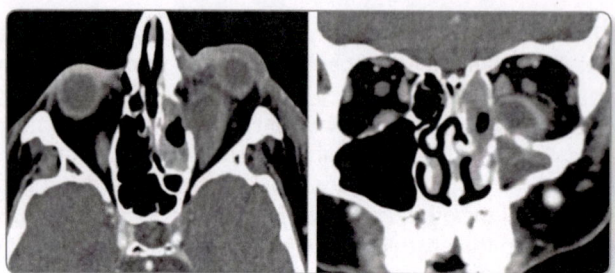

**Figure 3.16** Enhanced axial and coronal CT images of orbit show an acute subperiosteal abscess extending into postseptal space as a result of left ethmoid sinusitis. Note preseptal fat stranding as well. Urgent decompression of orbit required to save vision

(**Figure 3.16**), however; enhanced MRI is advantageous in the evaluation of the cavernous sinus and intracranial structures, or for subtle orbital enhancement. Contrast enhancement should be used in both techniques. CT bone algorithm images are useful to evaluate for subtle signs of infection or dehiscence within the paranasal sinuses, orbital walls and adjacent skull base. Sino-orbital infections arising from the frontal sinus will have a higher rate of intracranial involvement (**Figures 3.17 and 3.18**) shows more spread infections.

## Treatment

Medical treatment with aggressive intravenous antibiotic therapy may be sufficient in selective patients with limited abscess formation, with preservation of orbit function and minimal signs. Careful in-hospital observation is required if conservative treatment of orbital abscess is chosen. A significant percent of patients with orbital abscess present with signs requiring urgent imaging and surgical intervention to preserve vision and prevent cavernous sinus or intracranial extension.

## Specific orbital infections

Opportunistic infections such as aspergillosis should be considered in HIV patients. Herpes zoster ophthalmicus can occur along the ophthalmic (first) division of the trigeminal (V) cranial nerve, usually in elderly or immune-suppressed patients.

Imaging of the orbit 103

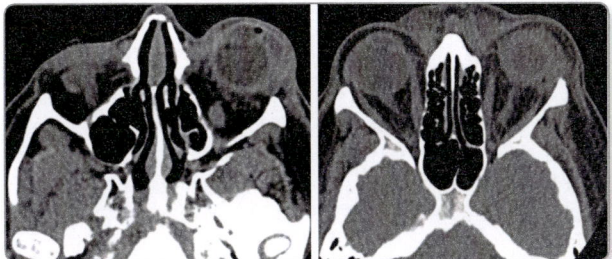

**Figure 3.17** Panophthalmitis: CT orbit of 48 males presented with swelling over left eye. Images show soft tissue swelling, mild proptosis, preseptal phlegmon and increased fluid trapped within left conjunctival sac. Minimal postseptal fat stranding. Note of thickening of the left globe sclera especially posteriorly and superiorly. Findings are in keeping with panophthalmitis

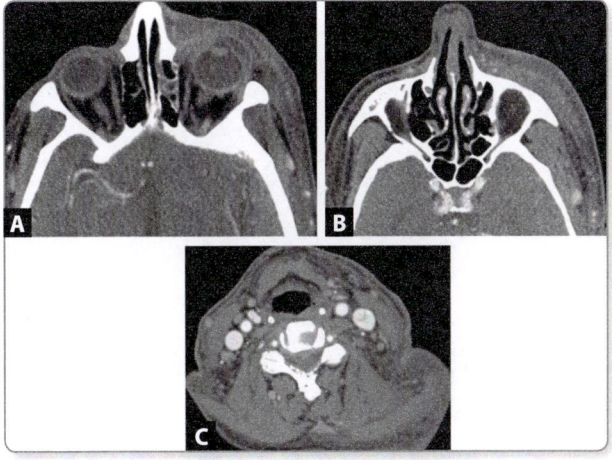

**Figures 3.18A to C** CT head and neck of 62 males with fever and swelling over left orbit. (A) Shows swelling and phlegmon over left orbit, including tear fluid trapped in conjunctival space behind left eyelid. Opacification of left ethmoid sinuses. (B, C) show swelling, soft tissue thickening and fat stranding extend over left face and lower in the neck

## Ocular infections

Posterior scleritis can be caused by bacteria, fungi, or viruses. Imaging shows thickening and enhancement of the eyeball, usually better visualized more posteriorly and superiorly (**Figure 3.19**).

Cytomegalovirus infection, the most common opportunistic infection in HIV patients, can involve the retina and choroid, and as a clue of its tendency to be a hemorrhagic infection, tends to offer ocular high attenuation on CT and variable signal on MR.

## Cavernous sinus thrombosis

Cavernous sinus thrombosis more frequently results from infections that have spread from infected areas (sinonasal cavities, orbits or mid face) that have venous drainage into the cavernous sinus. Septic thrombotic ophthalmic veins are a less common underlying cause. Patients with cavernous sinus thrombosis tend to be very ill and may present with ophthalmic, sinonasal, cavernous sinus, meningeal or cerebral findings as well as sepsis.

On contrast enhanced Imaging, the normal cavernous sinus shows homogenous diffuse enhancement outlining the contained

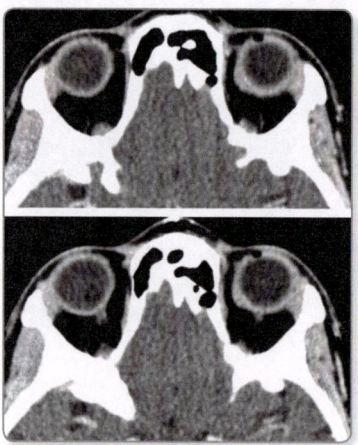

**Figure 3.19** CECT orbit for patient with left eye pain and diplopia. Images show thickening and enhancement of the posterior wall of the eye in keeping with scleritis

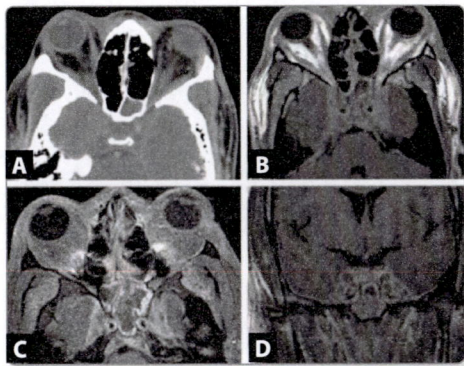

**Figures 3.20A to D** Cavernous sinus thrombosis: CT (A) and MRI (Axial T1WI) (B), Axial T1WI fat saturated after gadolinium (C), and Coronal T1WI fat saturated after gadolinium (D). The patient is 19-year-old male who had sinusitis and headache for 2 weeks and presented with acute onset severe face/orbit pain, swelling and right 3rd nerve ophthalmoplegia. Enhanced CT shows diffuse orbital infiltrate bilaterally with proptosis greater on right. Poor visualization of cavernous sinuses on CT necessitates MR imaging assessment. MR images show the diffuse inflitrate, propstosis with reduced caliber of supraclinoid ICA bilaterally and multiple filling defects (thrombi) in cavernous sinuses. Findings are in keeping with cavernous sinuses thrombosis followed sinusitis and orbital cellulitis

cranial nerves. With cavernous sinus thrombosis, the cavernous sinus will contain unenhanced foci of variable size or pattern, that may be subtle, as well as a fullness of that cavernous sinus. MR imaging is more sensitive in displaying these filling defects, with thrombi bright on T1- and T2-weighted images and as a filling defect within an otherwise enhanced cavernous sinus postgadolinium (**Figures 3.20A to D**).

# Orbital neoplasms

## Neural tumors of orbit

### Optic nerve glioma

Optic nerve glioma (ONG) is a slow growing, usually low grade astrocytic tumor, that arises from glial cells of the optic nerve. ONG may be unilateral or bilateral and may arise anywhere along the optic pathway. ONG may be isolated or associated with neurofibromato-

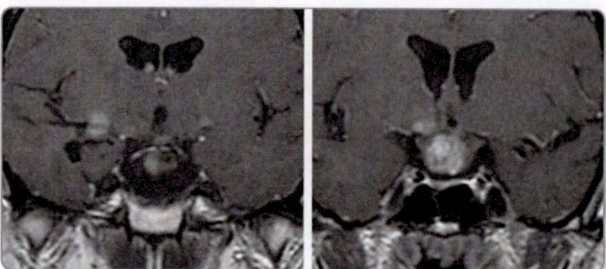

**Figure 3.21** Optic glioma: 20-year-old female with enhancing lesions on post gadolinium T1WI. The lesions involve the optic chiasma and extend along the optic tracts on both sides

sis type 1, particularly when bilateral or in young patients. Imaging usually shows a well-defined mass as a tubular or a fusiform enlargement of the optic nerve. Elongation of the optic nerve causing an anterior kink just posterior to the globe is a characteristic feature, when present. On MRI, ONG shows isointense signal to gray matter on T1, and hyperintensity on T2, with great variability and unpredictability in enhancement or growth patterns, especially if solitary and not associated with neurofibromatosis (**Figure 3.21**).

## Peripheral nerve sheath tumors

Peripheral nerve sheath tumors represent 4 percent of all orbital neoplasms. They arise from any neural elements of the orbit other than optic nerves which do not contain Schwann cells. Neurofibromas and schwannomas are benign, slow growing peripheral nerve sheath tumors that represent 2 percent of all orbital tumors. They are typically well demarcated enhancing round or fusiform lesions (**Figures 3.22 and 3.23**). Plexiform neurofibroma, as a vascular infiltrative tumor, represents the other 2 percent of orbital tumors. These latter tumors present in infancy or childhood and are considered pathognomonic for neurofibromatosis type one (NF1). The appearance of plexiform NF in infants and young children may be identical to that of capillary hemangioma. Malignant peripheral nerve sheath tumors (MPNST) are extremely rare. A clue to malignant etiology may be an accelerated growth rate.

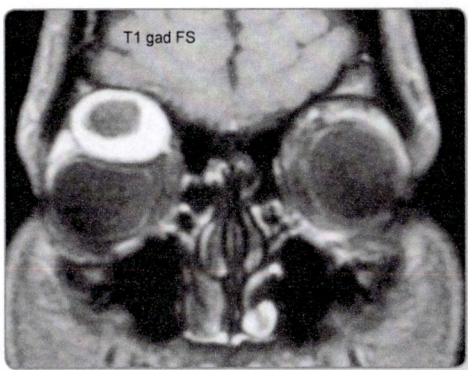

**Figure 3.22** Coronal T1 postgadolinium fat saturated image for patient with orbital schwannoma. The image shows a mass with a thick enhancing margin, displacing the right globe inferiorly and indenting its superior aspect. The mass causes subtle pressure erosions of the adjacent orbital roof

## Optic nerve sheath meningioma

Although not of neurogenic etiology, optic nerve sheath meningioma (ONSM) will be included here due to its close anatomic relationship to the optic nerve, its origin from the optic nerve sheath and to highlight its differentiating features from optic nerve glioma (ONG).

Meningioma (ONSM) is a benign tumor that arises from the meningoendothelial cells of arachnoid from the optic nerve sheath or rarely unrelated to the optic nerve. ONSM is more common in females and in an older age (fourth and fifth decades of life) compared to ONG or in children particularly in the first decade, and commonly in patients with neurofibromatosis type-2.

Imaging of perioptic meningioma may show eccentric, peripheral or circumferential thickening of the nerve sheath (on coronal imaging) that routinely enhances after contrast enhancement giving the so called tram track sign (axial imaging). When the meningioma is enlarged, it appears as a fusiform or even lobulated mass that enhances diffusely. As the ONSM enlarges, it may become more difficult to differentiate the nerve from its covering sheath; however the centrally positioned optic nerve can usually be differentiated, especially on the

**108   Introductory head and neck imaging**

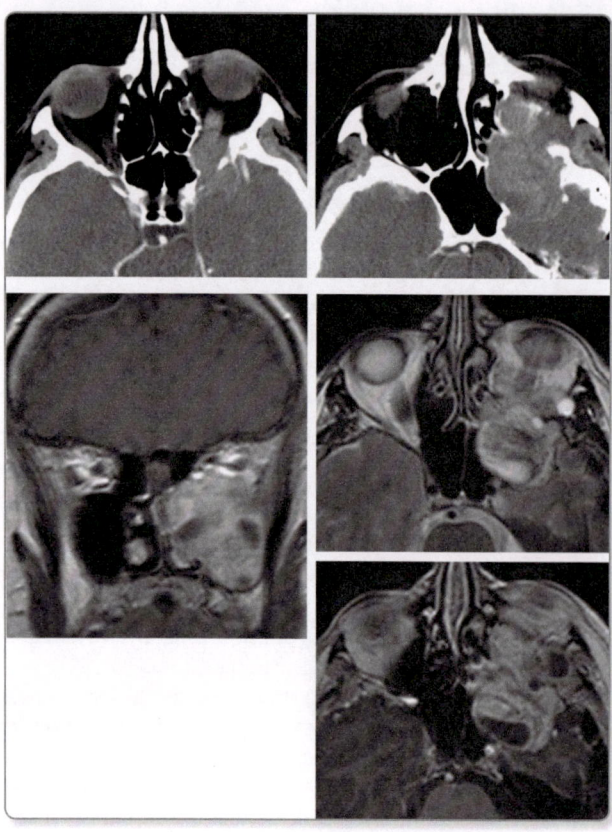

**Figure 3.23** CT scan of 50-year-old female with left V2 schwannoma. Large heterogenous mass involves left orbit, maxillary sinus with intracranial extension to left middle cranial fossa. MR (T2 and coronal and axial T1 postgadolinium) shows heterogenous signal of the mass and heterogenous enhancement after gadolinium

coronal image. The peripheral or outer margin of the mass may not be as well defined as for ONG. The presence of calcifications within the peripheral sheath is an important differentiating feature from optic nerve glioma. These calcifications appear as dense foci on CT and

Imaging of the orbit 109

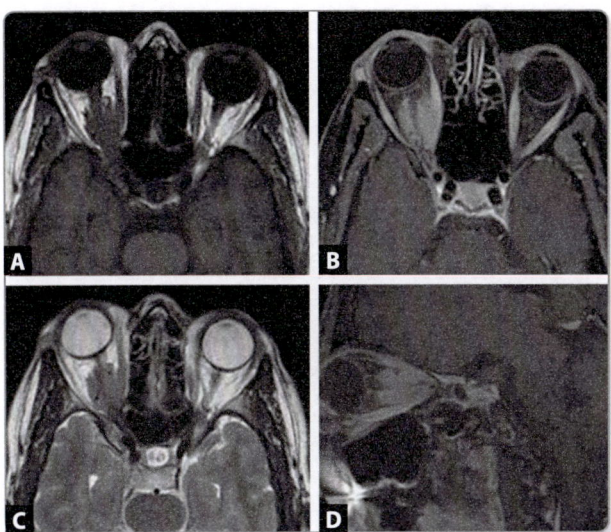

**Figures 3.24A to D** MRI orbit of 63-year-old female with right optic nerve sheath meningioma. Axial T1WI (A), Axial T1WI fat saturated after gadolinium (B), Axial T2WI (C), sagittal T1WI fat saturated after gadolinium (D). Images show circumferential mass surrounding the optic nerve which is isointense to the muscle on T1WI (A), slightly hyperintense on T2WI (B) and strongly enhanced after gadolinium (C, D). Note extension of the mass to the orbital apex along the optic nerve sheath (D)

signal void on MR imaging. The soft tissue component of the mass appears slightly dense on CT and hypointense on T1, and isointense to slightly hyperintense on T2-weighted images, due to the cellularity of the lesion. Hyperostosis of the adjacent bones may be seen on CT (bone window) at the orbit apex where the mass is adjacent to the bony walls of the optic canal and adjacent anterior clinoid process (**Figures 3.24 and 3.25**).

## Vascular tumors of orbit

### Cavernous hemangioma

Cavernous hemangioma is the most common orbital vascular tumor in adults and the most common retrobulbar mass in adults. These

## 110 Introductory head and neck imaging

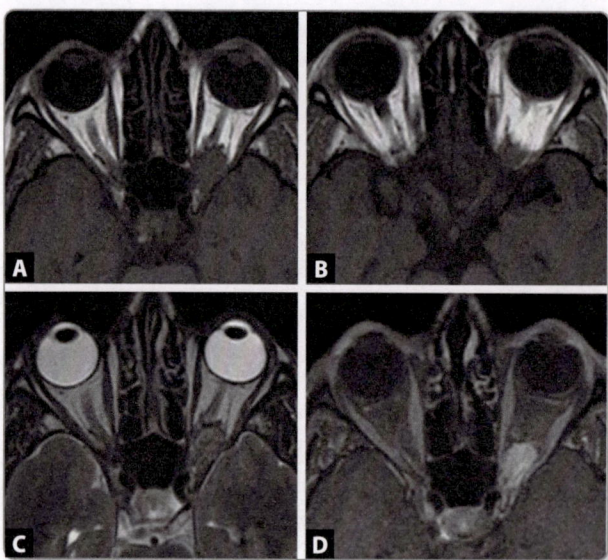

**Figures 3.25A to D** 50-year-old female with history of left eye blindness, diagnosed with left ONS meningioma. MR images axial T1 fat sat (A and B), T2WI fat sat (C) and postgadolinium T1 fat sat (D). Images show hypointense circumferential eccentric left ONS mass near to the apex on T1 (A,B), which is intermediate on T2 (C) and diffusely enhanced after gadolinium (D)

tend to occur from the second to fourth decades anywhere in the orbit. They gradually enlarge in size, and have smooth well-defined margins, round to ovoid configuration, with tendency to have slightly lobulated surface.

Cavernous hemangiomas are composed of large dilated vascular channels lined by thin attenuated endothelial cells. They may show minimal or patchy enhancement, especially on early phase post-contrast imaging, with a tendency to fill in later phase imaging (e.g. time –resolved or dynamic MRA) (**Figures 3.26A to D**). They tend to be less firm than other retrobulbar mass lesiones, (e.g. schwannoma, hemangiopericytoma) and tend to be indented by the globe, yet firm

Imaging of the orbit 111

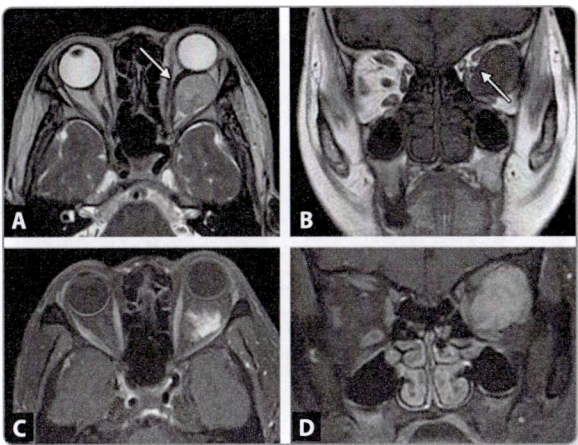

**Figures 3.26A to D** 64-year-old female with large well-defined slightly lobulated left retrobulbar mass that displaces the optic nerve (large white arrows) medially and slightly superiorly. There is left proptosis (A) axial T2, (B) coronal T1. Postgadolinium T1 fat suppressed early axial T1 (C) and late coronal T1 (D) show limited patchy enhancement early and diffuse more homogeneous enhancement on the later coronal image typical for cavernous hemangioma

enough to cause bone remodeling. They may contain foci of calcification.

### Capillary hemangioma

Capillary hemangioma is a synonym for benign hemangioendothelioma which is an infantile orbital endothelial cell neoplasm, most commonly seen in the superomedial extraconal location. It is the most common benign orbital tumor of infancy, presents in 1 percent of neonates with 30 percent at birth. It is characterized by a growth phase in the first year followed by involution. It appears as a lobular or infiltrative mass with intense enhancement after contrast due to its high vascularity (**Figure 3.27**). It has a heterogeneous or slightly hyperintense signal relative to muscle on T1 and high signal with flow voids on T2WI.

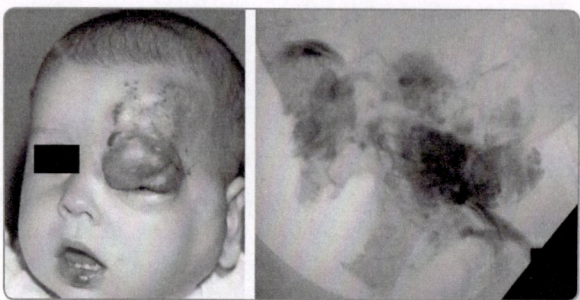

Figure 3.27 Infant with left orbital capillary hemangioma. Digital subtracted angiogram (DSA) was done for management planning and shows high vascularity of the lesion (*Courtesy*: Dr Karl Terbrugge, Professor and Chairman of Neuroradiology, University Health Network, University of Toronto) (*for color version see Plate 8*)

## Hemangiopericytoma

Hemangiopericytomas are rare vascular neoplasms that arise from pericytes of Zimmermann. About 50 percent of hemangiopericytomas are malignant and can metastasize. Early contrast blush related to high vascularity of the tumor or flow voids on MRI are a differentiating feature (**Figure 3.28**).

## Hematological malignancies

### Lymphoma

Lymphoproliferative tumors of the orbit range from benign lymphoid hyperplasia to malignant lymphoma. Lymphoid hyperplasia is a reactive benign disease that has good response to steroids. B-cell non Hodgkin's lymphoma has an extranodal predilection. Mucosa-associated lymphoid tissue (MALT) is the most common primary orbital non-Hodgkin's lymphoma. Due to its cellularity, lymphoma, on imaging, typically shows a soft tissue mass of uniform increased CT attenuation, and mild increased signal on T1WI and decreased signal on T2WI, as compared to muscle, with homogenous contrast enhancement (**Figure 3.29**). Lymphoma can involve any orbital structure with predilection for the preseptal tissues and lacrimal glands. Treatment of lymphoma includes radiotherapy and chemotherapy with variable

Imaging of the orbit

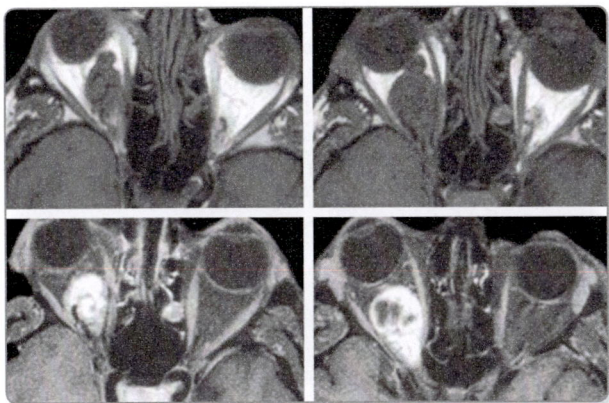

**Figure 3.28** MRI orbit: Axial T1 pregadolinium (top images) and T1WI fat saturated postgadolinium (lower images) of right orbital hemangiopericytoma. Images show right retrobulbar enhancing mass with signal void structures (vessels) indicating vascular nature

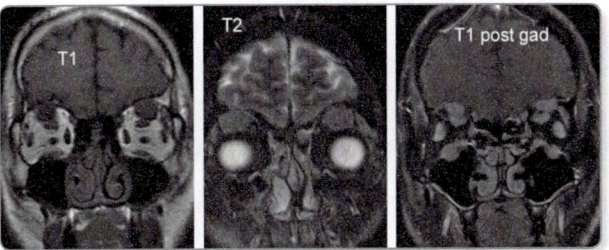

**Figure 3.29** MRI orbit of 47-year-old male with bilateral MALT lymphoma. Images show infiltrative masses in both orbits superiorly which are isointense to muscle on T1, slightly hypointense on T2 due to cellularity, and diffusely enhance after gadolinium

response based on the grade of the disease. Lymphoma tends to present as a painless mass in contrast to idiopathic orbital inflammatory disease (IOID) that often resembles lymphoma in appearance but has an element of pain in its presentation.

## Leukemia

Leukemia, one of the most common childhood malignancies, is classified into acute myelogenous leukemia (AML), acute lymphoblastic leukemia, chronic myelogenous leukemia and chronic lymphocytic leukemia. AML is the most common type and may present as granulocytic sarcoma (chloroma; a name related to its green color) with infiltration of the orbital structures by leukemic cells appearing as soft tissue mass that may involve the subperiosteum or orbital bones (**Figure 3.30**).

## Plasma cell tumors

Plasma cell tumors either arise purely from plasma cells (plasmacytoma) or from a mixture of plasma cells and lymphocytes (lymphoplasmacytic tumors). They may be isolated or part of systemic multiple myeloma. A soft tissue mass in the orbit may or may not involve the bony structures. Or the mass may arise from the paranasal sinuses and extends into the orbit (**Figure 3.31**).

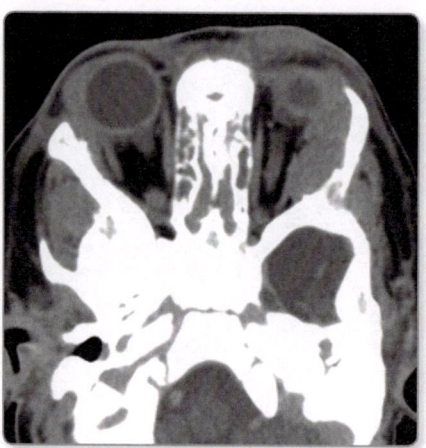

**Figure 3.30** CT brain study of 13-year-old with leukemia. Image shows homogenous soft tissue density in both orbits involving lateral extraconal spaces. Note opacification of sinuses

Imaging of the orbit 115

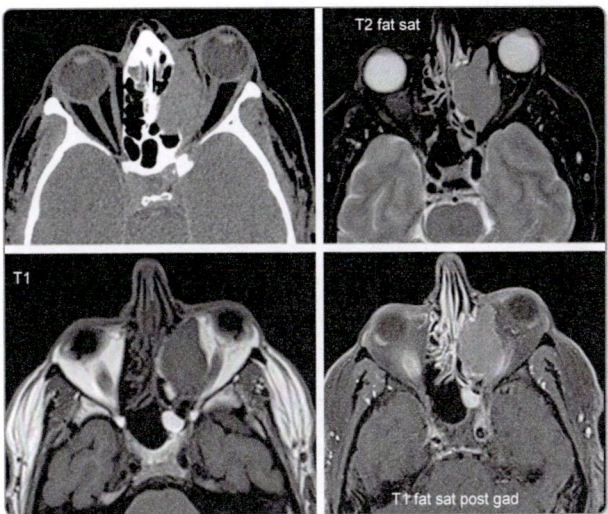

**Figure 3.31** Plasmacytoma: (A) CT orbit of 51-year-old female with history of left eye redness, discharge and proptosis. Image shows soft tissue mass involves left ethmoid sinus and extends to medial extraconal space encroaching but not invading the left intraconal left orbit compressing the left medial rectus muscle and approaching the optic nerve. MRI T2WI with fat saturation, T1WI, T1WI with fat saturation after gadolinium. Images show same mass with intermediate signal on T2 due to cellularity of the mass, with diffuse postgadolinium enhancement

## Malignant neoplasms in childhood

Rhabdomyosarcoma and retinoblastoma, in addition to leukemia and lymphoma, and metastatic disease mainly from neuroblastoma, constitute the main malignancies of orbit in the pediatric age group.

## Rhabdomyosarcoma

Rhabdomyosarcoma, although a rare childhood tumor, is still the most common primary malignancy of the orbit and the most common soft tissue malignancy in children. Although it may present at any age from birth to adulthood, it occurs primarily from 2 to 5 years of age. This malignant tumor, originating from embryonic muscle or mesenchymal tissues, is characterized by rapid progression. Rhabdomyosarcoma can arise primarily from the orbit, invade the orbit from adjacent structures or metastasize to the orbit. They have a variable imaging appearance ranging from a homogenous well-defined soft tissue mass to more invasive aggressive lesions that cause bone destruction. They show variable signal characteristics considering their bleeding tendency, usually low on T1, and high on T2 sequences, with contrast enhancement (**Figure 3.32**).

## Retinoblastoma

Retinoblastoma is a primary malignant retinal neoplasm and the most common intraocular malignancy in childhood. Children commonly present with leukokoria and visual loss. The tumor may grow into the vitreous or outward within the subretinal space causing retinal detachment and hemorrhage. Retinoblastoma is unilateral in 70 percent, bilateral in 25 to 30 percent of cases, trilateral when the pineal gland is involved or quadrilateral when pineal and pituitary are involved. Presence of punctate calcifications in a normal or enlarged globe is a typical feature on non-enhanced CT imaging (**Figure 3.33** Courtesy of Manohar Shroff, FRCPC). Contrast administration allows heterogeneous enhancement which helps to determine the extent of the mass. Chemotherapy is the first line in therapy. Advanced tumor may require radiation therapy or enucleation when vision cannot be preserved.

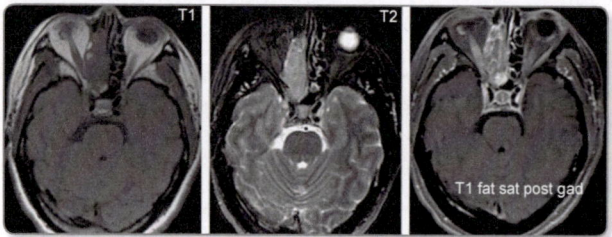

**Figure 3.32** Rhabdomyosarcoma: MRI of the paranasal sinuses and orbits of 53-year-old female with right ethmoidal sinus mass extends to the adjacent medial aspect of right orbit. Diagnosis of rhabdomyosarcoma was given on histopathology. Note intermediate signal on T2WI indicating cellularity of the tumor

Imaging of the orbit   117

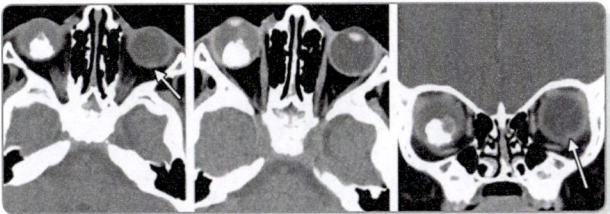

**Figure 3.33** CT orbits for a child with bilateral retinoblastoma. Images show large intraocular mass with dense calcification in the right orbit and small soft tissue on the left (white arrow) arising from the inner layer of the eye (retina) and bulge into the vitreous. (*Courtesy:* Dr Manohar Shroff, Associate Professor, Fellowship and Neuroradiology Program Director, Department of Medical Imaging, University of Toronto. Interim Chief of Radiology, Staff Neuroradiologist, Hospital for Sick Children, Toronto)

## Intraocular tumors

There are many benign and malignant tumors of the globe that mostly originate from the chorioretinal layers of the eye. Benign tumors include hamartoma which is associated with tuberous sclerosis, angioma in Von-Hippel-Lindau syndrome, hemangioma, and osteoma. Malignant tumors include retinoblastoma (see above) which is the most common childhood intraocular malignant tumor and ocular melanoma.

## Ocular melanoma

Melanoma is a primary malignant tumor of the uveal tract (choroid, ciliary body and iris) of which choroidal melanoma is the most common type representing about 85 percent of ocular melanomas. Typically, the tumor is solid, grows toward the vitreous and may elevate or detach the retina resulting in accumulation of blood under the lesion, then along the subretinal space. The tumor may metastasize to various parts of the body, commonly liver and lung.

Computed tomography scan shows a dense solid mass that enhances. MR imaging is more sensitive to detect the mass and the hemorrhage if present. The mass appears hyperintense on T1WI, isointense to slightly hypointense on T2WI and enhances after gadolinium.

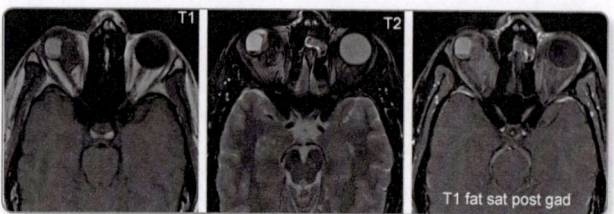

**Figure 3.34** MRI orbit (Axial T1WI, T2WI, and T1WI fat saturated after gadolinium) of 36-year-old female with right ocular melanoma. Images show heterogeneous mass with area of bright T1 due to melanin. The mass is heterogeneous slightly dark on T2 and enhancing after gadolinium. It extends to retrobulbar space

The hemorrhagic component is dense on CT and may liquefy over time, shows bright signal on T1 MR imaging, does not enhance after contrast on either CT or MR imaging, and should be differentiated from the tumor component (**Figure 3.34**).

## Metastasis of the orbit

Metastases occasionally involve the orbit. Breast and lung cancers are the main primary sites and may involve any structure within the orbit including the globe, optic nerve sheath complex, extraocular muscles or orbital bony walls. Blood born uveal metastases are more common in the posterior segment of the globe due to the rich blood supply from the posterior ciliary artery. Choroidal metastasis may cause retinal detachment and mimic uveal melanoma. MR Imaging of metastasis shows variable signals (**Figure 3.35**). Metastasis from breast cancer can be pathognomonic if there is a cicatrizing appearance (**Figure 3.36**). Atypical focal nodularity, single or multiple, within the extraocular muscles, suggests metastatic disease. Skin cancer may involve the orbit by direct invasion or metastatic spread.

## The lacrimal apparatus

Neoplasms of the lacrimal gland are divided into epithelial and nonepithelial tumors. The epithelial tumors have some similarity to tumors arising within the salivary glands, with glandular epithelial tumors, whether benign (pleomorphic adenoma) or malignant

Imaging of the orbit 119

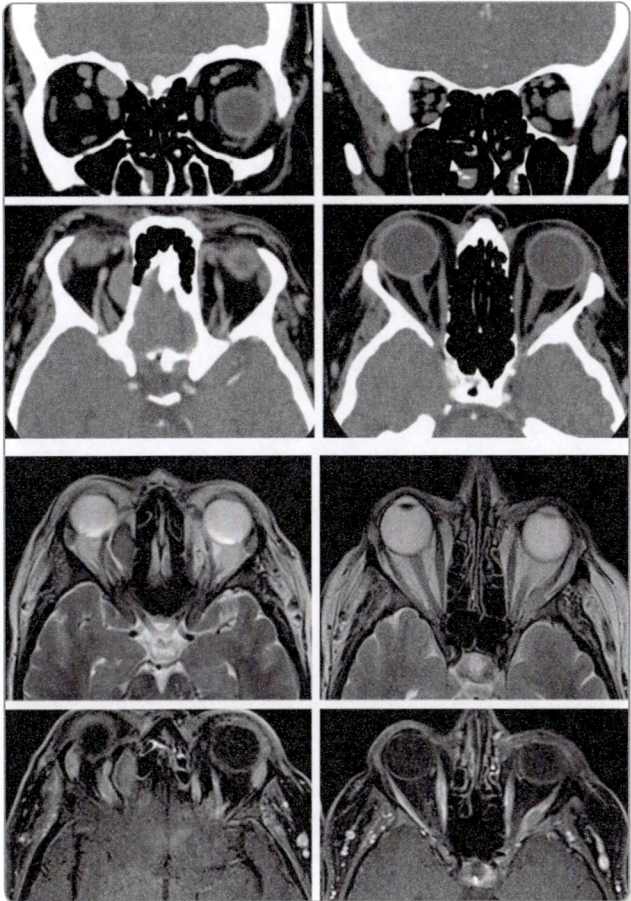

**Figure 3.35** Lung metastasis. 60-year-old female, newly diagnosed lung cancer. CT orbit shows focal enlargement of right superior oblique and left lateral rectus muscles. MR orbit shows that these lesions are distinguished from the muscles on T2WI (top images) with less enhancement than adjacent muscles after gadolinium (lower images). Imaging findings suggest bilateral metastases

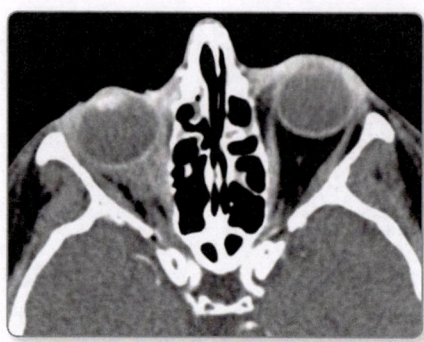

**Figure 3.36** Breast metastasis: Axial CECT of middle age female shows an ill-defined infiltrative right retrobulbar mass invading the medial rectus muscle and obscuring the optic nerve yet having enophthalmos indicating cicatrizing breast metastasis

(adenoid cystic carcinoma, mucoepidermoid carcinoma, acinic cell carcinoma, etc.) representing approximately 50 percent of lacrimal gland masses. These epithelial tumors are firmer, have more acute margins with the adjacent bone margins, cause pressure erosion of the bony margins of the lacrimal gland fossa, and may indent or displace the globe. Malignancy is suggested by infiltration or sclerosis of the adjacent bone structures or soft tissue infiltration of the adjacent orbital soft tissues. Pleomorphic adenoma is the most common epithelial benign tumor of lacrimal gland and is usually well circumscribed (**Figures 3.37A and B**). However, lack of aggressive features does not rule out malignancy, especially of a lower grade. These benign appearing epithelial masses typically show high signal on MR T2WI and homogeneous enhancement.

Approximately, 50 percent of lacrimal gland tumors will be lymphoid or inflammatory in nature, with lymphoma the most common non-epithelial neoplasm (**Figure 3.38**). Benign inflammatory entities, whether lymphoid or not, may resemble lymphoma and include idiopathic orbital inflammatory disease (Pseudotumor), sarcoidosis, Sjogren's or occasionally Wegener's. These non-epithelial lacrimal gland masses tend to be less firm than the glandular epithelial tumors with suggestive imaging findings

Imaging of the orbit 121

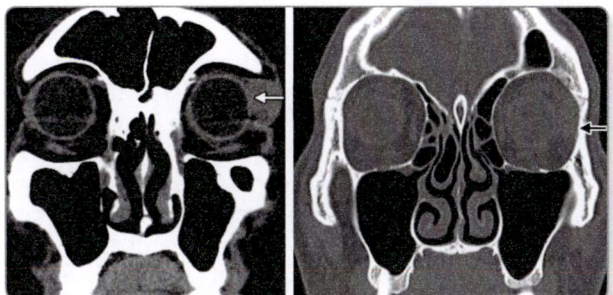

**Figure 3.37A** Epithelial tumors of lacrimal gland: CT orbit of 54 male with left orbital mass. Coronal soft tissue image shows a well defined mass in the superolateral aspect of left orbit involving the lacrimal gland (white arrow). Corresponding bone window shows scalloping of the adjacent bone (black arrow) indicating long standing benign tumor with nonaggressive features

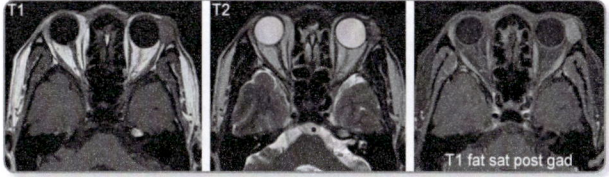

**Figure 3.37B** MRI orbit of the same patient showing same mass involving left lacrimal gland. The mass is hypointense on T1WI, predominantly hyperintense on T2WI with enhancement after gadolinium. Findings are in keeping with pleomorphic adenoma

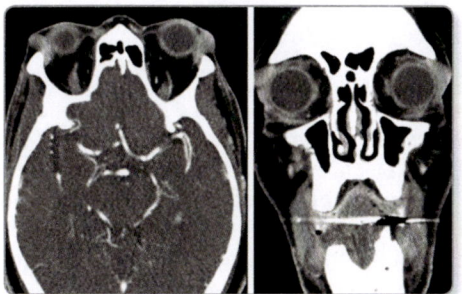

**Figure 3.38** CT orbit (axial and coronal) of 66-year-old male with bilateral lacrimal gland MALT lymphoma. Note enlargement and homogenous enhancement of both glands

when present including obtuse margins at the adjacent orbit walls, the mass indented by the globe, and lack of bone erosion by the mass. Lymphoma may be suspected in a painless lacrimal fossa mass that has a "lymphoid" configuration. IOID or acute inflammation of the lacrimal gland (dacryoadenitis) will be painful and have a rapid onset. Bilateral enlargement of the lacrimal glands suggest lymphoma with a differential of Sjogren's, sarcoidosis or, if painful, IOID. Uncommon nonepithelial tumors include mesenchymal tumors such as hemangiopericytoma and fibrous histiocytomas.

Tumors of the lacrimal sac are uncommon and include a variety of epithelial tumors (papillomas and carcinomas including salivary glandular tumors) and nonepithelial tumors (histiocytoma, hemangioma, lymphoma, and melanoma).

Swelling of the region of the inner canthus is more likely to be inflammatory/obstructive in etiology than neoplastic. Obstruction of the nasolacrimal drainage system is common, most often at the junction of the lacrimal sac and the proximal nasolacrimal duct, with resultant dilation of the lacrimal sac (lacrimal sac mucocele or dacryocystocele). Inflammation of the lacrimal sac is dacryocystitis and inflammation of an obstructed enlarged lacrimal sac may range from inflamed lacrimal sac mucocele to lacrimal sac pyocele to associated orbital cellulitis or orbital abscess.

# Inflammatory diseases of the orbit

## Idiopathic orbital inflammatory disease (IOID or orbital pseudotumor)

Idiopathic orbital inflammatory disease or pseudotumor is a nonspecific inflammatory process and the most common etiology of a painful orbital mass or infiltrate. IOID may involve any orbital structure with the extraocular muscles being the most common site (**Figures 3.39A to C**) followed by the lacrimal glands. A clue to diagnosis, in addition to the pain, may be the subtle presence of more than one site of involvement, including the retrobulbar orbit and optic nerve sheath complex. An intracranial variant of IOID involving the orbit apex, parasellar structures or the cavernous sinus, represents

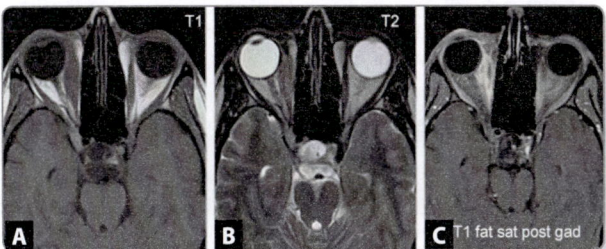

**Figures 3.39A to C** Idiopathic orbital inflammatory disease: MRI orbit of 35-year-old female with right orbital pseudotumor. (A, C) T1WI before and after gadolinium show an infiltrative isointense lesion involving right medial rectus muscle and adjacent extraconal fat which enhances after gadolinium. (B) T2WI shows same lesion with heterogenous signal, slightly brighter than muscles

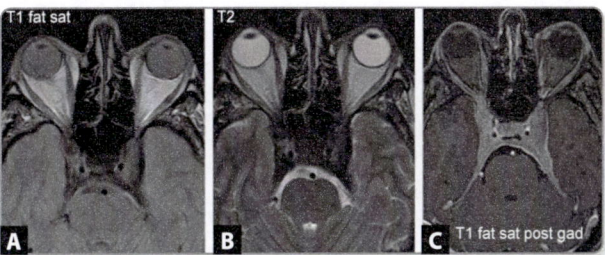

**Figures 3.40A to C** Tolosa-Hunt Syndrome: MRI head (Axial T1WI, T2WI and T1WI fat saturated after gadolinium) of 50-year-old male with cranial nerve palsies. Images show bilateral enlargement of cavernous sinuses (A), low signal on T2WI (B), with homogeneous enhancement extending to orbital apices (C). Note bilateral proptosis

the "Tolosa-Hunt syndrome" (**Figures 3.40A to C**). Treatment with systemic steroid is the first line of treatment for IOID.

Imaging findings include focal or diffuse infiltrative mass that strongly enhances. MR shows hypo to isointense lesion on T1WI as compared to muscles and isointense to slightly hyperintense on T2 sequences. Decreased T2 signal does not rule out this diagnosis, but suggests a fibrosing inflammatory variant that will also display diffuse enhancement. When involvement of the extraocular muscles

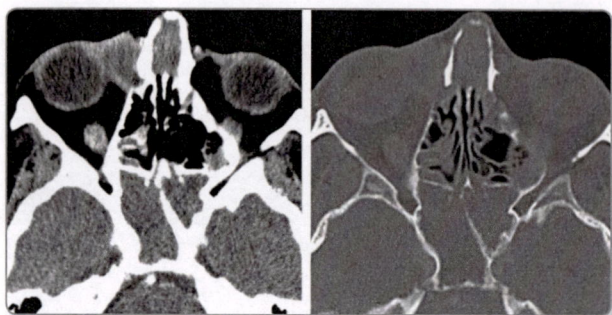

**Figure 3.41** Wegener's granulomatosis: CT scan of the orbit with contrast of 27-year-old female show enhancing soft tissue mass involving medial aspect- inner canthus of right orbit. Note opacification of nasal cavity anteriorly and sinuses due to involvement by Wegener's granulomatosis

(myositis) occurs, the anterior tendinous insertions of the muscles are typically involved in contrast to the sparing seen with thyroid orbitopathy.

## Wegener granulomatosis

Wegener granulomatosis is a multisystem disease characterized by respiratory system involvement, glomerulonephritis and necrotizing vasculitis (small vessels angiitis). Orbital involvement is the most common extrasinonasal site in the head and neck. The disease is characteristically bilateral and commonly spreads from sinonasal involvement (**Figure 3.41**). High titer antineutrophil cytoplasmic antibodies (C-ANCA) are highly indicative of the disease. Treatment with corticosteroid and cyclophosphamide is used in most cases.

## Sarcoidosis

Sarcoidosis, a noncaseating granulomatous inflammation, involves the orbits in approximately 25 percent of cases, especially diffuse enlargement of one or both lacrimal glands. Imaging findings include an enhancing mass or abnormal enlargement and enhancement of the involved orbital structure (**Figure 3.42**). When the optic nerve

Imaging of the orbit 125

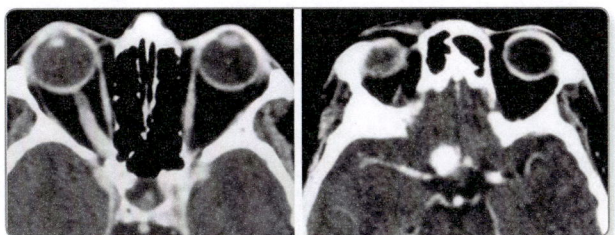

Figure 3.42 Axial enhanced CT orbit shows thickened and enhanced right optic nerve in its intraorbital and canalicular segments. Note dural thickening and enhancing suprasellar mass. Combination of findings very suggestive of sarcoidosis

is involved, leptomeningeal involvement of the optic nerve sheath (perioptic enhancement) may be seen, in addition to the thickening, signal change or enhancement of the nerve, best assessed by MR imaging.

### Langerhans cell histiocytosis

Langerhans cell histiocytosis (LCH) is a granulomatous disease, with a predilection for children between 1 to 4 years of age. Although a rare disease, orbital involvement is not uncommon, and is usually seen in those with the chronic forms of the disease, lesions in children are more commonly in bone or bone marrow. The frontal bone is most commonly involved, usually at the superior or superolateral aspect of the orbit more anteriorly. The pattern of bone destruction is nonspecific, usually solitary, and on CT or MR, resembles a soft tissue infiltrative mass suggestive of a malignant lesion (**Figure 3.43**). LCH also involves the hypothalamus causing diabetes insipidus.

### Sjögren syndrome

Sjögren syndrome is an autoimmune process characterized by keratoconjunctivitis sicca and xerostomia and may be associated with rheumatoid arthritis and systemic lupus erythematosus. The most common orbital manifestation is diffuse enlargement of one or both lacrimal glands, and may be associated with parenchymal changes in

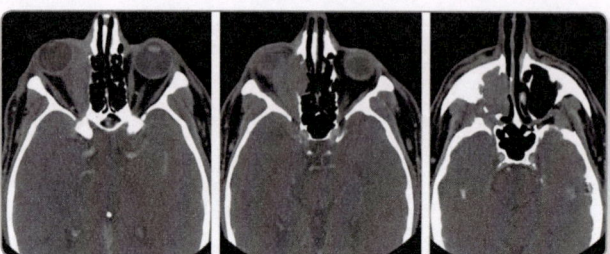

Figure 3.43 Langerhans cell histiocytosis: Enhanced axial CT head and neck of 46-year-old male with an infiltrative soft tissue mass involving the right orbit, ethmoid and maxillary sinuses and infiltrating the right lamina papyracea and right maxillary sinus posterior and medial walls. Tumor extends into the right pterygopalatine fossa

the salivary glands. The main differential of bilateral diffusely enlarged lacrimal glands includes lymphoma, sarcoidosis and Sjögren.

## Optic neuritis

Optic neuritis by definition signifies inflammation of the optic nerve that may be diffuse or segmental. Mild enlargement and slight enhancement of the optic nerve are appreciated best if imaged by MRI. Edema or acute inflammation may also be suggested by increased T2 signal and increased caliber of the optic nerve, best assessed on the coronal sequences. Fat suppression technique on these sequences allows for better detection of these changes, which may be subtle (**Figures 3.44 and 3.45**). Optic neuritis is most commonly seen in patients with multiple sclerosis and may be the first presentation in 15 percent of MS patients.

Other causes of optic neuropathies include infective, radiation and autoimmune optic neuropathies, such as in systemic lupus erythematosis, or compressive optic neuropathies due to adjacent mass lesions (e.g. sella) or aneurysms. Chronic optic neuropathies tend to have decreased optic nerve caliber and lack enhancement.

## Thyroid associated orbitopathy

Thyroid orbitopathy or Graves' dysthyroid ophthalmopathy is an orbital inflammatory disease associated with thyroid dysfunction and

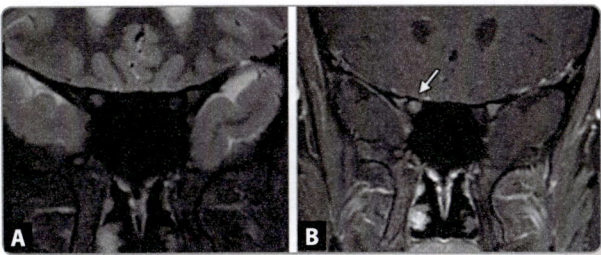

**Figures 3.44A and B** Optic neuritis: 30-year-old female with multiple sclerosis and right optic neuritis. (A) Coronal T2 Fat sat MR shows high T2 signal of optic nerve and thickening. (B) Postgadolinium coronal T1 with fat sat shows diffuse enhancement of the right optic nerve

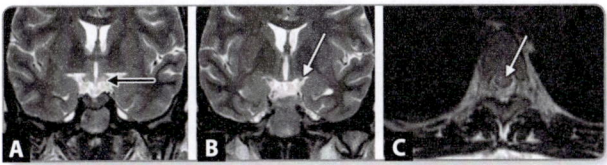

**Figures 3.45A to C** Optic neuritis with extensive chiasm involvement: 32-year-old female with Devic's disease. Coronal T2 with fat saturation shows high signal involving optic chiasma (A) and optic tracts (B) in keeping with neuritis. Note high signal abnormality of the cord on T2 Transverse MR of upper thoracic spine (C)

is the most common cause of unilateral or bilateral exophthalmos in the adult. Although thyroid orbitopathy usually occurs with a hyperthyroid state, it may be seen in hypothyroid or euthyroid states. The typical presentation is proptosis, eye swelling and restricted eye movement. Orbital extraocular muscle involvement is commonly bilateral and symmetrical; however thyroid orbitopathy has variable appearances. Classical imaging findings include enlargement of the extraocular muscles and increased intraorbital fat with resultant proptosis. In severe orbitopathy, the enlarged extraocular muscles and increased orbital fat may compress the optic nerve, especially at the orbit apex, causing visual loss (**Figures 3.46 and 3.47**). The disease has a predilection to involve the inferior rectus muscle, followed by medial,

## 128  Introductory head and neck imaging

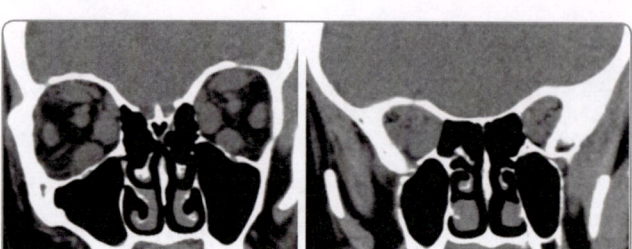

**Figure 3.46** CT orbit of 66-year-old female with thyroid ophthalmopathy. The extraocular muscles are enlarged bilaterally causing severe crowding of the optic nerve at the orbital apex

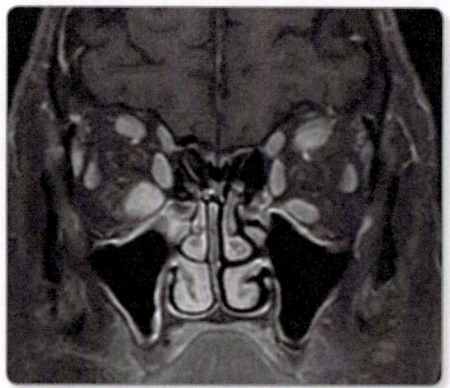

**Figure 3.47** Coronal T1 MRI of orbit after gadolinium with fat saturation: A 65-year-old female patient presented with proptosis and limited eye movement and found to have thyroid ophthalmopathy. Image shows enlargement and thickening of extraocular muscles bilaterally, sparing the lateral recti muscles which are typically the muscles least involved

superior and lateral recti, then oblique muscles, with characteristic sparing of the anterior inserting tendon of these muscles. Enlargement of lacrimal gland and engorgement of superior ophthalmic vein may be seen as well. The disease may be self limiting. However; follow-up with an endocrinologist may benefit patients with thyroid disease. Medical therapy with corticosteroid or even immunosuppressive drugs is considered initially since the disease is presumably related to an autoimmune process. Surgical decompression of the orbit is performed for severe conditions, compressive optic neuropathy or when vision is compromised.

The histopathology of thyroid orbitopathy consists initially of inflammatory cell infiltration, mucopolysaccharide deposition and increased water content. The extraocular muscles are infiltrated by lymphocytes and contain increased amount of hyaluronic acid, which binds to water, accounting for some of the orbital congestion. In the more chronic phase, the EOMs undergo muscle fiber degeneration and replacement fibrosis with resultant restrictive myopathy and lost elasticity.

The differential of multiple enlarged extraocular muscles is extensive and includes: thyroid orbitopathy, orbital inflammation-IOID (pseudotumor), orbital apex obstruction/congestion, carotid-cavernous fistula (CCF), endocrine (acromegaly), malignancy (metastases, lymphoma), systemic myositis (Crohn's and Wegener), infections such as sinusitis with secondary myositis, and trichinosis.

# Trauma of the orbit

Careful evaluation of traumatic injuries of the orbit is important. Fractures near the orbital apex can be displaced during surgical reduction, may encroach on the optic canal and cause blindness. It is important to recognize potential free floating bone fragments that are at danger of shifting or encroaching on the optic nerve, especially at the orbit apex- optic canal prior to their reduction. Fractures of the floor of anterior cranial fossa can result in CSF rhinorrhea and increase risks of infections.

Fractures of the orbital walls may be isolated or associated with other fractures of the facial bones such as naso-orbital fracture, Le Fort type II and III fractures, and trimalar (Zygomaticomaxillary) fractures. The middle third of orbital floor and lamina papyracea are the weakest aspects of the orbital walls, therefore more vulnerable to fractures.

Naso-orbital fractures typically result from a direct trauma to the nose and involve the medial orbital wall.

Le Fort type II fractures typically involve the base of the nose and extend to the medial orbital walls, then to the inferior orbit wall (floor) and lateral wall of the maxilla. The Le Fort III fracture involves medial, inferior and lateral orbital walls as well as the zygomaticomaxillary complex, with separation of the midface from the skull base. Le fort fractures can have unilateral, bilateral, symmetric or asymmetric components.

Trimalar or tripod fracture involves the zygomatic arch and separates the zygoma from adjacent bony structures by fracture or sutural diastasis (zygomaticofrontal, zygomaticosphenoid and zygomaticomaxillary sutures). The fracture will involve the lateral orbital wall, the inferior orbital wall commonly involving the infraorbital canal, and the zygomatic arch (**Figure 3.48**).

A "pure" orbit floor blow out fracture involves the inferior orbital wall (floor) but spares the inferior orbital rim. It typically results from a direct blow to the orbit with an object that is larger than the anterior orbital cavity such as a fist. This force causes increased intraorbital pressure resulting in fracture displacement and herniation of the structures inferiorly through the fracture into the maxillary sinus. An "impure" inferior blowout fracture involves the inferior orbital rim (**Figure 3.49**). When the fractured orbital floor segment herniated upward into the orbit, it is blow in fracture. It is important to assess the degree of displacement of the bony components, whether any muscle component or nerve is entrapped or impaled, the size of any bone dehiscence, the amount of tissues extending through that dehiscence and to assess for any visual pathway abnormality in order to assess treatment needs and assess for potential extraocular muscle dysfunction, potential enophthalmos or facial bone malalignment.

Blowout fracture of the medial orbital wall may result in herniation of intraorbital fat, the medial rectus and/or superior oblique muscles medially into the fracture site (**Figure 3.50**).

Computed tomography is the modality of choice in initial assessment of facial/ orbital trauma and the adjacent orbital or cerebral soft tissue injury (**Figure 3.51**).

## Imaging of the orbit 131

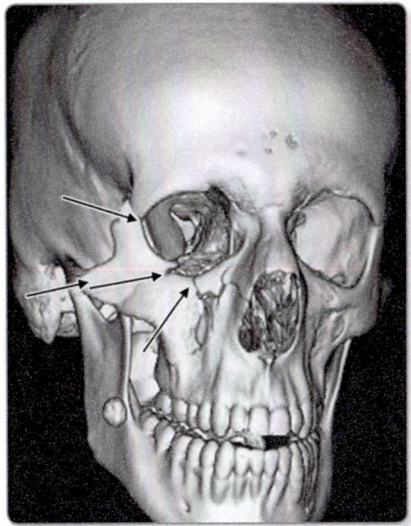

**Figure 3.48** Tripod fracture: 3-D reconstructed image from CT facial bone shows fracture of right zygomatic arch extends to zygomaticofrontal, zygomaticomaxillary, lateral and inferior orbital walls near infraorbital foramen

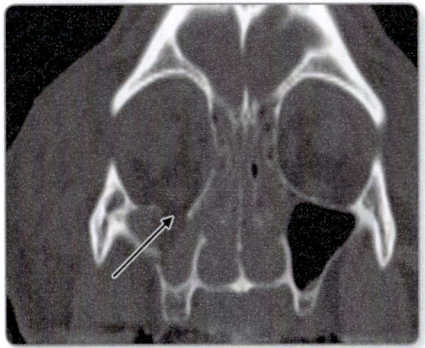

**Figure 3.49** Young male with history of trauma. CT shows fracture of right orbital floor involving orbital rim, with herniated orbital fat into maxillary sinus through the fracture. Note large soft tissue swelling over right orbit and face

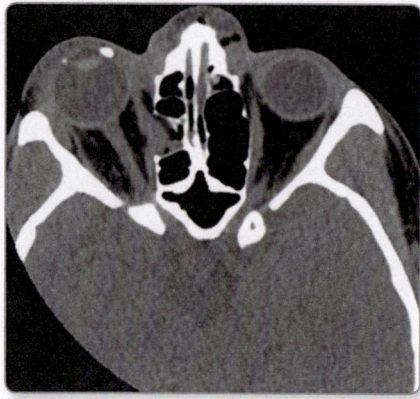

**Figure 3.50** CT of young male shows blowout fracture of medial wall of right orbit with medial rectus muscle herniated into the fracture defect. Note preseptal soft tissue swelling over right eye and nose with dense foreign bodies present

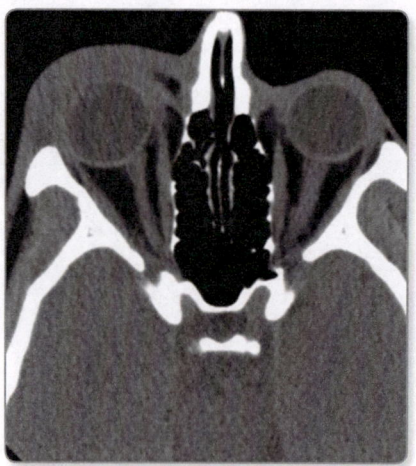

**Figure 3.51** CT of young male shows preseptal soft tissue swelling over right eye related to traumatic hematoma

Imaging of the orbit 133

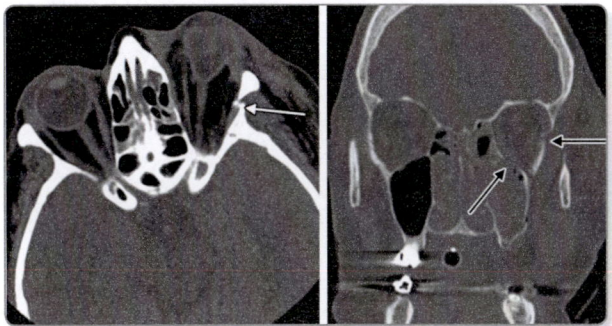

**Figure 3.52** CT scan (Axial soft tissue and coronal bone window) of 65-year-old female with direct trauma to left orbit. There is left exophthalmos and abnormal configuration of the eye in keeping with ruptured globe. Note overlying hematoma and fractures of lateral and inferior orbital walls (arrows)

Trauma of the orbit can be complicated by infection, foreign body, CSF leak, vascular injury or loss of vision including globe rupture, optic nerve injury (**Figure 3.52**) or intraorbital emphysema mass effect.

Urgent surgical intervention may be required in specific injuries to the orbit such as acute exophthalmos, entrapment or herniation of extraocular muscles or increased intraorbital edema/ hemorrhage requiring decompression of orbital contents or penetrating injuries.

# Intraocular detachments

Intraocular detachments can be divided into three groups; posterior hyaloid detachment (posterior vitreous detachment), retinal detachment and choroidal detachment.

The posterior hyaloid membrane is located between the vitreous and the retina, so when detached, it appears thickened and the hemorrhage occurs in the vitreous (**Figure 3.53**). This may also be seen with other conditions such as retinal detachment, persistent hyperplastic primary vitreous and myopia.

Retinal detachment occurs in a potential subretinal space as a result of separation between the two retinal layers: the sensory

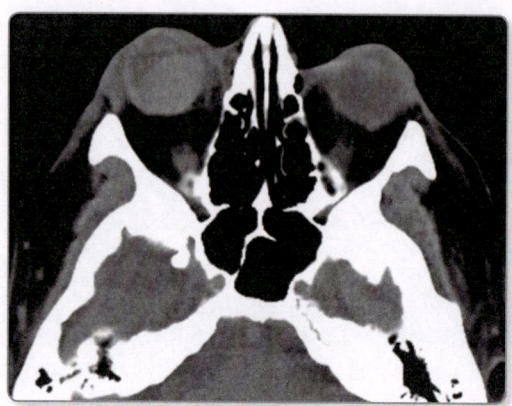

**Figure 3.53** Intraocular hemorrhage: CT head of 86-year-old female with vitreous hemorrhage followed anticoagulation

retina and pigmented epithelium. Malignant melanoma is the most common neoplasm to cause retinal hemorrhage. Retinal hemorrhage may also be seen associated with congenital coloboma. The hemorrhage occurs in the subretinal space and extends posteriorly to the optic nerve attachment giving a lentiform shape on imaging. When the hemorrhage is large enough to spread to both sides of optic nerve head/disc, there is a classic V shaped appearance (**Figure 3.54**).

Choroidal detachment occurs in a potential suprachoroidal space due to separation of choroid from sclera and is usually seen associated with blunt trauma or surgery to the eye and appears as a well-defined hematoma in the wall of the globe.

# Some overall thoughts about the orbit

## Organization of compartmentalizing the orbit

1. From anterior to posterior:
    - Preseptal tissues and orbital septum
    - Globe
    - Retrobulbar orbit

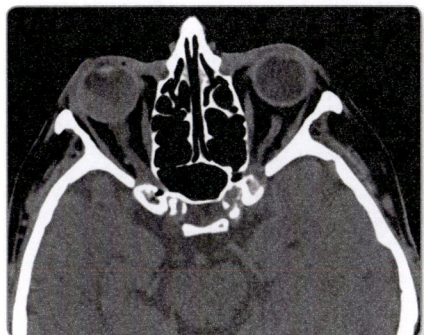

**Figure 3.54** CT head shows right intraocular hemorrhage in subretinal space, elevating the retina on both sides to optic nerve insertion. Findings in keeping with retinal detachment

- Orbit apex and foramina
- Cavernous sinus, parasellar and suprasellar tissues
2. From central to peripheral:
   - Globe
   - Optic nerve sheath complex
   - Perioptic tissues
   - Retrobulbar intraconal tissues
   - Conal tissues
   - Extraconal
   - Lacrimal gland
   - Nasolacrimal drainage system
   - Subperiosteal
   - Orbit walls
   - Extraorbital, e.g. paranasal sinuses
3. Imaging features to consider in assessing orbital lesions:
   - Margins: well-defined versus ill-defined
   - Lesion: attenuation, intensity, homogeneity versus heterogeneity
   - Patterns of enhancement or presence of flow voids
   - Presence of, and types of calcification(s), e.g. phleboliths
   - Rate of growth of mass: comparison with previous imaging

- "Soft" versus "Firm" mass: expansion or erosion of orbit walls/
- proptosis or displacement of orbital soft tissues
- Mass indents or indented by orbit structures
- Single versus multiple lesions
- Adjacent bone: infiltration versus expansion/ erosion

4. Imaging features interpreted in conjunction with clinical information:
   - Age and sex of patient
   - Known prior disease, e.g. neoplastic disease (primary or metastatic), systemic disease (e.g. metabolic, endocrine), previous surgery.
   - Presence or absence of pain/discomfort
   - Presence/type of visual change, associated cranial nerve abnormality, brain findings
   - Associated sinonasal signs/symptoms
   - Other systemic signs/symptoms, e.g. adenopathy, collagen disease

5. Causative possibilities- the usual etiologic categories and match to region of orbit
   - Congenital/ developmental
   - Inflammatory/ infectious
   - Allergic/autoimmune
   - Neoplastic (benign/malignant)
   - Traumatic
   - Drainage/obstructive
   - Vascular/congestive
   - Degenerative

## Some examples:

### Preseptal swelling

- Inflammatory (preseptal cellulitis)
- Post-traumatic: edema /contusion/hematoma
- Allergic response, e.g. insect bite, allergic exposure
- Neoplastic: basal cell carcinoma, squamous cell carcinoma, minor salivary epithelial carcinoma
- Postobstructive: cellulitis related to nasolacrimal duct obstruction

## Optic nerve sheath complex

Differential varies if longitudinal shape is parallel (tubular)/fusiform/globular

- Optic nerve/chiasm glioma
- Optic nerve sheath meningioma
- Optic neuritis/demyelination
- Nonspecific inflammation: sarcoid/Wegener/IOID, etc
- Vasoformative/congestive: CCF, arteriovenous malformation (AVM), venous thrombosis.
- Nonoptic pathway neoplastic: lymphoma/leukemia, metastases, etc.

## Retrobulbar orbit

- Masses: Neoplastic: hemangioma, schwannoma, lymphoma, hemangiopericytoma,
- Vascular: venous varix, etc
   Infiltrate: Neoplastic: lymphoma, leukemia, metastases
   Inflammatory: IOID, cellulitis, Wegener granulomatosis
   Vasoformative: CCF, AVM

## Final message

### Specific orbit imaging comments:

It is preferable to assess orbit structures with thin slice image acquisition and multiple planes of image acquisition/reconstruction, whatever modality (CT or MR) is utilized. Coronal images should be routine for all orbit studies. Sagittal or especially sagittal oblique imaging along the planes of the respective optic nerve sheath complexes in question are very advantageous in assessing involvement or extent. Sagittal imaging is very useful to assess aspects of the orbit immediately adjacent to the orbit floor or roof, or to assess the adjacent inferior brain, or paranasal sinuses and complements the coronal images for those circumstances where the axial plane may be lacking. The sagittal plane is also excellent to assess preseptal pathology, e.g. basal cell carcinoma for degree of orbit or bone infiltration. The best plane for axial imaging is parallel to the intraorbital course of the optic nerve, however if muscle cone information is of primary interest, imaging parallel to the medial rectus muscle may be satisfactory but will not show muscle cone compromise of the optic nerve at the orbit apex as well but the latter will be well shown by appropriate coronal images. For best assessment of vascular entities, dynamic vascular sequences are helpful, e.g. to assess "filling in" patterns of enhancement as seen in hemangioma, or CTA /MRA sequences to best show arteriovenous malformations or fistulae. The use of short fast image sequences during a performed Valsalva procedure may confirm a varix.

Initial decision of modality may be based on whether orbits alone (and immediate adjacent structures) will be imaged, or whether brain (e.g. optic neuropathy) will also be studied, or whether more extensive head and neck study is required, e.g. adenopathy, metastases to be assessed. Broader areas of coverage, assessment of sinonasal, craniofacial skeletal structures or presence of calcifications may favor CT as the initial mode of study as does need for extensive area of coverage.

Magnetic resonance imaging (MRI) offers greater tissue characterization, greater sensitivity to subtle tissue change or extent, greater assessment of enhancement within or beyond the orbit to include adjacent meninges, skull base, and upper deep neck or pharynx. Contrast enhancement will be used in the great majority of imaging exams with the exception of trauma (unless associated vascular injury to be assessed) or routine assessment of known thyroid orbitopathy. The relatively diffuse presence of orbital fat between the various orbital anatomic structures allows considerable information about the orbit mass/lesion, especially its extent, with contrast adding further information about the lesion or mass's characteristics that may not be required in various circumstances as mentioned above. Surgical planning requiring more detailed knowledge of the thin skeletal structures, such as the lamina papyracea, ethmoid roof or cribriform plate may be better assessed by CT than MR, with the signal void of cortical bone poorly visualized adjacent to air containing signal-lacking paranasal sinus structures. Only in those thicker orbital bone margins, containing medullary bone or bone components separate from air containing structures, does MR imaging become advantageous in assessing the osseous components.

# Bibliography

1. Al-Shafai LS, Mikulis DJ. Diffusion MR Imaging in a Case of Acute Ischemic Optic Neuropathy. AJNR Am J Neuroradiol 2006;27(2):255-7.
2. Azoulay R, Brisse H, Fréneaux P, Ferey S, Kalifa G, Adamsbaum C. Lacrimal location of sinus histiocytosis (Rosai-Dorfman-Destombes disease). AJNR Am J Neuroradiol 2004;25(3):498-500.
3. Carmody RF, Mafee MF, Goodwin JA, Small K, Haery C. Orbital and optic pathway sarcoidosis: MR findings. AJNR Am J Neuroradiol 1994;15(4):775-83.
4. Castillo M, Wallace DK, Mukherji SK. Persistent hyperplastic primary vitreous involving the anterior eye. AJNR Am J Neuroradiol 1997;18(8):1526-8.
5. Chan LL, Tan HE, Fook-Chong S, Teo TH, Lim LH, Seah LL. Graves ophthalmopathy: The bony orbit in optic neuropathy, its apical angular capacity, and impact on prediction of risk. AJNR Am J Neuroradiol 2009;30(3):597-602.
6. Finelli DA, Shurin SB, Bardenstein DS. Trilateral retinoblastoma: Two variations. AJNR Am J Neuroradiol 1995;16(1):166-70.
7. Fischer M, Kempkes U, Haage P, Isenmann S. Recurrent orbital myositis mimicking sixth nerve palsy: Diagnosis with MR imaging. AJNR Am J Neuroradiol 2010;31(2):275-6.
8. Flanders AE, Mafee MF, Rao VM, Choi KH. CT characteristics of orbital pseudotumors and other orbital inflammatory processes. J Comput Assist Tomogr 1989;13(1):40-7.
9. Galluzzi P, Hadjistilianou T, Cerase A, De Francesco S, Toti P, Venturi C. Is CT still useful in the study protocol of retinoblastoma? AJNR Am J Neuroradiol 2009;30(9):1760-5.
10. Hesselink JR, Weber AL. Pathways of orbital extension of extraorbital neoplasms. J Comput Assist Tomogr 1982;6(3):593-7.
11. Hoffmann KT, Hosten N, Lemke AJ, Sander B, Zwicker C, Felix R. Septum Orbitale: High-Resolution MR in Orbital Anatomy. AJNR Am J Neuroradiol 1998;19:91-4.
12. Hrach CJ, Quint DJ. Globe Tenting as a Result of Head Trauma. AJNR 1997;18:980–2.
13. Jackson A, Patankar T, Laitt RD. Intracanalicular optic nerve meningioma: A serious diagnostic pitfall. AJNR Am J Neuroradiol 2003;24(6):1167-70.
14. Jacobs DA, Galetta SL. Neuro-ophthalmology for neuroradiologists. AJNR Am J Neuroradiol 2007;28(1):3-8.
15. Jacquemin C, Bosley TM, Svedberg H. Orbit deformities in craniofacial neurofibromatosis type 1. AJNR Am J Neuroradiol. 2003;24(8):1678-82.
16. Johns TT, Citrin CM, Black J, Sherman JL. CT evaluation of perineural orbital lesions: Evaluation of the "tram-track" sign. AJNR Am J Neuroradiol 1984;5(5):587-90.
17. Judd CD, Chapman PR, Koch B, Shea CJ. Intracranial infantile hemangiomas associated with PHACE syndrome. AJNR Am J Neuroradiol 2007;28(1):25-9.
18. Kapur R, Sepahdari AR, Mafee MF, Putterman AM, Aakalu V, Wendel LJ, Setabutr P. MR imaging of orbital inflammatory syndrome, orbital cellulitis, and orbital lymphoid lesions: The role of diffusion-weighted imaging. AJNR Am J Neuroradiol 2009;30(1):64-70.

19. Lee JH, Lee MS, Lee BH, Choe DH, Do YS, Kim KH, Chin SY, Shim YS, Cho KJ. Rhabdomyosarcoma of the head and neck in adults: MR and CT findings. AJNR Am J Neuroradiol 1996;17(10):1923-8.
20. Mafee MF, Dorodi S, Pai E. Sarcoidosis of the eye, orbit, and central nervous system. Role of MR imaging. Radiol Clin North Am. 1999;37(1):73-87.
21. Ng E, Ilsen PF. Orbital metastases. Optometry 2010;81(12):647-57.
22. Ortiz O, Schochet SS, Kotzan JM, Kostick D. Radiologic-pathologic correlation: meningioma of the optic nerve sheath. AJNR Am J Neuroradiol 1996;17(5):901-6.
23. Pelton RW, Rainey AM, Lee AG. Traumatic subluxation of the globe into the maxillary sinus. AJNR Am J Neuroradiol 1998;19(8):1450-1.
24. Prayer D, Grois N, Prosch H, Gadner H, Barkovich AJ. MR imaging presentation of intracranial disease associated with Langerhans cell histiocytosis. AJNR Am J Neuroradiol 2004;25(5):880-91.
25. Provenzale JM, Allen NB. Wegener granulomatosis: CT and MR findings. AJNR Am J Neuroradiol 1996;17(4):785-92.
26. Provenzale JM, Weber AL, Klintworth GK, McLendon RE. Radiologic-pathologic correlation. Bilateral retinoblastoma with coexistent pinealoblastoma (trilateral retinoblastoma). AJNR Am J Neuroradiol 1995;16(1):157-65.
27. Rahangdale SR, Castillo M, Shockley W. MR in squamous cell carcinoma of the lacrimal sac. AJNR Am J Neuroradiol 1995;16(6):1262-4.
28. Razek AA, Castillo M. Imaging lesions of the cavernous sinus. AJNR Am J Neuroradiol 2009;30(3):444-52. Epub 2008 Dec 18.
29. RD Tien, PK Chu, Hesselink JR, Szumowski J. Intra- and paraorbital lesions: value of fat-suppression MR imaging with paramagnetic contrast enhancement. AJNR Am J Neuroradiol 1991;12(2):245-53.
30. Rodjan F, de Graaf P, Moll AC, Imhof SM, Verbeke JI, Sanchez E, Castelijns JA. Brain abnormalities on MR imaging in patients with retinoblastoma. AJNR Am J Neuroradiol 2010;31(8):1385-9. Epub 2010 Apr 22.
31. Saket RR, Mafee MF. Anterior-segment retinoblastoma mimicking pseudo-inflammatory angle-closure glaucoma: Review of the literature and the important role of imaging. AJNR Am J Neuroradiol 2009;30(8):1607-9.
32. Salvage DR, Spencer JA, Batchelor AG, MacLennan KA. Sarcoid involvement of the supraorbital nerve: MR and histologic findings. AJNR Am J Neuroradiol 1997;18(9):1785-7.
33. Simon EM, Zoarski GH, Rothman MI, Numaguchi Y, Zagardo MT, Mathis JM. Systemic sarcoidosis with bilateral orbital involvement: MR findings. AJNR Am J Neuroradiol 1998;19(2):336-7.
34. Sklar EM, Schatz NJ, Glaser JS, Post MJ, ten Hove M. MR of vasculitis-induced optic neuropathy. AJNR Am J Neuroradiol 1996;17(1):121-8.
35. Som P, Curtin H. Head and Neck Imaging. 5th edition. Elsevier/ Mosby 2011; 2(8-11):527-924.

36. Wasmeier C, Pfadenhauer K, Rösler A. Idiopathic inflammatory pseudotumor of the orbit and Tolosa-Hunt syndrome—are they the same disease? J Neurol 2002;249(9):1237-41.
37. William K Erly, Raymond F Carmody, Robert M Dryden. Orbital Histiocytosis X. AJNR 1995;16:1258-61.
38. Wycliffe ND, Mafee MF. Magnetic resonance imaging in ocular pathology. Top Magn Reson Imaging 1999;10(6):384-400.
39. Yousem DM, Atlas SW, Grossman RI, Sergott RC, Savino PJ, Bosley TM. MR imaging of Tolosa-Hunt syndrome. AJR Am J Roentgenol 1990;154(1):167-70.

# Imaging of the paranasal sinuses

chapter 4

David Ashton, Dzung Vu, Lalitha Shankar, Eugene Yu

### Abstract
Review of the anatomy of the paranasal sinuses, concepts behind functional endoscopic sinus surgery and important anatomic variants are discussed. Inflammatory and infectious sinus disease; sinonasal tumor imaging and staging are also covered.

### Keywords
Paranasal sinuses, nasal cavity, imaging, anatomy, Functional Endoscopic Sinus Surgery.

## Normal anatomy

### Lateral wall of the nasal cavity

All of the paranasal sinuses open into the lateral nasal wall. **Figure 4.1** shows a medial view of the right lateral wall of the nasal cavity. It shows the components of the ostiomeatal complex of which the ethmoid air cells are the cornerstone. The lateral mass (labyrinth) of the ethmoid articulates with the frontal, maxilla, lacrimal, palatine ('Pal' in **Figure 4.1**) and sphenoid bones.

The horizontal/axial section of the ethmoid shows that the lateral aspect of the ethmoid labyrinth — the lamina papyracea (LamPap in **Figure 4.1**), contributes to the medial wall of the orbit. The medial aspect of the labyrinth extends from the maxilla (anteriorly) to the palatine bone (posteriorly). It covers most of the maxillary hiatus and articulates inferiorly with the inferior turbinate bone. It carries the middle turbinate and the smaller superior turbinate, and occasionally a bony ridge called the supreme turbinate (of Zuckerkandl).

The turbinate's bones extend medially from the lateral nasal wall like awnings with "rolled-in" inferior borders. The spaces between the superior, middle and inferior turbinates and the lateral wall are called the superior, middle and inferior meatus respectively. In **Figure 4.1**,

Imaging of the paranasal sinuses 143

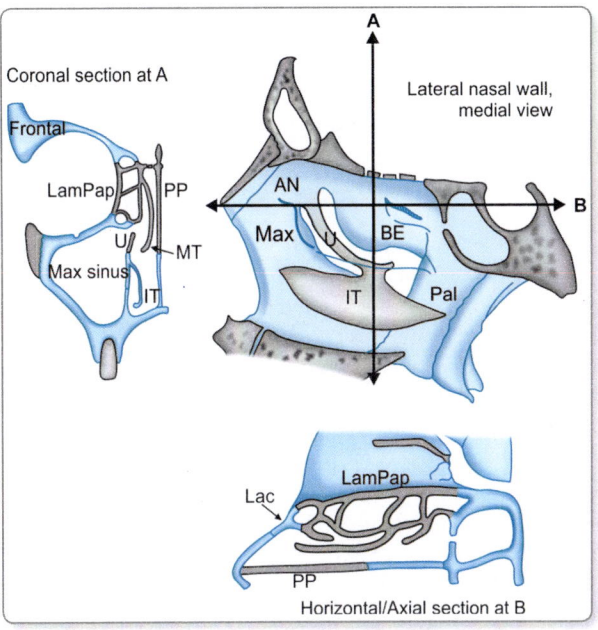

**Figure 4.1** Diagram of lateral nasal wall

the middle turbinate has been removed to show the two main bony features, the uncinate process and the bulla ethmoidalis.

## The uncinate process (Figure 4.1 'U')

The uncinate process is a thin hook-shaped plate, about 1.5 to 2 cm in length that runs inferoposteriorly from the roof of the ethmoid. In the coronal plane, it also runs in a superomedial direction. Anteriorly it is attached to the ethmoid crest of the maxilla where it is fused with the wall of the agger nasi cell (agger nasi cells are the most anterior ethmoidal air cells **Figure 4.1** 'AN'). Its posterosuperior free margin is parallel to the anterior surface of the bulla ethmoidalis. The two dimensional space between the free margin of the uncinate and the ethmoid bulla is the hiatus semilunaris. The infundibulum is the air passage that connects the maxillary sinus ostium through the hiatus semilunaris with the middle meatus. The posteroinferior margin of the uncinate articulates with the ethmoidal process of the inferior turbinate.

### The bulla ethmoidalis (Figure 4.1 'BE')

The bulla ethmoidalis is largest of the anterior ethmoid air cells which forms the posterior margin of the ethmoid infundibulum.

### The turbinates (Figure 4.1 middle MT and inferior IT turbinates)

The middle turbinate is suspended from the roof of the ethmoid by a vertical plate of bone. This is an important landmark during endoscopic sinus surgery as the cribriform plate, olfactory nerves and the ethmoid arteries are in close proximity. Removal of the vertical plate too close to the roof can result in CSF rhinorrhea or vascular injury. Inferior and lateral to the free portion of the middle turbinate lies the middle meatus. Posteriorly it attaches to a crest on the palatine bone. The middle turbinate has a complex configuration with three parts oriented in 3 planes. The anterior portion lies in a sagittal plane and inserts on the cribriform plate. The middle segment runs a horizontal plane through the labyrinth to insert onto the lamina papyracea; this middle portion is called the basal lamina and it acts to fix the middle third of the middle turbinate to the lamina papyracea and also divides the ethmoid air cells into anterior and a posterior group.

The superior turbinate is located posterior and superior to the middle turbinate. It is smaller and simpler in shape. Its posterior margin marks the posterior aspect of the ethmoid air cells.

It supreme turbinate (of Zuckerkandl) is present, it may appear as a simple bony ridge above and posterior to the superior turbinate.

The inferior turbinate is a separate bone and has no sinus opening. The nasolacrimal duct opens into the inferior meatus which is inferior to the corresponding turbinate.

### Drainage pathways of the paranasal sinuses

The term ostiomeatal complex or unit (OMU) consists of the maxillary sinus ostium, the ethmoid infundibulum, anterior ethmoid air cells and the frontal recess. This corresponds to the drainage path of the anterior sinuses.

## Ethmoid air cells

The basal lamina of the middle turbinate divides the ethmoid air cells into anterior and posterior groups. The anterior ethmoid air cells drain into the middle meatus while the posterior ethmoid air cells drain into the superior meatus.

Agger nasi air cells are the most anterior ethmoid air cells and are extramural in location (these are not confined by the ethmoid bone). On imaging, these cells are seen anterior to the anterior attachment of the middle turbinate.

Onodi air cells are posterior ethmoid air cells that extend lateral and superior to the sphenoid sinus and may abut the optic nerve canal.

## Maxillary sinus

The maxillary sinus presents a large triangular maxillary hiatus on the medial surface of the maxilla. This large opening is covered by contributions from the ethmoid bone, perpendicular portion of the palatine bone, the inferior turbinate and the lacrimal bone. The functional drainage of the maxillary sinus is through the maxillary ostium that opens into the infundibulum which in turn opens into the middle meatus.

## Frontal sinus

Uncinate attaching to ethmoid roof (short arrow), to lamina papyracea (long arrow) and **Figure 4.2B** to middle turbinate (dashed long arrows).

The frontal sinus lies between the anterior and posterior tables of the squamous part of the frontal bone and varies widely in its shape and extent. The frontal sinus drains through an hour-glass shaped frontal recess. The frontal recess courses inferiorly as a narrow passage bounded by the lamina papyracea laterally, the middle turbinate medially, and the agger nasi anteriorly. Its posterior limit is demarcated by the anterior ethmoid artery. The site of drainage of the frontal recess

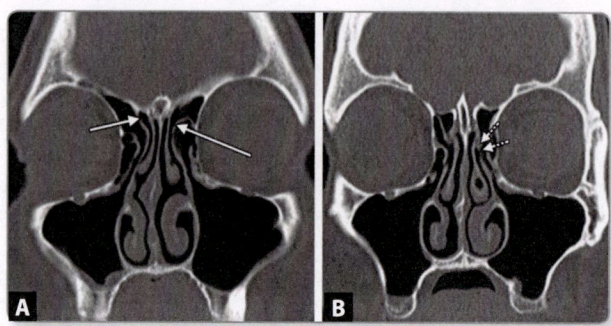

**Figures 4.2A and B** The variable superior attachment of the anterior aspect of the uncinate process. Uncinate attaching to ethmoid roof (short arrow), to lamina papyracea (long arrow) and to middle turbinate (dashed arrows)

will vary depending upon the uncinate. While the posterior margin of the uncinate is a "free margin", the site of attachment of the anterior portion of the uncinate can be variable. The anterior portion can attach to the skull base, lamina papyracea or the middle turbinate. As a result the frontal recess will drain inferiorly into the infundibulum when the uncinate process is attached to the ethmoid roof/skull base, or the middle meatus. When the uncinate process is attached to the lamina papyracea, the frontal recess will drain into the middle meatus and there will be a separation of the frontal recess and infundibulum (**Figures 4.2A and B**).

## Sphenoid sinus

The sphenoid sinus is generally paired but often symmetrical as its septum is rarely in the midline. The sinus drains via an ostium into the sphenoethmoidal recess, which lies between the nasal septum and the superior or supreme turbinate. Its ostia varies in its size and shape, and are the most posterior orifices and closest to the nasal septum.

# Paranasal sinus imaging anatomy

Paranasal sinus imaging anatomy as shown in **Figures 4.3 to 4.32**.

Imaging of the paranasal sinuses 147

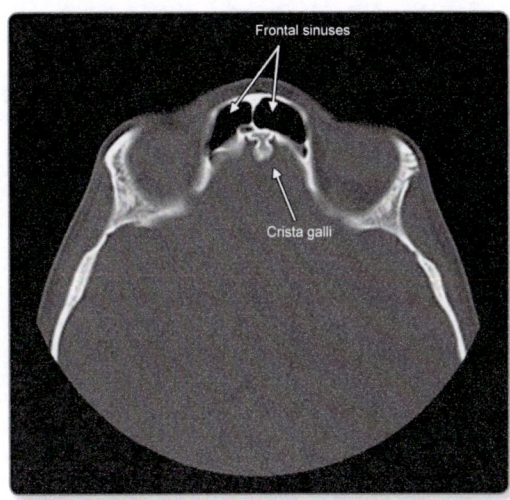

**Figure 4.3** Axial CT: Crista galli and frontal sinuses

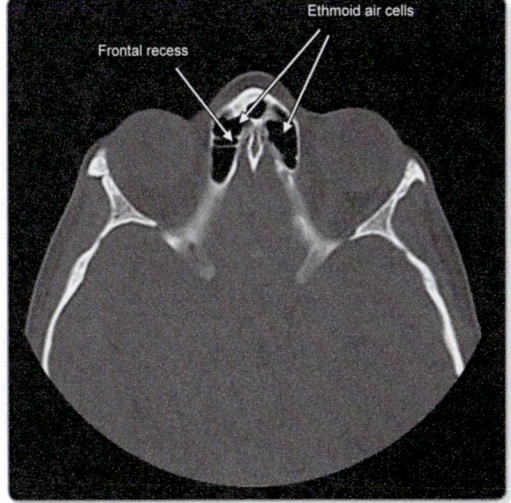

**Figure 4.4** Axial CT of frontal recess and ethmoid air cells

### 148 Introductory head and neck imaging

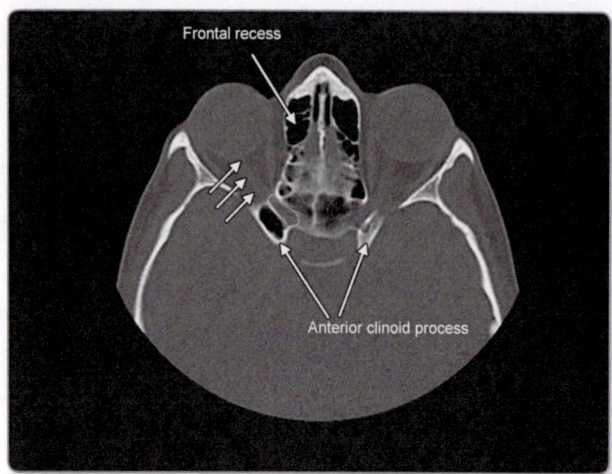

**Figure 4.5** Three short arrows: Optic nerve; shaded region; optic nerve canal

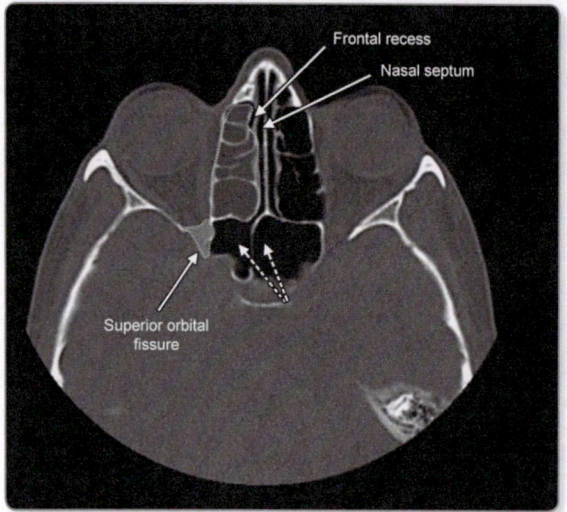

**Figure 4.6** Large shaded region: Ethmoid air cells (left); dashed arrows: Initial examination at this point suggest these are the sphenoid sinuses

Imaging of the paranasal sinuses  149

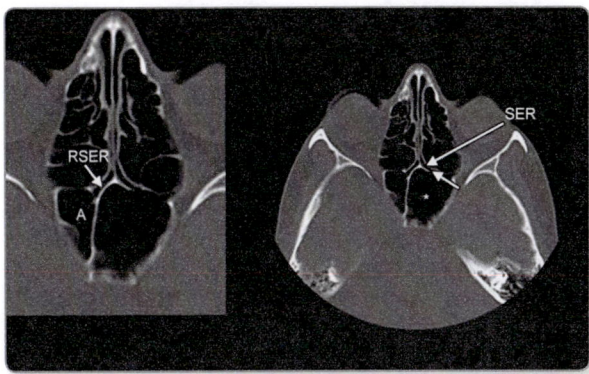

**Figure 4.7** Upon closer examination, the larger left sided air cell (*) communications with the sphenoethmoid recess (SER) on the left via the sphenoid ostium (short arrow). The magnified view shows that the air cell (A) does not communicate with the right sphenoethmoid recess (RSER) as there is a curvilinear septum separating the RSER from the air cell. At this point, it is still not possible to conclude that (A) is the right sphenoid sinus

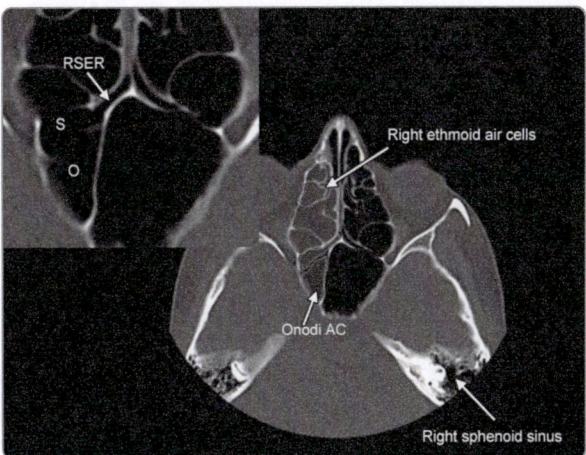

**Figure 4.8** Magnified view now shows communications between right sphenoethmoid recess (RSER) with the aire cell (S) which is the right sphenoid sinus. The larger air cell (O) located behind it is an Onodi air cell. Shaded green: Communication between RSER and right sphenoid sinus; Shaded blue: Right Onodi air cell (*for color version see Plate 8*)

## 150 Introductory head and neck imaging

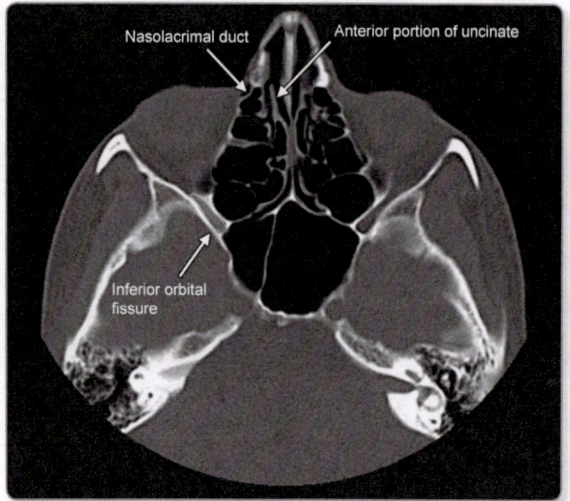

**Figure 4.9** Axial CT of nasolacrimal duct and inferior orbital fissure

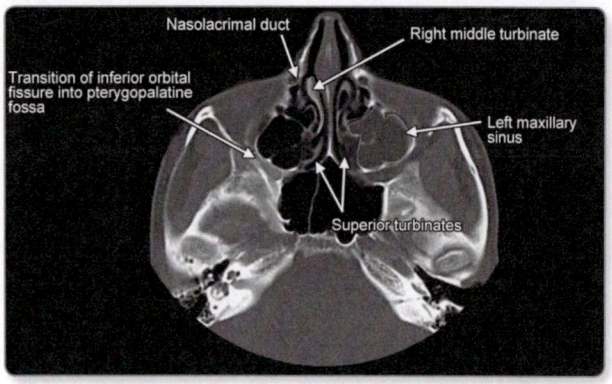

**Figure 4.10** Axial CT of nasolacrimal duct and inferior orbital fissure transition to pterygopalatine fossa

Imaging of the paranasal sinuses 151

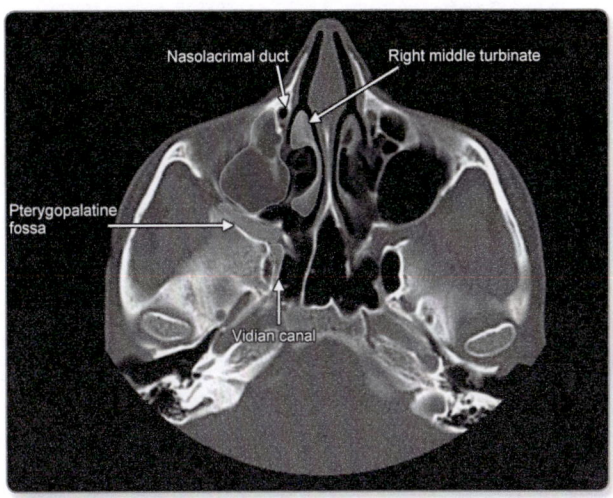

**Figure 4.11** Axial CT of pterygopalatine fossa

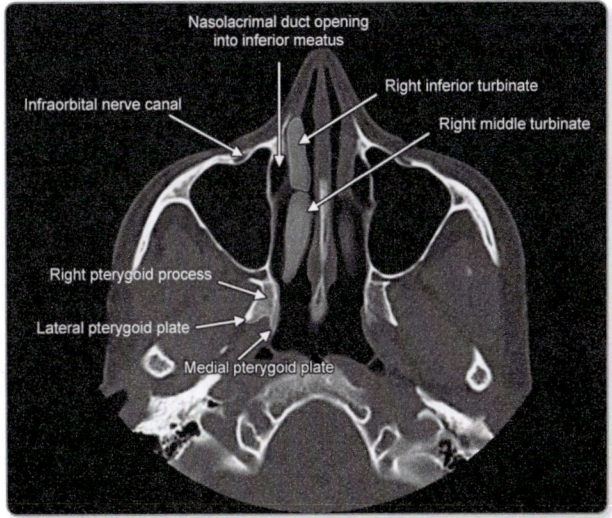

**Figure 4.12** Axial CT of pterygoid plates and inferior orbital canal

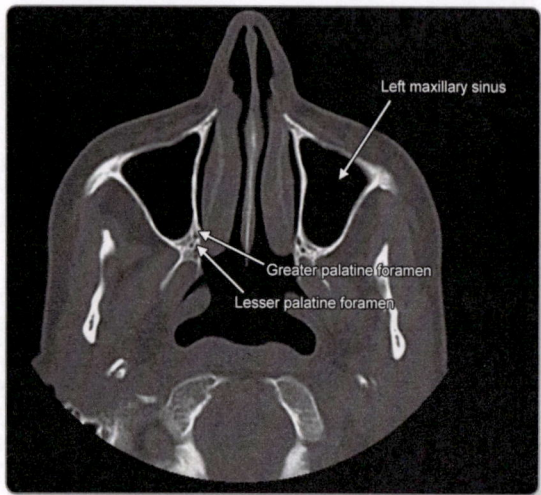

**Figure 4.13** Axial CT of pterygoid plates

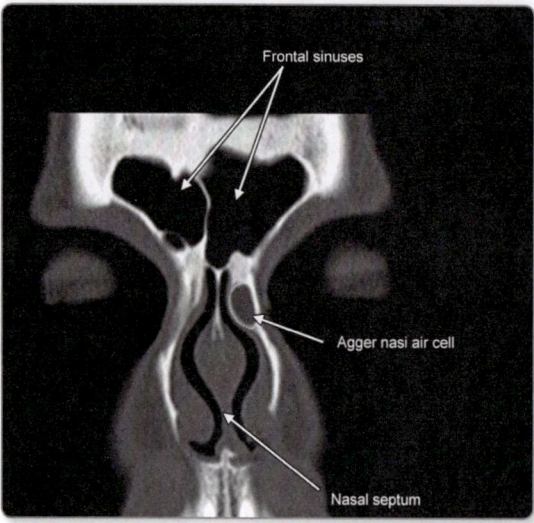

**Figure 4.14** Coronal CT through the anterior aspect of frontal sinuses and Agger nasi air cells

# Imaging of the paranasal sinuses 153

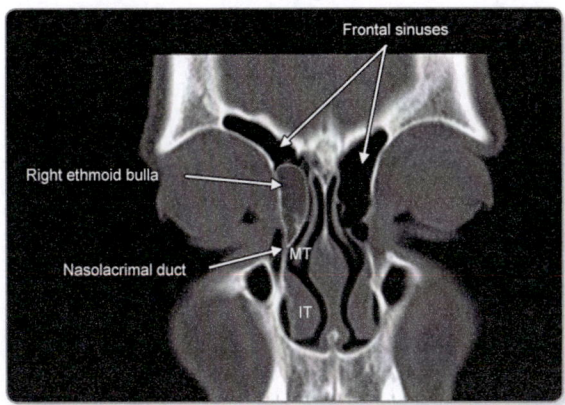

**Figure 4.15** MT: middle turbinate; IT: inferior turbinate; Red shaded: frontal recess (*for color version see Plate 9*)

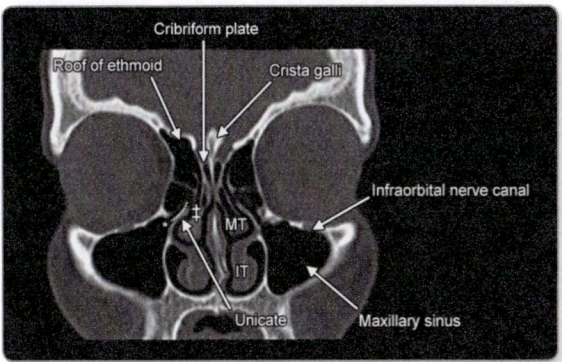

**Figure 4.16** ‡: Middle meatus; *: Maxillary sinus ostium; Dashed line: Infundibulum; MT: Middle turbinate with concha bullosa; IT: Inferior turbinate

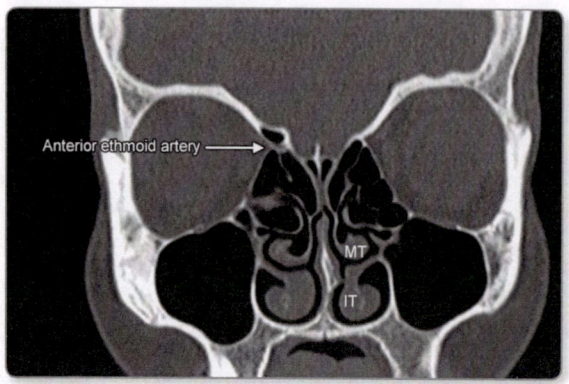

**Figure 4.17** Coronal CT through the course of the anterior ethmoid artery

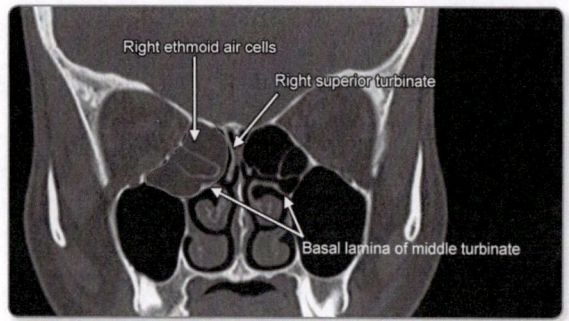

**Figure 4.18** Coronal CT of the ethmoid air cells and basal lamina

Imaging of the paranasal sinuses 155

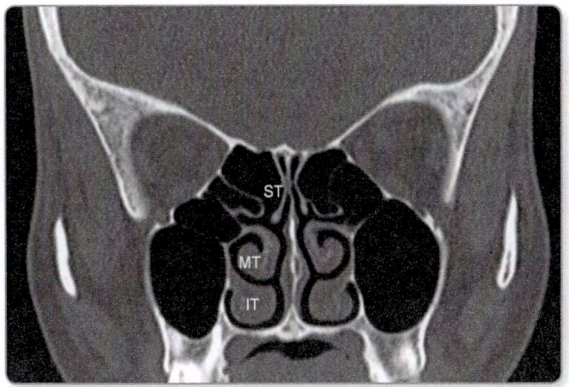

**Figure 4.19** ST: Superior turbinate; MT: Middle turbinate; IT: Inferior turbinate

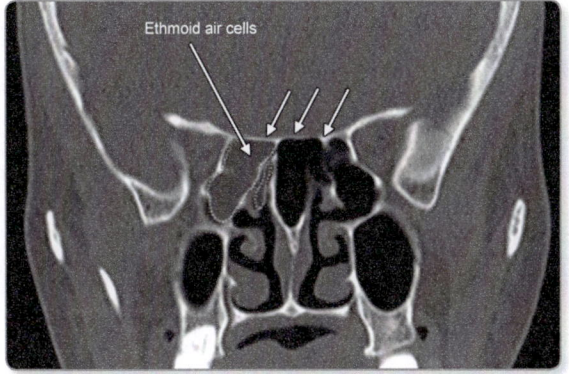

**Figure 4.20** Green shaded: Sphenoethmoid recess; Three short arrows: Planum sphenoidale (*for color version see Plate 9*)

**156 Introductory head and neck imaging**

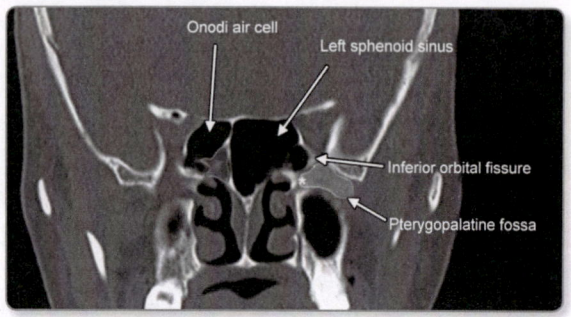

**Figure 4.21** Green shaded: Sphenoethmoid recess (*for color version see Plate 10*)

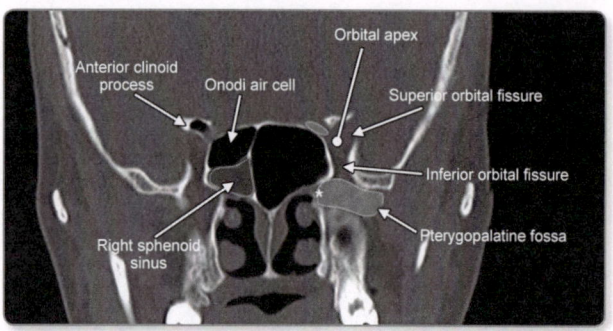

**Figure 4.22** Sphenopalatine foramen*, Oval shaded: Optic nerve canal

Imaging of the paranasal sinuses 157

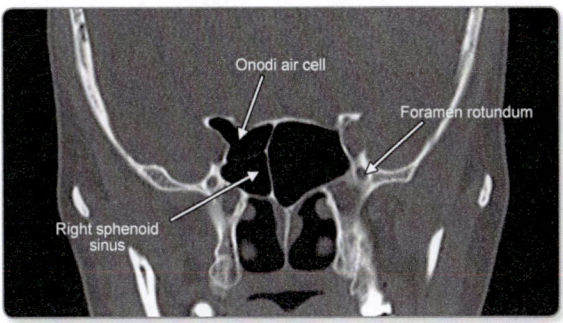

**Figure 4.23** Note right Onodi air cell is pneumatized into the right anterior clinoid process

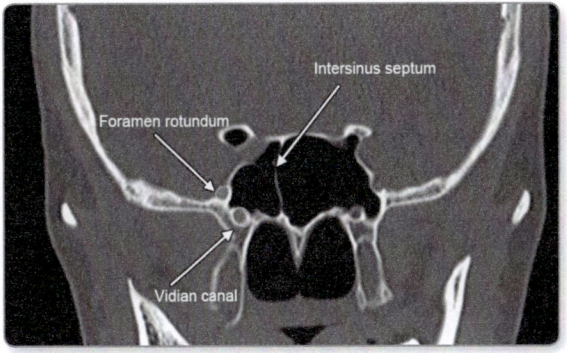

**Figure 4.24** Coronal CT of sphenoid sinus

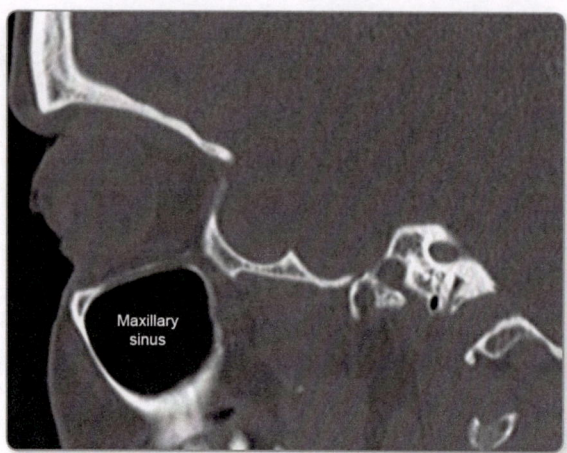

**Figure 4.25** Sagittal scan of maxillary sinus

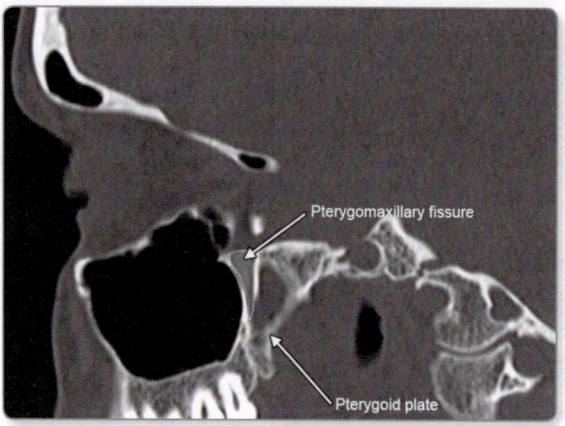

**Figure 4.26** Sagittal scan of the pterygomaxillary fissure

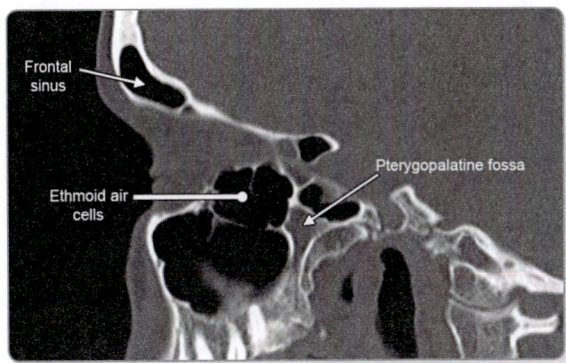

**Figure 4.27** Sagittal scan of the pterygopalatine fossa

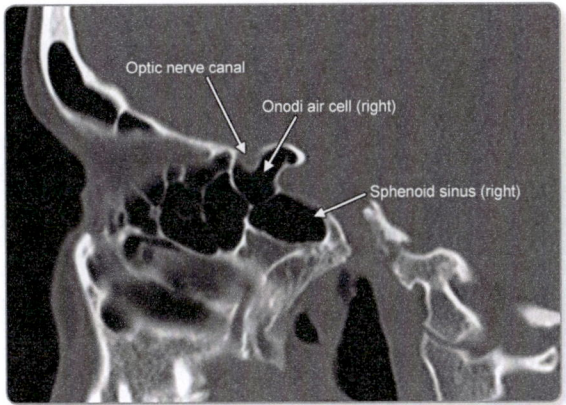

**Figure 4.28** Sagittal scan showing Onodi cell and its relation to the sphenoid sinus and optic nerve

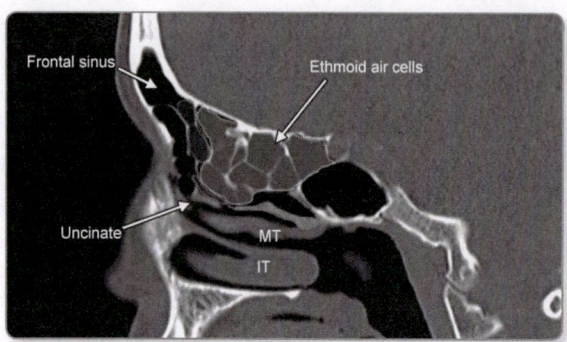

**Figure 4.29** Red shaded: Frontal recess; Blue shaded: Basal lamina of middle turbinate (*for color version see Plate 10*)

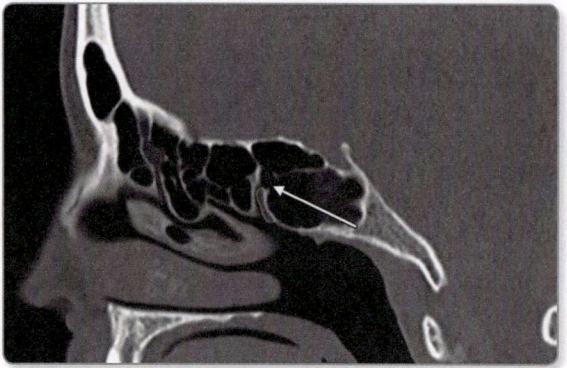

**Figure 4.30** Red shaded: Frontal recess; Green shaded: Sphenoethmoid recess; Arrow: Sphenoid ostium (*for color version see Plate 10*)

Imaging of the paranasal sinuses  161

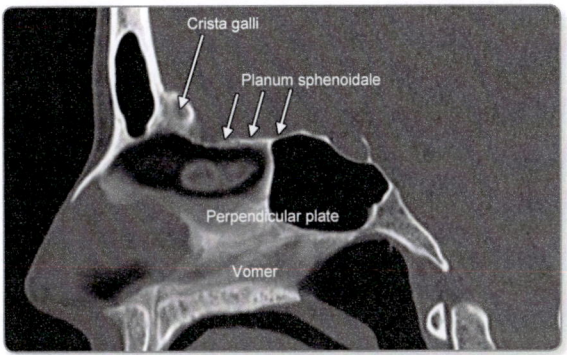

**Fig. 4.31** Sagittal scan of crista galli and planum sphenoidale

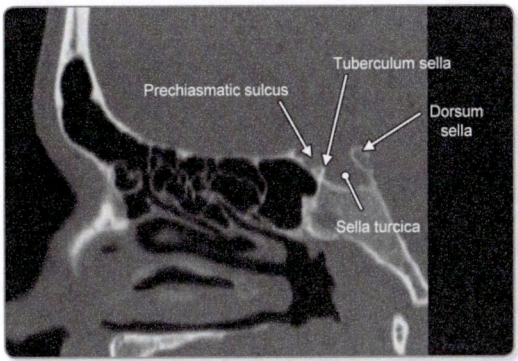

**Figure 4.32** Sagittal scan of sphenoid sinus and the nearby structures

## Functional endoscopic sinus surgery and anatomic variants

The three anatomic tight spots of the sinonasal cavities are the frontal recess (draining the frontal sinus), the ostiomeatal unit (draining the frontal recess, maxillary sinus and anterior ethmoid air cells), and the sphenoethmoid recess (draining the sphenoid sinus and posterior ethmoid air cells). The goal of functional endoscopic sinus surgery (FESS) is to re-establish normal ventilation and sinus drainage by removing obstructing bone and diseased mucosa. Prior surgical techniques, such as the inferior meatal antrostomy, attempted to create alternate pathways of drainage, which were not concordant with normal mucocililary function. These procedures were often less effective.

In FESS the nasal cavity and sinuses are accessed through the nostrils with a set of rigid fiberoptic endoscopes. The tip of the endoscopes will vary in angulation and various cutting and drilling instruments can be inserted along with the endoscope. CT data can be co-registered with the patient on the operating table to help triangulate the location of the various anatomic structures.

Ninety percent of patients have one or more anatomic variants. Some of these variants may be significant as they may limit surgical access and visualization, contribute to ostial obstruction or increase the risk of complications (hazardous variants). Anatomic variants that encroach on the OMU are noted to be just as common in the asymptomatic population as they are in patients with chronic rhinosinusitis (CRS). Thus, these variants are not considered a cause of CRS, which is a generalized mucosal disease. But in the presence of mucosal disease refractory to medical treatment, these variants may need to be addressed during FESS.

The actual FESS procedure will vary depending upon the location/pattern of mucosal disease. A complicated FESS procedure may involve uncinectomy, a wide meatal antrostomy involving the maxillary ostium, middle turbinectomy and total ethmoidectomy (**Figure 4.33**). A minimal procedure may include a complete uncinectomy, a small meatal antrostomy, and limited anterior ethmoidectomy including opening of the bulla or removal of a few ethmoid septations.

## Anatomic variants

The nasal septum may be deviated from the midline. This can be developmental or arise secondary to trauma. A septal spur can be an accompanying finding (**Figure 4.34**). A spur may contact and push the middle turbinate or lateral nasal wall and narrow the middle meatus. In such instances a septoplasty may need to be performed at the start of the FESS in order to facilitate access to the middle meatus. Pneumatizaiton of the septum may also narrow the OMU.

Imaging of the paranasal sinuses 163

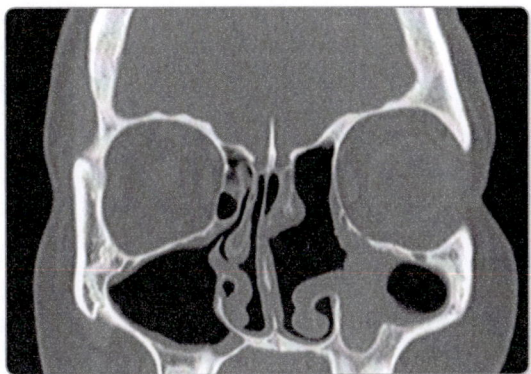

**Figure 4.33** Unilateral OMU FESS. There has been a left uncinectomy, antrostomy, turbinate head reduction and ethmoidectomy

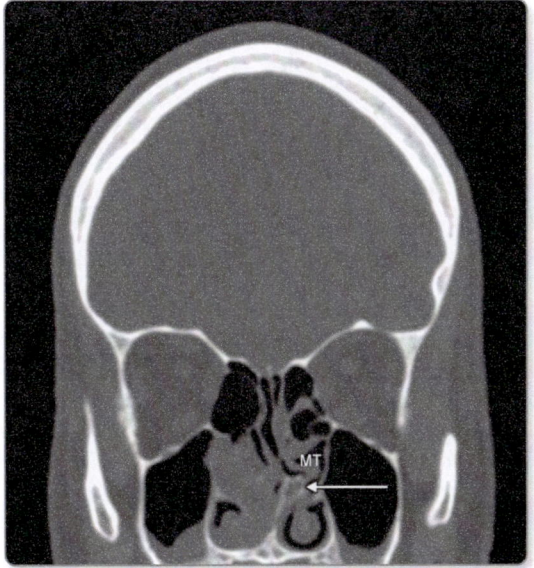

**Figure 4.34** Coronal CT demonstrates left septal deviation and a moderated sized septal spur (arrow) displacing the middle turbinate (MT) laterally and narrowing the middle meatus

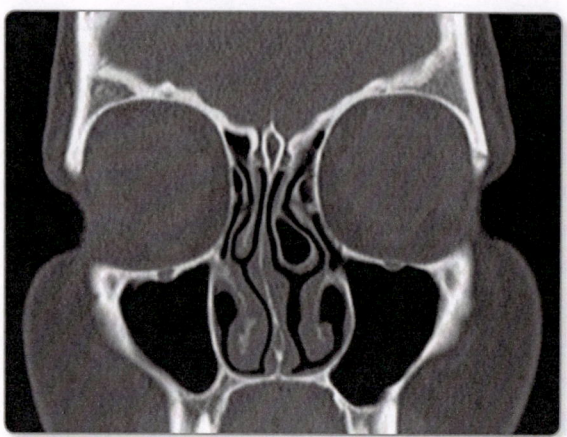

Figure 4.35 Concha bullosa of left middle turbinate

Pneumatization of the inferior bulbous portion of the middle turbinate is known as concha bullosa and is a common and usually asymptomatic variant (**Figure 4.35**). Bony or soft tissue hypertrophy can also occur within this strucure. If the resulting enlarged turbinate displaces the uncinate process, the infundibulum may be narrowed. Treatment may involve resection of the lateral lamellae and a turbinate head reduction. The residual turbinate may be sutured to the septum to prevent scarring and blockage of the lateral nasal wall.

A paradoxical middle turbinate refers to reversal of the normal medial convexity of the middle turbinate (**Figure 4.36**). This is found in 25 percent of the population and if large, may impair access to the middle meatus. Lateral deviation or pneumatization (**Figure 4.37**) of the uncinate process may cause obstruction of the ethmoid infundibulum and impair drainage of the maxillary sinus.

Ethmoid sinus variants related to the middle meatus include Haller cells. Haller cells are extensions of the anterior ethmoid cells beneath the orbital floor (**Figures 4.38 and 4.39**). If large, these may narrow the maxillary sinus ostium.

Imaging of the paranasal sinuses 165

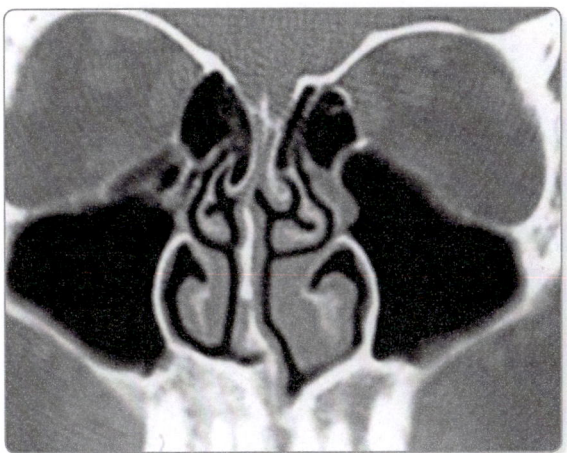

**Figure 4.36** Paradoxical middle turbinates

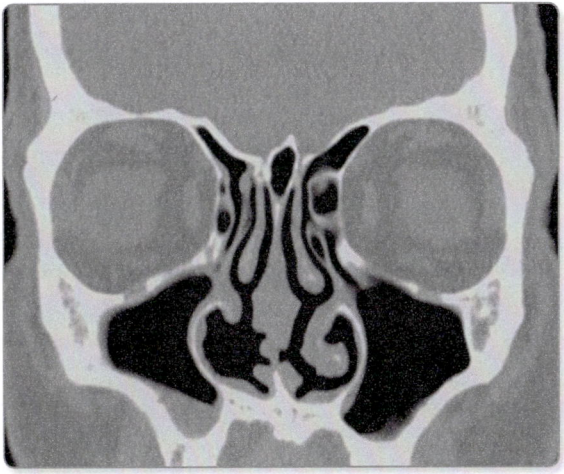

**Figure 4.37** Pneumatized left uncinate process. This can potentially narrow the hiatus semilunaris

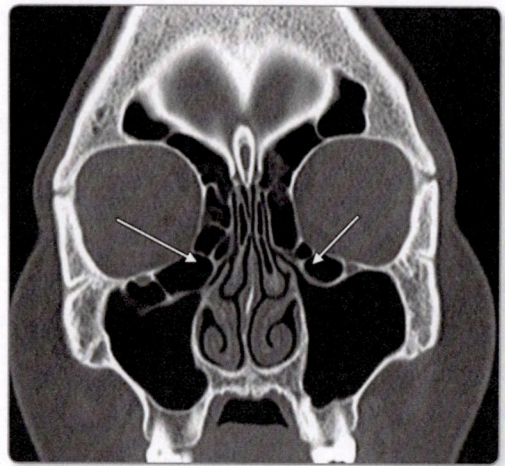

**Figure 4.38** Bilateral Haller air cells (arrows)

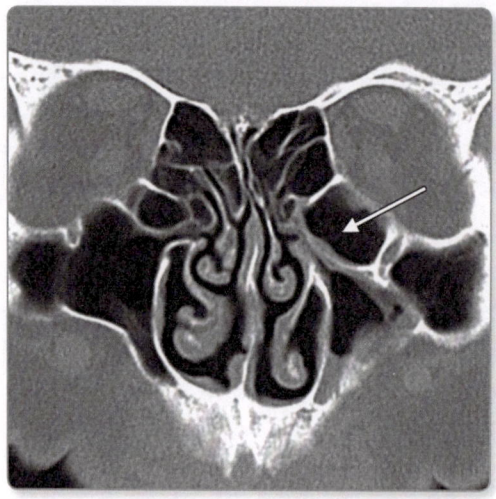

**Figure 4.39** The entire roof of the left maxillary sinus aerated by Haller cells

## Hazardous variants

Hazardous variants of the OMU involve the cribriform plate and lamina papyracea. The cribriform plate and fovea ethmoidalis of the frontal bone form the roof of the ethmoid bone (**Figure 4.40**). The lateral lamellae of the cribriform is thinner and less resistant to trauma than the adjacent bone. A longer lateral wall with a deeper olfactory fossa predisposes to perforation. This can lead to CSF leak, the risk of meningitis or meningocele formation. The Keros classification stratifies the depth of the olfactory fossa into three: Keros 1 (1–3 mm), Keros 2 (4-7 mm) and Keros 3 (8-16 mm). The greater the angle of the lateral lamellae as well as a greater degree of asymmetry in height of the olfactory fossa between the two sides will increase the risk of intracranial penetration.

Dehiscence or medial deviation of the lamina papyracea may be congenital or result from trauma. Lack of a firm bony margin will result in a greater risk of orbital penetration during FESS. Forceps or biting

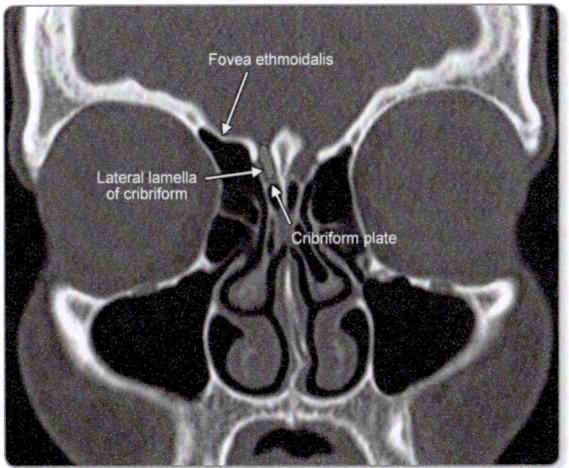

**Figure 4.40** The relationship of the fovea ethmoidalis and cribriform plate which together form the roof of the ethmoid air cells. Shaded area shows the olfactory fossa

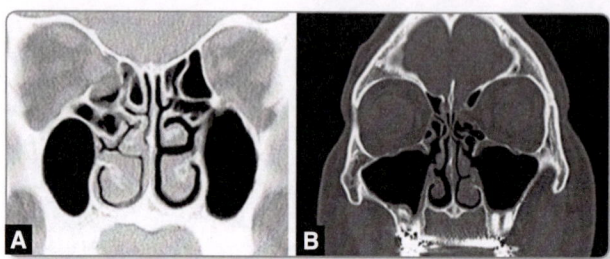

**Figures 4.41A and B** Dehiscence of the right (A) left (B) lamina papyracea with orbital fat protrusion

instruments may enter the orbit resulting in medial rectus laceration or orbital hematoma. Similarly, any medial deviation of the lamina papyracea (**Figures 4.41A and B**) will decrease the available space in the ethmoid region with which to maneuver the various surgical instruments during FESS.

The anterior ethmoid artery arises from the ophthalmic artery and traverses the ethmoid roof before penetrating the lateral lamellae of the cribriform plate to enter the olfactory groove. As a variant, the artery may be submucosal in its ethmoid course or traverse the upper nasal cavity within a small channel (**Figure 4.42**) placing it at potential risk for injury. A transected artery may retract into the orbit and result in hematoma formation.

The Onodi air cells as previously mentioned are posterior ethmoid air cells that are superolateral to the sphenoid sinus and may come into contact with the optic nerve canal (**Figure 4.43**). Such close contact will place the optic nerve at increased risk of injury.

Similarly, pneumatization into the anterior clinoid process (**Figure 4.44**) will also place the optic nerves at increased risk as only a thin layer of bone is all that is there to protect the nerve from any probing or cutting instruments.

The internal carotid arteries will often form a prominent "bulge" into the sphenoid sinus. Normally there is a good degree of bony coverage of this bulge. Care must be taken to alert the surgeon of instances where there is thinning or dehiscence of this protective covering (**Figures 4.45A and B**).

Imaging of the paranasal sinuses 169

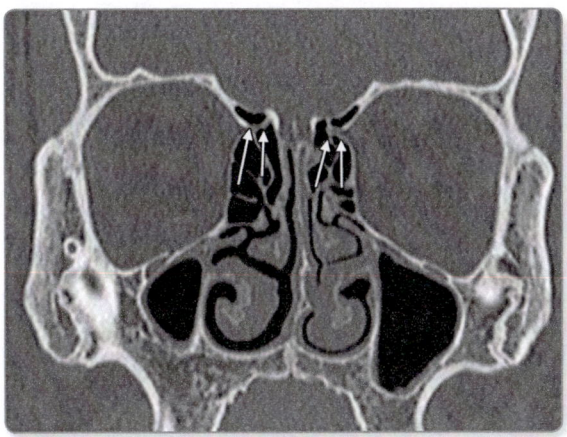

**Figure 4.42** Coronal CT shows the anterior ethmoid arteries (arrows) as they travel from the orbit into the anterior cranial fossa. "Exposure" of these arteries places them at potential risk for injury

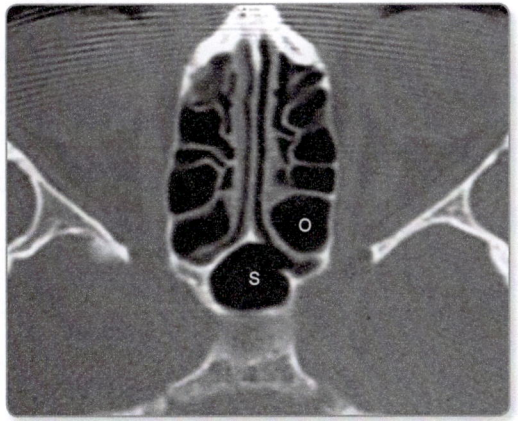

**Figure 4.43** Onodi air cell (O) is the largest posterior ethmoid air cell which can be closely related to the optic nerve. Sphenoid sinus (S)

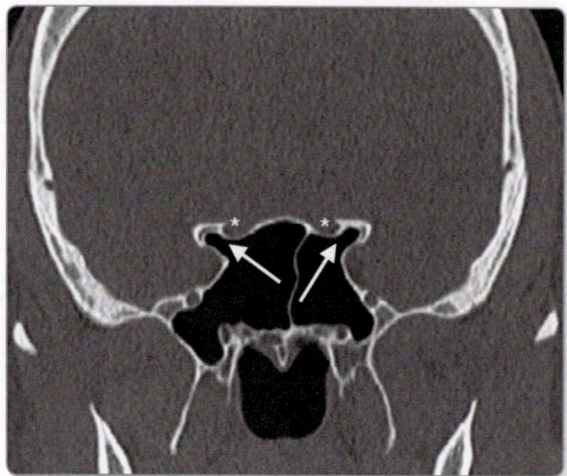

**Figure 4.44** Pneumatization of the anterior clinoid processes (arrows) also place the optic nerves (*) at greater risk

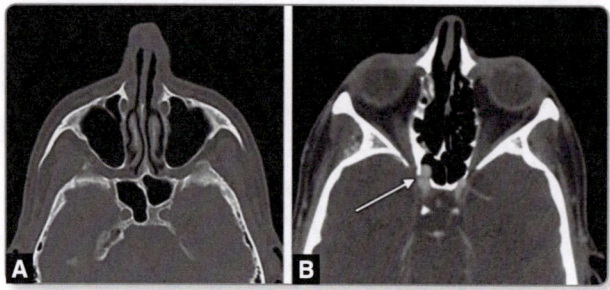

**Figures 4.45A and B** Internal carotid artery (ICA): Examples of the variability in the degree of bony coverage of the carotid as it travels along the sphenoid sinus. (A) Shows good bony separation of the artery and sinus. (B) ICA bony wall is dehiscent and the artery is bulging into the lumen

## Inflammatory diseases

### Acute rhinosinusitis

Acute rhinosinusitis (ARS) is defined as inflammation of the nose and paranasal sinuses lasting less than 12 weeks. Rhinitis and sinusitis usually coexist in most individuals and hence rhinosinusitis is the more appropriate terminology. Chronic rhinosinusits (CRS) persists for greater than 12 weeks despite medical management.

Acute rhinosinusitis (ARS) is most commonly a self-limited viral infection, lasting less than 10 days in duration and requiring only symptomatic treatment. Bacteria are the etiological agent in a minority of cases, usually as a complication of viral infection, dental sepsis or immunodeficiency. The most common bacterial organism is streptococcal pneumonia. Nosocomial bacterial rhinosinusitis with gram-negative organisms can be seen in the intensive care unit setting. It is difficult to distinguish bacterial and viral rhinosinusitis clinically. Worsening of symptoms after 5 days and illness duration longer than 10 days is suggestive of the former.

Acute rhinosinusitis (ARS) is characterized by the sudden onset of two or more of the following symptoms: nasal congestion, purulent discharge, facial pain and pressure, and anosmia. Anterior rhinoscopy, and or nasendoscopy will demonstrate mucosal edema and purulent secretions. The diagnosis is primarily clinical, based on the history and physical examination. Imaging is usually reserved in the event of a suspected complication. Imaging findings cannot distinguish between bacterial and viral etiologies.

Inflammation arising in ARS results in mucosal edema and increased sinonasal secretions. On CT, mucosal thickening manifests as circumferential soft tissue thickening. Secretions in the acute state are 95 percent water and hence show intermediate (10–25 HU) attenuation on CT. Ostial obstruction due to mucosal edema may result in a fluid level (**Figures 4.46A and B**). It may have a foamy aerosolized appearance. Mechanical trauma can also cause fluid levels, however the fluid is usually of increased density due to hemorrhage. Fluid levels can also be seen in the sphenoid sinus in nasally intubated patients due to a failure to clear secretions. MRI may show peripheral

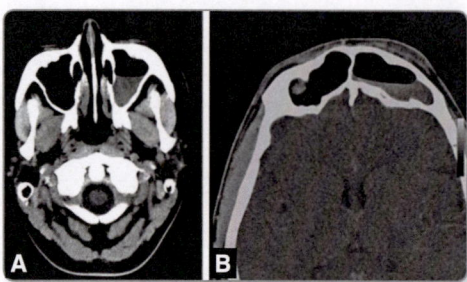

**Figures 4.46A and B** CT demonstrates fluid levels from sinusitis. (A) Left maxillary sinus in a patient with clinical findings of sinusitis. Note the edges of the fluid form a meniscus with the sinus wall. The fluid is of low density consistent with acute secretions. (B) Frontal sinusitis

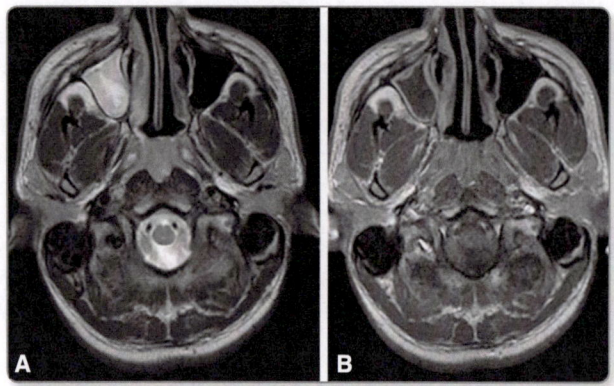

**Figures 4.47A and B** T2 and postcontrast T1 MRI of acute sinusitis. (A) Acute secretions are T2 hyperintense on MRI. The right maxillary sinus is opacified with T2 hyperintense secretions (B). Note linear mucosal enhancement at the periphery in the second image

enhancement along the sinus walls, corresponding to the inflamed mucosa (**Figures 4.47A and B**).

Imaging may be indicated in patients with clinical features such as periorbital edema, diplopia, ophthalmoplegia, decreased visual

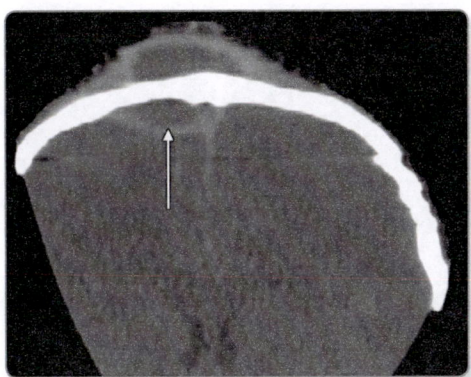

**Figure 4.48** Potts puffy tumor. Axial postcontrast CT demonstrates a frontal ring enhancing subperiosteal collection also known as a Potts Puffy tumor. There is also an epidural abscess present (Arrow)

acuity, severe frontal headache, frontal swelling, signs of meningitis, or focal neurologcial signs. These features suggest the presence of a complication arising from ARS. Complications can be classified as local, orbital and intracranial. Local complications include osteomyelitis, which most commonly involves the frontal bone. The sinus mucosa and bone marrow share venous drainage through the valveless diploic veins. Infection can spread into the diploic space and secondarily into the cortex of the inner and outer table of the skull. Perforation of the outer frontal table can result in a subperiosteal abscess known as a Pott's puffy tumor. CT will demonstrate bone destruction at the anterior table with a soft tissue ring enhancing collection (**Figure 4.48**).

## Orbital complications

Orbital complications include preseptal cellulitis, orbital cellulitis, subperiosteal abscess and cavernous sinus thrombosis. CT can distinguish between edema and abscess while MRI is better at assessing vascular complications. Ethmoid sinusitis with extension of infection through a normal, congential or traumtic dehiscence of the lamina papyracea is the most common source of orbital complications.

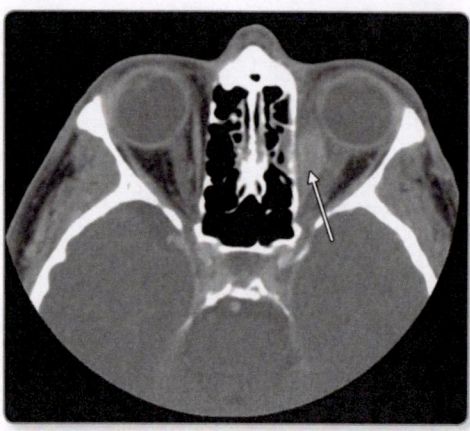

Figure 4.49 Axial postcontrast CT of a patient with orbital cellulitis. There is enlargement and increased enhancement of the medial rectus due to myositis (arrow). There is also increased density of the adjacent fat

Preseptal cellulitis involves the skin and subcutaneous tissue of the eyelid anterior to the orbital septum, and without involvement of the orbital cavity. CT demonstrates a diffuse increase in density of the lid and septum. Orbital cellulitis is a postseptal infection within the orbit with diffuse edema without abscess formation. CT with contrast shows increased density and enhancement of the intraorbital fat and occasionally involvement of the rectus muscles (**Figure 4.49**).

A subperiosteal abscess appears as an enhancing fluid collection most commonly in the medial orbit between a breached lamina papyracea and the periosteum (**Figure 4.50**). The globe may be displaced anteriorly with proptosis, compression and stretching of the optic nerve. CT will demonstrate enhancing collections, and osteomyelitis of the orbital walls as well as associated orbital cellulitis. Delay in treatment is associated with coalescence of orbital cellulitis into an orbital abscess with the enhancing collection within the intraconal space or extraocular muscles (**Figures 4.51A and B**).

Imaging of the paranasal sinuses  **175**

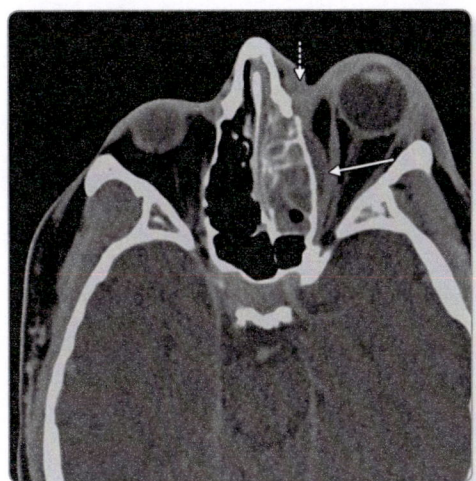

**Figure 4.50** There is a medial subperiosteal abscess (arrow) secondary to ethmoid sinusitis. The abscess is displacing the medial rectus muscle laterally. Also note increased density of the preseptal tissues, consistent with preseptal cellulitis (Broken arrow)

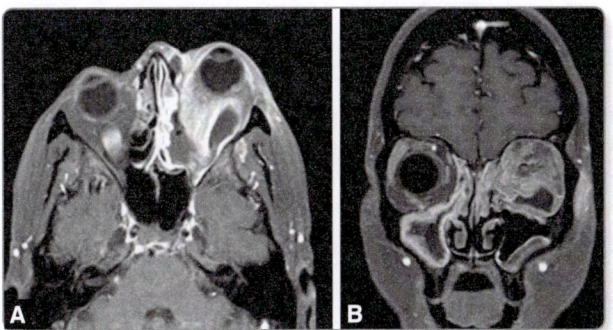

**Figures 4.51A and B** Axial (A) and coronal (B) fat saturated postgadolinium MRI of orbital cellulitis and abscess. There is diffuse enhancement of the orbital fat with coalescence into an orbital abscess. Note proptosis of the globe

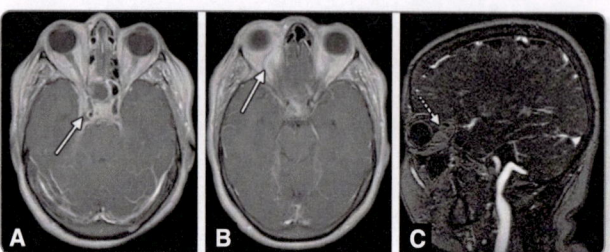

**Figures 4.52A to C** Axial postgadolinium MRI (A, B) show enlargement and lateral convexity of the right cavernous sinus. A filling defect in the posterior cavernous sinus is consistent with thrombosis. Middle image shows a clot within the right ophthalmic vein (arrow). Sagittal contrast MRV (C) confirms thrombosis of the superior ophthalmic vein (dashed arrow). This arose secondary to sphenoid sinusitis (arrow)

Cavernous sinus thrombosis may arise secondary to orbital cellulitis or directly from sinusitis. It is most commonly seen with infection of the sphenoid and ethmoid sinuses (**Figures 4.52A to C**). The septic process spreads from the orbit or sinus via the valveless venous system into the superior and inferior ophthalmic veins and then to the cavernous sinus. Intercavernous spread between the right and left cavernous sinus can also occur. On postcontrast imaging, filling defects in the ophthalmic veins and cavernous sinus can be seen.

## Intracranial complications

Intracranial complications include meningitis, epidural, subdural and cerebral abscess, and cavernous and superior sagittal sinus thrombosis. Due to the proximity of the sinuses to the intracranial compartment, direct intracranial extension can also occur through any sinus wall defects that may be present. Indirect spread via shared venous drainage of the dura and sinus walls is more common.

Meningitis most commonly arises from sphenoid and ethmoid sinus disease. Postgadolinium T1 MRI sequences may show dural or leptomeningeal enhancement, and inflammatory exudate in the subarachnoid space. Epidural, subdural and cerebral abscess is most often of frontal sinus origin (**Figures 4.53A to C**). Epidural abscess

Imaging of the paranasal sinuses 177

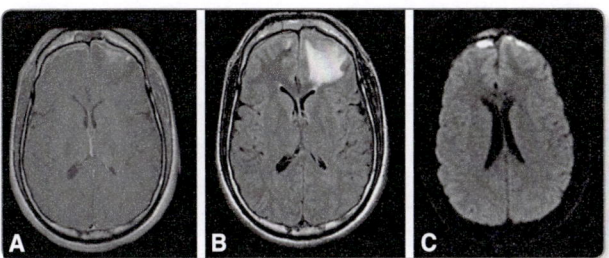

**Figures 4.53A to C** Intracranial complications of sinusitis. (A) an axial postcontrast T1 MRI showing the presence of subdural abscess over the frontal convexity. There is also patchy enhancement in the left frontal lobe consistent with cerebritis (B) is a diffusion image showing restriction within the collection (C)

accumulates between the dura and bone and is visible on both MRI and CT. Infections within the subdural space are not constrained by any dural attachments to the skull and hence can spread diffusely over the convexity and along the tentorium (**Figure 4.54**).

Cerebral edema and infarction are complications that can also arise secondary to the presence of inflammation and venous thrombosis.

## Chronic rhinosinusitis

In chronic rhinosinusitis (CRS), inflammation persists for longer than 12 weeks despite medical treatment. Diagnosis is based on clinical symptoms combined with evidence of mucosal disease on endoscopy and/or CT. Symptoms must include 2 of the following: nasal blockage, congestion or stuffiness, nasal discharge, facial pain or pressure and headache, and loss of smell.

Chronic rhinosinusitis is classified into 3 subtypes: CRS without nasal polyposis (60-65%), CRS with nasal polyposis (20-35%) and allergic fungal sinusitis (8-12%).

Objective evidence of mucosal disease can be obtained on endoscopy of the nasal cavity and middle meatus. The presence of polyps, edema and discharge, are positive findings. CRS is primarily a clinical diagnosis with a limited role for imaging but CT is considered the modality of choice when imaging is deemed necessary. Imaging

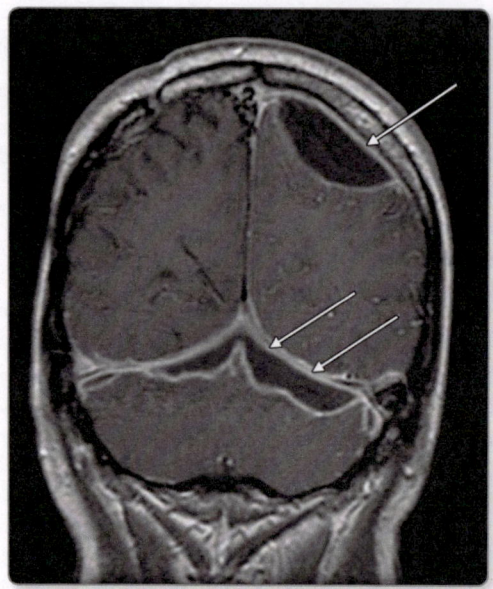

**Figure 4.54** Coronal postgadolinium MRI demonstrates large supratentorial (arrow) and infratentorial subdural abscesses (double arrow). As infection is not constrained by the dural attachment to the skull, it can spread diffusely through the subdural space

can help define extension of mucosal disease into the sphenoid, ethmoid and frontal sinuses, which may be hidden from endoscopy. It also depicts bony anatomy and any anatomic variations that may be present. Such information is critical for surgical planning. It must be remembered however, that CT imaging has to be interpreted in the context of the clinical symptoms and endoscopic findings as 30 percent of asymptomatic adults will have incidental CT mucosal abnormalities.

## Chronic rhinosinusitis without nasal polyposis

CRS without nasal polyposis is the most common form of CRS. Characteristic features of the other two subtypes, namely polyps and allergic mucin are absent. CRS without nasal polyps is a complex

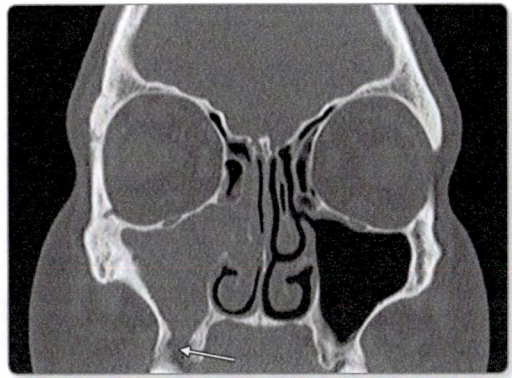

**Figure 4.55** Coronal CT shows lucency around the root of the right molar tooth (arrow) with spread of inflammation superiorly into the antrum. Opacification and sclerosis of the right maxillary sinus is consistent with chronic odontogenic sinusitis

inflammatory disorder of unknown etiology. Although bacteria play a role, it is not a simple chronic bacterial infection. Contributing factors include allergic and nonallergic rhinitis, smoking, postsurgical scarring, and occasionally immunodeficiency. Dental infection is an important etiologic factor in around 10 percent of cases of maxillary sinusitis (**Figure 4.55**).

Computed tomography findings in CRS include diffuse or focal mucosal thickening resulting in partial or complete opacification of the paranasal sinuses. Chronic secretions demonstrate increased attenuation with Hounsfield unit measurements of 30 to 60. Care must be taken as this degree of CT attenuation may obscure the density of an underlying neoplastic process. MRI is even more sensitive to the presence of mucosal thickening (**Figures 4.56A and B**). MRI is performed if an underlying mass or intracranial complication is suspected. Acute sinonasal secretions are 95 percent water and 5 percent protein. Chronic entrapped secretions demonstrate increased protein with decreased free water due to water reabsorption. Varying MRI signal intensities will result depending upon the protein concentration with four patterns described:

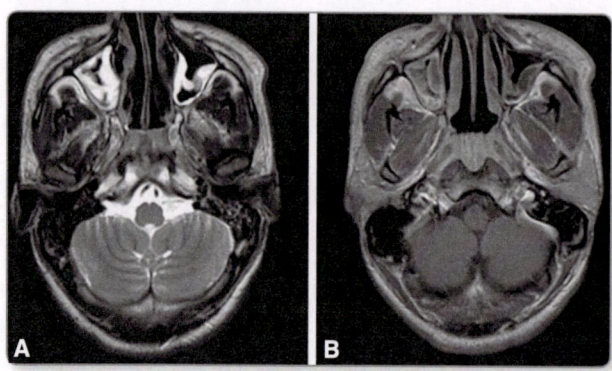

**Figures 4.56A and B** (A) Axial T2 MRI showing mucosal thickening and edema as peripheral T2 hyperintensity. (B) Postgadolinium MRI demonstrates enhancing mucosa and nonenhancing submucosal edema

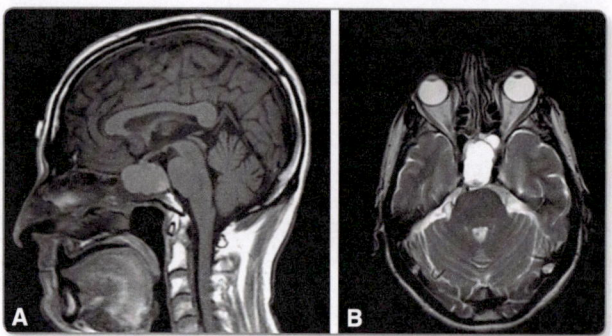

**Figures 4.57A and B** High T1 and T2 signal within sphenoid sinus secretions

1. Hypointense on T1 and hyperintense on T2 with a protein concentration less than 9 percent
2. Hyperintense on T1 and hyperintense on T2 at a protein concentration of between 20 and 25 percent (**Figures 4.57A and B**)
3. Hyperintense on T1 and hypointense on T2 at a protein concentration of between 25 and 30 percent

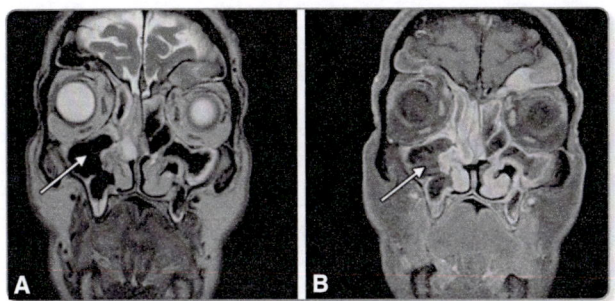

**Figures 4.58A and B** Protein concentrations in inspissated secretions above 30% results in very low T2 and T1 signal (arrows)

4. Hypointense on T1 and T2 with protein concentrations greater than 30 percent (**Figures 4.58A and B**)

Increases in protein concentration up to 30 percent lead to T1 and T2 shortening with resultant T1 and T2 hyperintensity. With protein concentration above 30 percent, there is no remaining free water in the inspissated secretions and there is a resultant marked decrease in T2 and T1 signal. This is particularly evident on T2 imaging, which may mimic an aerated sinus. Peripheral rim enhancement is appreciated on both CT and MRI but may unapparent on CT if there are hyperdense secretions present.

Linear peripheral calcification can also be rarely seen in CRS.

## Chronic rhinosinusitis with nasal polyposis

Chronic rhinosinusitis (CRS) with nasal polyposis is characterized by the presence of polyps in the nasal cavity or paranasal sinuses. Polyps are composed of edematous hyperplastic submucosal connective tissue containing a predominance of eosinophils. Large polyps may be visible though the nares and are distinguished by their pale yellow color, due to their avascular nature, and lack of sensation. CRS with nasal polyposis is associated with aspirin sensitivity and asthma. Polyps are usually bilateral and involve the anterior ostiomeatal units including the ethmoid infundibulum and uncinate process.

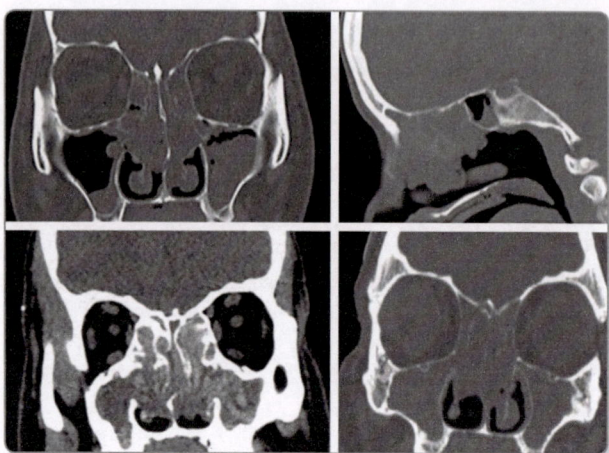

**Figure 4.59** CT imaging of nasal polyposis. First two images show multiple lobulated opacities in the ethmoid and nasal cavity. The third image shows a "cascading" appearance within the nasal cavity. Fourth image shows rarefaction of the ethmoid septations secondary to pressure effect and deossification

On CT polyps are of soft tissue density and similar to thickened mucosa (**Figure 4.59**). They have a rounded or lobulated configuration and will often protrude into the nasal cavity. If the nasal vault or sinus is completely opacified, their presence may not be easily appreciated. Secretions may become entrapped within crevices between the polyps leading to increased density on CT. A "cascading" pattern of high density secretions and low density mucosa can occur. Bone changes associated with sinonasal polyposis include expansion, deossification, sclerosis and occasionally erosion. Widening of the infundibulum is characteristic. Unlike other polypoid processes such as antrochoanal polyps, or inverted papillomas, the widening is bilateral and associated with extensive sinusitis. Lateral bulging of the lamina papyracea may occur. Truncation of the bulbous part of the middle turbinate is a specific sign and like deossification of the ethmoid trabeculae, is likely due to mechanical pressure erosion and hyperemia from mucosal inflammation. The signal intensity of polyps

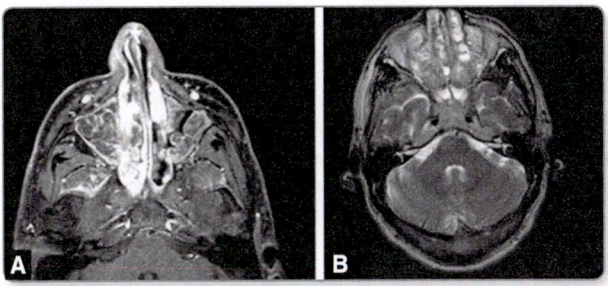

**Figures 4.60A and B** MRI of nasal polyposis. First image, axial postcontrast MRI shows multiple polyps within the maxillary sinuses, nasal cavity and nasopharynx. Most of the polyps demonstrate peripheral enhancement. Second image, axial T2 MRI shows inspissated hypointense secretions between the T2 hyperintense polyps

on MRI varies according to edematous, cystic and fibrous stages. Most commonly they are hyperintense on T2 and show peripheral mucosal enhancement on postgadolinium sequences (**Figures 4.60A and B**).

## Allergic fungal sinusitis

Allergic fungal sinusitis (AFS) is a subtype of CRS characterized by the presence of allergic mucin, which is a thick inspissated mucous containing eosinophils and fungal hyphae. AFS occurs in immunocompetent patients and results from allergic inflammation to colonizing fungus. Criteria for the disease include:
Evidence of type1 hypersensitivity/IgE to one or more fungi on:
- Skin testing or serology
- Nasal polyposis.
- Characteristic CT findings.
- Eosinophilic mucus.

Positive fungal stain of mucin removed during surgery with no fungal tissue invasion.

Surgery is required for diagnosis to confirm the presence of allergic mucin. Mucosal biopsy shows an eosinophil-predominant inflammatory process similar to CRS with nasal polyposis.

Computed tomography findings include unilateral or bilateral opacification of multiple paranasal sinuses with sinus expansion, erosion and intrasinus high attenuation foci (**Figures 4.61A and B**). Hyperattenuating areas on unenhanced CT are due to calcium and magnesium salts deposited within the necrotic areas of mycelium and fungus infected mucus, combined with inspissated secretions. The ethmoid and maxillary sinuses are most frequently affected.

Bone erosion is associated with expansion and occurs in 20 percent of patients (**Figure 4.62**) and is thought to result from pressure atrophy or inflammatory mediators related to allergic mucin. It is not

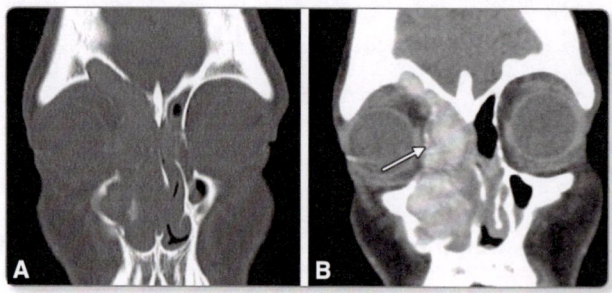

**Figures 4.61A and B** Allergic fungal sinusitis. Coronal bone and soft tissue CT shows is unilateral opacification and expansion of the right frontal, ethmoid and maxillary sinuses with high attenuation material. There is erosion of the lamina papyracea with extension into the orbit (arrow)

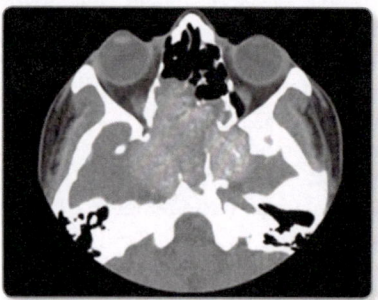

**Figure 4.62** Allergic fungal sinusitis. Axial Soft tissue CT demonstrates expansion of the posterior ethmoid and sphenoid sinuses, including the lateral recesses with high attenuation material in a patient with allergic fungal sinusitis and visual loss

Imaging of the paranasal sinuses 185

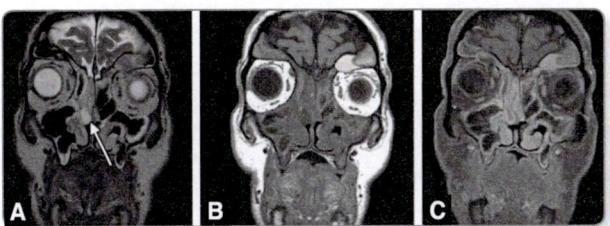

**Figures 4.63A to C** MRI of allergic fungal sinusitis. (A) Coronal T2 MRI shows hypointense signal voids in the maxillary, ethmoid and right frontal sinuses due to lack of free water and susceptibility effects. This could be mistaken for a normal aerated sinus. There is a polyp in the right nasal cavity, which is a common associated finding (arrow). (B) Coronal T1 imaging reveals hypointensity within the sinuses that corresponds to areas of very low T2 signal. This helps confirm that the T2 "signal void" is in fact not a truly aerated sinus. (C) Coronal T1 with gadolinium. There is peripheral sinus enhancement postgadolinium

related to fungal invasion, which does not occur in AFS. In patients with bilateral advanced disease, orbital and intracranial extension can arise via penetration through the lamina papyracea and posterior wall of the frontal sinus respectively.

MRI shows decreased signal on T1, markedly decreased signal on T2 imaging. Signal voids can be seen due to a lack of free water and susceptibility effects in the presence of iron, manganese and calcium (**Figures 4.63A to C**). Peripheral enhancement is noted in the affected sinus. Hyperdensity on unenhanced CT and a lack of central enhancement help differentiate AFS from tumor. AFS is refractory to medical treatment and surgery is required to remove inspissated secretions and restore sinus ventilation.

## Sinochoanal polyp

A choanal polyp is a solitary lesion that arises in a sinus cavity and extends through the ostium in to the nasal cavity. The most common type is the antrochonal polyp, which protrudes through the ethmoid infundibulum into the middle meatus (**Figures 4.64A to D**). It may extend posteriorly to reach the choana and protrude into the nasopharynx. Ethmochoanal and sphenochoanal polyps are other rare types (**Figure 4.65**). A sphenochoanal polyp traverses the sphenoid

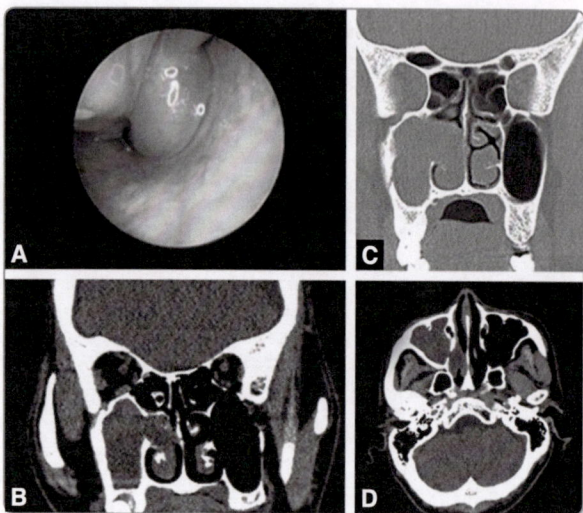

**Figures 4.64A to D** Antrochoanal polyps. This polyp is extending through a widened accessory maxillary sinus ostium to protrude into the right nasal cavity (*for color version of Figure 4.64A see Plate 11*)

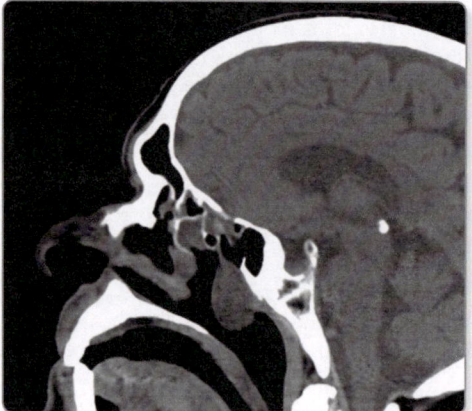

**Figure 4.65** Sagittal CT shows an ethmochoanal polyp extending from the ethmoid sinus into the nasal cavity and choana. Note low "mucoid" density on CT

Imaging of the paranasal sinuses 187

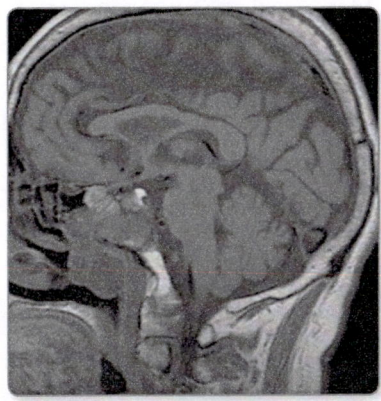

**Figure 4.66** Sagittal MRI demonstrates a polyp in the sphenoid sinus, which passes through the sphenoid ostium into the sphenoethmoidal recess, nasal cavity and nasopharynx. T1 hyperintensity within the superior sphenoid sinus represents proteinacious secretions. If the sphenoid origin of the polyp is not recognized, postsurgical recurrence will occur

ostium and extends into the sphenoethmoidal recess, and nasopharynx. Narrowing of the polyp as it passes through the ostia results in a dumbbell appearance (**Figure 4.66**).

Polyps appear as well defined lesions demonstrating mucoid density on CT and hyperintense on T2 signal. Polyps may show peripheral rim enhancement. Vascular compromise due to constriction of its neck at the sinus ostium may lead to central enhancement of the intranasal component. It is important to properly identify the sinus of origin when one is considering surgical excision. Incomplete resection of the polyp will lead to recurrence.

## Mucous retention cyst

A mucous retention cyst (MRC) develops secondary to blockage of the duct of a minor serous or mucinous salivary gland within the lining of the paranasal sinuses. They are common incidental findings in asymptomatic individuals. On imaging it may be difficult to distinguish

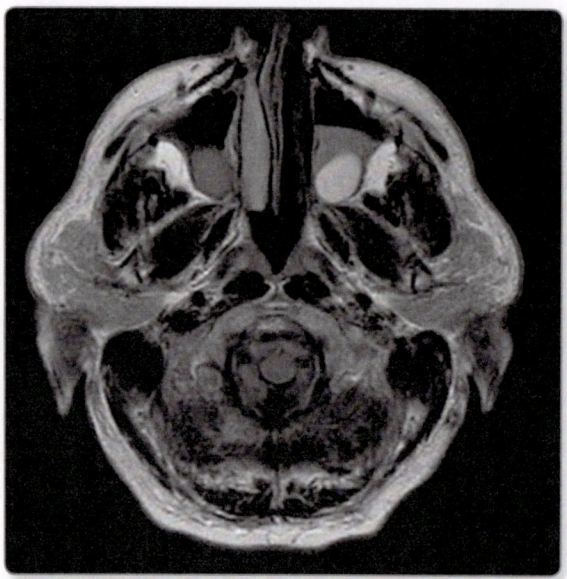

**Figure 4.67** Mucous retention cyst

a mucous retention cyst from a polyp. MRC are smoothly marginated and dome shaped and most often arise from the alveolar recess of the maxillary sinus (**Figure 4.67**). Serous MRC are of water attenuation and intensity on CT and MRI, whereas mucous types show soft tissue density on CT, and T1 signal greater than water on MRI. Unlike polyps they do not have a stalk or/and do not demonstrate contrast enhancement.

## Mucocele

A mucocele is a chronic cystic expansile lesion of the sinus that is lined by the sinus mucosa. They result from obstruction of a sinus ostium or a compartmentalized portioin of a sinus. It can arise secondary to CRS, polyposis, trauma, surgery or tumor (**Figures 4.68 and 4.69**). In decreasing order of frequency is involvement of the frontal, ethmoid,

Imaging of the paranasal sinuses

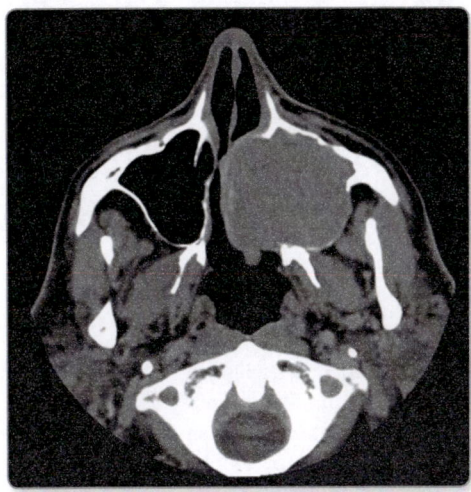

**Figure 4.68** Left maxillary sinus mucocele. Note expansion of the sinus with thinning and remodelling of the walls

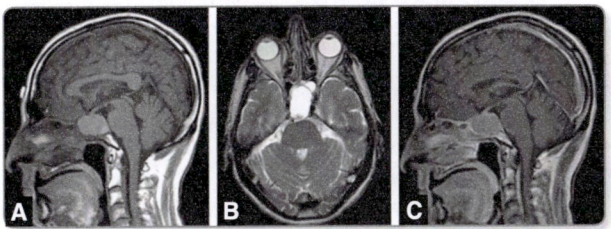

**Figures 4.69A to C** MRI of a sphenoid sinus mucocele. The sinus is expanded and the contents are bright on T1- and T2-weighted imaging due to the presence of proteinaceous secretions. Peripheral rim enhancement is present on the third image

maxillary and sphenoid sinuses. Frontal and ethmoid mucoceles may expand into the orbit with resultant diplopia and proptosis. Sphenoid mucoceles can compress the optic pathway and cause ocular palsy.

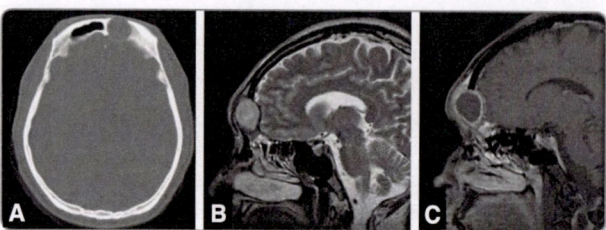

**Figures 4.70A to C** Mucopyocele within the left frontal sinus. Thick peripheral rim enhancement is present as adjacent soft tissue swelling and enhancement

A diagnosis of mucocele will require the affected sinus to be expanded. CT density and MRI intensity of a mucocele will depend on the degree of desiccation of the sinus contents, thus, T1 and T2 signals may be hyperintense or hypointense. CT demonstrates a thin rim of remodeled/expanded bone with possible focal dehiscence as well as sclerosis. Peripheral mucosal rim enhancement is seen on MRI and CT. Thick peripheral enhancement with or without involvement of surrounding soft tissues can be seen with superinfection (mucopyocele) (**Figures 4.70A to C**). Nodular or central enhancement can suggest the presence of an underlying tumor.

## Silent sinus syndrome

Obstruction of the maxillary sinus drainage can lead to atelectasis of the sinus with resultant enophthalmos and diplopia. The mechanism is thought to be a result of recurrent episodes of chronic obstruction of the maxillary ostium leading to negative antral pressure and bony demineralization. There is resultant in-drawing of the sinus walls. Inferior bowing of the orbital floor/maxillary roof results in an increase in orbital volume and resultant enophthalmos. CT findings include obstruction of the infundibulum as the uncinate is drawn superiorly and medially to come into close approximation to the inferomedial bony orbital margin. Concavity of the sinus walls and opacification of the antrum are also evident. Coronal imaging will demonstrate inferior retraction of the orbital floor (**Figures 4.71A and B**).

Imaging of the paranasal sinuses 191

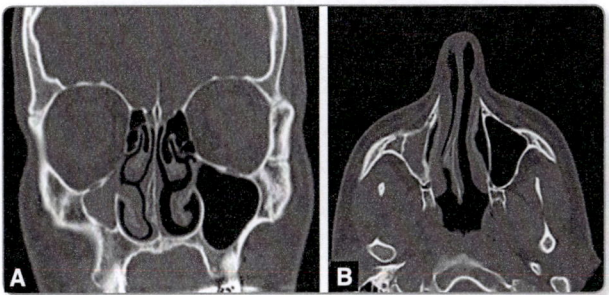

**Figures 4.71A and B** Silent or atelectatic sinus syndrome involving the right maxillary sinus. There is opposition of the right uncinate to the inferomedial orbital margin. In-drawing of the right natural walls are noted and there is a depression of the floor of the right orbit

## Fungal sinusitis

The spectrum of fungal sinusitis ranges from asymptomatic localized saprohytic colonization and growth to fulminant rhino-orbital-cerebral fungal infection. Fungal rhinosinusitis can be classified into invasive and noninvasive types based on the presence of sinus mucosal invasion. Allergic fungal sinusitis is considered a form of CRS and was discussed above.

## Noninvasive fungal sinusitis

This type of fungal sinusitis involves fungal colonization of a sinus cavity. Fungi are ubiquitous organisms and their spores are frequently inhaled into the sinuses where they can be detected by culture in healthy asymptomatic adults without visible disease. In immunocompetent patients, often in association with impaired sinus drainage due to CRS or polyps, fungal mycelia can proliferate to occupy available space with the sinuses and form dense fungal concretions called "fungal balls". The term mycetoma should be avoided as the term refers to invasion of subcutaneous tissue by bacteria or fungi. The term aspergilloma should also be used cautiously as it is not the only etiologic agent.

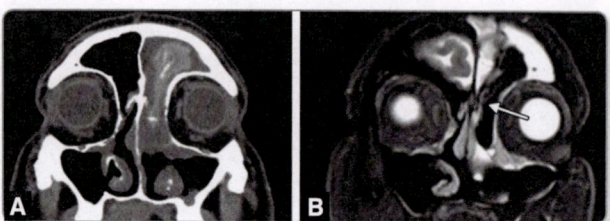

**Figures 4.72A and B** Fungal colonization in the left frontoethmoid region. The fungal ball is of high CT attenuation (A) with small foci of calcification. The corresponding T2 MRI (B) shows the classic black signal void (arrow)

Imaging shows diffuse opacification of a single sinus, most frequently the maxillary sinus, with high attenuation material on CT. Small foci of punctate calcific density are often seen at the center of the sinus (**Figures 4.72A and B**). There is enhancement of the sinus periphery corresponding to inflamed mucosa and sclerosis of the sinus walls. Fungus balls can have a thick cheesy consistency or may be solid. On MRI, they appear as signal voids. Such signal voids are especially evident on T2-weighted imaging and reflects a lack of hydration and the presence of paramagnetic elements such as iron and manganese.

Patients may be asymptomatic or complain of a pressure sensation from the affected sinus, or have symptoms of CRS. Treatment would involve endoscopic surgical removal.

## Invasive fungal sinusitis

Invasive fungal sinusitis includes acute fulminant invasive and chronic invasive fungal infections.

### Acute fulminant invasive fungal sinusitis

Acute fulminant invasive fungal sinusitis is a rapidly progressive disease seen mostly in immunocompromised patients. The etiologic fungi include the Zygomycetes class of fungus such as Mucor and the Ascomycetes class such as Aspergillus. These fungi colonize the sinonasal cavities in normal individuals but can become pathogenic in immunocomprised patients, particularly in those with impaired neutrophil function. Predisposing disorders include hematologic malignancy, diabetes, AIDS, organ transplantation and iatrogenic immunosuppression with chemotherapeutic agents. In these susceptible hosts, the fungus will invade the mucosa, submucosa and bone. Invasion of blood vessels can result in ischemic necrosis. The infection can spread directly across the sinus wall into the adjacent soft tissues. Passage through the bony sinus walls can also occur through perivascular channels. This can lead to invasion of the adjacent brain and orbit. Spread into the cavernous sinus and intracranial compartment can also occur via the orbital apex. Angioinvasion may cause thrombosis of the carotid artery and cavernous sinus with resulting infarction.

Typical clinical scenarios would include a fever of unknown origin in an immunocompromised patient. The patient may have associated sinonasal symptoms. Clinical examination may reveal white or black discoloration of the nasal mucosa indicating invasion and subsequent necrosis. The diagnosis requires histopathological evidence of hyphae invading tissue, which can be confirmed by culture. CT and MRI are useful for preoperative planning and in the assessment of orbital and intracranial spread.

Early CT findings may be nonspecific and show thickening of the nasal cavity mucosa and soft tissue edema. The nasal mucosal changes are usually unilateral and of greater severity than expected in CRS. The involved sinus may be filled with soft tissue density. Unlike other fungal diseases, hyperattenuation of sinus contents is not a common feature. The ethmoid and maxillary sinuses are most frequently involved. Bone erosion and extrasinus extension can also develop. In the maxillary sinus, there may be a loss of the periantral fat planes following invasion (**Figures 4.73A to C**). Postcontrast CT imaging can detect occlusion of the ophthalmic veins and artery if the orbital apex is involved. Cavernous sinus thrombosis may arise.

MRI will show variable signal intensity within the sinuses on T1 and T2 sequences. Fungal elements may show a decreased T2 signal. Infarcted mucosa may show restricted diffusion and decreased enhancement on postgadolinium T1 sequences. Intracranial and

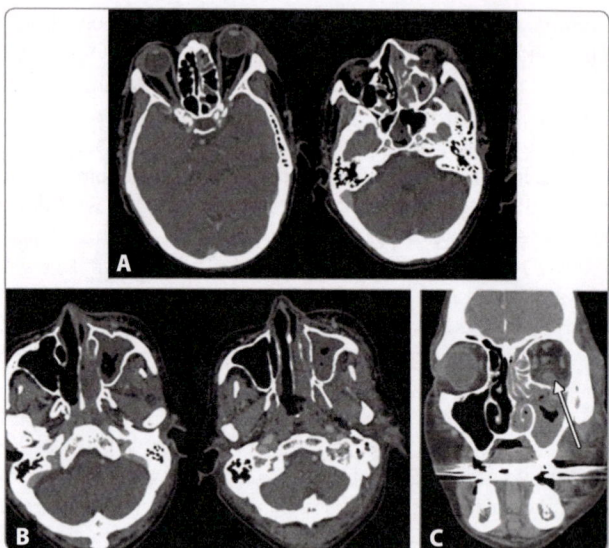

**Figures 4.73A to C** Invasive aspergillosis in a bone marrow transplant patient. The left ethmoid and maxillary sinuses are affected. The presence of significant soft tissue swelling in the premalar and retroantral soft tissues suggests an aggressive infection. Coronal CT shows inflammatory changes extending into the left orbit (arrow)

extra-sinus involvement is better assessed with MRI. Extrasinus soft tissue invasion is hyperintense on T2 imaging and will enhance. Intracranial findings include cerebral infarction, leptomeningeal enhancement, cerebritis and cerebral abscess (**Figures 4.74 and 4.75**).

## Chronic invasive fungal sinusitis

Chronic invasive fungal sinusitis may arise in patients with milder degrees of immunodeficiency, such as in the diabetic population or in patients on low dose corticosteroids. Chronic invasive fungal sinusitis is a chronic indolent process that may persist for several weeks. Common organisms include Mucor, Rhizopus and Aspergillus. There may be a several month history of CRS symptoms before the

Imaging of the paranasal sinuses 195

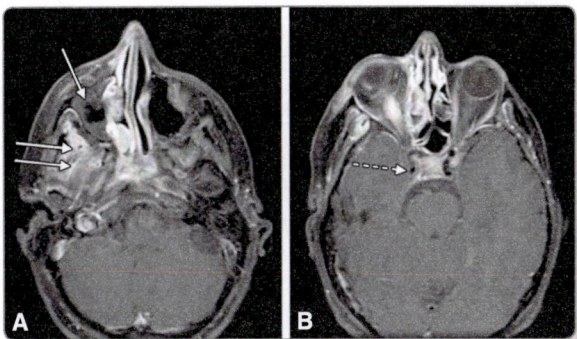

**Figures 4.74A and B** Axial T1 fat saturated postgadolinium MRI. Note the lack of normally present enhancement of the right maxillary sinus mucosa due to infarction from angioinvasion (arrow). There is also abnormal enhancement of the right masticator space consistent with extrasinus extension (double arrows). The second image shows a lack of enhancement in the right cavernous sinus consistent with cavernous sinus thrombosis (dashed arrow)

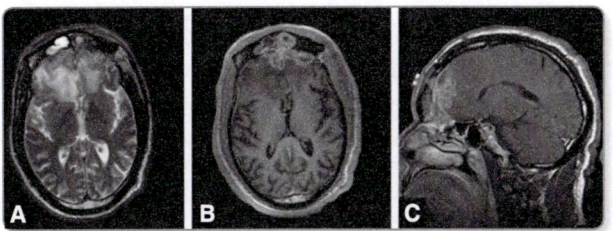

**Figures 4.75A to C** Intracranial extension of aspergillus sinusitis. Axial T2 (A) and axial (B) and sagittal (C) enhanced MRI shows abnormal heterogeneous soft tissue extending from the frontal sinus through the frontal bone to invade the frontal brain parenchyma

development of orbital or brain involvement. Invasion of the orbital apex results in decreased vision and ocular immobility. Unenhanced CT may show the presence of a hyperdense mass, representing hyphae within one or more sinuses with bony erosion and soft tissue extension. On MRI the fungal mass again may show decreased signal intensity on T1 and T2. Hyperdensity of the sinus contents, in addition to the time course, helps distinguish the disease from the acute invasive form.

## Granulomatous sinusitis

Granulomatous diseases include various infectious, autoimmune, and idiopathic processes.

Wegeners granulomatosis is a systemic vasculitis of the medium and small arteries, venules, and arterioles. It causes a granulomatous inflammation of the upper and lower respiratory tract, and a necrotizing glomerulonephritis. It is associated with the presence of antineutrophil cytoplasmic antibodies (ANCAs). Sinonasal involvement presents with sinusitis, bloody discharge, and nasal crusting and ulceration. The diagnosis is suggested by the clinical findings combined with laboratory ANCA levels. Confirmation is usually required with biopsy of an active site of disease. Sinonasal biopsies often only demonstrate nonspecific inflammation and a more invasive lung or renal biopsy may be needed.

Initially on imaging, the disease may appear as nonspecific mucosal thickening within the sinuses that may be indistinguishable from CRS. In more advanced disease obliteration of small arteries causes bone destruction, which begins in the midline affecting the septum and turbinates before spreading into the medial maxillary wall. Progressive involvement of the sinuses leads to erosion of the ethmoid septa, lamina papyracea and cribrifom plate (**Figures 4.76 and 4.77**). In 50 percent of patients there is concomitant new bone

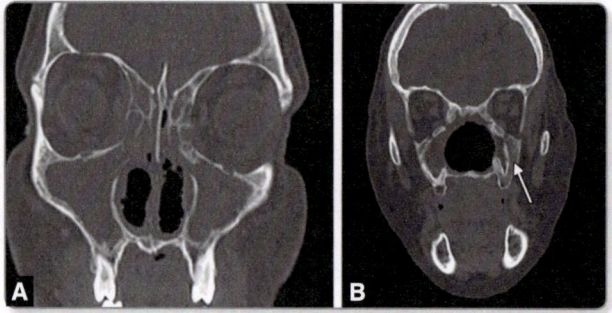

**Figures 4.76A and B** Wegeners granulomatosis. (A) Coronal CT shows diffuse opacification of the sinuses. (B) Coronal CT of advanced Wegeners granulomatosis. Note destruction of the nasal septum and lateral nasal walls. There is erosion of the ethmoid septations. New bone formation with a "tram line" appearance is also evident (arrow)

Imaging of the paranasal sinuses

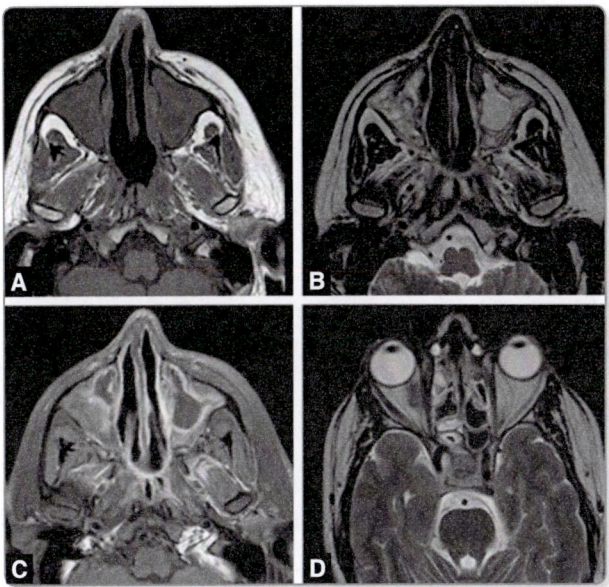

**Figures 4.77A to D** MRI of sinonasal Wegeners granulomatosis. (A) Axial T1 MRI shows T1 hyperintense cancellous bone within the posterior wall of the maxilla, between the hypointense cortex, resulting from new bone formation. (B) Axial T2 MRI. The maxillary sinus demonstrates peripheral T2 hypointensity due to the formation of submucosal granulomas. (C) Axial postgad fat saturated MRI shows enhancement of the mucosa. (D) Axial T2 MRI of the orbit. There is a T2 hypointense mass in the right orbit, representing extrasinus disease

formation of the sinus walls, with relatively hypodense cancellous bone apparent between a dense outer and inner cortex, giving rise to a 'tram line' effect.

On MRI, mucosal thickening is initially T2 hyperintense. The formation of submucosal granulomas results in T1 and T2 mucosal hypointensity, which enhances (**Figures 4.77A to D**). New bone formation may be detectable within the sinus wall as T1 hyperintense fatty marrow. Extrasinus extension most commonly occurs in the orbit and is seen in 30 percent of cases.

Sarcoidosis is another granulomatous disorder, which also can affect the nasal cavity. Septal mucosal thickening and permeative erosive changes with the nasal bones are described. Opacification of sinuses is usually secondary to obstruction rather than direct involvement.

Infectious agents resulting in granulomatous inflammation within the sinuses include mycobacteria, leprosy, fungal infections and syphilis.

## Sinonasal tumors

Malignancy of the sinonasal cavities accounts for approximately 3 to 4 percent of head and neck neoplasms and 0.5 percent of all malignancy. Benign neoplasms have a similar incidence. The presence of multiple types of epithelium and mesenchymal elements in the sinonasal cavity leads to a multitude of different possible tumor histologies. Squamous cell carcinoma accounts for 70 to 80 percent of all malignancies and adenocarcinoma (10%) is the next most common. Additional rare histologies include esthesioneuroblastoma, undifferentiated carcinoma, melanoma and lymphoma. 50 to 60 percent of tumors arise in the maxillary sinus with the remainder localized mainly in the nasal cavity and ethmoid sinuses. Tumor originating within the frontal and sphenoid sinuses is rare.

Early tumors of the paranasal sinuses are often asymptomatic or may present with nonspecific symptoms such as rhinorrhea, nasal obstruction, facial pain and hyposmia. Consequently, patient's often present with advanced stage disease, with the majority of patients demonstrating extension through at least one sinus wall.

In patients with operable disease, surgical resection is the primary treatment. Surgery however, may be complicated by the involvement of important surrounding structures such as the orbit, anterior skull base and carotid arteries. The role of imaging is to evaluate the status of these various compartments. Radiation therapy is employed to decrease locoregional recurrence, which is the most common cause of treatment failure and death. Survival rates in node negative patients are around 50 percent at 5 years for squamous carcinoma and adenocarcinoma.

Imaging of the paranasal sinuses 199

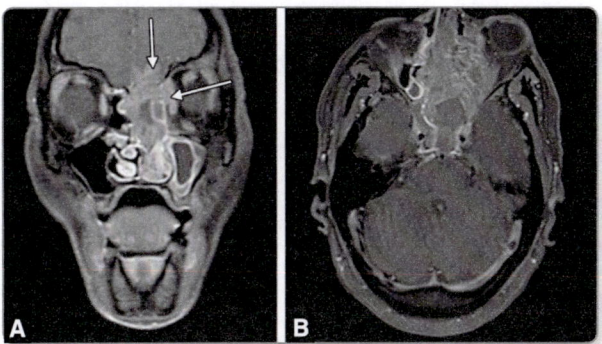

**Figures 4.78A and B** Nasoethmoidal patterns of spread. (A) Coronal fat saturated T1 post gadolinium. Squamous cell carcinoma in the left ethmoid sinus/nasal cavity with spread superiorly (short arrow) into the anterior cranial fossa and laterally into the orbit (long arrow). (B) Axial fat saturated postgadolinium MRI. Alveolar rhabdomyosarcoma invading the orbit and orbital apex, passing through the orbital fissure into the middle cranial fossa

## Patterns of tumor spread

Sinonasal neoplasms can extend into adjacent structures directly through the sinus walls or via perineural spread. The pattern of tumor spread is based upon the epicenter of the primary tumor. Important regions to assess in sinonasal malignancy include the orbits, anterior cranial fossa and sphenoid sinus (**Figures 4.78A and B**). Nasoethmoid tumors can spread superiorly through the cribriform plate and fovea ethmoidalis into the anterior cranial fossa. Medal extension through the lamina papyracea into the orbit may require an orbital exenteration. Lesions at the orbit apex may spread into the middle cranial fossa.

Tumors involving the maxillary sinus can extend through the posterior wall into adjacent masticator space and pterygopalatine fossa, as well as superiorly into the orbit (**Figures 4.79A to D**). Disease involving the pterygopalatine fossa and masticator space can result in further direct or perineural spread into the orbit and intracranial compartments. Inferomedial spread into the palate and nasal cavity are relatively easier to resect with a maxillectomy.

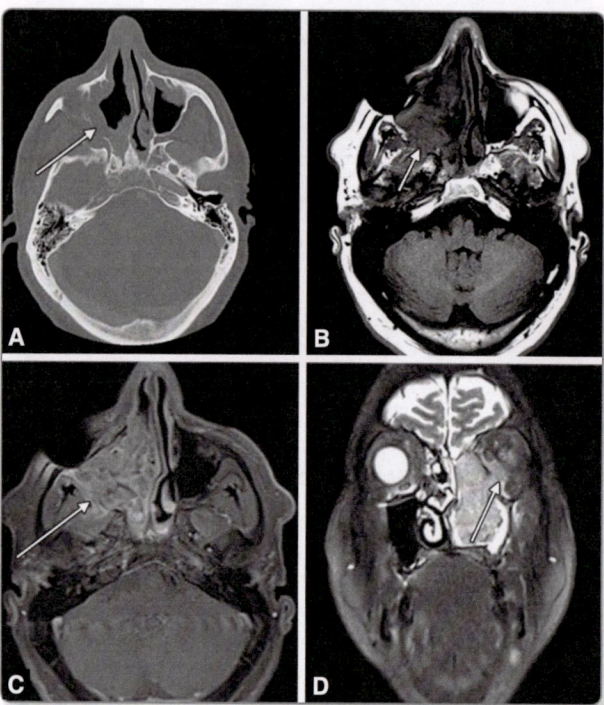

**Figures 4.79A to D** Patterns of tumor spread from the maxilla. (A) Axial CT shows destruction of the right posterolateral maxillary wall (long arrow). (B) Axial T1 MRI. There is loss of the normal T1 hyperintensity in the right pterygopalatine fossa due to tumor infiltration (short arrow). (C) Postgadolinium T1. Tumor extension into the lateral pterygoid of the masticator space is more evident with contrast (arrow). Note extension through medial wall of maxilla and sphenopalatine foramen into nasal cavity. (D) Coronal T2 fat saturated MRI in another patient. SCCa of nasal cavity with extension into the orbit (arrow)

## Imaging

The imaging appearance of sinonasal tumors is often nonspecific and endoscopic examination is required to assess local extent and provide biopsy material. The main role of imaging is to precisely map the deep extent and tumor margins. The anatomic extent provides prognostic information and determines whether or not the tumor is resectable and will help guide the surgical approach. The planning of radiation portals also relies on precise tumor mapping, as does the assessment of treatment response to chemotherapy and radiotherapy. Accurate tumor delineation also facilitates preservation of important uninvolved structures.

MRI and CT have complementary roles in the assessment of tumor and both may be performed in the radiologic work up. CT provides better evaluation of the bony margins of the sinuses, orbits and anterior cranial fossa. Fibro-osseous lesions are also better characterized with CT. MRI gives superior soft tissue delineation of tumor and is very helpful in the assessment of perineural tumor spread.

## Appearance of tumor

The majority of tumors are of low to intermediate signal intensity on T1 and T2 images. This is due to the dense cellularity and a high nuclear to cytoplasmic ratio within these lesions. Hemorrhage may result in areas of high T1 signal. There may be intralesional foci of T2 hyperintensity, representing areas of necrosis or cystic change. In contrast, entrapped secretions, inflamed mucosa and polyps are often usually extremely and uniformly, hyperintense on T2 imaging. This feature helps in the differentiation of secretions and mucosa from tumor (**Figures 4.80A to C**). Chronic secretions with increasing protein and decreased water content demonstrate increased T1 and decreased T2 signal (**Figures 4.81A to C**).

Around 5 percent of tumors, including minor salivary gland, nerve sheath tumors and inverted papilloma demonstrate T2 hyperintensity. In these tumors, postgadolinium T1 MRI can help differentiate tumor from inflammatory change. Sinonasal tumors demonstrate heterogeneous or less commonly homogenous enhancement which is brighter than normal muscle. Inflamed mucosa enhances more avidly than tumor and is located around the peripheral bony margin of the sinus. Interruption of this uniform peripheral enhancement can be seen as the tumor extends outside the sinus. Secretions will not enhance.

On CT tumors demonstrate mild enhancement. However, very frequently, it can still be very difficult to differentiate tumor from entrapped secretions on CT.

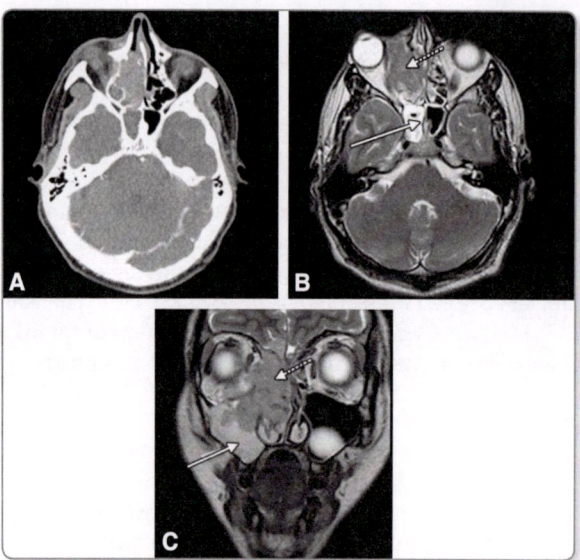

**Figures 4.80A to C** Appearance of sinonasal tumors. (A) Postcontrast CT. The exact posterior extent of the nasoethmoial squamous cell carcinoma is not entirely clear. (B and C) T2 axial and coronal MRI. The tumor is of intermediate signal (dashed arrows) and can be easily distinguished from very hyperintense trapped secretions in the maxillary and sphenoid sinuses (arrows)

## Bone involvement

Bone involvement by tumor can manifest as erosions, remodeling, sclerosis and new bone formation. Bony change is best assessed with CT. Bony erosion is commonly seen with malignancies including squamous cell carcinoma, undifferentiated carcinoma, metastases and sarcoma (**Figure 4.82**). Aggressive infections however can also erode bone and give rise to a sinonasal "mass".

A slowly growing tumor may cause pressure erosion of the adjacent bone while allowing time for new bone formation to develop at the outer margin. This can lead to expansion and remodeling of the sinus. While this is more typical of benign pathologies such as mucoceles and polyps, it may also be seen (with or without erosive

# Imaging of the paranasal sinuses

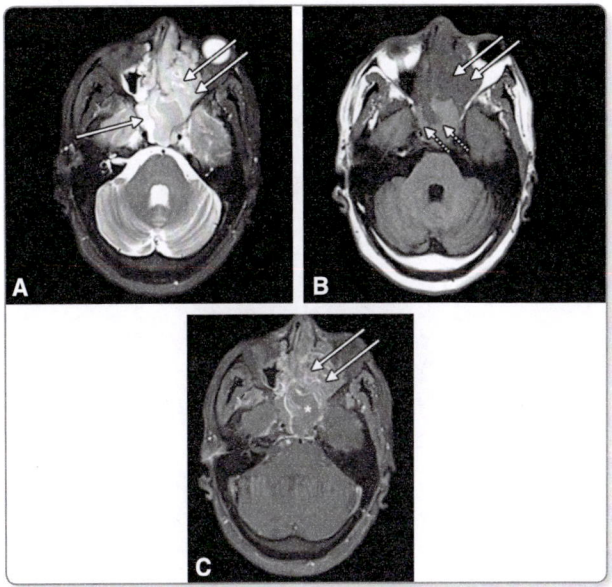

**Figures 4.81A to C** Tumor and entrapped secretions. (A) Axial T2 MRI. There are three different T2 signal intensities in the this image. On the right, very high T2 hyperintensity is unlikely to represent tumor and consistent with secretions (arrow). Intermediate signal intensity region (double arrow) is consistent with tumor. The left sphenoid sinus is slightly more hypointense and its composition is uncertain on T2 imaging alone. (B) Axial T1 MRI. The right and left sphenoid sinus demonstrates homogenous T1 hyperintensity (dashed arrows) – this is consistent with proteinaceous sections. The tumor is of low T1 signal (double arrows). (C) Axial T1 postcontrast. The tumor demonstrates heterogenous low level enhancement (double arrows). The secretions in the sphenoid sinuses do not enhance (*)

change) in malignant salivary gland tumors, lymphoma, melanoma and esthesioneuroblastoma.

Thin cortical bone, such as the cribriform plate, has a limited ability to remodel, and hence benign lesions such as polyps can cause pressure-related deossification and mimic a destructive process.

Reactive sclerosis is seen more commonly with chronic rhinosinusitis but it can also occur in response to obstruction of a sinus ostium secondary to tumor (**Figure 4.83**). Osteosarcoma causes bone

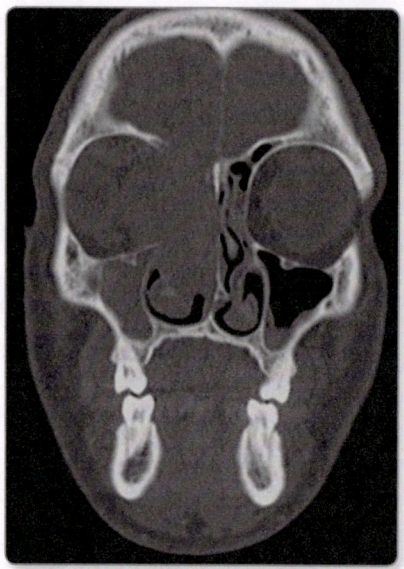

**Figure 4.82** Bone erosion due to tumor. Coronal CT demonstrates erosion of the ethmoid roof and extension through the frontal sinus into the anterior cranial fossa. There is also destruction of the medial wall of orbit

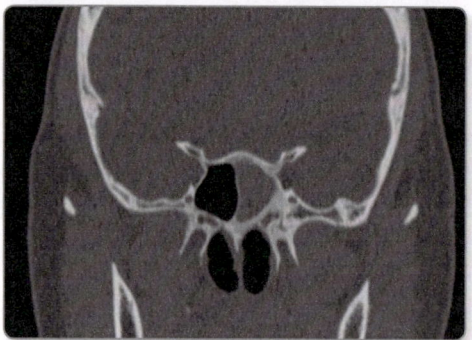

**Figure 4.83** Coronal CT demonstrates sclerosis of the walls of the left sphenoid sinus due to chronic sinusitis following left sphenoid ostial obstruction by an inverted papilloma (not shown)

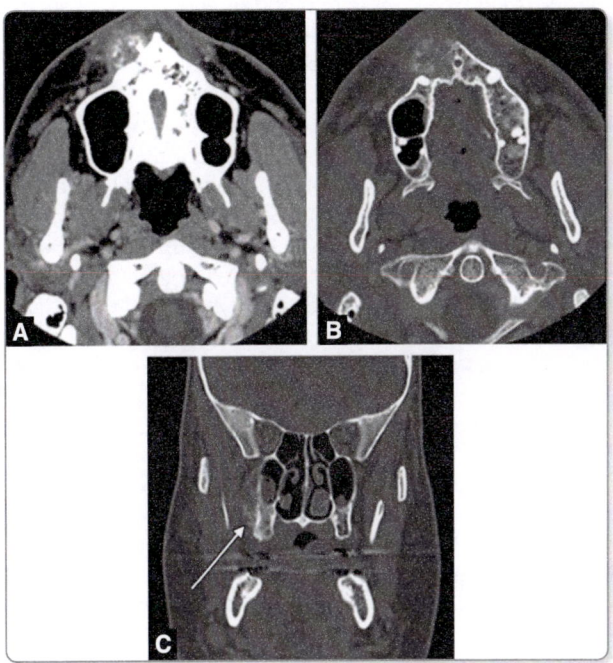

**Figures 4.84A to C** Osteosarcoma. (A and B) Patient with osteosarcoma of the premaxilla showing characteristic spiculated bony matrix. (C) Another patient with osteosarcoma involving the right maxillary alveolus and lower maxillary sinus shows similar fluffy spiculated bone formation laterally (arrow)

destruction with associated aggressive appearing new bone formation that can have a spiculated appearance (**Figures 4.84A to C**).

## Skull base and intracranial extension

Nasoethmoidal and less frequently, maxillary tumors, may extend into the anterior cranial fossa. The cribriform plate and fovea ethmoidalis are thin cortical bones, which together with the dural lining, forms the skull base over the ethmoid sinuses. As a tumor advances superiorly, it will first invade the bony floor of the anterior cranial fossa. Further growth leads to extension into the epidural space and the dura. Advanced tumor may pass through the dura into the subarachnoid space and finally into the brain parenchyma. Localized parenchymal brain involvement may still be amenable to surgical resection. However, involvement of the optic chiasm, extensive bony skull base infiltration, extensive brain parenchymal invasion, pituitary gland and cavernous sinus involvement are considered contraindications to surgery.

Involvement of the skull base and the depth of invasion will guide the surgical approach. For tumor confined to the ethmoid sinus, a medial maxillectomy is performed with an en bloc ethmoidectomy. If the skull base is invaded, then in addition to transfacial surgery, a subfrontal approach is required to facilitate access to the anterior cranial fossa. If the dura or frontal lobes are involved, they are resected and the dural defect repaired with a fascial or pericranial graft. When the dura is uninvolved, the olfactory roots are divided at the cribriform plate. The involved skull base is then resected and reconstructed with a pericranial flap.

Preoperative imaging with a combination of CT and MRI can help assess the depth of invasion. On T1 and T2 MRI sequences, the ethmoid and orbital roofs appear as signal voids. Bone infiltration can be detected when the intermediate signal tumor disrupts the signal void of the cortex. CT provides better definition of cortical bone and is superior in the assessment of invasion of the cribriform plate (**Figures 4.85 and 4.86**).

Bones such as the clivus, with significant fatty marrow, are hyperintense on T1 sequences. Infiltration by tumor leads to replacement of fat with resultant T1 hypointensity. Fat saturated postgadolinium sequences will suppress normal marrow signal and help to delineate enhancing tumor. MRI is superior at demonstrating marrow involvement and dural and intracranial extension. Nodular enhancement and thickening of the dura or smooth thickening of more than 5 mm is considered 100 percent specific for dural invasion and 75 percent sensitive (**Figures 4.87A to C**). Linear dural enhancement less than 5 mm is more commonly regarded as a reactive nonneoplastic response to tumor rather than direct tumor invasion. The presence

Imaging of the paranasal sinuses 207

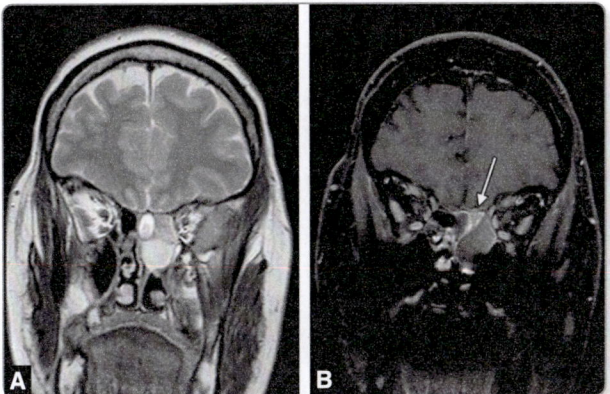

**Figures 4.85A and B** Inverted papilloma in the ethmoid region. The tumor extends up to the floor of the anterior cranial fossa. Coronal T2 MRI (A) shows an intact dark line representing the intact bony floor. Coronal postcontrast scan shows thin dural enhancement consistent with a dural reaction (arrow) (B)

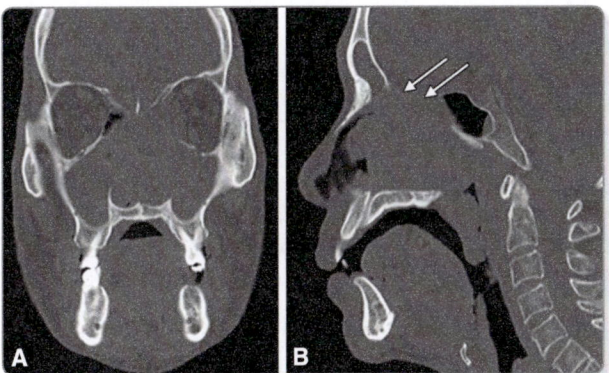

**Figures 4.86A and B** Coronal (A) and sagittal (B) CT in a patient with a sinonasal SCCa. Imaging shows erosion of the cribriform plates bilaterally. Sagittal image shows a fairly long segment of bony erosion (arrows). Coronal scan also shows left orbital invasion

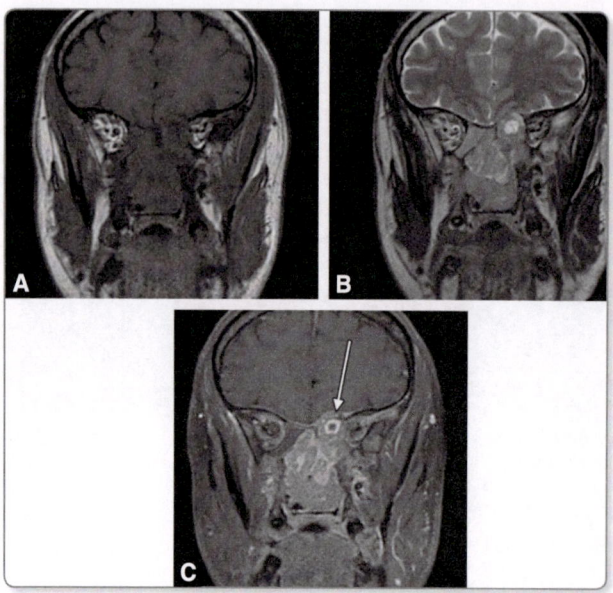

**Figures 4.87A to C** Tumor extension into the epidural space and dura on MRI. (A and B) Coronal T1 and T2 image of an SCCa shows loss of the signal void of the floor of the fovea and cribriform plate. (C) Coronal T1 postgadolinium better demonstrates the intracranial component of the tumor. Thickened dural enhancement is more consistent with dural invasion (arrow)

of cerebral T2 hyperintensity may be a manifestation of mass effect and displacement of the brain but may also indicate the presence of parenchyma invasion (**Figures 4.88A and B**).

## Orbital invasion

The periorbita is the condensed periosteum of the seven bones comprising the orbit and is continuous with the dura at the optic foramen and orbital fissures. It is a resilient barrier to tumor spread into the orbit. If tumor does not extend through the periorbita, orbital preservation with periosteal resection yields similiar survival to orbital exenteration, and maintains a functioning eye.

Imaging of the paranasal sinuses  209

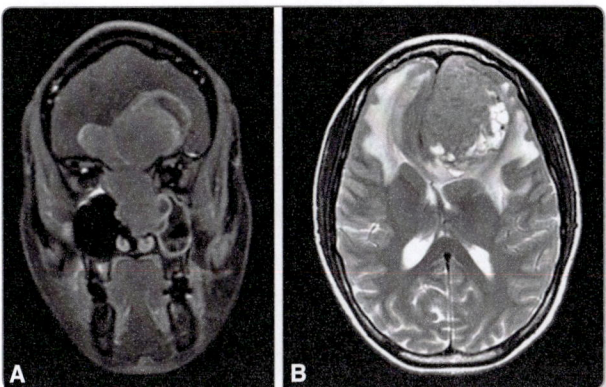

**Figures 4.88A and B** Coronal postcontrast T1 (A) and axial T2 (B) MRI of an esthesioneuroblastoma. The mass involves both the nasal cavity and anterior cranial fossa. The axial image shows significant T2 hyperintensity in the adjacent frontal lobe brain parenchyma. At surgery, no brain parenchymal invasion was present. The signal change represented reactive brain edema

Erosion of the medial and inferior bony orbital walls is accurately demonstrated with CT (**Figures 4.89A to C**). Assessment of the perorbita is difficult as the tumor may displace the periorbita and extraconal fat without invading it. The periorbita is also not visualized on CT. Frank Infiltration of the orbital fat, a nodular tumor/orbit interface, and enlargment of the extraocular muscles are reliable but late signs of periorbital extension (**Figures 4.90 and 4.91**).

On MRI, cortical bone and periorbita cannot be reliably distinguished as both demonstrate T1 and T2 hypointensity. However, invasion beyond the inner periorbita is of more importance. Sinonasal tumors are reliably hyperintense to periorbita and complete periorbital invasion is seen when the hypointense line, representing the combined bone/periorbita layer is not detected and tumor extends into the fat. Both CT and MRI are accurate at predicting periorbital invasion but lack sensitivity to exclude invasion. Definitive assessment is obtained at surgery with intraoperative frozen section.

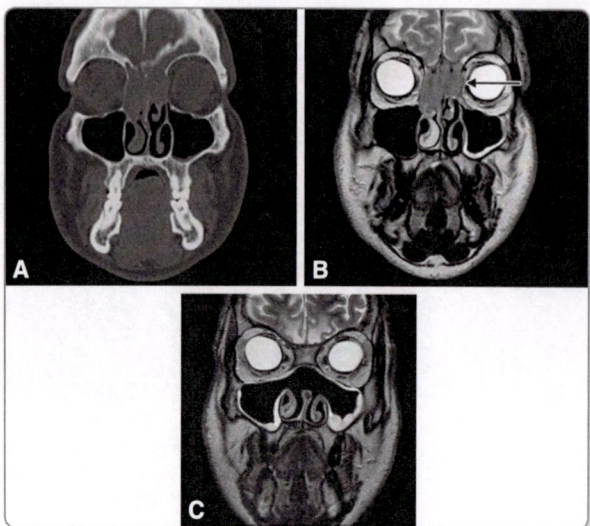

**Figures 4.89A to C** Assessment of orbital invasion. (A) Coronal CT demonstrates thinning and slight lateral bowing of the left medial orbital wall. (B) Coronal T2 MRI. A hypointense line is seen between the tumor and orbital contents, consistent with displaced but intact periorbita (arrow). (C) Coronal T2 after orbit preserving craniofacial resection. The periorbita was intact on frozen section and orbital exenteration was not required

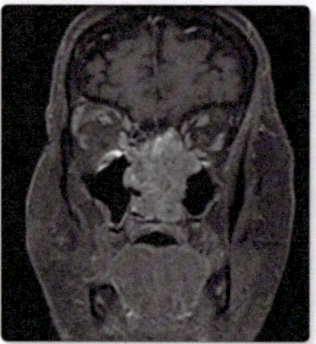

**Figure 4.90** Adenoid cystic carcinoma of the sinus. Coronal postcontrast scan shows an early bulge along the left inferomedial wall of the left orbit consistent with remodelling and an intact periorbita

Imaging of the paranasal sinuses 211

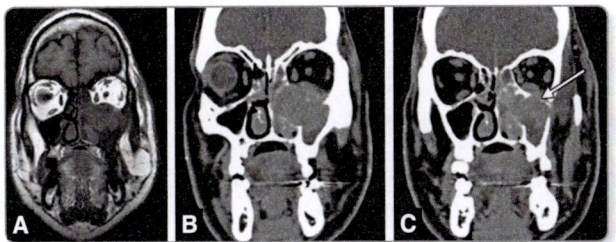

**Figures 4.91A to C** Coronal T1 MRI (A) and CT (B, C) of an adenocarcinoma. The tumor has breached the bony left orbital floor and has come into intimate contact with the inferior rectus muscle. Ill defined soft tissue is also infiltrating the orbital fat (arrow). Imaging is consistent with orbital invasion

## Perineural tumor spread

Perineural tumor invasion refers to microscopic tumor extension into any of the three layers of the nerve: perineurium, epineurium, endoneurium. It is not an extension along lymphatic channels but rather is the direct contiguous spread of tumor in microscopic continuity with the primary tumor mass. It is a common complication of sinonasal malignancy and tumors with a propensity to perineural spread include adenoid cystic carcinoma, squamous cell carcinoma, mucoepidermoid carcinoma, melanoma and sarcoma. Perineural tumor invasion provides another mechanism whereby sinonasal tumors can extend into the intracranial compartment. It is associated with decreased survival and increased locoregional recurrence. Its presence tumor can dramatically alter the patient's treatment plan as it usually renders the disease unresectable. As up to 40 percent of patients are clinically asymptomatic, radiological detection of disease is crucial.

Perineural tumor spread refers to the radiologic appearance of gross perineural tumor extension. Perineural tumor spread is covered in the chapter 10.

## Tumor subtypes

Some of the more common sinonasal lesions are reviewed below.

## Malignant lesions

### Squamous cell carcinoma

Squamous cell carcinoma is a malignant epithelial tumor demonstrating squamous differentiation. It is graded according to how well it resembles normal squamous epithelium and accounts for 60 to 80 percent of all malignancies. Around 50 to 60 percent arise in the maxillary sinus, with 15 to 20 percent in the nasal cavity, and 10 to 20 percent in the ethmoid sinus. Tumors arising from the frontal and sphenoid sinus constitute only 2 percent of cases.

Risk factors include occupational exposure to a variety of dust and chemicals including nickel, mineral oils, and chromium. Smoking is not a significant etiological factor. There are no specific imaging findings on CT or MRI. Imaging reveals a mildly enhancing soft tissue mass that is intermediate on T1- and T2-weighted imaging. Bony erosion is commonly seen.

### Adenocarcinoma

Adenocarcinomas (AC) are malignant neoplasms of glandular origin or tumors which demonstrate a gland-like cellular arrangement. They are the second most common sinonasal malignancy, accounting for 10 to 20 percent of cases. Histologically, they are classified into four categories: intestinal type AC, minor salivary gland, seromucinous and low grade not-otherwise-specified. They most commonly occur in the ethmoid sinuses and occupational exposure to wood dust is a strong risk factor.

Mucoepidermoid and adenoid cystic carcinomas are the most common salivary gland histological types. Adenoid cystic carcinoma is a slowly growing tumor with a propensity for perineural spread with high rates of local recurrence and distant metastases.

## Melanoma

Sinonasal melanomas constitute approximately 5 percent of malignant neoplasms and arise from melanocyte precursors normally present in the mucosa. Melanoma most often arises in the nasal cavity, along the anterior nasal septum, lateral nasal wall and inferior

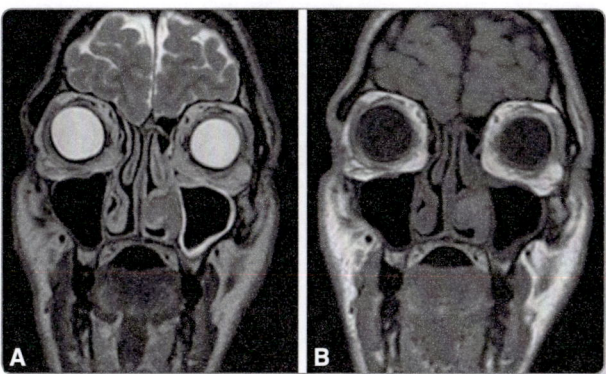

**Figures 4.92A and B** Coronal T2 (A) and T1 (B) MRI of sinonasal melanoma. There is a polypoid mass enlarging the inferior turbinate and involving the lower left lateral nasal wall. T1 hyperintensity is due to the presence of melanin

turbinate. On CT it appears as a lobular mass with bone remodeling. Melanotic melanomas demonstrate T1 hyperintensity and T2 hypointensity due to the presence of melanin and hemorrhage (**Figures 4.92A and B**). Amelanotic melanoma has a nonspecific appearance. Pigmentation of the lesion can be visualized at endoscopy.

## Olfactory neuroblastoma (Esthesioneuroblastoma)

Olfactory neruoblastoma is a rare malignant tumor derived from the specialized olfactory neuroepithelium of the upper nasal cavity. The tumor may spread to the ipsilateral ethmoid sinus and progress to invade the orbit and cross into the anterior cranial fossa. The bulk of the tumor may be intracranial and have a "dumbbell" shape due to focal narrowing as it extends through the cribriform region (**Figures 4.88 and 4.93**). Diffuse seeding of the dural and subdural space may occur. Cervical lymph node metastases occur in 5 percent at presentation and increase to 10 to 15 percent at 6 months. The Kadish clinical staging system is the most commonly used:

*Stage A*: Confined to the nasal cavity

*Stage B*: Involvement of one or more paranasal sinuses

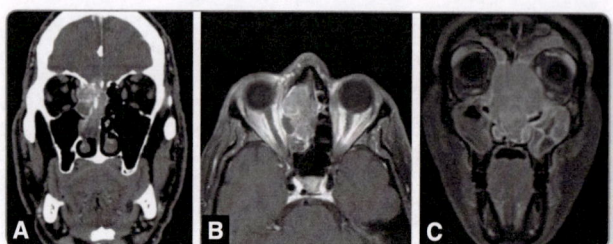

**Figures 4.93A to C** Esthesioneuroblastoma. (A and B) Coronal CT and axial contrast enhanced MRI shows a heterogeneous mass in the right nasal cavity. There is remodelling of the medial orbital wall on the right. The tumor has extended superiorly into the anterior cranial fossa. (C) A larger tumor filling the nasal cavity in another patient. Mild outwards bulge of both medial orbital walls is noted. Secondary retained secretions are present in the frontal and maxillary sinuses

*Stage C*: Extension beyond the nasal cavity and paranasal sinuses

*Stage D*: Regional lymph nodes or distant metastases.

On MRI, the tumor is isointense to hyperintense to gray matter on T1 and isointense to hyperintense on T2 imaging. There is heterogeneous enhancement. When present, T2 hyperintense cysts along the intracranial margin are highly suggestive of the diagnosis (See **Figures 4.88A and B**). CT may show both benign remodeling and erosive change.

## Sinonasal undifferentiated carcinoma

Sinonasal undifferentiated carcinoma (SNUC) is a poorly differentiated malignancy thought to arise from the Schneiderian mucosa of the sinonasal cavities. It is composed of undifferentiated pleomorphic cells arranged in nests with wide trabeculae. Some cases demonstrate neuroendocrine differentiation on immunohistochemistry. The disease is highly aggressive with a poor prognosis. There are no distinguishing imaging features.

# Benign lesions

## Inverted papilloma

Inverted papillomas are benign but locally aggressive epithelial neoplasms arising from the ectodermally derived mucosa of the nasal cavity and sinuses. They have a characteristic endophytic growth pattern with in-folding of the mucosa into the underlying stroma. Histology reveals the presence of nonkeratinized squamous, mucinous and surface ciliated cells. Treatment is frequently complicated by recurrence. In 5 percent of cases, there is an associated squamous carcinoma that may be present initially or develop later.

These tumors most commonly arise along the lateral nasal wall and spread into the adjacent sinuses. Despite their large volume, they are focally attached at their point of origin in the sinonasal cavity and in 90 percent of cases this can be identified on CT as an area of focal hyperostosis (**Figure 4.94**). Identification of the site of origin preoperatively may prevent unnecessary resection and decrease recurrence. Other CT findings include bone remodeling erosion. Small residual

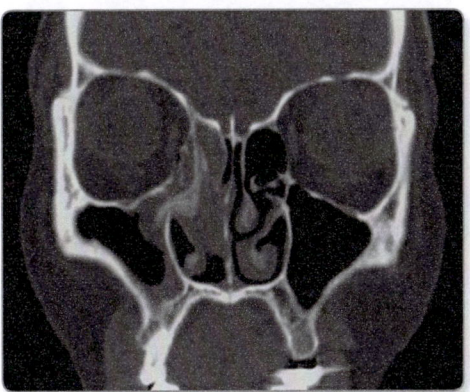

**Figure 4.94** Coronal CT of inverted papilloma. Note the focal area of hyperostosis along the lateral nasal wall extending into the maxillary sinus. This represented the site of origin of the inverted papilloma

bony fragments representing the remnants of resorbed bone may also be seen (**Figures 4.95A and B**). Extensive bone destruction is suspicious for an associated squamous carcinoma. The tumor appears as a nonspecific polypoid mass on CT.

On MRI, inverted papilloma may show a characteristic striated appearance. The epithelial tumor component appearing as a hypointense striation (due to its high cellularity) that alternates with the edematous hyperintense stroma (**Figures 4.96 and 4.97**). Another characteristic MRI finding is that of a cerebriform or crenulated appearance (**Figures 4.98A and B**).

## Angiofibroma

Juvenile angiofibroma is a rare benign unencapsulated vascular tumor that occurs exclusively in adolescent males. The lesion is composed of thin walled vessels without smooth muscle, in a fibrous stroma. Although benign, the tumor is locally aggressive. Nasal obstruction and epistaxis are the most common presenting symptoms. CT and MRI are important to assess tumor extent prior to surgery and detect recurrence.

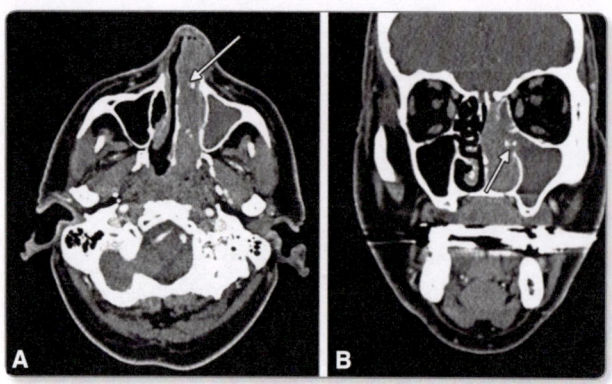

Figures 4.95A and B Inverted papilloma mass in the nasal cavity with obstructive left maxillary sinusitis demonstrating calcifications (arrows)

Imaging of the paranasal sinuses    **217**

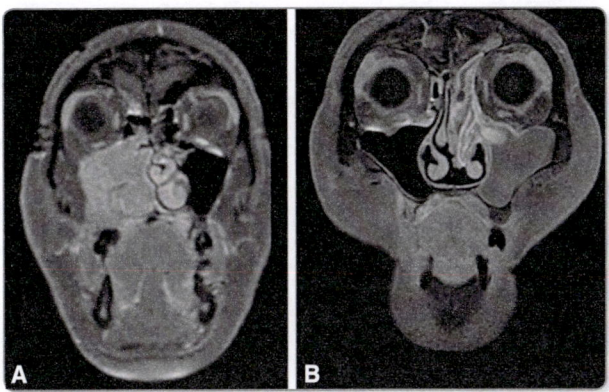

**Figures 4.96A and B** Inverted papilloma. (A) Shows an enhancing mass that involves the right nasal cavity and maxillary sinus. (B) Another patient showing a striated appearance of a left nasal cavity inverted papilloma

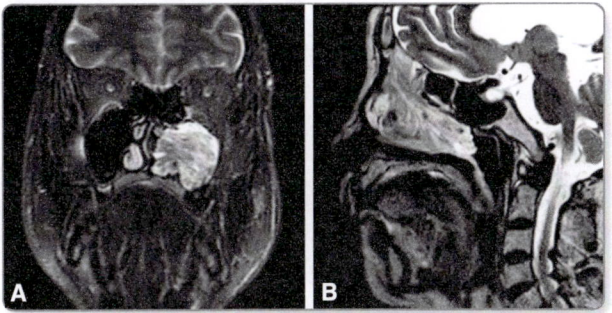

**Figures 4.97A and B** Two different patients demonstrating the striated appearance of inverted papilloma

The origin of the lesion is in the sphenopalatine foramen or adjacent pterygopalatine fossa. Tumor often can extend into the nasal cavity and possibly the nasopharynx via the sphenopalatine foramen (**Figure 4.99**). Laterally, the tumor can also directly invade the masticator space or invade anteriorly into the maxillary sinus (**Figures 4.100 and 4.101**). Tumor may also enter the orbit via the inferior orbital

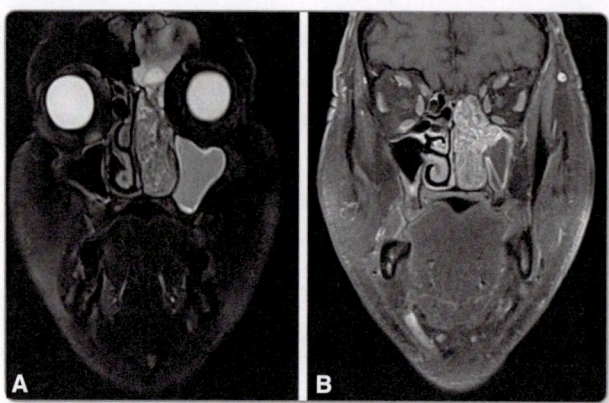

**Figures 4.98A and B** Coronal T2 and postcontrast T1 scans showing the cerebriform or cernulated appearance of a left nasal cavity inverted papilloma

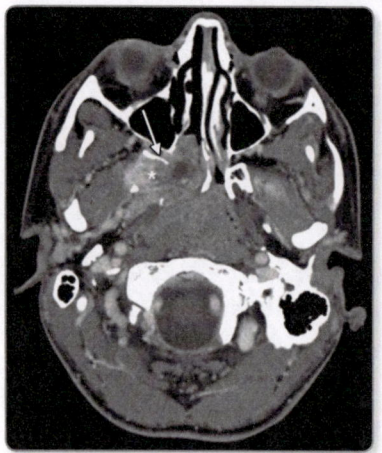

**Figure 4.99** Angiofibroma. Contrast CT shows an enhancing mass involving the right nasal cavity with extension laterally through the sphenopalatine foramen into the pterygopalatine fossa (arrow). Masticator space invasion is also present (*)

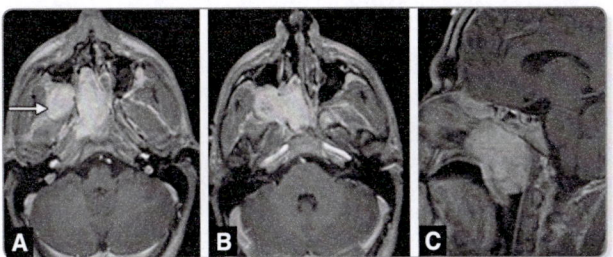

**Figures 4.100A to C** Axial (A, B) and sagittal (C) contrast MRI showing an enhancing mass involving the right nasal cavity and extending through a widened sphenopalatine foramen into the right masticator space (arrow)

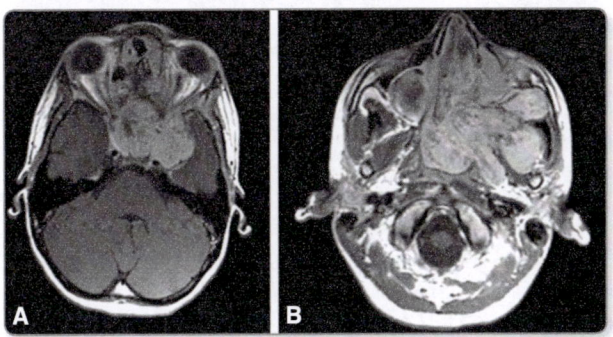

**Figures 4.101A and B** Very large angiofibroma with extension into the nasal cavity, sphenoid sinus and left masticator space. The left cavernous sinus is also infiltrated

fissure and the middle cranial fossa via the superior orbital fissure or by direct extension (**Figures 4.102A and B**). Juvenile angiofibroma can also cause simple pressure erosion and remodeling at the base of the pterygoid process. It can also invade into the body and greater wing of sphenoid. Intracranial extension can occur via extension along neuroforamina or through direct bony invasion.

CT shows an enhancing tumor with an epicenter at the sphenopalatine foramen that extends laterally into the pterygopalatine

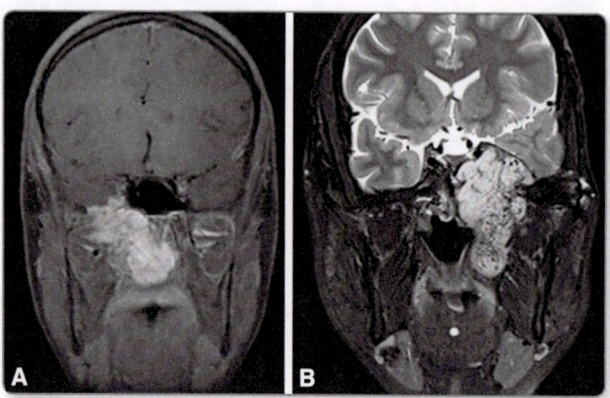

**Figures 4.102A and B** Two coronal images showing intracranial extension via direct superior infiltration through the floor of the middle cranial fossa. Note flow void signals on the MRI image

fossa and masticator space. The lesion characteristically shows avid enhancement due to its inherent vascularity. On MRI, flow voids may also be seen. Invasion into the sphenoid bone marrow be demonstrated on postcontrast fat saturated T1 images (**Figure 4.102**). Catheter angiography will show a vascular supply via the internal maxillary artery (**Figure 4.103**).

## Fibro-osseous lesions

Osteomas are benign bone-forming tumor. They are the most common tumor of the sinonasal cavities, found in 3 percent of all CT sinus examinations 80 percent occur in the frontal sinus. They arise from the sinus wall and project into the available space of the lumen (**Figures 4.104A to C**). There are two categories of osteoma: cortical and fibrous. Cortical osteomas are highly mineralized, resembling cortical bone while fibrous types have a ground glass density. They are asymptomatic unless they obstruct the sinus ostium or extend into adjacent structures. Possible complications can include secondary mucocele formation, CSF leak and pneumocephalus. CT can easily

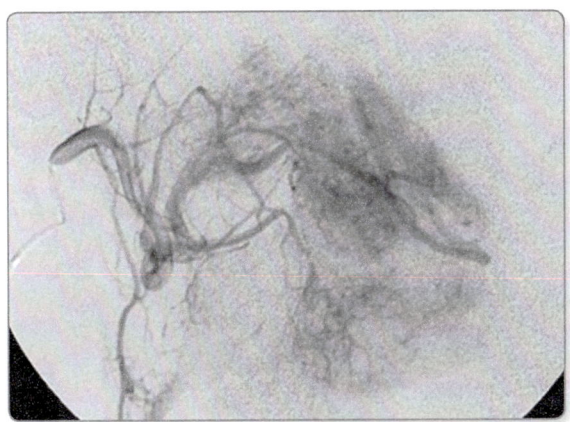

**Figure 4.103** Catheter angiography of angiofibroma. Injection of the internal maxillary artery shows large vascular tumor blush

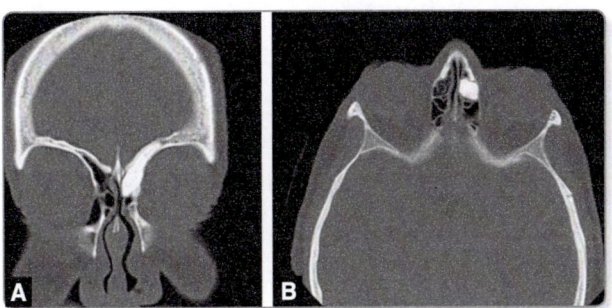

**Figures 4.104A and B** Osteoma. Coronal and axial CT image showing a dense cortical osteoma in the left frontal sinus that projects into the frontoethmoid recess

identify the presence of osteomas and nicely depicts the degree of mineralization. On MRI, cortical osteomas appear as signal voids and may be difficult to detect.

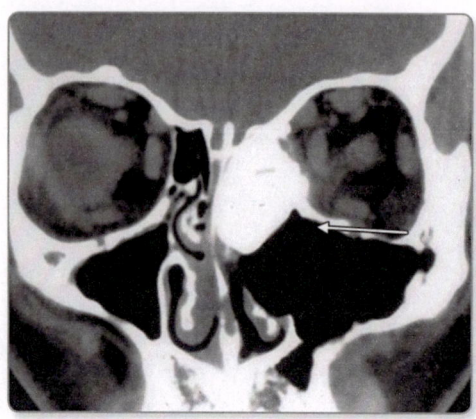

**Figure 4.104C** Benign osteoma of the ethmoid sinus with medial orbital periosteitis

## Fibrous dysplasia

Fibrous dysplasia is a non-neoplastic, developmental disorder of bone characterized by replacement of medullary bone with fibrous tissue and immature woven bone. Involvement of a single bone or multiple bones may occur. While osteomas project into the lumen of the sinus and are surrounded by normal sinus walls, fibrous dysplasia manifests as an expansion of the diplopic space of the sinus wall. Obstruction of ostiomeatal channels may result.

On CT, the density will vary according to the degree of mineralization of the fibrous tissue. Areas of lucency and the characteristic ground glass mineralization on CT are evident. On MRI, signal intensity is generally low to intermediate on T1 and T2, with T2 hyperintense foci corresponding to fibrous tissue with poor mineralization. These fibrous components often enhance avidly, resulting in a heterogeneous appearance on postgadolinium T1 sequences that can be mistaken for malignant tumor if CT correlation is not available (**Figures 4.105 and 4.106**).

Imaging of the paranasal sinuses 223

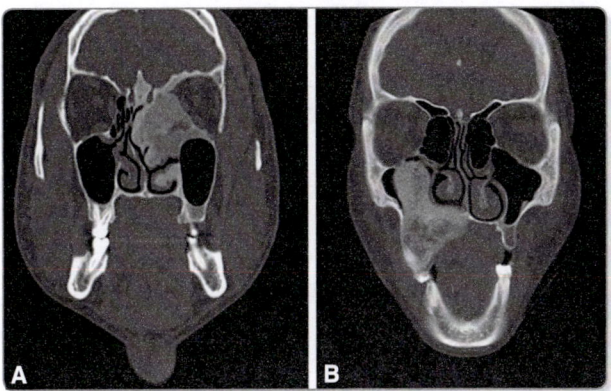

**Figures 4.105A and B** Coronal CT in two different patients with fibrous dysplasia. The scan shows characteristic bony expansion with an internal ground glass matrix. First image shows involvement of the left ethmoid and nasal cavity. The crista galli and supraorbital roof are also involved. The second patient has involvement of the right maxillary alveolus and hard palate

## Congenital disorders

### Congenital frontonasal masses

Congenital midline nasal masses are rare, occurring in 1/20000 to 1/40000 births. They result from failure of separation of neural and surface ectoderm during development of the nasofrontal region. In early life, there is transient separation between the nasal and frontal bones called the fonticulus nasofrontalis. A prenasal space temporarily separates the posterior margin of the nasal bone from the anterosuperior nasal cartilage. A foramen cecum also exists. This is a small opening between the frontal and ethmoid bones. A dural diverticulum extends from the anterior cranial fossa, through the foramen cecum and into the prenasal space. This tract reaches skin at the nasal bridge-osteocartilaginous junction. This dural diverticulum normally regresses. Abnormal regression of this tract may lead to frontonasal masses including nasal dermal sinus and congenital inclusion cyst, frontoethmoidal cepahalocele or nasal glioma. These abnormalities may be intranasal, extranasal or both.

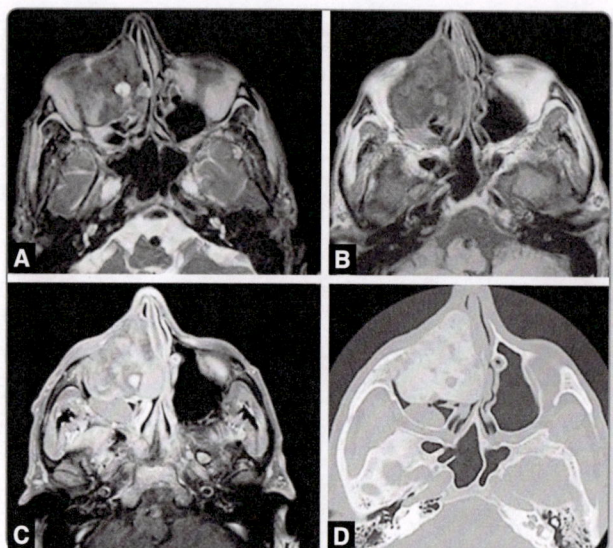

**Figures 4.106A to D** MRI and CT of fibrous dysplasia. (A to C) Axial T2, T1 and postcontrast MRI shows the large heterogenous mass filling much of the right maxillary antrum. Areas of cystic change are evident. The MRI appearance would not be out of keeping with an aggressive neoplasm. (D) CT scan demonstrates the mass to be fibrous dysplasia. Characteristic bony expansion and internal ground glass density are highly consistent with FD

MRI is the imaging modality of choice as it is able to delineate brain, CSF and cartilage. Sagittal and axial T1 and T2 are the most useful sequences, and slice thickness should be 3 mm or less with a FOV of 12 to 14 cm. Diffusion imaging aids in the detection of epidermoid cysts.

## Nasal dermal sinus

The regressing dural diverticulum may pull skin into the prenasal space resulting in an epithelial lined tract that has variable extension from the skin towards the crista galli. A dermoid (**Figures 4.107A to C**) or epidermoid cyst may occur along the course of the sinus in 50 percent of cases. Intracranial extension occurs in 20 percent of cases.

Imaging of the paranasal sinuses 225

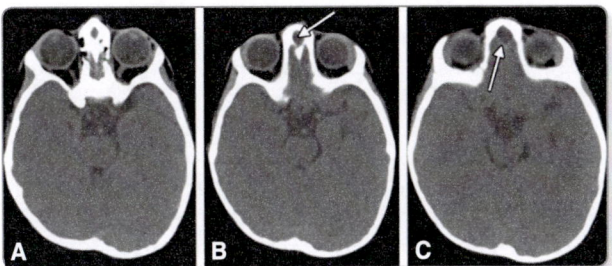

**Figures 4.107A to C** Axial CT images shows the presence of a frontonasal region dermoid (arrows). *Courtesy* of Dr Suzanne Laughlin, Hospital for Sick Children, Toronto, Canada

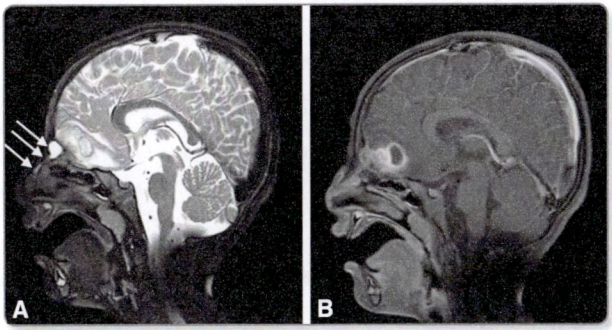

**Figures 4.108A and B** Sagittal T2 and postcontrast T1 imaging shows a nasal dermal sinus (arrows) complicated by a frontal lobe abscess. *Courtesy* of Dr Suzanne Laughlin, Hospital for Sick Children, Toronto, Canada

Affected patients will be at risk of meningitis and cerebritis (**Figures 4.108A and B**). The objective of imaging is to determine the extent of the tract to guide surgical therapy, and identify an associated dermoid or epidermoid cyst.

On MRI, a nasal dermal sinus is seen as a linear T1 hypointensity and T2 hyperintensity extending from the subcutaneous tissue of the nasal bridge into the prenasal space. Cysts within the tract, demonstrating restricted diffusion is consistent with an epidermoid. Dermoid cysts contain fatty components that are T1 hyperintense and suppress on T2 fat saturated imaging. An intracranial dermoid or epidermoid cyst may enlarge the foramen cecum or result in a bifid crista gall that can be seen on CT.

## Nasal gliomas

Nasal gliomas are not true neoplasms but are composed of dysplastic neurogenic tissue that become isolated from the subarachnoid space during dural regression. They have no connection to the intracranial compartment and present as an extranasal subcutaneous mass on the dorsum of the nose, or as an intranasal mass involving the lateral nasal wall more commonly than the septum. On MRI they are non-enhancing, rounded or polypoid lesions that are T1 iso/hypointense and T2 hyperintense to gray matter.

## Frontoethmoidal encephaloceles (Figure 4.109)

Nonseparation of neural and surface ectoderm during development can secondarily result in mesodermal defects. Encephaloceles are herniations of brain parenchyma and dura through a defect in the skull with a persistent connection to the subarachnoid space. Meningoceles are herniations of CSF. Frontoethmoidal encephaloceles are either nasofrontal or nasoethmoidal. Nasofrontal encephaloceles project through the nasofontanelle between the nasal and frontal bones into the glabellar region. Nasoethmoidal encephaloceles herniate through the foramen cecum into the prenasal space and nasal cavity. MRI demonstrates the herniated parenchymal tissue, which is isointense to gray matter on T1 and hyperintense on T2 and in continuity with the brain.

## Choanal atresia (Figures 4.110A and B)

Choanal atresia refers to obliteration of the posterior aperture of the nasal cavity and occurs in 1 to 7000 to 8000 live births. In 90 percent of cases, the narrowing is osseous due to incomplete canalization of the choanae. Membranous obstruction is due to failure to reabsorb epithelial plugs that fill the nasal cavity during development. Bilateral atresia presents at birth with respiratory distress as neonates are

Imaging of the paranasal sinuses 227

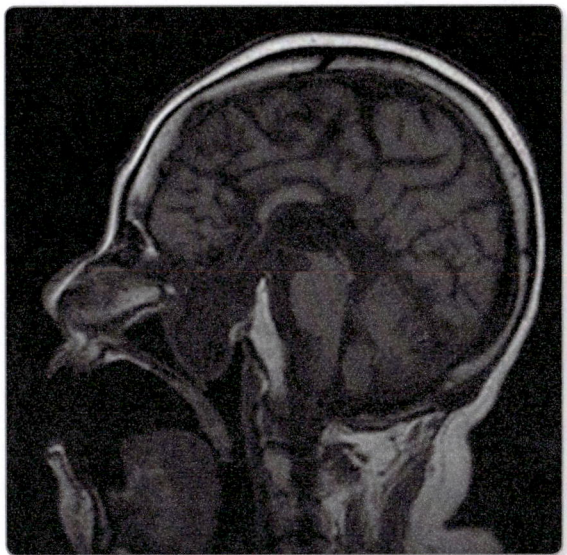

**Figure 4.109** Sagittal T1-weighted image shows a large inferiorly protruding CSF collection. There is a large defect in the floor of the sella and sphenoid body. Sphenoid meningocele

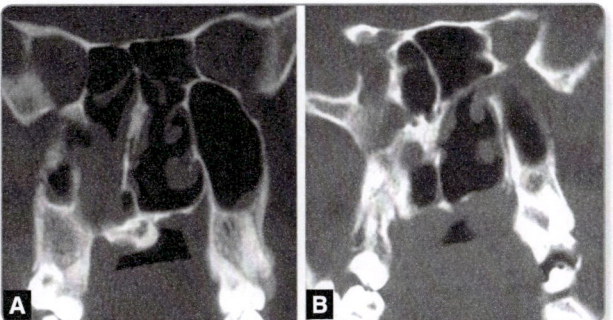

**Figures 4.110A and B** Bony and choanal atresia. Asymmetry of the right nasal cavity lumen with narrowing of the bony aperture and membranous remnants in the lumen is seen

obligate nose breathers. 50 percent of cases have unilateral disease which presents later in life with nasal obstruction.

The diagnosis is suggested by failure to pass a catheter more than 32 mm from the nose to the oropharynx and is confirmed with CT. Images should be obtained at 1mm slice thickness or less with measurements taken on the bone algorithm reformations angled 5 to 10 degrees to the hard palate. The choanal airspace is measured from the lateral wall of the nasal cavity to the vomer and values less than 0.34 cm in children under 2 years, is diagnostic. Other findings include hypertrophy of the vomer and thickening and in-drawing of the posterior maxilla.

# Bibliography

1. Chong VF, et al. Functional endoscopic sinus surgery (FESS): What radiologists need to know. Clinical radiology 1998;53(9):650-8.
2. Hoang JK, et al. Multiplanar sinus CT: A systematic approach to imaging before functional endoscopic sinus surgery. AJR. American journal of roentgenology 2010;194(6):W527-36.
3. Kubal WS. Sinonasal imaging: malignant disease. Seminars in ultrasound, CT and MR 1999;20(6):402-25.
4. Mafee MF, JM Chow, R Meyers. Functional endoscopic sinus surgery: Anatomy, CT screening, indications, and complications. AJR. American journal of roentgenology 1993;160(4):735-44.
5. Raghavan P, Phillips CD. Magnetic resonance imaging of sinonasal malignancies. Top Magn Reson Imaging 2007;18(4):259-67.
6. Shankar L, Evans K. An atlas of the imaging of the paranasal sinuses, Second edition- Informa Health Care Publisher, 2006.
7. Som PM, et al. Sinonasal tumors and inflammatory tissues: Differentiation with MR imaging. Radiology 1988;167(3):803-8.
8. Stammberger HR, Kennedy DW. Paranasal sinuses:anatomic terminology and nomenclature. The Anatomic Terminology Group. The Annals of otology, rhinology & laryngology. Supplement 1995;167:7-16.

# Diseases of the nasopharynx

**chapter 5**

Manas Sharma, Eugene Yu, Peter Yang

**ABSTRACT**
Review of inflammatory, infectious and neoplastic entities that affect the nasopharynx are covered.

**KEYWORDS**
Nasopharynx, anatomy, CT, MRI.

## Anatomy

The nasopharynx (NP) is the most superior part of the aerodigestive tract. It is bounded superiorly by the floor of the sphenoid sinus and clivus and inferiorly by the plane of the palate (**Figure 5.1**). Laterally, the parapharyngeal space separates the NP from the masticator space while the posterior aspect is bounded by the prevertebral musculature. The plane of the posterior choana separates the NP from the nasal cavity. The nasopharyngeal mucosa predominantly consists of squamous epithelium and is reinforced by a muscular and fascial sling consisting of the superior constrictor muscle and the buccopharyngeal fascia (BPF) which is derived from the middle layer of the deep cervical fascia. Another fascia called the pharyngobasilar fascia (PBF) extends from the upper free edge of the superior constrictor muscle to the skull base. A defect in the PBF called the sinus of Morgagni allows for the passage of the Eustachian tube and the intrapharyngeal portion of the levator veli palatini muscle on either side. On cross sectional imaging one of the main anatomic imaging landmarks is the torus tubarius (TT) or the cartilaginous portion of the eustachian tube. The torus tubarius appears as a protrusion along the posterolateral wall on either side of the nasopharynx. The fossa of Rosenmüller or the lateral pharyngeal recess is situated just medial to the TT.

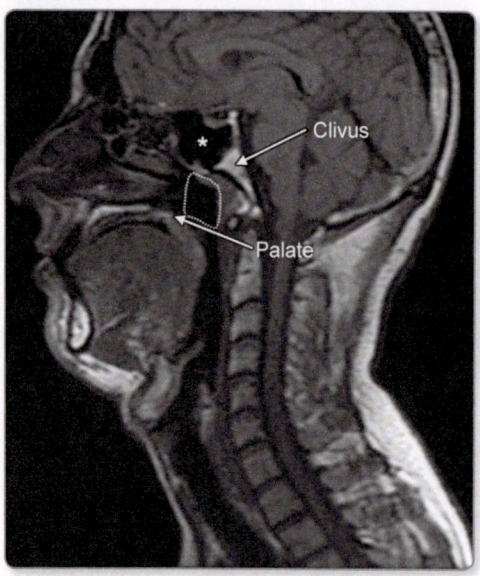

**Figure 5.1** Sagittal T1 weighted image shows the outline of the nasopharynx which is delineated superiorly by the sphenoid sinus (*) and clivus. The inferior margin is the plane of the palate

---

# Imaging of the nasopharynx

The central location of the nasopharynx allows for the possibility of disease extension into several key adjacent anatomic areas such as the bony central skull base, the cavernous sinus as well as the parapharyngeal and masticator spaces. These adjacent anatomic spaces can be difficult to evaluate clinically and therefore imaging plays an important role in the accurate delineation the various disease processes that can involve the nasopharynx.

CT and MRI are complementary for imaging of the nasopharynx. Multiplanar reconstructions of volumetric CT data acquired on modern multidetector CT provides not only excellent bony detail but also a good overview of the nasopharyngeal soft tissues. MRI also provides excellent soft tissue detail and is vital in the delineation of disease extent. MRI can also show subtle bone marrow signal alterations that can reflect early disease involvement.

Imaging protocols for NP assessment will differ from institution to institution and are influenced by the individual preferences of radiologists. CT protocols for evaluating the nasopharynx and central skull base at our center consists of axial postcontrast imaging of the head and neck with sagittal and coronal soft tissue and bone reformations. MRI is performed routinely with a head and neck coil and consists of sagittal, axial and coronal T1, axial and coronal fat saturated T2 imaging. Gadolinium enhanced, fat saturated T1 weighted images are acquired in the axial and coronal planes. The level of coverage for both modalities extends from the level of the lateral ventricles down to the aortic arch.

# Diseases of the nasopharynx

The nasopharynx can be affected by a variety of diseases. Some of the more common entities are discussed:

## Nasopharyngitis

Nasopharyngitis is inflammation of the soft tissues of the NP. It can arise as a complication of the common cold. In its acute form it is usually a self-limiting mucosal inflammatory condition while more chronic nasopharyngitis may result from infection of hypertrophied tissue in the nasopharyngeal cavity. Nasopharyngitis can also arise secondary to the ingestion or exposure to caustic agents (**Figure 5.2**). It can also arise secondary to radiation therapy. Imaging of nasopharyngitis will reveal the presence of enhancement and edema of the NP.

# Nasopharyngeal cysts

## Retention cysts

These are simple, submucosal cysts located in the midline or off midline. They are often visualized incidentally on imaging and are usually asymptomatic. They may be single or multiple.

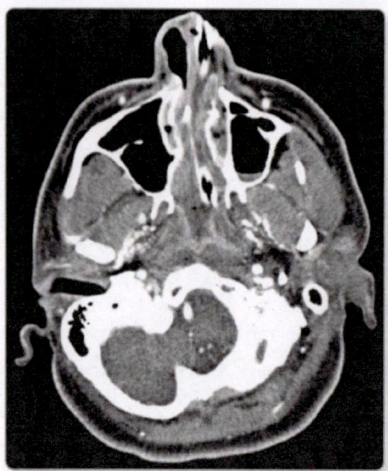

**Figure 5.2** Contrast CT scan demonstrating nasopharyngitis in a patient who ingested acid during an attempted suicide. The nasopharyngeal mucosa is inflamed as evidenced by enhancement and edema

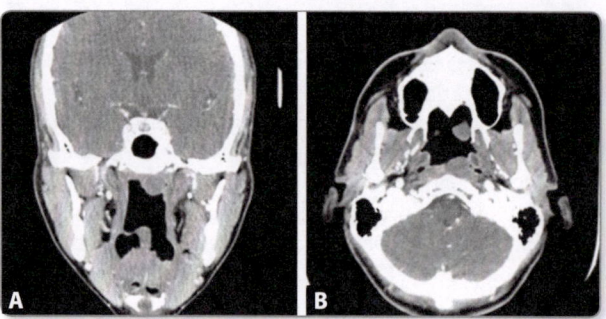

**Figures 5.3A and B** Off-midline simple cystic lesion along the nasopharyngeal mucosa is more suggestive of retention cyst

On imaging, they appear as a non-enhancing or rim-enhancing simple cyst (**Figures 5.3A and B**). Usually, they are T1 hypo- and T2 hyperintense. The presence of proteinaceous cystic content may result in T1 hyperintensity. Cysts may appear pear-shaped if located in the lateral pharyngeal recess.

## Tornwaldt cysts

Also called a pharyngeal bursa, these posterior midline cystic lesions are often detected incidentally on cross-sectional imaging for other purposes. They are most commonly detected in the second or third decades, with no sexual predilection. In a review of reports of thousands of CT and MRI exams, investigators found an incidence of Tornwaldt cyst in 0.01 percent of CT's and 0.1 percent of MRI's.

Developmentally, the pharyngeal bursa represents a potential space where the notochord retains its union with the pharyngeal ectoderm. Adenoidectomy has also been implicated as a possible etiologic factor. Presumably this is due to injury to the pharyngeal duct orifice with resulting inflammation that may progress to infection and subsequent cyst development.

Tornwaldt cysts can become symptomatic should they become infected and give rise to fever, pharyngeal pain and swelling. Other symptoms may include postnasal drip, halitosis, headaches, and neck pain. Middle ear symptoms due to Eustachian tube dysfunction can also arise.

An imaging differential diagnosis would include retention cysts, encephalocele, and meningocele. Imaging reveals a low density lesion in the midline along the posterior roof of the nasopharynx on CT (**Figure 5.4**). MRI can show high signal intensity within the cyst on both T1 and T2 weighted images. High T1 signal and or low T2 signal within the cyst suggests the presence of proteinaceous material or hemorrhage. An uncomplicated cyst shows no surrounding soft tissue changes (**Figures 5.5A to D**). Intracystic calcification may also be visualized (**Figure 5.6**).

# Lymphoid hyperplasia/hyperplastic adenoid

Adenoid hyperplasia is the excessive enlargement of the lymphoid tissue located posteriorly in the nasopharyngeal wall. This tissue is a part of the Waldeyer's ring. The adenoids normally become quite

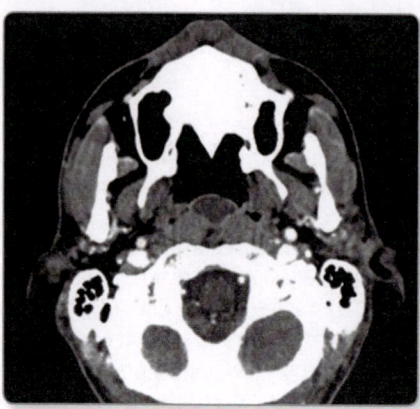

**Figure 5.4** Hypoattenuating posterior midline cyst in the nasopharynx

large during the first year of life and reach their greatest size in mid-childhood receding thereafter. When enlarged in reaction to foreign bodies and infective processes, the adenoids can potentially obstruct the airway and effect breathing and voice. Chronic infection, either viral or bacterial, can keep adenoids enlarged for years even in adults.

Primary causes of the adenoid hyperplasia include various bacterial and viral infections and allergy. Symptoms that may develop include mouth breathing and a change in voice. Grossly enlarged adenoids may obstruct the Eustachian tubes and result in secondary otitis media. Sinusitis may also develop as a complication.

Cross-sectional imaging will show the enlarged lymphoid tissue as a lobulated a soft tissue mass confined to the nasopharynx. The mass may have a somewhat "crenulated" or striated appearance and have small interspersed foci of trapped air (**Figures 5.7A and B**).

Treatment for adenoid hyperplasia is symptomatic and may also involve the use of antibiotics and adenoidectomy.

## Juvenile angiofibroma

Juvenile angiofibroma (JAF) is a benign, vascular, non-encapsulated, locally invasive nasopharyngeal mass found almost exclusively in

Diseases of the nasopharynx 235

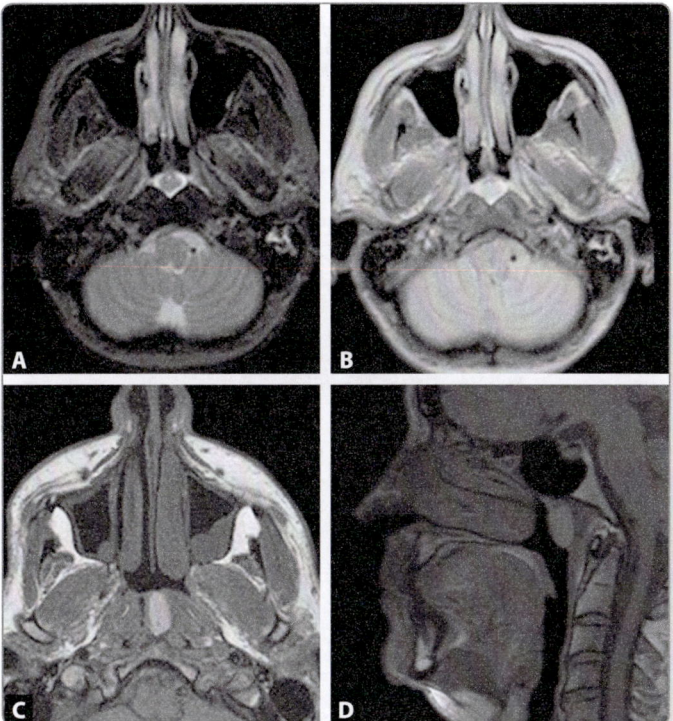

**Figures 5.5A to D** Axial T2 (A) postcontrast T1 (B) and unenhanced T1 (C) imaging showing examples of Tornwaldt cysts. The high T1 signal is compatible with proteinaceous cystic content. (D) Sagittal T1 image of a high signal Tornwaldt cyst

adolescent males. It comprises 0.5 percent of all head and neck neoplasms. The tumor can be locally aggressive with extension into adjacent anatomic compartments including the skull base.

The JAF presents in an adolescent male with unilateral nasal obstruction in 90 percent of patients and epistaxis in 60 percent. Pain, unilateral swelling, proptosis, nasal voice, discharge, serous otitis media, anosmia are other potential complications.

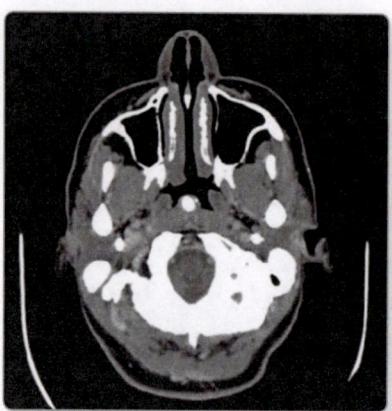

**Figure 5.6** Calcified Tornwaldt cyst

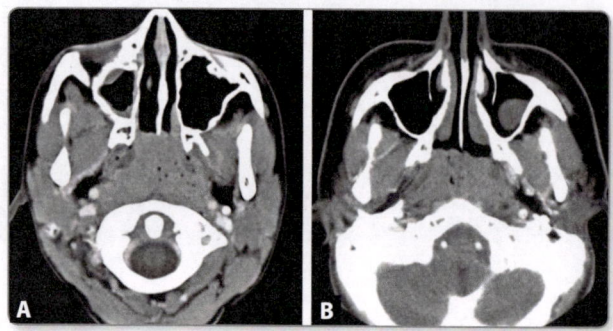

**Figures 5.7A and B** Two CT examples of lymphoid hyperplasia. The young age of the patient and the presence of interspersed foci of air are imaging clues suggestive of lymphoid hyperplasia

The JAF is a highly vascular tumor and biopsy should to be performed with extreme caution due to the risk of hemorrhage. Preferred treatment consists of complete surgical resection. Adjuvant radiation can also be used in instances of incomplete resection. Preoperative embolization is helpful to reduce blood loss.

# Diseases of the nasopharynx

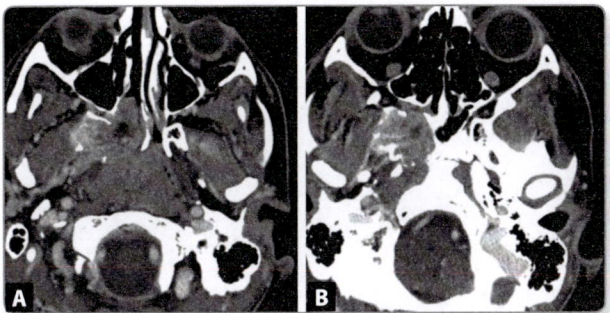

**Figures 5.8A and B** Contrast enhanced CT of a 14-year male patient with an eccentrically located enhancing vascular nasopharyngeal mass. Note the lateral extension into the right masticator space

On imaging, JAF appears as an enhancing mass centered at the sphenopalatine foramen (**Figures 5.8A and B**) and extending into the posterior nasal cavity, nasopharynx and pterygopalatine fossa with or without extension into the skull base. There is a propensity for early involvement of upper medial pterygoid lamina with extension into the sphenoid sinus in 60 percent. The lesion may infiltrate into the maxillary and ethmoid sinuses, masticator space, and inferior orbital fissure or even to the middle cranial fossa via the vidian canal or foramen rotundum (**Figures 5.9A to E**).

MRI reveals an avidly enhancing, heterogeneous mass on T1 weighted imaging. JAF shows intermediate to high T2 signal and the presence of punctate and serpentine flow voids. Postcontrast coronal T1 imaging with fat saturation is helpful to delineate involvement the cavernous sinus and skull base.

On angiography, an intense capillary blush fed by enlarged feeding vessels from the external carotid artery is seen (**Figure 5.10**).

## Nasopharyngeal tuberculosis

Tuberculous involvement of the nasopharynx may be primary, without involvement of any other system, or secondary to pulmonary or

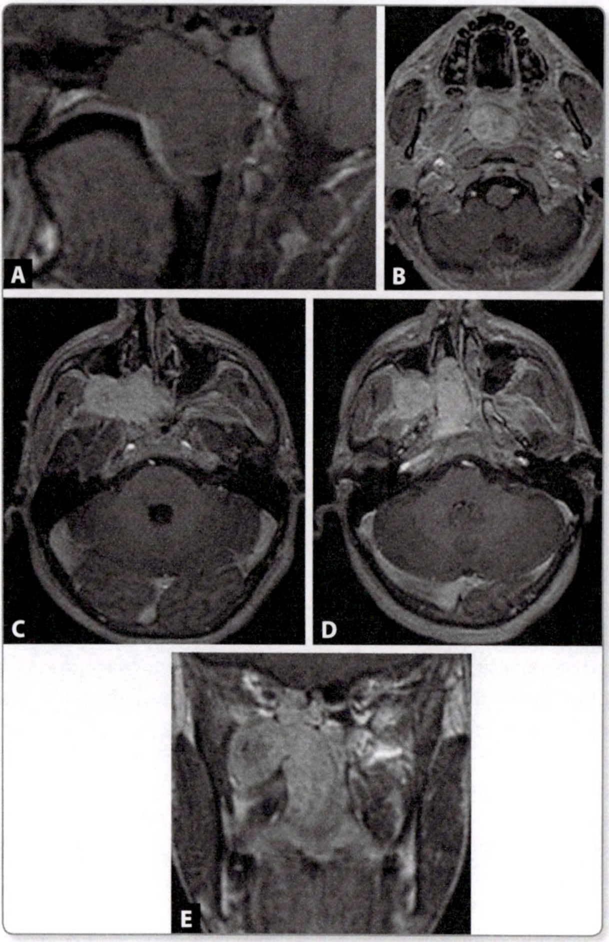

**Figures 5.9A to E** Juvenile angiofibroma appears as a homogeneous mass with isointense T1 signal (A). The lesion shows avid enhancement on the postgadolinium images (B–E). The tumor epicenter is in the region of the sphenopalatine foramen but extends laterally into the pterygopalatine fossa and masticator space and medially into the nasopharynx

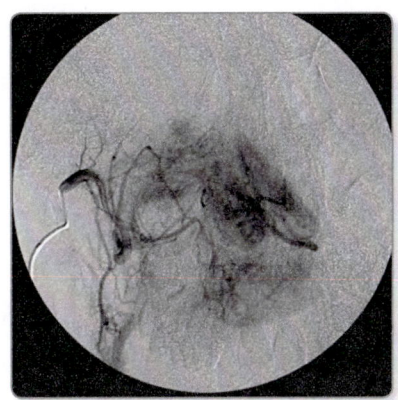

**Figure 5.10** Intense vascular blush seen on this selective angiogram of the right internal maxillary artery

extrapulmonary disease. Primary involvement is more common and can arise due to reactivation of dormant acid-fast bacilli in the adenoids or direct mucosal infection after inhalation of the bacilli. Secondary infection can arise via hematogenous or lymphatic spread from a primary focus or during bacillary expectoration.

Presenting features can include nasal obstruction, mouth breathing and snoring. ESR is elevated and the Mantoux test is usually strongly positive. Chest imaging may show evidence of pulmonary tuberculosis. On clinical examination a pink, glistening polypoidal mass or a mucosal plaque with or without ulceration is noted.

CT imaging reveals a nonspecific, moderately enhancing mucosal mass with preservation of surrounding fat planes. The adjacent bony structures are usually not involved. Cervical lymphadenopathy is common.

MRI can show a focal enhancing mucosal mass or mucosal thickening. Moderate contrast enhancement is present (**Figures 5.11A to C**).

Differential considerations would include nasopharyngeal carcinoma, lymphoma or Wegener's granulomatosis. Syphilis, leprosy and fungal diseases although rare, may give rise to a similar appearance.

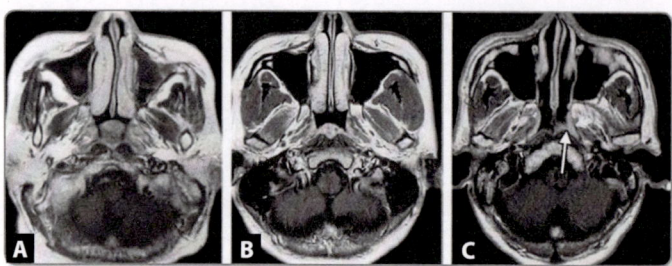

**Figures 5.11A to C** Axial gadolinium enhanced imaging from three different patients with proven nasopharyngeal tuberculosis. (A, B) The presence of an enhancing nasopharyngeal mass. (C) An area of focal mucosal thickening and enhancement along the left lateral and posterolateral wall (arrow). These features can mimic nasopharyngeal carcinoma. *Courtesy*: AD King, AT Ahuja, GMK Tse, ACA van Hasselt, ABW Chan. MR Imaging Features of Nasopharyngeal Tuberculosis: Report of Three Cases and Literature Review. AJNR 2003;24(2), 279-82, © American Society of Neuroradiology (Images used with permission of the ASNR)

Tuberculosis can also coexist with malignancy. Although diagnosis can be made by PCR or by isolation of Mycobacterium tuberculosis, biopsy is required to exclude malignancy.

## Nasopharyngeal carcinoma

Nasopharyngeal carcinoma (NPC) is the most common neoplasm to affect the nasopharynx. NPC is a locally aggressive neoplasm that has a high incidence of neck adenopathy. It is most common in the Asian population and is endemic in southern China with a yearly incidence between 15 to 50 cases per hundred thousand people.

The NPC arises secondary to an interplay between genetic and environmental factors. N-nitrosodimethylamines present in the southern Asian diet is considered a likely contributory carcinogen. An association with Epstein-Barr virus has also been well documented. There are three histological subtypes of NPC: Type 1 is the least common, and occurs in non-endemic and endemic areas and is similar to the squamous carcinoma affecting other locations in the pharyngeal mucosal space. Type II is a nonkeratinizing carcinoma. Type III consists of undifferentiated epithelial cells mixed with nonmalignant T lymphocytes.

The NPC can be asymptomatic or present with the development of a neck mass related to lymph node enlargement. Nasal obstruction and eustachian dysfunction leading to otitis media are also common presentations. Advanced disease can also present with cranial nerve dysfunction, trismus and headache. NPC has a propensity for perineural spread mostly along the mandibular division of the trigeminal nerve. NPC has the highest incidence of distant metastasis among the head and neck cancers, with bone, lung and liver disease being the most commonly affected areas.

Treatment primarily consists of radiation therapy with adjuvant chemotherapy also used in higher stage disease. Imaging is critical for accurate staging and thereby guiding treatment. MRI is the current modality of choice, although CT scan can help provide additional information as to the status of the bony skull base. MRI is usually better in assessing the primary tumor extent, cavernous sinus extension, retropharyngeal adenopathy and perineural disease.

Nasopharyngeal carcinoma appears as a mildly T2 hyperintense and T1 intermediate signal mucosal based mass. Early disease often arises in the lateral pharyngeal recess (**Figures 5.12 to 5.14**). Tumor can extend laterally and disrupt the pharyngobasilar fascia and thereby extend into the adjacent parapharyngeal space (**Figures 5.15A and B**). As tumors enlarge, they will also extend into the more laterally located masticator space. Nodal metastases are present in 90 percent of cases at presentation, with retropharyngeal and upper cervical adenopathy seen most commonly.

Bony invasion is evident by marrow signal alterations in the clivus and sphenoid sinus floor on MRI (**Figures 5.16A and B**). More extensive disease can also extend back to involve the longus musculature, occipital condyles and C1 and C2 vertebral bodies (**Figure 5.17**). Thin slice CT is helpful for the assessment of bony erosions. Both sclerosis and or lytic change can be seen on CT.

Disease that has extended into the masticator space can also invade and spread along the V3 division of the trigeminal nerve

## 242 Introductory head and neck imaging

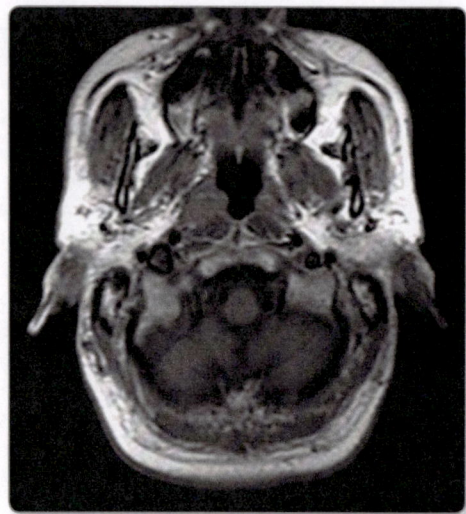

**Figure 5.12** Axial T1 weighted image shows a small isointense mass in the right lateral pharyngeal recess

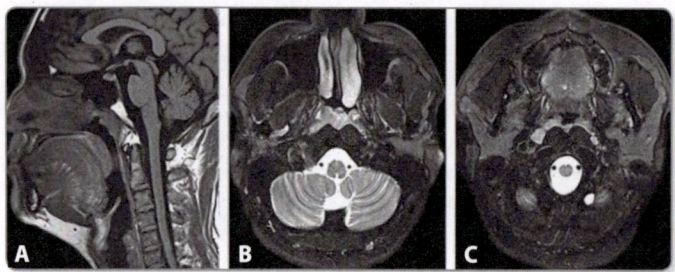

**Figures 5.13A to C** Sagittal T1 (A) weighted image showing an irregular mucosal based T1-isointense mass with hyperintense appearance on T2 axial images (B, C) typical of nasopharyngeal carcinoma. Note the presence of bilateral retropharyngeal adenopathy

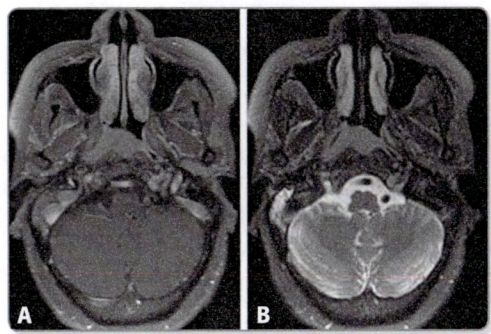

**Figures 5.14A and B** Typical appearances of nasopharyngeal carcinoma showing mild enhancement (A) and mild T2 hyperintensity (B)

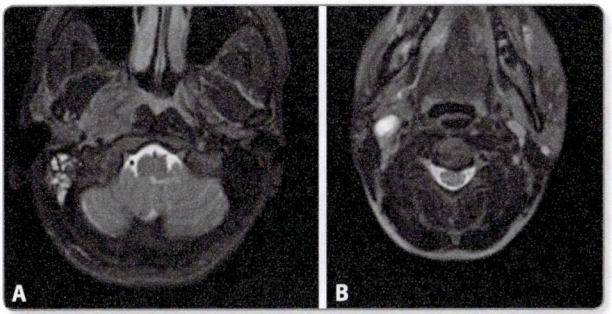

**Figures 5.15A and B** Nasopharyngeal carcinoma with deeper extension across the pharyngobasilar fascia and involving the right parapharyngeal space fat and the carotid (post styloid-parapharyngeal space) (A). Necrotic right level 2 lymph node is also visible (B). Fluid within the right mastoid is secondary to eustachian tube dysfunction

(**Figures 5.18 and 5.19**). Perineural disease will manifest as enhancement and enlargement of the nerve. Tumor infiltration into the cavernous sinus can arise secondary to direct tumor spread superiorly as well as via perineural spread along V3 nerve. Due to the central location of

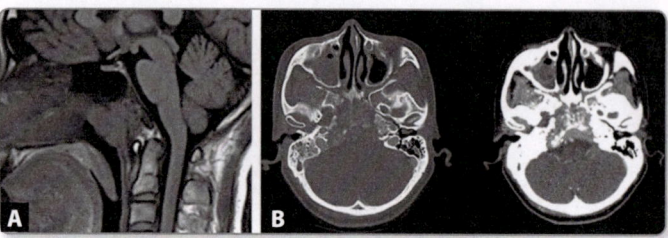

**Figures 5.16A and B** (A) Sagittal T1-weighted image showing isointense nasopharyngeal tumor along the roof with involvement of the skull base along the clivus. Bone marrow signal alterations along the base of skull are well detected on sagittal and coronal unenhanced T1 images. (B) Axial CT images in a patient with NPC showing diffuse permeative destruction of the clivus and right petrous apex

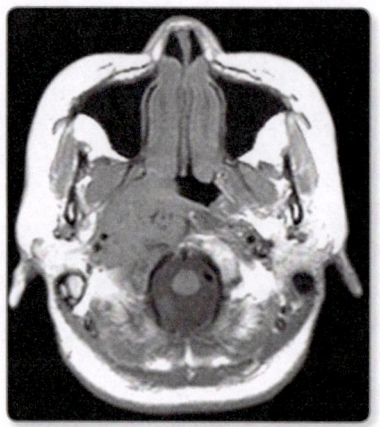

**Figure 5.17** Axial T1 weighted image shows a right sided NPC with extension laterally to encase the neurovascular bundle. Also note the abnormal signal in the right prevertebral musculature and right occipital condyle

the nasopharynx and the infiltrative nature of NPC, disease can also extend into several key anatomic locations such as the sella and orbit (**Figures 5.20 and 5.21**).

## Diseases of the nasopharynx 245

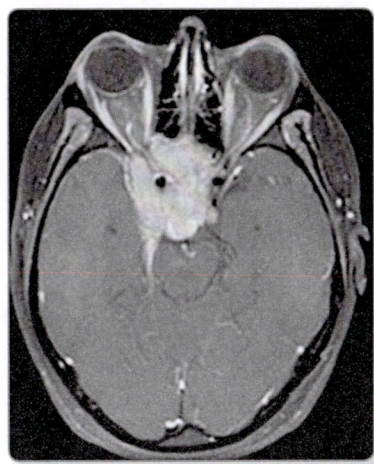

**Figure 5.18** Postcontrast study shows invasion into the right cavernous sinus, clivus and filling the sphenoid sinus. Cavernous sinus invasion can arise via direct tumor infiltration from below

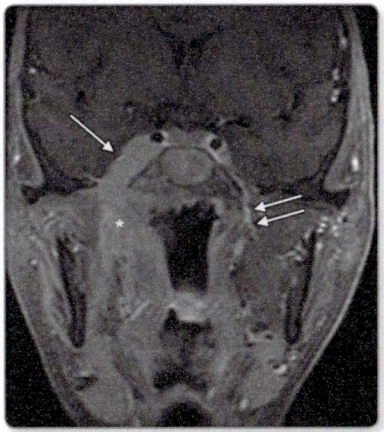

**Figure 5.19** Nasopharyngeal carcinoma (NPC) with invasion into the right masticator space (*) and subsequent extension along V3, through a widened foramen ovale into the markedly thickened cavernous sinus (arrow). Double arrows show the normal V3 on the left side

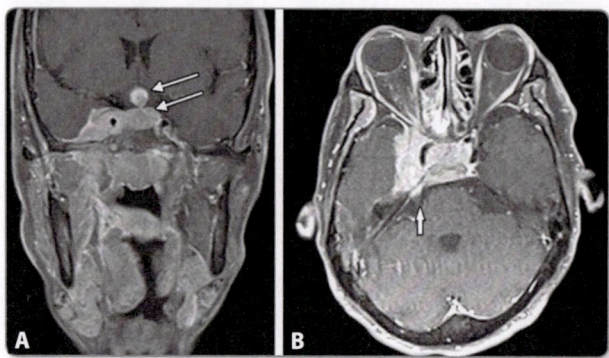

**Figures 5.20A and B** Coronal (A) and axial (B) gadolinium enhanced MRI showing NPC extension through the floor of the right middle cranial fossa and central sphenoid to infiltrate the pituitary gland and infundibulum (thin arrows in [A]). Infiltration of the right cavernous sinus has also led to further retrograde perineural tumor extension along the right main trigeminal nerve trunk (thick arrow)

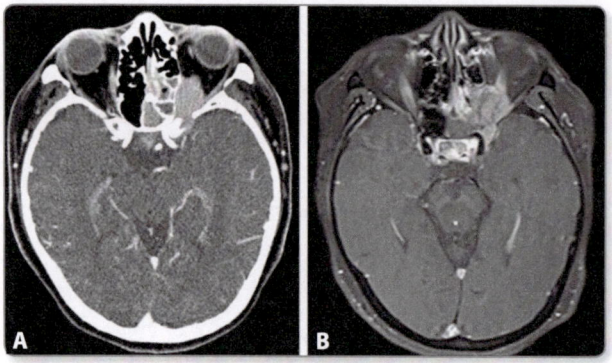

**Figures 5.21A and B** Contrast enhanced axial CT (A) and MRI (B) imaging showing tumor extension into the left posterior orbit

Differential considerations from an imaging perspective may include adenoid hyperplasia, lymphoma, nasopharyngeal tuberculosis, minor salivary gland malignancies, and other rare lesions such as rhabdomyosarcoma and pseudotumor.

### Nasopharyngeal carcinoma staging (Table 5.1)

The 7th Edition of the American Joint Committee on Cancer (AJCC) tumor, node, metastases (TNM) staging system was updated and revised on January 1, 2010.

## Lymphoma

Non-Hodgkin's lymphoma (NHL) accounts for 5 percent of malignancies of the head and neck. Within the head and neck, NHL is most frequently found involving the Waldeyer's ring. The nasopharynx is the second most commonly affected site after the tonsil, accounting for 24 percent of cases. Lymphoma within the nasopharynx can be either the primary or secondary site of involvement. Primary nasopharyngeal lymphomas are extranodal non-Hodgkin's lymphomas that are often grouped together with nasal lymphoma in the literature. It is not clear if these are different biological entities. They are rare in the western population and are found to be more prevalent in people of Asian, Mexican and South American descent. Males seem to be affected more with increasing age and with peak incidence seen in the seventh decade.

Patients commonly present with symptoms such as nasal obstruction, nasal discharge, epistaxis, conductive hearing loss, neck nodal swelling/mass and weight loss. There may also be concurrent symptoms from other sites of involvement within the Waldeyer's ring or the nasal cavity.

The CT appearances are usually that of a homogenous mucosal or submucosal based mass within the nasopharynx with mild enhancement (**Figures 5.22 and 5.23**). On MRI, lymphoma demonstrates intermediate signal intensity on T1 and T2 weighted sequences with mild to moderate enhancement following gadolinium administration. There may be diffuse involvement of the walls, with a large exophytic

|  | TNM stage | Description |
|---|---|---|
| Primary tumor (T) | Tx | Primary tumor cannot be assessed |
|  | T0 | No evidence of primary tumor |
|  | Tis | Carcinoma *in situ* |
|  | T1 | Tumor confined to the nasopharynx, or tumor extends to oropharynx and/or nasal cavity without parapharyngeal extension |
|  | T2 | Tumor with parapharyngeal extension |
|  | T3 | Tumor involves the bony structures of skull base and/or paranasal sinuses |
|  | T4 | Tumor with intracranial extension and/or involvement of cranial nerves, hypopharynx, orbit, or with extension to the infratemporal fossa/masticator space |
| Regional lymph nodes (N) | Nx | Regional nodes cannot be assessed |
|  | N0 | No regional lymph node metastases |
|  | N1 | Unilateral metastasis in cervical lymph node(s) ≤ 6 cm in its greatest dimension above the supraclavicular fossa, and/or unilateral or bilateral, retropharyngeal lymph nodes ≤ 6 cm in its greatest dimension |
|  | N2 | Bilateral metastases in cervical lymph node(s) ≤ 6 cm in greatest dimension above the supraclavicular fossa |
|  | N3 | Metastasis in a lymph node(s) > 6 cm and/or to supraclavicular fossa |
|  | N3a | > 6 cm in dimension |
|  | N3b | Extension to the supraclavicular fossa |
| Metastases (M) | Mx | Distant metastasis cannot be assessed |
|  | M0 | Absence of distant metastasis |
|  | M1 | Presence of distant metastasis |

**Table 5.1:** Nasopharyngeal carcinoma staging

## Diseases of the nasopharynx 249

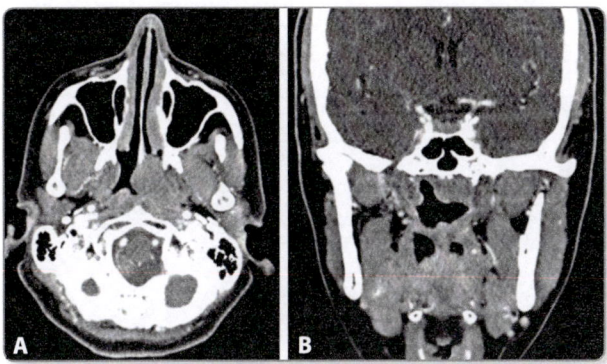

**Figures 5.22A and B** Contrast CT imaging shows a lobulated soft tissue mass protruding into the nasopharynx in a patient with nasopharyngeal lymphoma

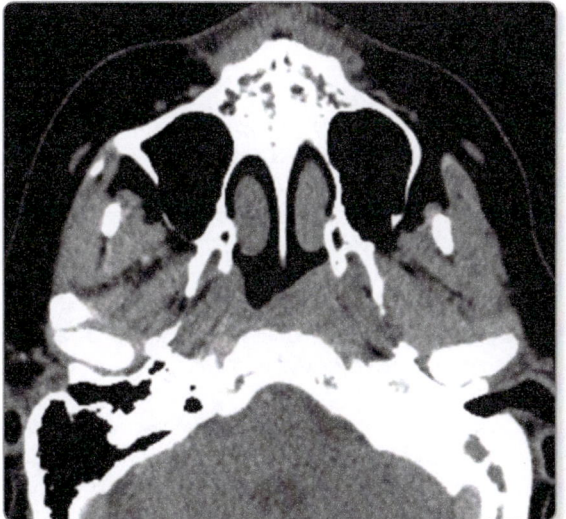

**Figure 5.23** 59-year-old female with a left sided nasopharyngeal mass. Tissue sampling revealed lymphoma. This patient presented with left sided ear symptoms

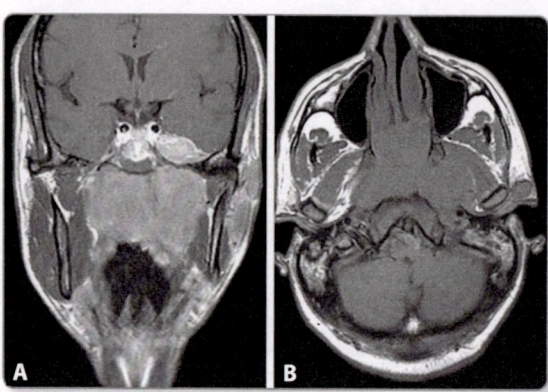

**Figures 5.24A and B** Coronal (A) enhanced and axial (B) unenhanced MRI shows a large mass involving the nasopharynx diffusely with infiltration into the left cavernous sinus the dura along the left middle cranial fossa and the left masticator space. The axial scan nicely shows abnormal intermediate signal within the clivus as well as encasement of the left neurovascular bundle. Anterior extension into the posterior nasal cavity is also present

mass filling the nasopharyngeal airway. Deep infiltration of tumor may arise with extension to the prevertebral tissues, parapharyngeal fat, pterygoid processes and skull base (**Figures 5.24A and B**). Perineural spread can also arise. Mostly, tumor tends to extend superficially along the pharyngeal wall to involve the nasal cavity and palatine tonsil.

Retropharyngeal and cervical nodal involvement, either unilateral or bilateral, is common at presentation or during the course of the disease. Effusions of the middle ear and mastoids are common secondary to eustachian tube dysfunction.

The imaging differential diagnosis includes NPC, adenocarcinoma, adenoid cystic carcinoma, melanoma, plasmacytoma, and sarcomas such as rhabdomyosarcoma and metastasis. Lymphoma is usually considered when a large tumor is found without or with minimal deep tumor extension, or extension along the pharyngeal wall into the nasal cavity or tonsil. Inferior tumor extension to involve the tonsil without skull base invasion may be more suggestive of nasopharyngeal lymphoma.

## Other rare nasopharyngeal disorders

Adenocarcinoma, adenoid cystic carcinoma, melanoma and metastatic deposits are seen sometimes within the nasopharynx. There have been case reports in the literature on a range of other benign and malignant neoplasms and tumor-like lesions in the nasopharynx. The nasopharyngeal mucosal space can also be affected by other benign and malignant conditions such as:
- Postradiation mucositis
- Hemangioma
- Benign mixed tumor
- Minor salivary gland tumor
- Rhabdomyosarcoma
- Teratoma
- Lipoma/liposarcoma
- Kaposi's sarcoma
- Amyloidosis
- Inflammatory pseudotumor
- Extra osseus chordoma
- Nasopharyngeal encephalocele/menigoencephalocele.

Postradiation mucositis is often seen as thick inflamed enhancing mucosa in patients undergoing radiotherapy and this may cause difficulty in assessing the primary lesion on follow-up. Minor salivary gland tumors can also occur within the nasopharynx. Radiographically, these may be difficult to distinguish from more common tumors such as NPC. Proper assessment of the extent of disease is very important especially with tumors such as adenoid cystic carcinoma which have a higher incidence of perineural spread.

A moderately vascularized, aggressive mass seen in the nasopharynx in a child should raise the possibility of rhabdomyosarcoma. These tumors have a propensity for aggressive local invasion and neck adenopathy. Intracranial as well as orbital invasion is common (**Figures 5.25A to E**).

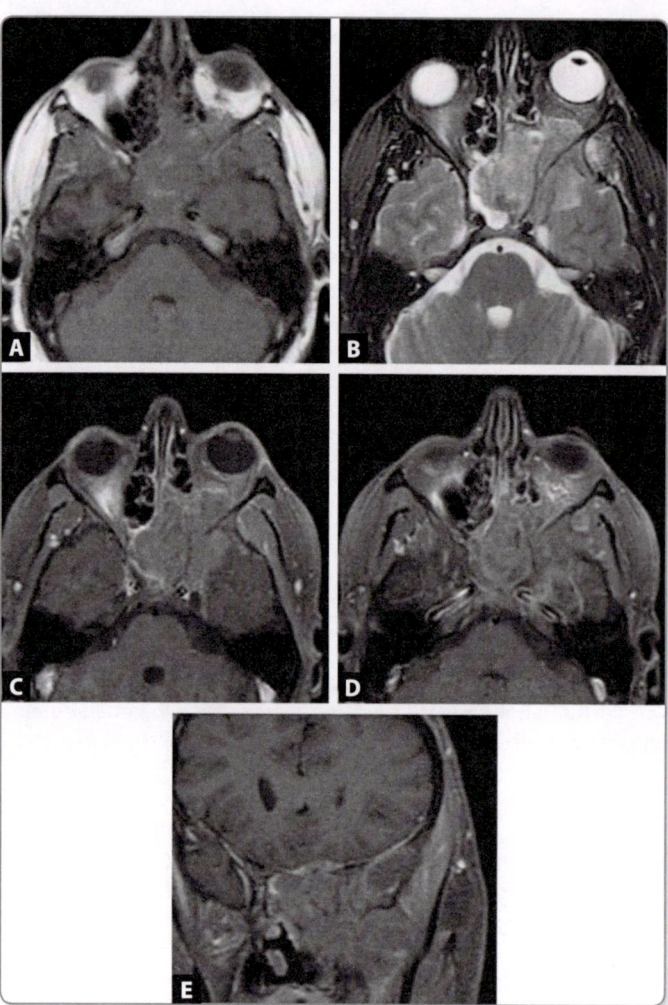

**Figures 5.25A to E** 22-year-old male patient with a heterogenous, lobulated, enhancing mass within the nasopharynx extending into the left orbit, masticator space and floor of the left middle cranial fossa. This lesion was rhabdomyosarcoma

Nasopharyngeal encephaloceles are very rarely reported. MRI imaging is very helpful in the assessment of these lesions with the key being the demonstration of a connection to the intracranial compartment (**Figure 5.26**).

Occasionally, chronic inflammatory changes of the nasopharyngeal lymphoid tissue can simulate a neoplasm clinically and radiologically. These inflammatory pseudotumors (IPT) have been described in various locations of the body including the nasopharynx (**Figures 5.27A to C**). When they involve the cavernous sinuses and causes painful ophthalmoplegia it is known as Tolosa-Hunt syndrome. Skull base and nasopharyngeal involvement have been rarely reported. IPT may show aggressive behavior with bony erosion and cranial neuropathy. IPT may be radiologically indistinguishable from an invasive neoplasm. In a case series of seven patients of nasopharyngeal IPT, it was found that IPT was located submucosally within the nasopharynx and showed direct extension to the carotid space, without abnormal thickening of the mucosa. This is in contrast to NPC which is more mucosal based. ICA encasement and narrowing are also more common in IPT than in NPC. Associated pachymeningeal thickening may be seen in IPT, while lymphadenopathy is less common.

# Conclusion

Acute inflammatory conditions involving the NP do not have much of a role for imaging and are dealt with clinically. Most of the common incidentally or otherwise discovered cystic lesions such as retention cysts or Tornwaldt cysts, can be easily differentiated radiologically from each other as well as from neoplasms. It is usually not difficult to diagnose juvenile angiofibroma due to the characteristic age, sex and clinical presentation and imaging features.

The accurate imaging of NPC is important to help delineate tumor extent and the detection of adenopathy. Lymphoid hyperplasia and lymphoma can be difficult to distinguish from each other as well as from NPC and the presentation including patient age may be helpful.

## 254  Introductory head and neck imaging

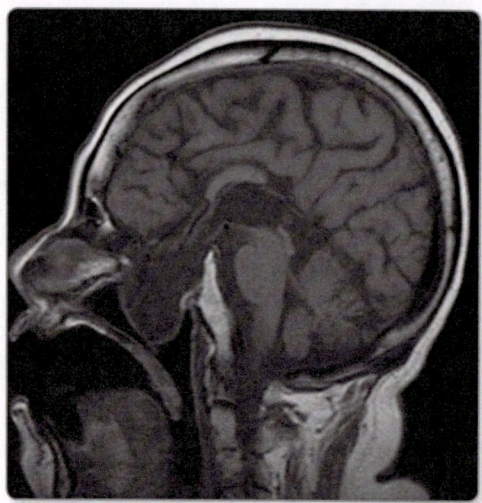

**Figure 5.26** Sagittal T1 weighted image shows a large meningocele protruding inferiorly across a central skull base defect, into the nasopharynx

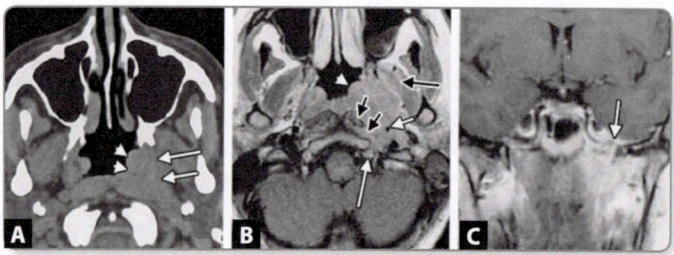

**Figures 5.27A to C** The images are from a 16-year-old female showing a focal mass in the left nasopharynx with extension to the longus musculature and the left neurovascular bundle. The coronal image shows extension through the left foramen ovale and thickening of the dural along the floor of the middle cranial fossa. *Courtesy*: S De Vuysere, R Hermans, R Sciot, I Crevits, G Marchal. Extraorbital Inflammatory Pseudotumor of the Head and Neck: CT and MR Findings in Three Patients. AJNR 1999;22(6):1133-9, © American Society of Neuroradiology

# Bibliography

1. Kösling S, Knipping S, Hofmockel T. Imaging of nasopharyngeal diseases. Review. German. Radiologe 2009;49(1):17-26.

*Adenoid hyperplasia:*

2. Gates G. Sizing up the adenoid. Arch Otolaryngol Head Neck Surg 1996; 122(3):239-40.

*Tornwaldt Cyst:*

3. Ben Salem D, Duvillard C, Assous D, Ballester M, Krausé D, Ricolfi F. Imaging of nasopharyngeal cysts and bursae. Eur Radiol 2006;16(10):2249-58. Epub 2006 Apr 26.
4. Moody MW, Chi DH, Mason JC, Phillips CD, Gross CW, Schlosser RJ. Tornwaldt's cyst: incidence and a case report. Ear Nose Throat J 2007;86:45-7.
5. Woo EK, Connor SEJ. Computed tomography and magnetic resonance imaging appearances of cystic lesions in the suprahyoid neck: a pictorial review. Dentomaxillofac Radiol 2007;36:451-8.

*Tuberculosis:*

6. Ann D King, Anil T Ahuja, Gary MK Tse, Andrew CA van Hasselt, Amy BW Chan. MR Imaging features of nasopharyngeal tuberculosis: report of three cases and literature review. Am J Neuroradiol 2003;24:279-82.
7. Percodani J, Braun F, Arrue P, et al. Nasopharyngeal tuberculosis. J Laryngol Otol 1999;113:928-31.

*Lymphoma:*

8. King AD, Lei KIK, Richards PS, Ahuja AT. Non-Hodgkin's Lymphoma of the nasopharynx: CT and MR imaging. Clinical Radiology 2003;58:621-5.
9. Lei KI-K, Suen JJS, Hui P, Tong M, Li W, Yau SH. Primary nasal and nasopharyngeal lymphomas: A comparative study of clinical presentation and treatment outcome. Clinical Oncology 1999;11:379-87.
10. Michael MC Cheung, John KC Chan, WH Lau, William Foo, Paddy TM Chan, CS Ng, Roger KC Ngan. Primary Non-Hodgkin's lymphoma of the nose and nasopharynx: clinical features, tumor immunophenotype, and treatment outcomes in 113 patients. Journal of clinical oncology, 1988;16(1)70-7.

*Nasopharyngeal carcinoma:*

11. Goh J, Lim K. Imaging of Nasopharyngeal Carcinoma. Ann Acad Med Singapore 2009;38(9):809-16.
12. King AD, Lam WW, Leung SF, Chan YL, Teo P, Metreweli C. MRI of local disease in nasopharyngeal carcinoma: tumour extent vs. tumor stage. Br J Radiol 1999; 72(860):734-41.
13. King AD, Vlantis AC, Tsang RK, et al. Magnetic resonance imaging for the detection of nasopharyngeal carcinoma. Am J Neuroradiol 27(6):1288-91.
14. King AD, Ahuja AT, Leung SF, et al. Neck node metastases from nasopharyngeal carcinoma: MR imaging of patterns of disease. Head Neck 2000;22(3):275-81.
15. Lee AW, Au JS, Teo PM, et al (Eds). Clin Oncol (R Coll Radiol) 2004;16(4):269-76.

16. Mao YP, Xie FY, Liu LZ, et al. Re-evaluation of 6th edition of AJCC staging system for nasopharyngeal carcinoma and proposed improvement based on magnetic resonance imaging. Int J Radiat Oncol Biol Phys 73(5).
17. Sanguineti G, Geara FB, Garden AS, et al. Carcinoma of the nasopharynx treated by radiotherapy alone: determinants of local and regional control. Int J Radiat Oncol Biol Phy 1997;37(5),985-96.
18. Staging of nasopharyngeal carcinoma: suggestions for improving the current UICC/AJCC Staging System. In: 7th edition of the International Union Against Cancer (UICC) Manual.
19. Yu E, O'Sullivan B, Kim J, Siu L, Bartlett E. Magnetic Resonance Imaging of Nasopharyngeal Carcinoma. Expert Rev. Anticancer Therapy 2010;10(3).

***Inflammatory Pseudotumor:***
20. Garg V, Temin N, Hildenbrand P, Silverman M, Catalano PJ. Inflammatory pseudotumor of the skull base. Otolaryngol Head Neck Surg 2010;142(1):129-31.
21. Lu CH, Yang CY, Wang CP, Yang CC, Liu HM, Chen YF. Imaging of nasopharyngeal inflammatory pseudotumours: differential from nasopharyngeal carcinoma. Br J Radiol 2010;83(985):8-16. Epub 2009 May 26.

# Imaging of the masticator and parapharyngeal spaces

### chapter 6

Dorothy Lazinski

**ABSTRACT**

This chapter begins with a comprehensive review of the imaging anatomy of the parapharyngeal and masticator spaces. Common infectious and neoplastic conditions are covered.

**KEYWORDS**

Parapharyngeal, masticator space, CT, MRI.

## Part I: The masticator space

## Anatomy

The masticator space encompasses the muscles of mastication including the medial and lateral pterygoid, masseter and temporalis muscles and the intervening bony buttress consisting of the mandible. The zygomatic arch serves as a second bony buttress and landmark for further subdivision into the suprazygomatic compartment comprised of the temporalis muscle as well as an infrazygomatic compartment which is comprised of the remaining muscles.

The masticator space has an intimate relationship with the skull and skull base allowing access for the spread of disease. The mandible articulates with the skull base via the temporomandibular joint. The muscles have a relationship with the calvarium and skull base by means of their sites of origin. The medial pterygoid muscle arises from the medial surface of the lateral pterygoid plate of the sphenoid bone and attaches to the medial surface of the mandibular ramus to the angle of the mandible. The lateral pterygoid muscle arises from the lateral surface of the lateral pterygoid plate and attaches to the neck of the mandibular condyle while a smaller component attaches to the disc and capsule of the TM joint. The temporalis muscle arises as a broad fan-shaped sheet along the temporal squamous bone and tapers inferiorly under the zygomatic arch attaching to the coronoid process and inferiorly along the anterior ramus to the level of the third molar. The masseter muscle has a dominant superficial head which extends from the anterior inferior margins of the zygomatic arch and overlies the ramus to the angle of the mandible. The deeper smaller head arises from the posterior zygomatic arch and extends to the upper mandibular ramus and coronoid process.

Innervation of the muscles is via corresponding muscular branches of the third (mandibular) division of the trigeminal nerve. The lingual nerve also resides within the space. These branches provide a conduit for potential distal perineural spread of disease.

The arterial vascular supply is primarily from the external carotid artery via maxillary artery branches in addition to smaller contributions from the superficial temporal artery branches.

Venous drainage is primarily into a vast network of veins which form the pterygoid plexus. It receives venous branches from the corresponding arterial branches. This plexus communicates with the cavernous sinus, pharyngeal venous plexus as well as facial and ophthalmic veins. Additional venous channels include those which correspond to the superficial temporal artery branches.

All of these structures within the masticator space are invested by the superficial layer of the deep cervical fascia which constitutes the superficial fascia of the neck. This fascia attaches from the lower neck to the inferior margins of the mandible where it divides into two. The lateral slip of fascia extends over the masseter muscle, attaches to the zygomatic arch and then extends over the temporalis muscle. The medial slip extends along the medial margins of the medial pterygoid muscle to its origin along the medial margins of the lateral pterygoid plate of the sphenoid bone medial to foramen ovale. Foramen ovale can be considered functionally to be the roof of the masticator space through which disease can enter the intracranial compartment.

Imaging of the masticator and parapharyngeal spaces 259

# Imaging anatomy

## Masticator space: superior (Figure 6.I.1)
Suprazygomatic masticator space (shaded), temporalis (t) muscle.

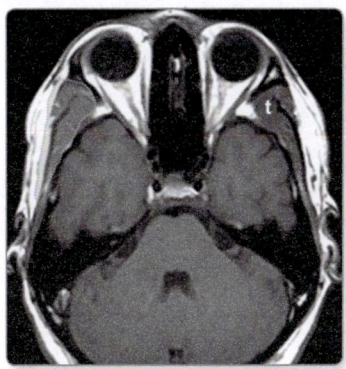

**Figure 6.I.1** *(for color version see Plate 11)*

## Masticator space: mid (Figure 6.I.2)

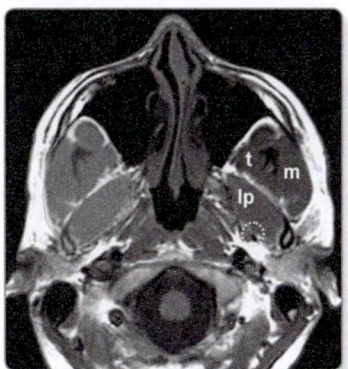

**Figure 6.I.2** *(for color version see Plate 11)*

**Figures 6.I.1 and 6.I.2** Infrazygomatic masticator space (shaded) includes the inferior temporalis (t), lateral pterygoid (lp) and masseter (m) muscles. The muscles, temporomandibular joint and the mandibular division of the trigeminal nerve, V3, (yellow circle) are invested in the superficial layer of the deep cervical fascia

## Masticator space: inferior (Figure 6.I.3)

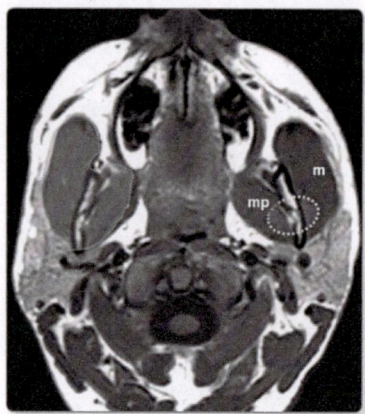

**Figure 6.I.3** Infrazygomatic mastication (lower section): medial pterygoid (mp) and masseter (m) muscles, intervening mandible and mandibular division of V3 (yellow oval) are invested in the superficial layer of the deep cervical fascia (*for color version see Plate 12*)

## Masticator space: anterior (Figure 6.I.4)

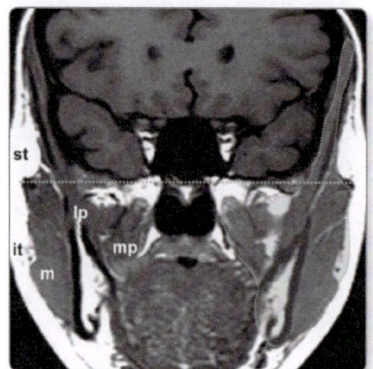

**Figure 6.I.4** Supra-(st) and infra-zygomatic temporalis (it) muscles (zygomatic boundary-dotted line), medial (mp) and lateral pterygoid (lp) and masseter (m) muscles as well as mandible and mandibular division of V3 are invested in the superficial layer of the deep cervical fascia (*for color version see Plate 12*)

Imaging of the masticator and parapharyngeal spaces   261

## Masticator space: mid section coronal (Figure 6.I.5)

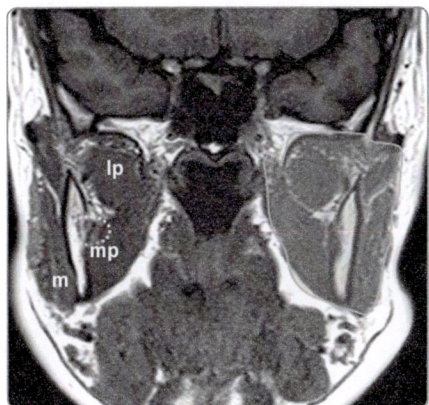

**Figure 6.I.5** Masseter (m), medial (mp) and lateral pterygoid (lp) muscles with intervening mandible and mandibular division of V3 (yellow oval) invested in the superficial layer of the deep cervical fascia (*for color version see Plate 13*)

## Masticator space: posterior (Figure 6.I.6)

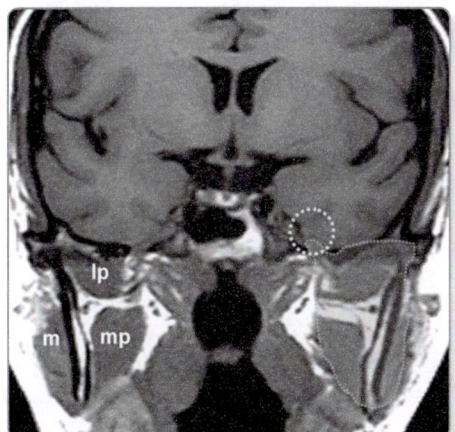

**Figure 6.I.6** Medial (mp) and lateral (lp) pterygoid and masseter (m) muscles as well as V3 at level of foramen ovale (yellow circle) invested in fascia (*for color version see Plate 13*)

## Pathology

Disease processes involving the masticator space are generally of infectious, inflammatory or neoplastic etiologies.

The imaging characteristics and pattern of disease involvement of a particular structure/s within the confines of this space allows one to generate a limited differential diagnosis.

## Muscles of mastication

Myositis affecting the muscles of mastication is often secondary to trauma, infection or inflammation within adjacent structures or spaces. It is most often reactive due to a contiguous dental source of infection involving the mandible, secondary to parotitis or parapharyngeal infiltration from deep spread of infection from the oropharynx, typically from tonsillar/peritonsillar abscess. It is manifest by enlargement and/or edema of the affected muscles. Occasionally, there may be evolution of intramuscular abscess.

On CT, edema may be manifest as an enlarged muscle with diminished attenuation. Edema appears as a diffuse area of T2 signal hyperintensity on MRI. An abscess would be characterized as localized rim-enhancing fluid collection (**Figures 6.I.7 to 6.I.10**).

Primary benign and malignant tumors arising within the muscles are uncommon. Lipoma, hemangioma and lymphangioma are such examples (**Figures 6.I.11A and B**). They may be multi-compartmental. Rhabdomyomas are rare as are rhabdomyosarcomas which occur more commonly in younger patients. The imaging characteristics of these lesions parallel those found elsewhere in the body.

Secondary metastatic lesions to muscle do occur but are rare (**Figure 6.I.12**). Extranodal manifestation of lymphoma (**Figures 6.I.13A and B**) either as a focal mass or diffuse infiltrative process involving the muscles is more common and should be considered in the differential especially if there are additional characteristic sites of involvement including the parotid and lacrimal glands, mucosal involvement of Waldeyer's ring as well as lymphadenopathy.

Most commonly however, the muscles of mastication are secondarily involved by direct tumor infiltration from adjacent oral

Imaging of the masticator and parapharyngeal spaces 263

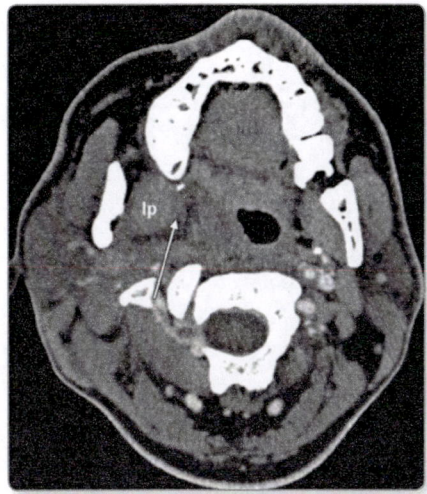

**Figure 6.I.7** Inflammatory myositis: CT showing edema (long arrow) and inflammatory stranding within the left parapharyngeal fat with enlargement of the lateral pterygoid (lp) muscle. These changes are secondary to an inflammatory process originating within the tonsil, peritonsillar abscess (not shown)

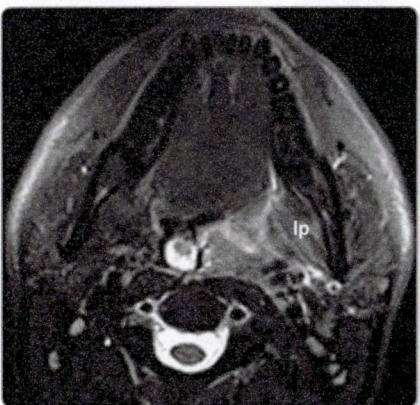

**Figure 6.I.8** Inflammatory myositis: Axial T2-weighted MRI demonstrating diffuse edema within the lateral oropharyngeal wall, parapharyngeal space and lateral pterygoid (lp) muscle as a consequence of peritonsillar abscess

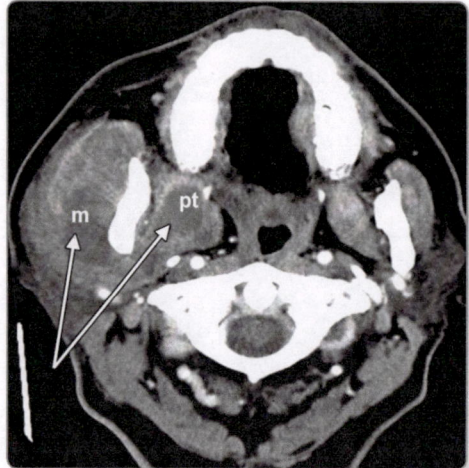

**Figure 6.I.9** Dental-related rim-enhancing abscess (arrows) formation within the right masseter (m) and pterygoid (pt) muscles

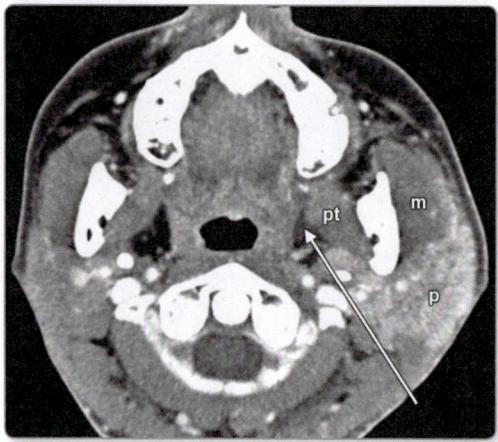

**Figure 6.I.10** Inflammatory myositis with diffuse enlargement and edema of the left masseter (m) and pterygoid (pt) muscles secondary to parotitis (p). There is increased attenuation of the parapharyngeal fat (arrow) due to inflammatory stranding

Imaging of the masticator and parapharyngeal spaces 265

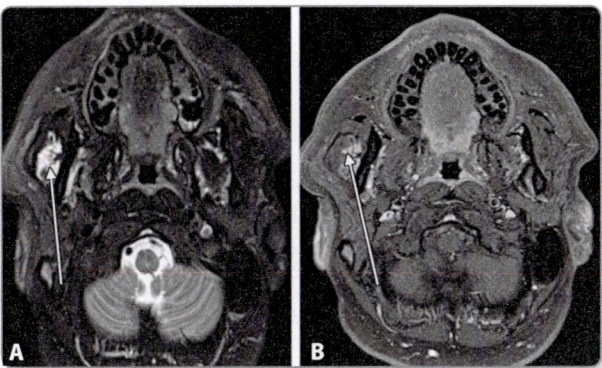

**Figures 6.I.11A and B** Primary tumor: T2-weighted and postgadolinium axial MRI images demonstrating hemangioma (arrow) within the right masseter muscle. A T2-hyperintense lobulated lesion with patchy enhancement which fills in on delayed images is characteristic

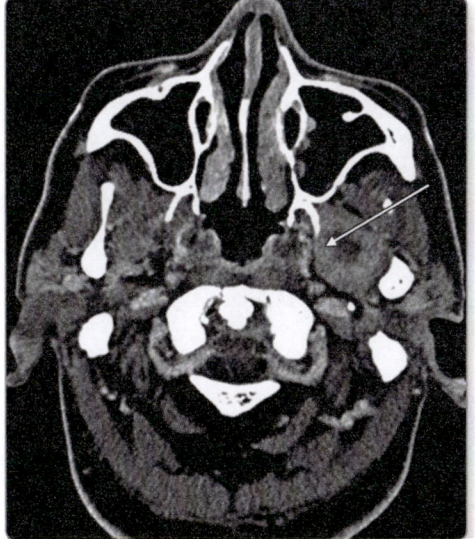

**Figure 6.I.12** Secondary tumor: Carcinoma of the lung metastasis (arrow) to lateral pterygoid muscle

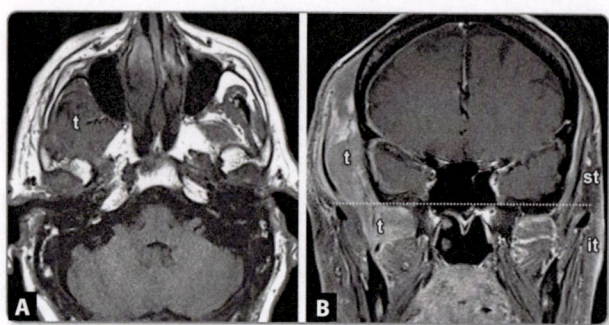

**Figures 6.I.13A and B** Secondary tumor: Lymphoma, within the supra- (st) and infrazygomatic (it) masticator space with diffuse involvement of the temporalis (t) muscles

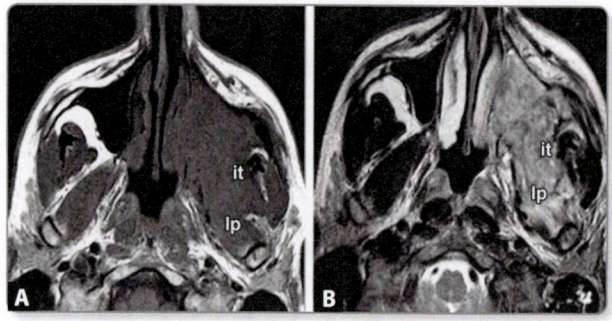

**Figures 6.I.14A and B** Secondary tumor: Aggressive maxillary sinus carcinoma extending posteriorly to transgress the retromaxillary fat and directly invading the infrazygomatic temporalis (it) and lateral pterygoid (lp) muscles

cavity and oropharyngeal squamous cell carcinoma (**Figures 6.I.14A and B**). Gingival mucosal tumors including retromolar carcinoma can invade the mandible and secondarily infiltrate the muscles of mastication which have an intimate relationship to the mandible. Lateral nasopharyngeal, posterior sinus, as well as lateral oropharyngeal tumors including tonsillar, lateral soft palate, oropharyngeal wall and tongue base tumors can transgress fascial planes and fat containing spaces such as the parapharyngeal and retromaxillary spaces and invade the masticator space. If the tumor is very large and effaces the parapharyngeal fat, it may be difficult to determine if the muscles are involved as they may be displaced due to mass effect. MRI may be more helpful in defining the tissue planes and confirming muscle involvement. Clinically, trismus is a feature of muscle involvement.

## Mandible

Mandibular lesions are often odontogenic in origin, manifest as infectious processes including focal abscess or osteomyelitis, dental-related cysts or tumors.

Infection may arise following tooth extraction or untreated periapical abscess. The infection decompresses itself into the surrounding tissues forming subperiosteal fluid collection/abscess. There can be secondary spread to involve the adjacent muscles as well as distal spread along fascial planes along the path of least resistance to the suprazygomatic space along the temporalis muscle and inferiorly to the submandibular space and floor of mouth. Clinically, cellulitis, fever and trismus are prominent features.

Osteomyelitis is characterized by bone resorption, edema within the fat overlying the bone and reactive thickening of the soft tissues (**Figures 6.I.15A and B**). The bony changes are best appreciated and characterized on CT. A sequestrum may be visualized and periosteal reaction may be present. On MRI, there is replacement of the normal T1 fat marrow signature due to increased inflammatory cellularity and edema. Chronic osteomyelitis is associated with less exuberant soft tissue changes. There is frequently, mild overlying soft tissue swelling and underlying sclerosis of the mandible associated with bone loss.

Although many forms of dental origin cysts exist, the two most common cysts seen on imaging include the radicular (periapical) and dentigerous cysts respectively (**Figures 6.I.16 and 6.I.17**). The radicular cyst appears as a small round well defined lucency associated with the root of a tooth. It arises as a consequence of an infected tooth resulting in periapical inflammation and granuloma formation which evolves into a cyst. A dentigerous cyst is a developmental cyst with

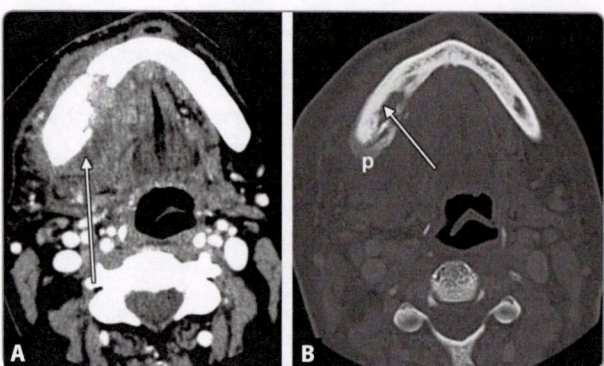

**Figures 6.I.15A and B** Soft tissue swelling and enhancement, low density collection along the lingual mandibular margins (arrow) associated with bone destruction and periosteal new bone formation (p) and sequestrum (arrow) characterizing abscess formation and osteomyelitis of the mandible

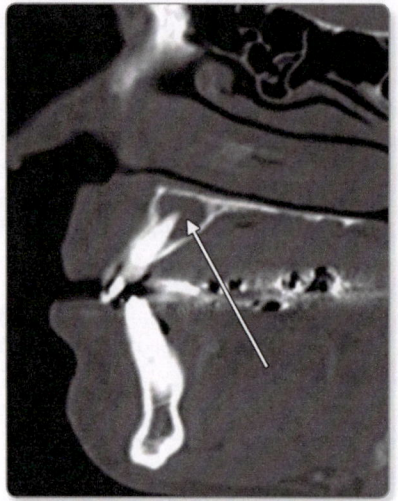

**Figure 6.I.16** Radicular (periapical) cyst: Well defined oval lucency surrounding the root of the tooth (arrow)

Imaging of the masticator and parapharyngeal spaces 269

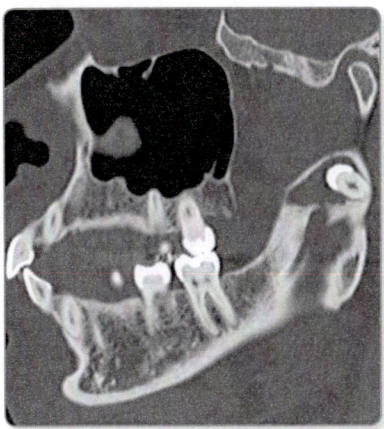

**Figure 6.I.17** Dentigerous cyst: Well-defined expansile cystic lucency associated with the crown of an unerupted third mandibular molar

smooth corticated margins surrounding the crown of an unerupted tooth. It is often an incidental imaging finding. It is benign and painless but can grow and then come to clinical attention due to mass effect.

## Odontogenic tumor

Ameloblastoma is a benign odontogenic tumor of epithelial origin. It occurs most frequently in the third to fifth decades and most commonly occurs in the ramus and posterior body of the mandible. It usually presents as painless swelling of the mandible. On imaging, it appears as an expansile, usually multiloculated or multiseptated "soap-bubble" cystic lesion (**Figures 6.I.18A to C**) with some solid components which can mimic an odontogenic keratocyst. It can be locally aggressive, cause tooth resorption and displacement and extend into the adjacent soft tissues with perforation of the cortex. It has a high recurrence if incompletely excised.

The mandible is also a site of nonodontogenic tumors including primary bone tumors such as osteosarcoma, chondrosarcoma, Ewing's sarcoma, lymphoma, plasmacytoma as well as secondary

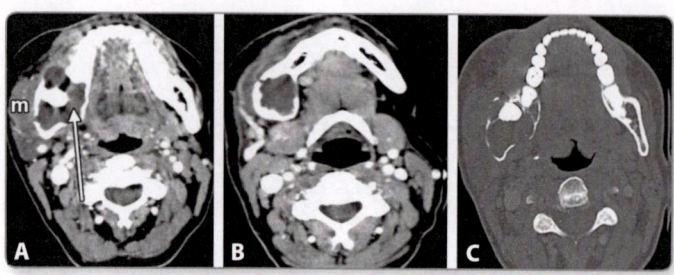

**Figures 6.I.18A to C** Ameloblastoma: Expansile cystic and septated lesion (arrow) within the angle of the right mandible with extension into the overlying masseter (m) muscle

tumors which may arise from metastases or direct invasion from oral cavity mucosal tumors, typically, squamous cell carcinomas (**Figures 6.I.19A and B**).

Osteosarcoma in the head and neck comprises 6 percent of all osteosarcomas. It most frequently involves the mandible and may be lytic, blastic or mixed. Most frequently, it has a poorly defined aggressive pattern of bone destruction associated with dense osteoid matrix or calcification and characteristic sunburst periosteal reaction (**Figures 6.I.20A and B**). Chondrosarcoma is rarer and is characteristically associated with the temporomandibular joint. Cellular tumors including Ewing's sarcoma and lymphoma show no pathognomonic imaging features. There is typically a permeative pattern of bone loss on CT, soft tissue mass and enhancement reflective of cellularity. Plasmacytoma presents as a focal well defined lytic lesion with soft tissue mass (**Figures 6.I.21A to D**). A small percentage may develop multiple myeloma. Metastatic involvement by any tumor is not infrequent and widespread lesions as well as knowledge of known primary malignancy is helpful. The lesions reflect the primary tumor and may be lytic, blastic or mixed.

Osteonecrosis of the jaws (ONJ) is a very challenging diagnosis. It often is a clinical diagnosis. Osteoradionecrosis (ORN) (**Figures 6.I.22A and B**) is a consequence of radiation tissue injury with devitalized bone unable to mount a reparative response to injury. It may share

Imaging of the masticator and parapharyngeal spaces **271**

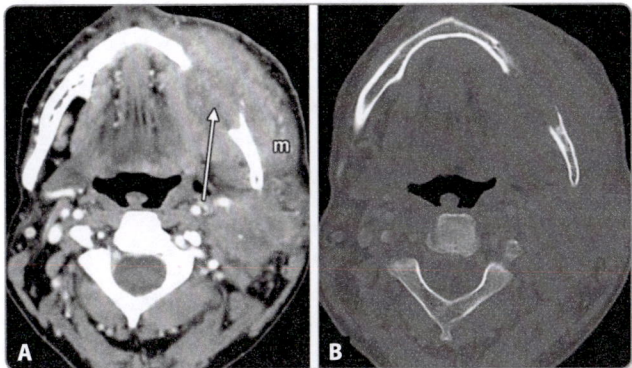

**Figures 6.I.19A and B** Secondary involvement of the mandible and muscles of mastication by a primary mucosal squamous cell carcinoma of the alveolus. The soft tissue mass (arrow) is invading into the masseter (m) and floor of mouth with associated lytic destruction of the underlying mandible

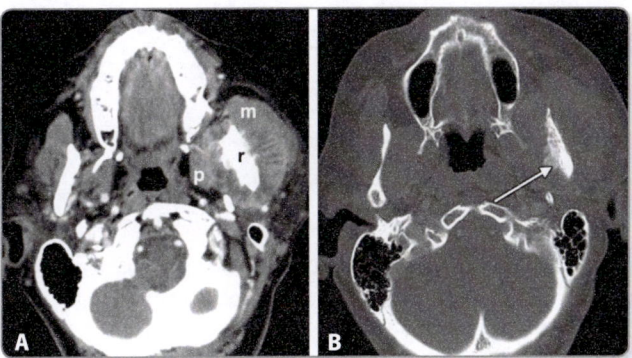

**Figures 6.I.20A and B** Osteosarcoma of the mandible. Aggressive bony lesion with sclerosis of the left mandibular ramus (r), sunburst periosteal reaction (arrow) and soft tissue mass with few small calcific/osteoid foci. The mass invades into the masseter (m) muscle and displaces the pterygoid muscle (p)

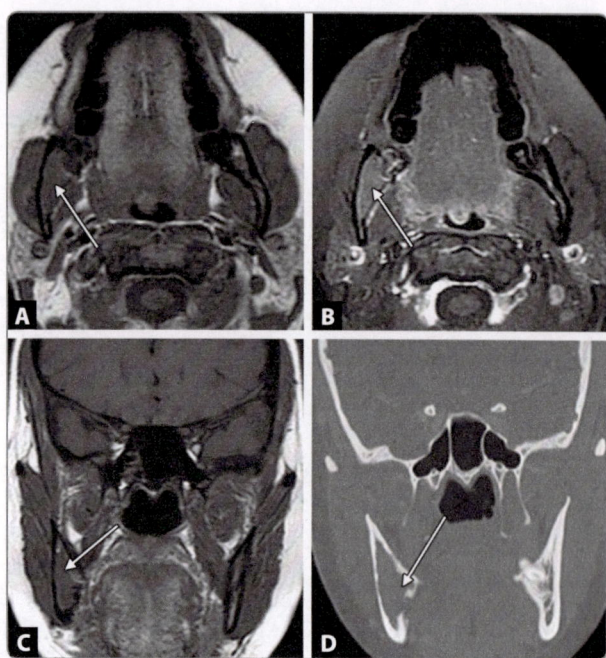

**Figures 6.I.21A to D** Plasmacytoma. Axial T1-weighted pre- and postgadolinium images through the mandible demonstrates an expansile enhancing lesion replacing the normal fat marrow signal intensity (arrow). Coronal T1-weighted MRI and corresponding coronal CT images demonstrate the expansile lesion with disruption of the lingual cortex

features of infection as well as tumor and either or both can coexist with this condition in the setting of previous radiation treatment for tumor. Some disease states such as underlying sickle cell disease and bisphosphonate therapy in advanced cancer treatment also predispose to the ONJ.

Osteonecrosis of the jaw (ONJ) is characterized on CT by bony loss, fragmentation, sclerosis and adjacent soft tissue thickening. Gas may be present. Patients present with pain and swelling and clinically, there is exposed bone possibly complicated by infection with draining sinus

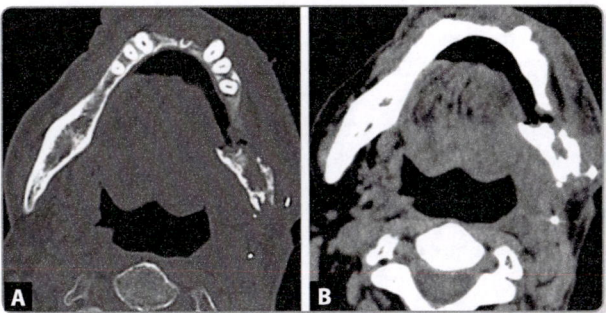

**Figures 6.1.22A and B** Radionecrosis of the mandible. Unenhanced axial CT images demonstrate bone exposure, sclerosis, bone loss and fragmentation of the left angle of the mandible following radiation for parotid carcinoma

and fistula formation. On MRI, there is diminished T1 signal intensity characterizing replacement of the normal fat marrow signature while T2 signal characteristics and enhancement pattern are variable and not pathognomonic. They do however, demonstrate the extent of the abnormality. Bone scan may be helpful in the initial phase which typically shows a decrease in radionuclide uptake. PET may also show a similar pattern. Increased uptake is however seen with infection, tumor as well as the later reparative phase. There may be periosteal reaction and extension into the soft tissues. These features are often shared with infection thus making it difficult to establish the diagnosis. While biopsy may be helpful to exclude recurrent tumor, it is subject to sampling error. In addition, sampling is to be avoided if ONJ due to bisphosphonate use is suspected as it can exacerbate the condition. Therefore, the diagnosis is frequently based on clinical grounds with CT and MRI showing the extent of the abnormality and used to monitor for serial change.

# Neurogenic lesions

Primary nerve sheath lesions can arise along the course of the lingual or mandibular divisions of the trigeminal nerve within the masticator space and can be symptomatic for the branch involved. Neurofibromas can occur as isolated lesions but are more frequently associated with NF 1. On imaging, they are also well defined, ovoid or fusiform in morphology, but may differ from schwannomas in their signal and enhancing characteristics. More frequently, they appear as lower density lesions on CT due to a component of fatty infiltration and necrosis. They may be associated with dystrophic calcifications. Enhancement is generally weak, typically with scant peripheral rim enhancement (**Figures 6.I.23A to C**). On imaging, schwannomas are well defined, fusiform and enhance avidly and heterogeneously. They may appear cystic. In general MRI characteristics are similar to lesions found outside the head and neck (**Figures 6.I.24A to C**) with fairly bright T2 signal and avid enhancement. Cystic change can also occur.

Granulomatous and malignant processes within the masticator space can directly involve nerve branches with risk for secondary perineural spread of disease. Patients will complain of numbness or dysesthesia in the nerve root distribution. On imaging, this process is identified by observing thickening of the nerve, effacement of the fat within the foramina through which the nerves traverse and linear enhancement along the nerve. Enhancement of the nerve may be contiguous or present as skip lesions (**Figures 6.I.25A and B**).

Perineural spread of disease within the masticator space can spread into the intracranial compartment through foramen ovale into Meckel's cave (**Figures 6.I.26A and B**) with potential for further

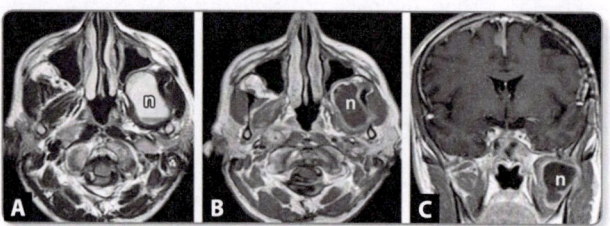

**Figures 6.I.23A to C** Patient with NF 1. Axial T2 and postcontrast axial and coronal T1 weighted imaging of a neurofibroma (n). The lesion appears as a cystic (low T1 and high T2 signal intensity), peripherally enhancing lobulated mass in the left masticator space displacing the pterygoid muscles

Imaging of the masticator and parapharyngeal spaces 275

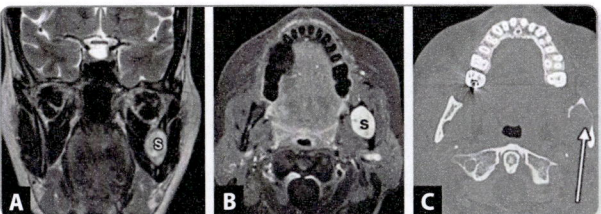

**Figures 6.I.24A to C** Mandibular schwannoma. Coronal T2-weighted and axial T1-weighted fat suppressed postgadolinium series through the masticator space. The schwannoma appears as a T2 hyperintense lesion (s) with intense enhancement. It is centered on the inferior alveolar canal of the mandible and is indenting the medial pterygoid muscle. The axial CT image shows smooth bony expansion and remodeling of the inferior alveolar canal (arrow)

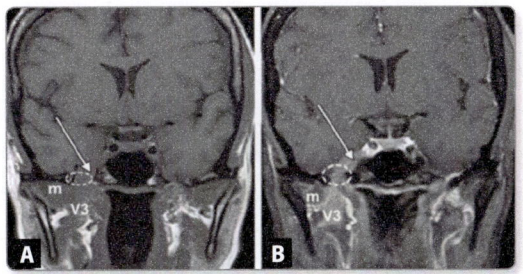

**Figures 6.I.25A and B** Perineural disease secondary to lymphoma. Coronal T1-weighted pre- and fat suppressed postgadolinium images demonstrating thickening of the third division of the trigeminal nerve (V3) coursing from the masticator space (m) through a widened foramen ovale (dashed oval) into Meckel's cave (arrow)

retrograde spread to the brainstem nerve root entry zone. As such, the entire course of the nerve including its retrograde and anterograde branches must be evaluated. Adenoid cystic carcinoma in particular has a predilection for perineural pattern of disease but other tumors including, squamous cell carcinoma, mucoepidermoid carcinoma and lymphoma can also behave in such a fashion.

Foramen ovale along with the greater sphenoid wing forms the roof of the masticator space separating the intra- and extracranial

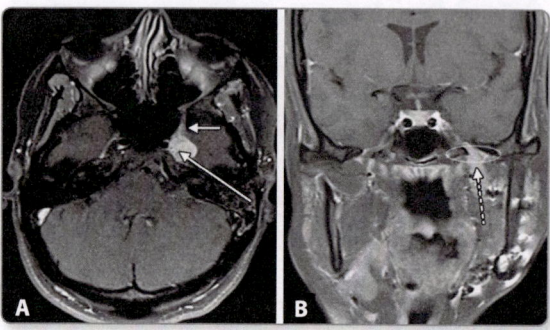

**Figures 6.I.26A and B** Patient with angiosarcoma of the mandible that presented with facial pain and tingling in the chin two years following surgical resection and reconstruction. Postgadolinium fat-suppressed T1-weighted series demonstrating thick enhancement along V3 from the surgical bed (dotted arrow) in the masticator space to foramen ovale (oval) into Meckel's cave (long white arrow) as well as anterograde extension along foramen rotundum (short white arrow)

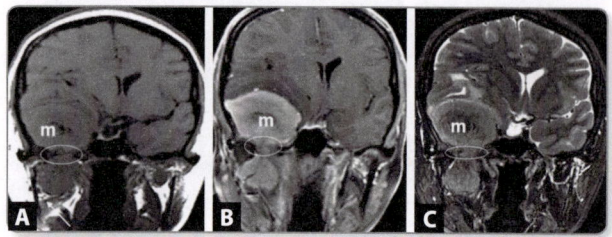

**Figures 6.I.27A to C** Coronal T1-weighted pre- and postgadolinium and coronal T2-weighted images demonstrate an intracranial dural based meningioma (m) applied along the floor of the right middle cranial fossa. The tumor is gaining access into the masticator space below through foramen ovale

compartments. Foramen ovale can serve as a potential conduit for spread of disease between the masticator space and the intracranial compartment. Both primary neurogenic lesions such as schwannoma and secondary lesions such as perineural disease can traverse the foramen. Extracranial extension of primary intracranial lesions such as meningioma can also extend inferiorly via foramen ovale (**Figures 6.I.27A to C**).

Imaging of the masticator and parapharyngeal spaces   277

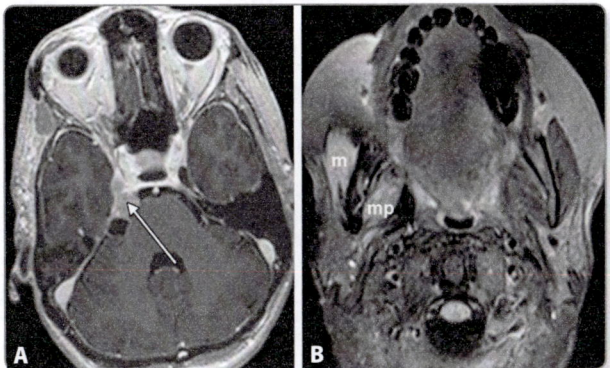

**Figures 6.I.28A and B** Masticator space muscle denervation. Postgadolinium fat suppressed T1-weighted series demonstrate a trigeminal schwannoma (arrow) involving Meckel's cave and the right prepontine cistern. The right medial pterygoid (mp) and masseter (m) muscles demonstrate volume loss and enhance in the subacute phase of denervation

A disease process or injury affecting the motor division of (V3) anywhere along its course from brainstem to target tissue can result in denervation of the muscles of mastication. Systemic diseases including polymyositis and myasthenia gravis can also result in denervation changes. In the initial phase of active muscle resorption, acute denervation appears as mass-like enlargement of the muscles of mastication due to edema and should not be interpreted as the site of local pathology. Involved muscles typically enhance in the acute and subacute phases. A search for the offending lesion should be made (**Figures 6.I.28A and B**).

On the other hand, chronic denervation results in fatty atrophy and asymmetry of the affected muscles in the case of a unilateral lesion and caution should be exercised to avoid misconstruing the contralateral unaffected muscles as abnormal as they will appear asymmetrically larger in volume (**Figures 6.I.29A and B**).

## Summary

The masticator space is invested as a compartment by the superficial layer of the deep cervical fascia. Pathology can arise within or involve

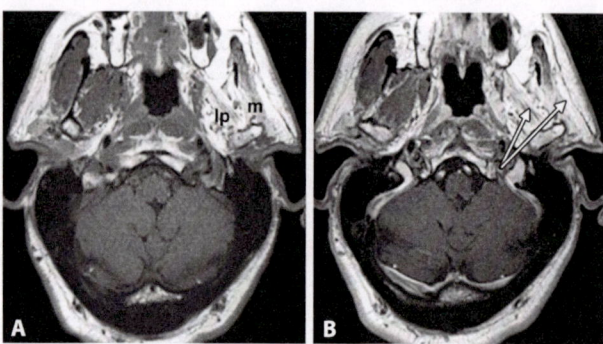

**Figures 6.I.29A and B** Chronic denervation: Pre- and postgadolinium axial T1 weighted series. Fatty infiltration and atrophy of the left muscles of mastication (arrows); lateral pterygoid (lp) and masseter (m)

one or all of the components of this space: the muscles of mastication, the bony buttress as well as the nerves. Infectious, inflammatory and malignant processes can affect each of these components. It will be the imaging characteristics of the lesion and the pattern of disease spread which will allow for an appropriate differential diagnosis to be generated.

# Bibliography

1. Chiandussi S, Biasotto M, Dore F, Cavalli F, Cova MA, Di Lenarda R. Clinical and Diagnostic Imaging of Bisphosphonate-associated Osteonecrosis of the Jaws. Dentomaxillofacial Radiology. 2006;35:236-43.
2. Curtin Hugh D. Separation of the Masticator Space from the Parapharyngeal Space. Radiology. 1987;163:195-204.
3. Davic Steven B, Matthews Vincent P, Williams Daniel W. III. Masticator Muscle Enhancement in Subacute Denervation Atrophy. AJNR. 1995;16:1292-4.
4. Garcia-Ferrer Luis, Bagan Jose V, Martinez-Sanjuan Vicente, Hernandez-Bazan Sergio, Garcia Raquel, Jimenez-Soriano Yolanda, Hervas Vicente. MRI of Mandibular Osteonecrosis Secondary to Bisphosphonates. AJR. 2008;190:949-55.
5. Lewin Jonathan S, Park Jung K. Imaging of the Parapharyngeal and Masticator Spaces. In: William W. Orrison, Jr. (Ed.). Neuroimaging, Volume 2, Chapter 33: 1193-1202. WB Saunders Company, Philadelphia; 2000.
6. Russo CP, Smoker WRK, Weissmann JL. MR Appearance of Trigeminal and Hypoglossal Motor Denervation. AJNR. 1997;18:1375-83.

# Part II: The parapharyngeal space

## Anatomy (Figures 6.II.1A and B)

Conceptually, the parapharyngeal space (PPS) is a simple compartment to visualize. It is described as a pyramidal shaped space with the base abutting the skull base tapering to its apex at the superior cornua of the hyoid bone. On axial imaging, it appears triangular in shape.

Analysis of the space becomes more complex when defining the fascial boundaries. It occupies a central position bordered laterally by the superficial layer of the deep cervical fascia separating it from the masticator space. Medially, it is bordered by the middle (buccopharyngeal) layer of the deep cervical fascia, overlying the deep pharyngobasilar fascia and pharyngeal constrictors, thereby separating it from the mucosal/visceral compartment. Posteriorly, it lies anterior to the prevertebral compartment which is invested by the deep layer of the deep cervical fascia. Inferiorly, there is no true fascia existing between the parapharyngeal space and posterior aspect of the submandibular space allowing for ready communication and trans-compartmental spread of disease. An understanding of these fascial boundaries is necessary as the pattern of transgression of these fascial boundaries in relationship to the parapharyngeal space allows

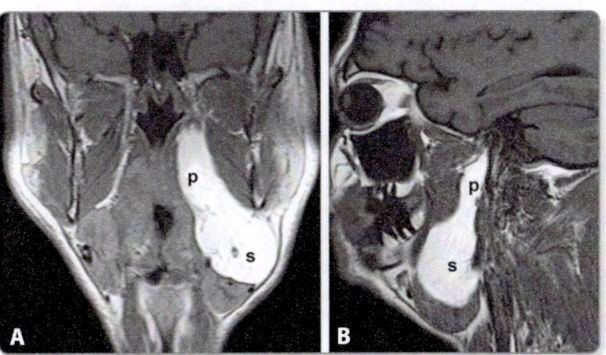

**Figures 6.II.1A and B** Parapharyngeal space (p) communicates with the submandibular space (s): coronal and sagittal T1 weighted MRI images demonstrate a lipoma arising in the left parapharyngeal space extending inferiorly into the submandibular space

one to determine or predict the site of origin of a disease process and offer a reasonable, limited and more accurate differential diagnosis.

The parapharyngeal space can be further subdivided into prestyloid and retrostyloid compartments. This division is created by the tensor vascular styloid fascia which is associated with the tensor veli palatini, styloid process and styloid musculature. This fascia helps separate the anterolateral prestyloid compartment (which borders the masticator space) from the posteromedial retrostyloid compartment that borders the paravertebral and visceral spaces.

The prestyloid parapharyngeal space is largely occupied by fat, the pterygoid plexus and traversing small vessels and nerves including a branch of the fifth cranial nerve. Small congenital rests of salivary gland tissue can also be found.

The retrostyloid space contains the carotid artery, jugular vein, cranial nerves IX to XII and the posterior sympathetic chain. In some textbooks, this retrostyloid compartment is referred to as the "carotid" space.

## Parapharyngeal space: superior (Figure 6.II.2)

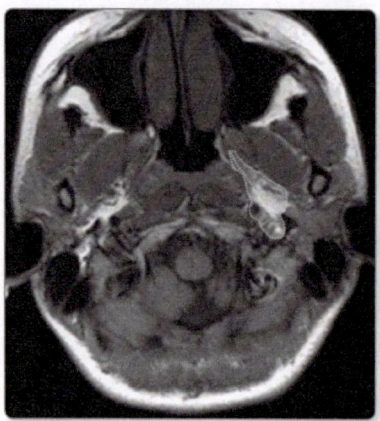

**Figure 6.II.2** Shaded region corresponds to the parapharyngeal space on axial imaging (outlined by yellow dotted line). It can be further subdivided into the prestyloid space (anterolateral to white dashed line) and retrostyloid space (posteromedial to white dashed line). White dashed line corresponds to the tensor vascular styloid fascia (*for color version see Plate 14*)

Imaging of the masticator and parapharyngeal spaces 281

## Parapharyngeal space: inferior (Figures 6.II.3A and B)

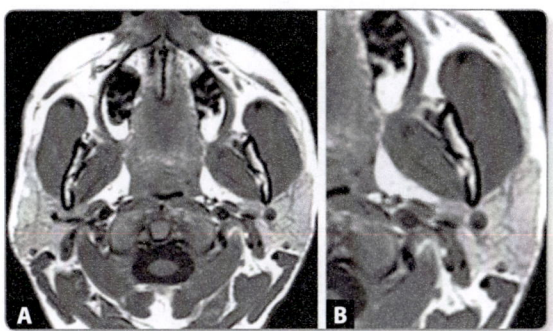

**Figures 6.II.3A and B** Triangular shaped area of fat (outlined in yellow) bordered by the masticator space laterally, visceral space medially and parotid space posterolaterally. This corresponds to the prestyloid portion of the PPS. The red shaded area corresponds to the retrostyloid component which some refer to as the carotid space (*for color version of Figure 6.II.3B see Plate 14*)

## Parapharyngeal space: anterior (Figure 6.II.4)

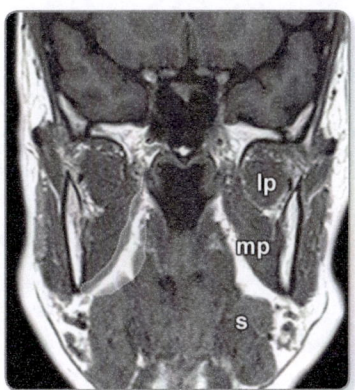

**Figure 6.II.4** Fat-filled space (yellow shaded area) medial to the muscles of mastication, [medial pterygoid (mp) and lateral pterygoid (lp) muscles] (*for color version see Plate 14*)

## Parapharyngeal space: posterior (Figures 6.II.5 and 6.II.6)

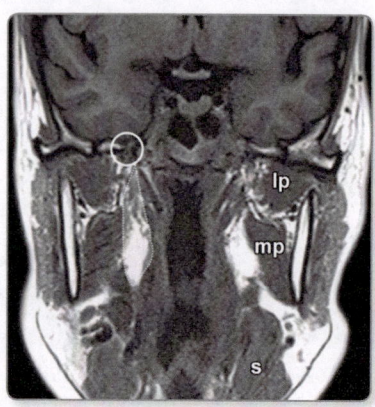

**Figure 6.II.5** Fat-filled space (yellow shaded area) tapering superiorly at skull base medial to foramen ovale (circle); [lateral pterygoid (lp) and medial pterygoid (mp) muscles] (*for color version see Plate 15*)

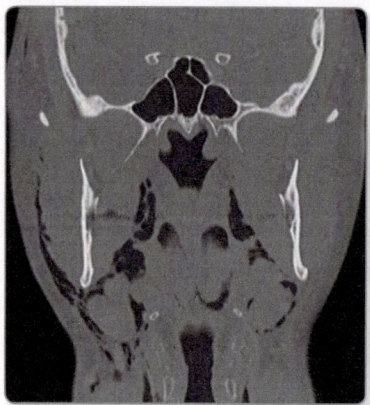

**Figure 6.II.6** Soft tissue emphysema within the neck following a dental procedure. Air is dissecting along and delineating the parapharyngeal space along either side of the pharynx. On the right, air is also outlining the masseter muscle in the masticator space

# Pathology

## Prestyloid parapharyngeal space

A mass within the prestyloid parapharyngeal space is often clinically occult until it has reached sufficient size to generate mass effect on adjacent structures. This typically is in the form of displacement and apparent intraoral fullness of the palate and lateral oropharyngeal wall and tonsil. This pattern of growth is due to the relative fixed constraints of the bony structures laterally (mandible) and superiorly (skull base).

Given the paucity of contents within the prestyloid parapharyngeal space, primary pathology originating in this compartment is limited. Typically, salivary gland origin tumors both benign and malignant, nerve sheath lesions, vascular malformations and rarer lesions such as lipomas, dermoids and second branchial cleft cysts can be found. More often this space is secondarily involved by processes, typically infection and tumor within the adjacent masticator space laterally, visceral space medially, parotid space posterolaterally, and retrostyloid space posteromedially. Focal metastases can occur rarely.

By analyzing the relationship between the lesion and the parapharyngeal fat, one can often establish the lesions' site of origin. This simplifies diagnostic considerations. A lesion within the parapharyngeal space is characteristically surrounded by fat on all sides. If large, it will encroach upon and displace the structures of adjacent spaces depending on its pattern of growth. Lesions arising outside the parapharyngeal space, will distort the fat within the space. For example, a lesion within the masticator space will encroach upon the prestyloid anterolateral parapharyngeal fat displacing the fat predominantly medially as well as possibly, anteriorly and posteriorly dependent on its tumor volume. A lesion within the parotid space will widen the stylomandibular tunnel and displace the fat predominantly anteriorly and medially. A lesion within the visceral space will displace the fat laterally while a lesion within the posteromedial retrostyloid space will displace the prestyloid fat predominantly anteriorly.

# Patterns of parapharyngeal fat displacement (Figures 6.II.7 to 6.II.11)

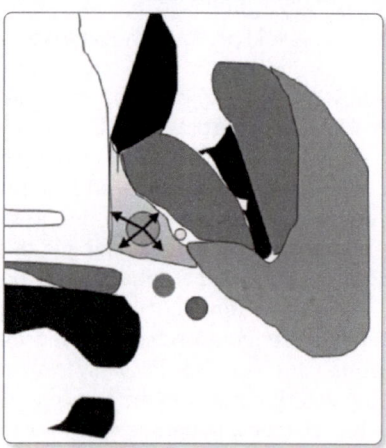

**Figure 6.II.7** A lesion centered within the parapharyngeal space is surrounded by fat. An uninterrupted rim of fat will confirm its parapharyngeal origin. As the lesion enlarges, it will efface the fat according to its direction of growth (*for color version see Plate 15*)

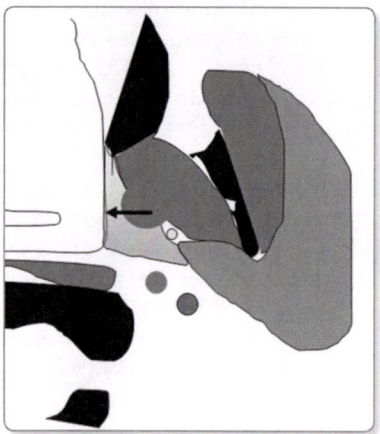

**Figure 6.II.8** A lesion centered within the masticator space will displace and compress the parapharyngeal fat predominantly medially (*for color version see Plate 15*)

Imaging of the masticator and parapharyngeal spaces 285

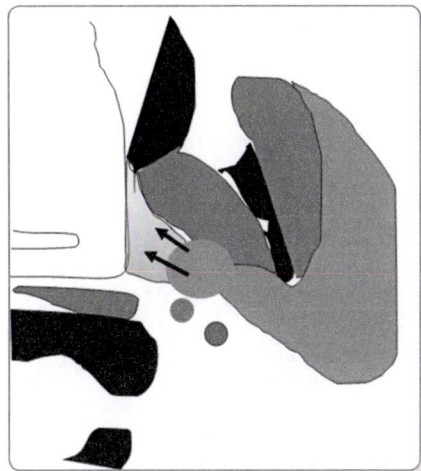

**Figure 6.II.9** A lesion centered within the parotid space widens the stylomandibular tunnel and will displace and compress the parapharyngeal fat anteriorly as well as medially (*for color version see Plate 16*)

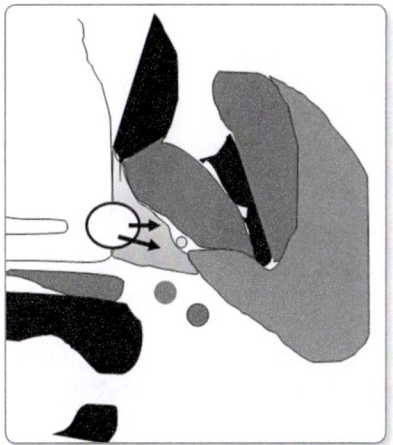

**Figure 6.II.10** A lesion centered within the visceral space will displace and compress the parapharyngeal fat predominantly laterally (*for color version see Plate 16*)

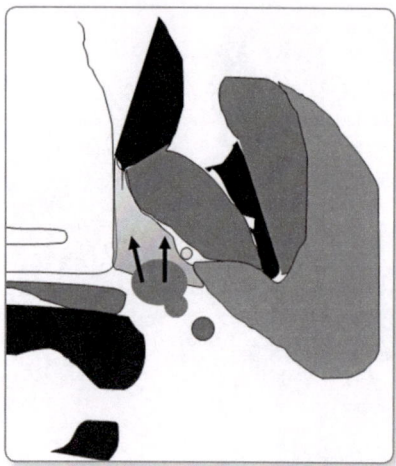

**Figure 6.II.11** A lesion centered within the retrostyloid parapharyngeal space will displace and compress the parapharyngeal fat anteriorly (*for color version see Plate 16*)

## Infection

Clinically, parapharyngeal infection presents with fever, facial cellulitis and intraoral fullness with more ominous signs including dysphagia, difficulty breathing, trismus and cranial nerve dysfunction indicative of deeper spread of disease.

Axial CT with multiplanar reformats is the imaging modality and technique of choice in the acute setting to localize the source of infection, depict its extent and detect complications alerting to potential life threatening conditions including retropharyngeal extension, venous thrombophlebitis or carotid erosion or pseudoaneurysm formation. It allows for treatment decision and surgical approach to drainage.

On imaging, parapharyngeal spread of infection, depending on its severity, may manifest as inflammatory stranding of the fat, infiltrative (phelgmonous) fluid attenuation which has not matured into a discrete collection, or localized uni- or multiloculated irregular rim-enhancing abscess formation with potential spread to adjacent masticator, submandibular, parotid, carotid or retropharyngeal spaces. Involvement of these spaces manifests with edematous enlargement of the involved structures with obliteration of the fat-tissue planes (**Figures 6.II.12 and 6.II.13**). Overlying cellulitis appears as thickening of the skin and platysma with stranding of the subcutaneous fat.

## Tumors

The majority of solitary tumors within the prestyloid parapharyngeal space are benign. The most common benign tumor is of salivary gland origin, the pleomorphic adenoma. On imaging, it is well circumscribed, frequently lobulated with a heterogeneous appearance, particularly when large in size. Often it has cystic components and occasionally may hemorrhage if large. A useful sign is the presence of calcifications

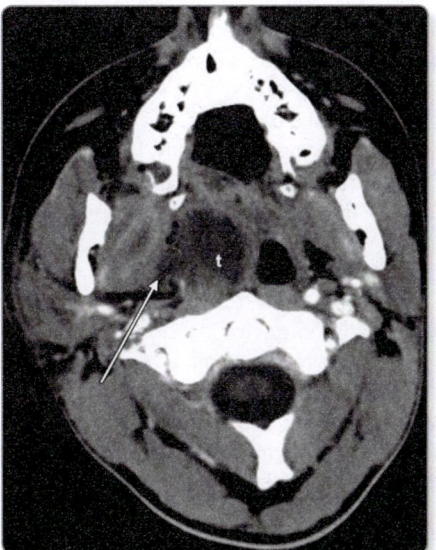

**Figure 6.II.12** Contrast-enhanced axial CT demonstrating tonsillar abscess (t) decompressing laterally into the parapharyngeal space (arrow)

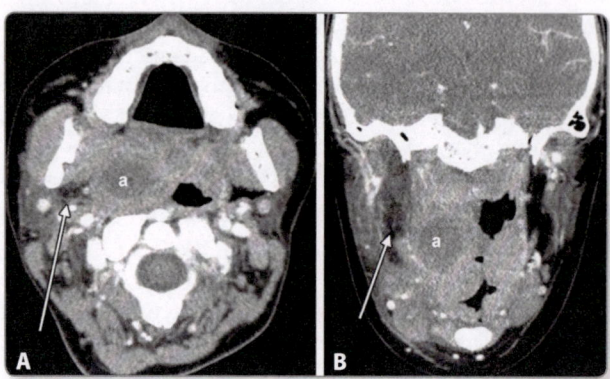

**Figures 6.II.13A and B** Axial contrast-CT and coronal reformat demonstrating tonsillar abscess (a) with lateral parapharyngeal fat infiltration (arrow)

which are best visualized on CT. On MRI, pleomorphic adenomas exhibit similar morphological features as on CT and are characterized by low to intermediate T1 and variably increased T2 signal intensities (**Figures 6.II.14A to E**).

Well defined margins of a lesion are not confidently reliable in conferring a benign diagnosis as roughly two-thirds of minor salivary gland origin malignancies including mucoepidermoid (most common), adenoid cystic and acinic cell carcinomas may have well defined margins. They are however, much more rare than pleomorphic adenomas. Ill-defined margins however, do suggest a more aggressive lesion.

MRI is useful in demonstrating the margins of a lesions and confirming a complete fat tissue plane surrounding a primary parapharyngeal mass. Analyzing the margins may be helpful in excluding an exophytic tumor arising from the deep lobe of the parotid gland which can mimic a primary parapharyngeal origin tumor. The fascial layer between the deep lobe of the parotid gland and prestyloid parapharyngeal space is often incomplete allowing for easy extension of disease. Sometimes, this differentiation is not possible if the tumor is large and the tissue plane between the lesion and margins of the deep lobe of the parotid are effaced or partially effaced. A sign which

Imaging of the masticator and parapharyngeal spaces 289

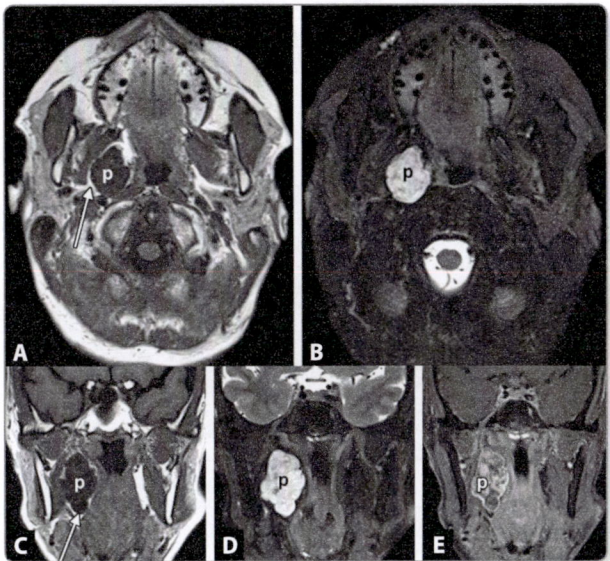

**Figures 6.II.14A to E** Pleomorphic adenoma. Axial and coronal T1 and T2-weighted images demonstrate a solitary well circumscribed lobulated mass (p) in the right parapharyngeal space surrounded by fat (arrow). Postcontrast coronal series demonstrate patchy enhancement

may be helpful in characterizing a parotid lesion is widening of the stylomandibular tunnel (**Figures 6.II.15 to 6.II.17**). It is important to differentiate if possible, a deep lobe parotid lesion from a parapharyngeal lesion, as the surgical approach differs for a parotid lesion in order to preserve facial nerve function. For surgical planning, if this distinction cannot be made, a planned parotid surgery approach is undertaken to minimize the risk of facial nerve injury.

Given the presence of traversing nerves through the prestyloid parapharyngeal space, the differential diagnosis for a well defined, ovoid or tubular, enhancing lesion in the prestyloid parapharyngeal space may suggest a lesion of nerve sheath origin. Imaging characteristics parallel those found elsewhere (**Figures 6.II.18A to C**).

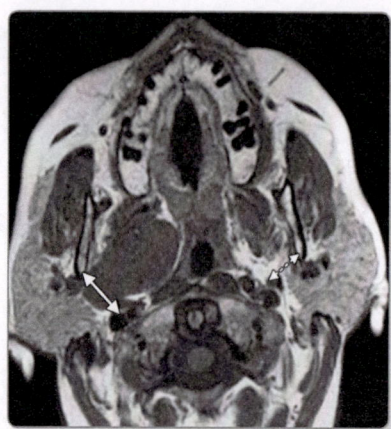

**Figure 6.II.15** Axial T1-weighted image demonstrating well defined lobulated mass within the right parapharyngeal space encroaching upon the parotid space. Although it appears that there is an intact fat tissue plane between the deep parotid tissue and the lesion, there is uncertainty as to its origin given that the right stylomandibular tunnel is widened (long arrow). Such widening is an imaging feature suggestive of a deep lobe parotid lesion. The origin of the lesion is considered indeterminate. It remains possible that the lesion could be arising from a small slip of deep parotid lobe tissue and occupying the parapharyngeal space. In such a case, a planned parotid surgery would be undertaken. Short dashed arrow shows contralateral stylomandibular tunnel

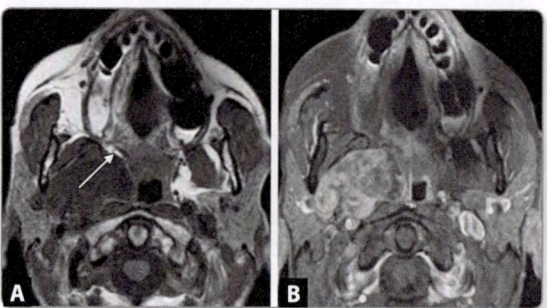

**Figures 6.II.16A and B** Parotid pleomorphic adenoma. Axial T1-weighted pre- and postgadolinium images demonstrate a pleomorphic adenoma clearly arising from the deep lobe of the right parotid gland, projecting into the parapharyngeal space characteristically widening the stylomandibular tunnel. It displaces the parapharyngeal fat anteromedially (arrow)

Imaging of the masticator and parapharyngeal spaces   291

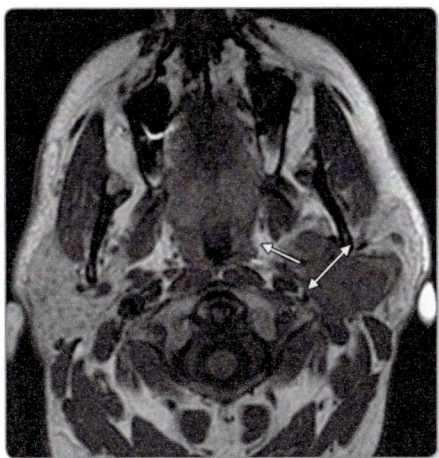

**Figure 6.II.17** Parotid acinic cell carcinoma. Axial T1-weighted image demonstrates an infiltrative lesion involving the superficial and deep lobes of the left parotid gland widening the stylomandibular tunnel (double headed arrow) and anteromedially displacing the parapharyngeal fat (short arrow)

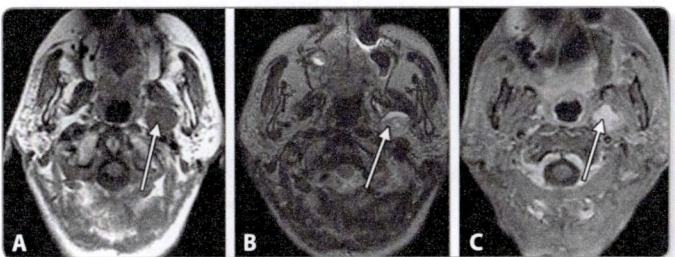

**Figures 6.II.18A to C** Parapharyngeal space schwannoma. Axial T1-, T2-weighted and postgadolinium fat suppressed T1-weighted images demonstrate a well circumscribed avidly enhancing ovoid lesion (arrow) with intact surrounding fat tissue plane within the left parapharyngeal space mildly indenting the deep lobe of the parotid gland. Imaging characteristics parallel those of nerve sheath lesions presenting elsewhere in the body

Lipomas of the parapharyngeal space are uncommon (**Figure 6.II.19**). The imaging features parallel fat density on CT and fat signal intensity on all MRI pulse sequences with homogeneous fat suppression.

Malignancies particularly involving the naso- and oropharynx as well as masticator and parotid spaces can transgress fascial borders and secondarily involve the parapharyngeal space. This is particularly more common in the spread of disease from nasopharyngeal carcinomas which violate the pharyngobasilar fascia and infiltrate laterally into the parapharyngeal space (**Figure 6.II.20**). There may be frank invasion of the space or subtle fat infiltration of the fat in the early phase. Similarly, lateral oropharyngeal wall and tonsillar tumors can transgress the pharyngeal constrictor muscle and extend into the parapharyngeal space (**Figure 6.II.21**). Parapharyngeal extension may be clinically silent as this space is largely comprised of fat. Imaging is therefore crucial in the staging of these malignancies which border the parapharyngeal space. MRI, given its superb tissue contrast resolution and anatomical detail, is the preferred imaging modality for assessing the extent of parapharyngeal space involvement.

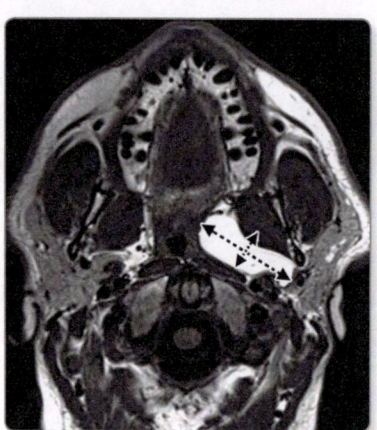

**Figure 6.II.19** Fatty mass occupies the central parapharyngeal space with displacement of the lateral oropharyngeal wall, pterygoid muscle, prevertebral muscle and parotid gland (arrows). Lipoma was found at surgery

Imaging of the masticator and parapharyngeal spaces 293

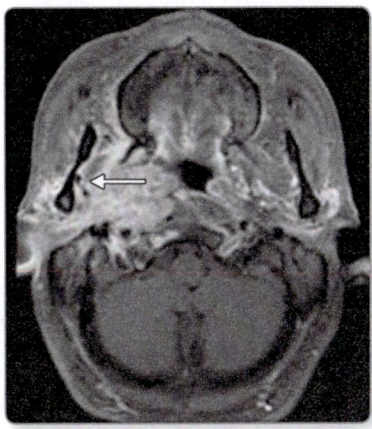

**Figure 6.II.20** Nasopharyngeal carcinoma. Axial T1-weighted postgadolinium fat-suppressed image demonstrating a nasopharyngeal carcinoma infiltrating laterally into the prestyloid parapharyngeal space (arrow) as well as posterolaterally into the retrostyloid parapharyngeal space and posteriorly, into the prevertebral musculature

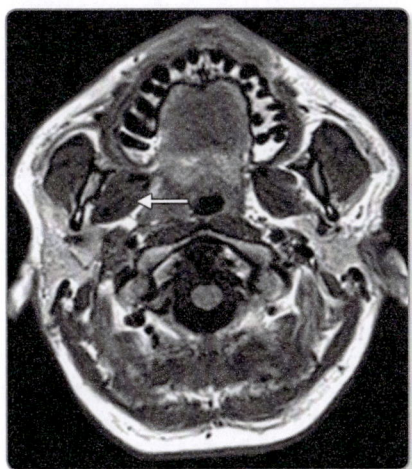

**Figure 6.II.21** Tonsillar carcinoma. Axial T1-weighted image demonstrating subtle lateral infiltration of a tonsillar carcinoma into the parapharyngeal space (arrow)

Focal metastases within the prestyloid parapharyngeal space can occur but are very rare.

# Retrostyloid parapharyngeal space

Processes within the retrostyloid parapharyngeal space lie medial to the styloid process and displace the parapharyngeal fat predominantly anteriorly as well as medially. The space is occasionally referred to as the suprahyoid carotid space. Masses within the retrostyloid parapharyngeal compartment are largely related to vascular or neurogenic structures associated with the carotid sheath bundle at and below the skull base to the level of the hyoid. Secondary involvement of this space may be due to extension of tumor, nodal disease or inflammatory process.

Involvement of the neurovascular bundle can produce distinct clinical signs which implicates pathological involvement of a particular structure directly or secondarily due to mass effect from adjacent structures given the intimate physical relationship of these structures in a confined space.

The syndrome of Vernet may result with paralysis of the ninth, tenth and eleventh cranial nerves. Involvement of the glossopharyngeal (IX) nerve may result in vasodepressor syncope syndrome and Horner's syndrome may result from involvement of the sympathetic chain.

Vascular lesions include thrombosis of the carotid artery or jugular vein which can mimic a necrotic mass or adenopathy and but can be readily sorted out by the tubular morphology in the expected location.

Dissection of the internal carotid artery with partial thrombosis or pseudoaneurysm formation can be a cause of Horner's syndrome or hypoglossal palsy due to mass effect on the sympathetic chain or hypoglossal nerve at the skull base respectively. This can be recognized by asymmetrical segmental or focal enlargement of the vessel with narrowing of the native lumen associated with increased, typically eccentric, intraluminal density on CT characterizing the thrombus within the false lumen contained by the flap. On MRI, the eccentric

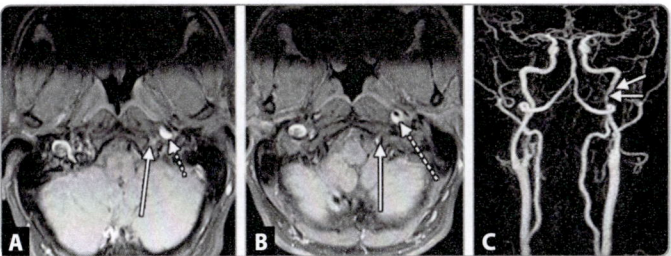

**Figures 6.II.22A to C** Carotid artery dissection. Axial T1-weighted fat suppressed images at skull base demonstrate eccentric T1 signal hyperintensity associated with the internal carotid artery flow void. This signal hyperintensity represents methemoglobin consistent with subacute blood clot within the wall of the vessel (dashed arrow) following a carotid dissection. The contrast angiogram demonstrates a short segment of irregular narrowing of the internal carotid artery (double paired arrows) representing the dissection. The dissection has occurred just anterior to the hypoglossal canal affecting the nerve root as it exits (solid arrow). The patient presented with hypoglossal palsy

clot within the false lumen may be seen to encroach upon the flow void within the native lumen if patent. A flap may or may not be visualized. The clot, if subacute, will demonstrate T1 signal hyperintensity characteristic of methemoglobin. This finding is more conspicuous on T1-weighted images acquired with fat-suppression technique (**Figures 6.II.22A to C**). It is therefore, prudent to evaluate the carotid sheath structures when a patient presents with neurological findings exhibiting features of Horner's syndrome or hypoglossal palsy. Images should be extended below the skull base to capture the neurovascular bundle within the neck.

## Tumors

The most common primary tumors within the retrostyloid parapharyngeal space are benign glomus and neurogenic tumors.

Glomus tumors arise from cells which function as homeostatic chemoreceptors responding to hypoxic conditions. They are hypervascular and are most commonly located at the carotid bifurcation and skull base associated with the jugular foramen (glomus jugulare), tympanic cavity (glomus tympanicum) or along the vagus nerve within the neck and mediastinum (glomus vagale). They are frequently multicentric, initiating a search for multiple lesions. They are frequently silent biochemically but may be active with the most common actively secreting lesion being the glomus vagale. Catecholamine release may characteristically cause labile hypertension, tremor, palpitations and sweating. A small percentage may be malignant associated with metastatic disease. Approximately 10 percent of patients with glomus tumors have a hereditary form. Approximately 10 to 20 percent of glomus tumors are bilateral or multiple.

Glomus jugulare and glomus tympanicum tumors may be a cause of tinnitus, a frequent complaint which often initiates imaging workup. Glomus jugulo/tympanic lesions can clinically present as a red pulsatile retrotympanic mass. On CT, the glomus tympanicum appears as an avidly enhancing lesion overlying the cochlear promontory associated with Jacobson's nerve. Glomus jugulare (**Figures 6.II.23A and B**) centered on the jugular foramen associated with Arnold's nerve, is a slowly expansile vascular mass with permeative pattern of bone loss. This tumor can invade the jugular vein.

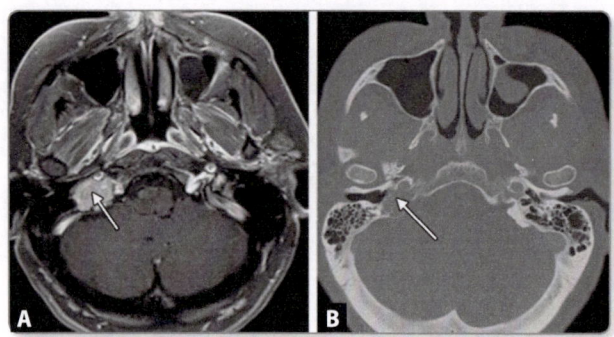

**Figures 6.II.23A and B** Glomus jugulare. Axial T1 weighted postgadolinium MRI image and corresponding CT axial image displayed on bone algorithm demonstrating an enhancing mass centered on the right jugular fossa and associated with permeative pattern of bone loss

Glomus vagale tumor may be asymptomatic or present with signs of vagus nerve dysfunction such as vocal cord palsy or secondarily, due to the close proximity to the hypoglossal canal and nerve, hypoglossal palsy. The internal carotid artery is displaced anteriorly and often medially (**Figures 6.II.24A and B**).

The glomus tumors all share similar imaging characteristics of well circumscribed, occasionally lobulated masses with avid enhancement and a "salt and pepper" matrix on MRI. The "salt" representing areas of hemorrhage and the "pepper" corresponding to vascular flow voids (**Figures 6.II.25A and B**). Dynamic enhancement with rapid initial accumulation of contrast is strongly suggestive of this lesion and is helpful in differentiating from a nerve sheath lesion such as schwannoma which also frequently enhances avidly but in a slightly delayed diffuse fashion.

Neurogenic lesions include schwannomas and neurofibromas, arising from the IX to XII cranial nerves arising from the sympathetic chain. The signal and enhancing characteristics of schwannomas are similar to those found elsewhere. They are well circumscribed, ovoid or fusiform in morphology. Vagal schwannomas are the most common of

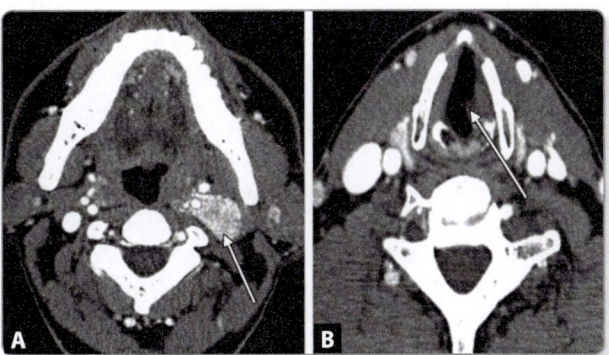

**Figures 6.II.24A and B** Glomus vagale. Axial postcontrast CT images demonstrating an avidly enhancing mass associated with the left carotid sheath structures. It is largely posterior to the artery and partially surrounds it. There is a corresponding left vocal cord palsy with medial deviation of the left vocal cord

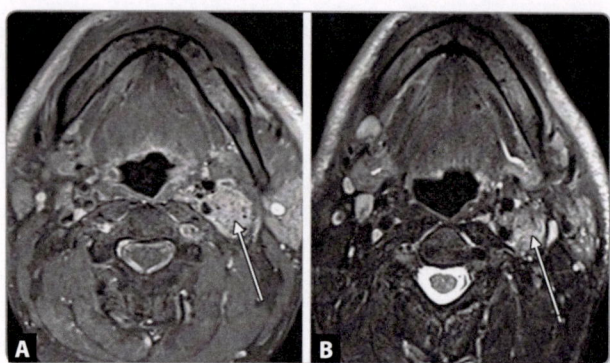

**Figures 6.II.25A and B** Glomus vagale. Axial T1-weighted postgadolinium fat suppressed image on the left demonstrates a mass situated posterior to the left internal carotid artery which avidly enhances with a stippled pattern (arrow). The axial T2-weighted fat suppressed axial image on the right demonstrates stippled areas of flow void characterizing the salt and pepper appearance of these lesions due to areas of slow and high flow within the lesion

these tumors. They, as well as the glomus vagale, usually present with vocal nerve palsy and displace the internal carotid artery anteriorly and medially. When they extend to the jugular foramen at the skull base however, they cause smooth scalloping of the bony margins as apposed to the permeative bone loss seen with glomus jugulare.

The hypoglossal schwannoma (**Figures 6.II.26A and B**) presents with weakness of the ipsilateral tongue musculature reflecting denervation. This is characterized on imaging as posterior displacement of the involved side of the tongue and often, atrophy of the tongue muscles. Posterior displacement of the tongue results in apparent asymmetrical fullness of the tongue which should not be interpreted as tumor but rather recognized as characteristic displacement of the hemi-tongue associated with ipsilateral palsy or paresis. Atrophy of the muscles support the finding of hypoglossal palsy. This is in contrast to tumor which results in the presence of a visible tumor mass with infiltration of normal fat planes (**Figures 6.II.27A and B**).

Imaging of the masticator and parapharyngeal spaces 299

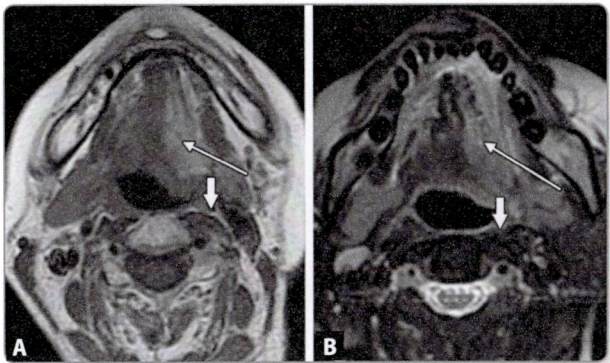

**Figures 6.II.26A and B** Tongue denervation. Axial T1 and T2-weighted images through the tongue demonstrate fatty atrophy (thin arrow) and posterior displacement of the ipsilateral tongue base (thick arrow) as a consequence of motor denervation from the hypoglossal schwannoma at the skull base

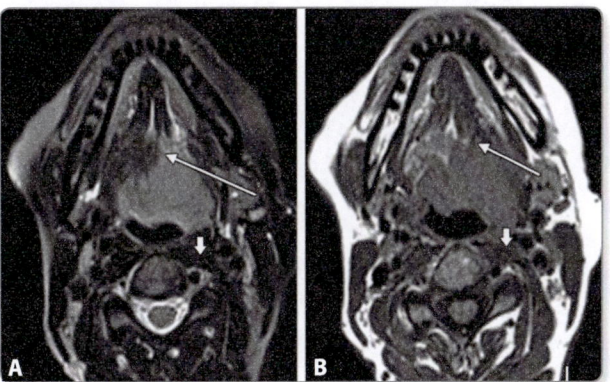

**Figures 6.II.27A and B** Tongue carcinoma. Axial T1 and T2-weighted images demonstrate posterior displacement of the tongue (thick arrow) but this is due to large infiltrative tumor (thin arrow) resulting in greater volume of tissue

## 300 Introductory head and neck imaging

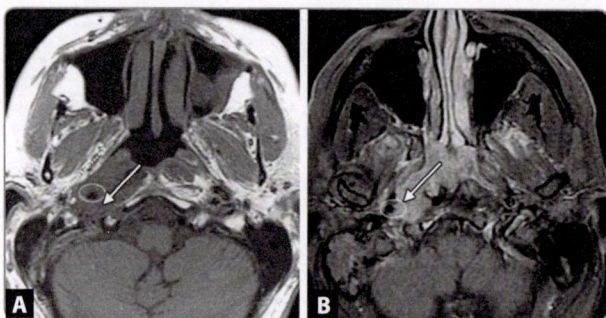

**Figures 6.II.28A and B** Nasopharyngeal carcinoma. Axial T1- and T2-weighted MRI images demonstrate a right sided nasopharyngeal carcinoma which infiltrates posterolaterally (arrow) into the retrostyloid parapharyngeal space (medial to dashed line) and encasing the internal carotid artery (oval)

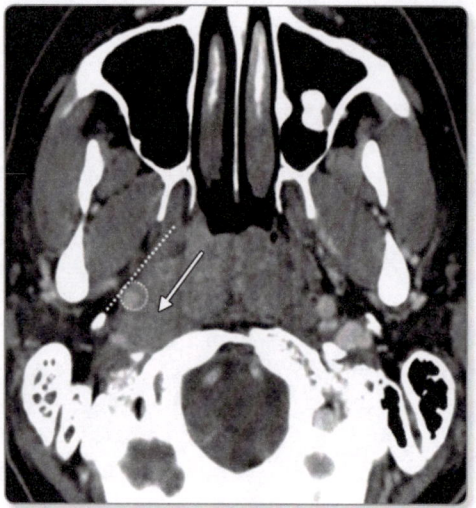

**Figure 6.II.29** Corresponding postcontrast axial CT image demonstrating posterolateral infiltration of the nasopharyngeal carcinoma (arrow) into the retrostyloid parapharyngeal space (medial to dashed line) and encasing the internal carotid artery (circle)

Malignant tumors within the retrostyloid parapharyngeal space are most frequently observed with direct posterolateral extension of naso- and oropharyngeal carcinomas (**Figures 6.II.28 and 6.II.29**). This infiltration results in loss of the fat tissue planes separating the neurovascular components. Occasionally, extracapsular spread of nodal disease may infiltrate into this space.

## Summary

The parapharyngeal space occupies a central deep compartment within the suprahyoid neck bordered by compartments invested by fascial layers. Pathologies can arise primarily within the parapharyngeal space but more often, the space is involved secondarily by disease processes which have transgressed fascial borders. By examining the relationship of the lesion or disease process with the pattern of parapharyngeal fat displacement or involvement, the origin of the lesion can frequently be suggested and a reasonable differential diagnosis generated.

## Bibliography

1. Curtin Hugh D. Separation of the Masticator Space from the Parapharyngeal Space. Radiology. 1987;163:195-204.
2. Lewin Jonathan S, Park Jung K. Imaging of the Parapharyngeal and Masticator Spaces. In William W. Orrison, Jr. (Ed.). Neuroimaging, Volume 2, Chapter 33: 1175-1193. WB Saunders Company, Philadelphia; 2000.
3. Shin Ji Hoon, Lee Ho Kyu, Kim Sang Yoon, Choi Choong Gon, Suh Dae Chul. Pictorial Essay. Imaging of Parapharyngeal Space Lesions: Focus on the Prestyloid Compartment. AJR. 2001;177:1465-70.
4. Som PM, Sacher M, Stollman AR, et al. Common Tumors of the Parapharyngeal Space: Refined Imaging Diagnosis. Radiology. 1988;169:81-5.
5. Tom BM, Rao VM, Guglielmo F. Imaging of the Parapharyngeal Space: anatomy and pathology. Crit Rev Diagn Imaging. 1991;31:315-56.

# Radiographic anatomy and pathology of the oral cavity

chapter 7

Claudia Kirsch, Kristin McNamara

**Abstract**

The cross-sectional anatomy of the oral cavity is covered. A comprehensive review of oral cavity cancer is then presented followed by a discussion of congenital and inflammatory conditions.

**Keywords**

Oral cavity, tongue, CT, MRI.

## Introduction

The oral cavity is the most anterior portion of the head and neck containing a wide variety of tissues in a relatively small region. The first important distinction is separating the oral cavity from the oropharynx. The posterior oral cavity is delineated from the oropharynx by an imaginary line along the circumvallate papillae, anterior tonsillar pillars, and junction of the hard and soft palate (**Figures 7.1A and B**). This distinction is clinically relevant because carcinomas in the oral cavity and oropharynx are different in both presentation and prognosis. The remaining boundaries of the oral cavity include: the lips anteriorly; the cheeks laterally; the hard palate superiorly, superior and inferior alveolar ridges, and the mylohyoid muscle inferiorly. Contained within these margins are the lips and their vermillion border, the anterior two thirds of the oral tongue, floor of mouth, buccal mucosa, upper and lower gingiva, hard palate, anterior tonsillar pillar and retromolar trigone. Tumors and various pathologies can arise from any of the tissues within the oral cavity including the gingival, lingual and buccal mucosal linings, bone, teeth, muscles, nerves, blood vessels, and salivary glands.

Radiographic anatomy and pathology of the oral cavity 303

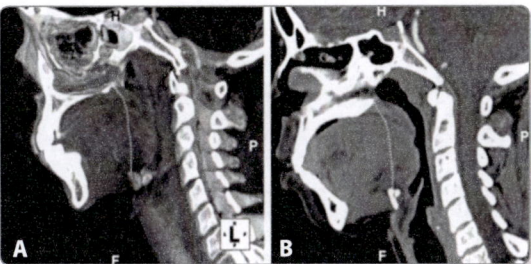

**Figures 7.1A and B** Sagittal CT of the normal oral cavity anatomy in 3D reconstruction and sagittal plane. The dotted line shows the posterior margin of the oral cavity. It marks the posterior margin of the hard palate and the circumvallate papillae. The oral tongue is anterior to the line and the tongue base is posterior (*for color version of Figure 7.1A see Plate 17*)

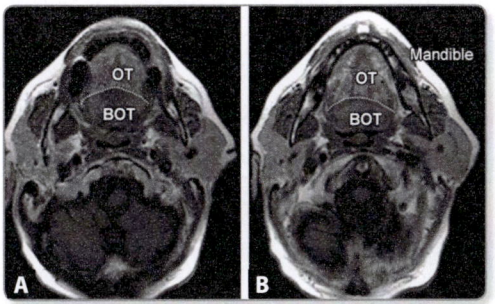

**Figures 7.2A and B** Axial T1-weighted MRI series through the oral cavity. Dotted line represents the circumvallate papillae separating the oral tongue (OT) and the base of tongue (BOT). Shaded area outlines the sublingual space

# Cross-sectional anatomy of the oral cavity

Cross-sectional anatomy of the oral cavity is shown in **Figures 7.2 to 7.6**.

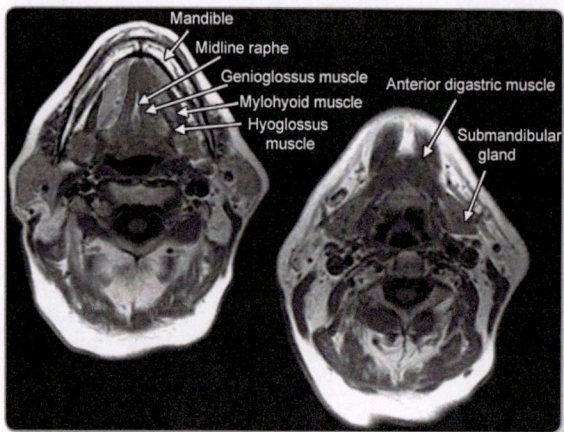

**Figure 7.3** Axial T1-weighted images showing tongue musculature

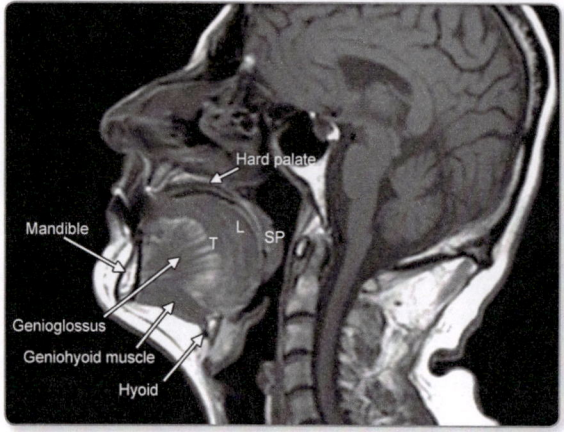

**Figure 7.4** Sagittal T1-weighted image. SP – soft palate, L – longitudinal intrinsic muscle of tongue, T – transverse intrinsic muscle of tongue

Radiographic anatomy and pathology of the oral cavity 305

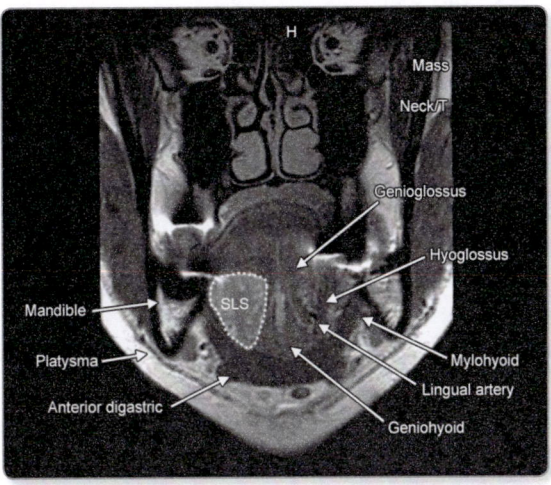

**Figure 7.5** Coronal T1-weighted image of the oral cavity. Shaded area SLS – sublingual space, shaded area SMS – submandibular space

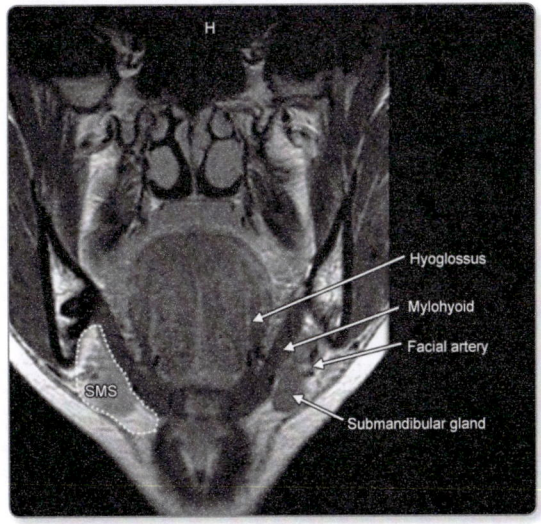

**Figure 7.6** Coronal T1-weighted image of the oral cavity

## The lips and gingiva

The outer covering of the lips is composed of stratified squamous epithelium. This differs from inner surface which is lined by non-keratinizing stratified squamous mucosa. The space between the mouth and cheeks is the vestibule, which is lined by buccal mucosa arising from the teeth and gums. The parotid (Stensen's) duct curves along the buccal fat pad and drains into the vestibule opposite the second maxillary molar. The medial lingual mucosa and lateral buccal surfaces along the alveolar mandible and maxilla are called the gingiva. The junction point between the gingival and buccal mucosa is the gingivobuccal sulcus, which is an important potential site for oral cavity squamous cell carcinoma. The mucosa overlying the pterygomandibular raphe just posterior to the last mandibular molar is the retromolar trigone. The lips are innervated by motor divisions of CN VII. Lymphatic drainage is predominately to submental (level 1A) and submandibular (level 1B) lymph nodes.

## The floor of mouth

The floor of mouth (FOM) is the U-shaped region of tissue that is situated along the anterior and sides of the tongue. The FOM is located between the surface mucosa and the mylohyoid muscle which forms the "floor" for the floor of mouth. The mylohyoid muscle is best visualized in the coronal plane. The mylohyoid also divides the oral cavity into a superior sublingual space and inferior submandibular space. The mylohyoid muscle originates from the mylohyoid ridge or line along the inner mandible and extends posteriorly to the level of the posterior molar root. The posterior medial mylohyoid fibers insert on the hyoid bone and the posterior margin of the muscle is a free margin. The submandibular gland wraps around the free edge of the posterior mylohyoid and sits partially in the posterior sublingual space and the submandibular space. The mylohyoid muscle is innervated by the motor mylohyoid branch of the trigeminal nerve (CN V3).

## The oral tongue

The mobile oral tongue has a dividing fibrous lingual septum or midline raphe. The tongue is composed of intrinsic and extrinsic muscle fibers. The four interdigitating intrinsic muscles comprise the majority of the tongue. These muscles are the superior and inferior longitudinal, transverse and the oblique muscles. The extrinsic muscles originate from bony attachments external to the tongue with their distal fibers interdigitating into the intrinsic musculature. The extrinsic tongue muscles include the genioglossus, styloglossus, hyoglossus and palatoglossus muscles. Both intrinsic and extrinsic tongue muscles receive motor innervation from the hypoglossal nerve (CN XII), which is located between the mylohyoid and hyoglossus muscles in the oral cavity. In addition, the palatoglossus receives innervation from the pharyngeal plexus. The sensory axons of the anterior two thirds of the tongue converge to form the lingual nerve, which is a branch of the mandibular division (V3) of the trigeminal nerve (CN V). The chorda tympani nerve is a division of the facial nerve (CN VII) and extends through the petrotympanic fissure and joins with the lingual nerve. These two nerve bundles then travel distally along the lateral border of the oral cavity. The parasympathetic fibers of the CN VII synapse in the submandibular ganglion, which is suspended from the lingual nerve adjacent to the hypoglossal nerve.

The genioglossus is the largest extrinsic muscle and is a paired muscle with fibers separated by the midline lingual fatty septum. The genioglossus originates from a tendon arising from the genial tubercle along the inner mandible.

The styloglossus muscle originates from the styloid process and stylomandibular ligament. The fibers extend between the internal and external carotid arteries and superior and inferior constrictor muscles along the lateral oral tongue and divide into two sets of fibers. The muscle's longitudinal fibers insert along the side of the tongue anterior to the hyoglossus muscle. The posterior styloglossus fibers interdigitate with the hyoglossus muscle. The palatoglossus muscle arises from the soft palate and inserts on the lateral tongue with distal fibers inserting into the styloglossus muscle. The palatoglossus muscle and surrounding mucosa create the anterior tonsillar pillar or palatoglossal arch, and is considered part of the oral cavity.

## The hard palate

The hard palate is formed by the palatine process of the maxilla and horizontal plates of the palatine bones. The hard palate is bounded both anteriorly and laterally by the alveolar processes and gingiva. Within the hard palate just posterior to the incisor teeth is the incisive foramen allowing passage for the nasopalatine nerves and arteries. This nerve an important nerve which needs to be anesthetized during upper dental work. In the posterior hard palate just medial to the posterior third molar are the greater and lesser palatine foramen through which travels the greater and lesser palatine arteries and nerves (**Figure 7.7**). The greater palatine artery and nerve supplies the tissues of the hard palate while the lesser palatine artery and nerve supplies the soft palate.

## Maxilla and mandible

The maxilla and mandible are affected by a diverse range of pathologic processes. Many developmental, metabolic, neoplastic, inflammatory, and traumatic lesions or disorders which affect the skeleton can

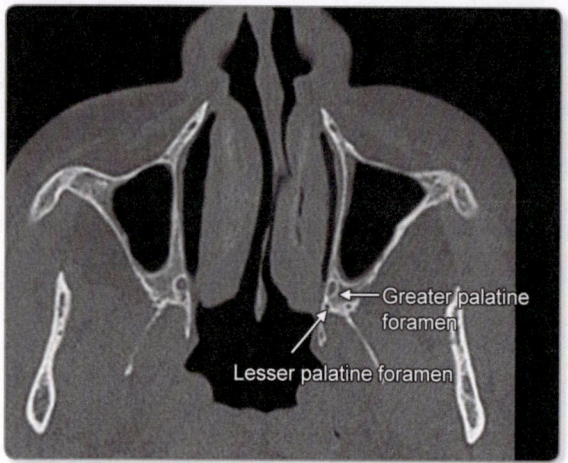

Figure 7.7 Axial CT image shows the greater and lesser palatine foramen

present in the jaws. In addition, numerous benign and malignant soft tissue tumors as well as metastatic malignancies may present centrally within the maxilla or mandible. However, given the presence of teeth and associated structures, there are also a variety of pathologies which are unique to the jaws. Teeth can be a source of infection and inflammatory processes and can give rise to odontogenic cysts and tumors from tissues involved in tooth formation. The goal of imaging in this region is not only to determine the extent of disease, but also to characterize the radiographic features as an aid in generating a differential diagnosis and treatment planning. Assessment of lesion shape, borders, internal architecture, relationship and effects on surrounding teeth, expansion or perforation of cortical plates, and extension to soft tissue are fundamental to radiographic analysis.

## Imaging of the oral cavity with CT and MRI

MRI and CT imaging of the oral cavity are complementary. CT offers excellent visualization of bony detail and lends itself well in the evaluation of fracture and cortical erosion by tumor. MRI has advantages in its ability to resolve soft tissue anatomy. Both MRI and CT allow for multiplanar reconstruction. Protocols for MRI of the oral cavity carcinomas will defer from institution to institution. Ideally, MRI should be performed with a dedicated neck coil. Imaging in the sagittal, axial and coronal planes are obtained generally with a slice thickness of 4 mm or less. At our institution, we perform sagittal and coronal imaging with fields of view on T1-weighted sequences in the axial plane ranging from 16 to 18 cm, and on T2-weighted sequences ranging from 18 to 20 cm. Pre- and post-contrast T1-weighted images after intravenous administration of gadolinium should be performed in the same planes, allowing for differentiation of fat and proteinaceous fluids. A noncontrast T1 is used for delineating the anatomy and determining the status of the various normal fat and muscle planes. These imaging features are helpful when evaluating for tumor infiltration. Postcontrast T1 images with fat saturation are also useful in the assessment of perineural tumor spread. Having patients puff their cheeks during CT imaging can be performed. This would help in delineating masses within the buccal vestibule along the buccal or gingival surfaces. This technique is limited in MRI due to the greater time needed during image acquisition.

# Pathology

## Vascular

Vascular lesions of the oral cavity include any of the vascular lesions of the head and neck and can be classified either into two broad categories: hemangiomas or vascular malformations (VM). Hemangiomas are true neoplasms demonstrating actual cell proliferation. These present during infancy and will enlarge then involute as the patient matures. Vascular malformations are congenital lesions. They may manifest during infancy and childhood and will not regress. Vascular malformations can be subdivided into capillary, arterial, venous, lymphatic and mixed (**Figures 7.8A and B**). A full discussion of these lesions is included in the Chapter 14 on Vascular Lesions of the Head and Neck.

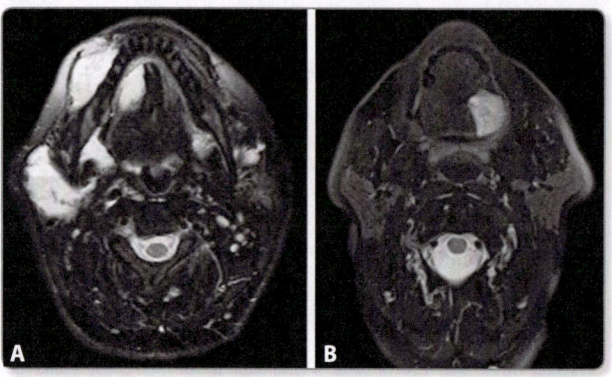

**Figures 7.8A and B** Venous vascular malformation (VVM) in two different patients. (A) Shows an extensive lesion that involves the right sublingual space (SLS) as well as the right and left parotid, masticator space and the soft tissues over the right mandible. (B) Shows a localized VVM involving the left posterior oral tongue. VVM are readily apparent as very high signal masses on these fat saturated T2-weighted images

## Infectious

Infection is the most common pathology seen in the oral cavity and may be secondary to poor oral hygiene, immunosuppression, or from treatments such as radiation therapy that can alter the normal salivary pH resulting in an increased likelihood of dental disease. Imaging is critical for the assessment of the airway, the spaces involved, and detecting abscess formation. CT bone window images also allow for evaluation of periapical lucency around the teeth, suggestive of odontogenic disease. Ludwig's angina refers to a cellulitis of the FOM usually secondary to an infected mandibular molar. The bacterial agents are usually the oral flora. The tissues can undergo gangrenous necrosis with minimal pus. If untreated, FOM abscess can develop (**Figures 7.9A to C**).

## Neoplastic

In Western societies, oral cancer accounts for approximately 0.6 to 5.0 percent of all cancers in societies such as the US, Europe and Australia. Oral cavity carcinoma is the sixth leading cause of cancer in the world. Risk factors include alcohol and tobacco (they are synergistic), sun exposure, and human papilloma virus (HPV). Current research implicates HPV in nearly 14 percent of cases. Other research in familial aggregates of cancer reveals a possible genetic component

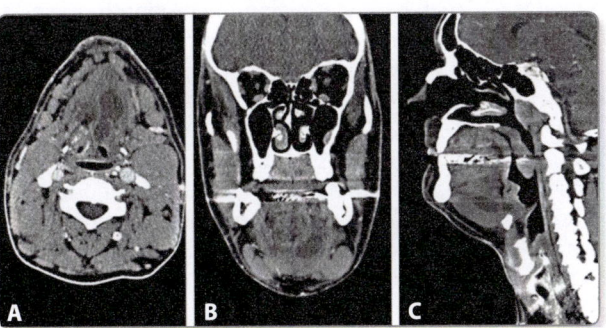

**Figures 7.9A to C** Floor of mouth abscess. *Courtesy*: Dr Eric Bartlett

in the development of oral cancer in younger patients. Another risk factor is the chewing of betel nut by males and females in India. As a result, oral cavity carcinoma is extremely prevalent in that country, representing nearly 45 percent of all cancers. The vast majority of oral cancers are squamous cell carcinomas (SCCA), which comprise 90 percent of all oral malignant lesions. Additional carcinomas include salivary gland tumors such as adenoid cystic or mucoepidermoid carcinomas, lymphoma, melanoma and the rare sarcomas or bone tumors.

Imaging plays a critical role in tumor staging is needed in evaluating the full deep extent of infiltration. This is necessary when assessing for the feasibility of surgical resection and/or radiation therapy and planning.

Oral cavity tumors are classified by site of origin. Awareness of a tumor's location and behavior is essential for adequate radiographic analysis as both tumor spread and the treatment options are variable. This section presents imaging examples of carcinoma and additional pathologies occurring in major sites including the floor of mouth, oral tongue, buccal mucosa, bony upper alveolus, hard palate, and retromolar trigone.

## Neoplastic — critical imaging findings

In oral cavity cancers, tumor origin is important in determining its propensity to spread along certain pathways. Many papers discuss the multifactorial effects determining the prognosis in oral cavity cancers, however on imaging there are five major features that play a key prognostic role: tumor size and thickness, perineural invasion, bone marrow invasion, and lymph node involvement with extracapsular spread.

Multiple studies have demonstrated that increased tumor size is associated with decreased overall survival, thus the important T-factor on the AJCC chart. The T-factor affects both the five-year survival rates and rates of positive cervical lymphadenopathy. The comparative effects of the T-size with both survival rates and rates of metastatic lymphadenopathy, in a study by Tytor et al., for oral cavity SCCa are listed below:

T1 - tumor 2 cm or smaller: 91 percent survival rate - 14 percent rate of positive lymph nodes

T2 - tumor > 2 cm < 4 cm: 63 percent survival rate - 37 percent rate of positive lymph nodes

T3 - tumor > 4 cm: 60 percent survival rate - 57 percent rate of positive lymph nodes

In the oral tongue, tumor thickness is an important prognostic factor in the risk of local recurrence, the presence of nodal metastasis, and overall patient morbidity and mortality. MRI allows for adequate measurement of the tumor thickness and often helps in assisting physicians/patients in treatment planning.

An additional important prognostic factor is tumor invasion of the perineural sheath or epineurium. A study by Brown et al. noted an incidence of regional metastatic disease in 71 percent of patients with perineural invasion. This number is nearly double the incidence of metastatic disease which was found in only 36 percent of patients with oral cavity carcinomas with no perineural invasion. Local control rates also drop from 78 percent in patients without perineural invasion to 38 percent if perineural invasion was present. Thus, perineural invasion is strongly associated with decreased survival and increased local recurrence requiring aggressive treatment.

Bone marrow invasion is a finding on the AJCC chart that upstages a lip carcinoma to a T4. CT is very sensitive in assessing for cortical bony invasion. MRI can provide further information as to the status of the central marrow space in affected bones.

The presence or absence of lymphadenopathy is often considered one of the most important prognostic factors. This is discussed separately in the chapter 11 on cervical lymph nodes of the neck.

## Lip carcinoma

Carcinomas of the lip usually arise from the vermillion border and may spread to involve adjacent skin or underlying muscles of the mouth such as the orbicularis oris. Small early lesions are often easier to detect on clinical examination. The role of imaging comes into play when the lesion may be more advanced and the margins indeterminate. The goal of imaging is to determine the full extent of the lesion, including possible perineural spread and the integrity of the adjacent bone (**Figures 7.10 and 7.11**). CT is very sensitive to assess for subtle bony

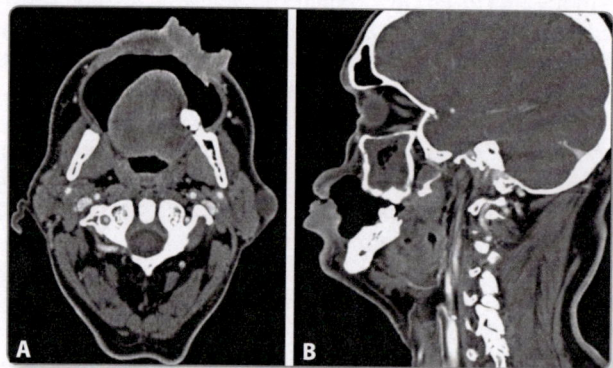

**Figures 7.10A and B** Axial and sagittal CT imaging of a large ulcerated mass involving the left lower lip. This scan was performed with a puffed cheek technique. This helps distend the gingivolabial sulcus and shows that there is no tumor extension onto the mandible

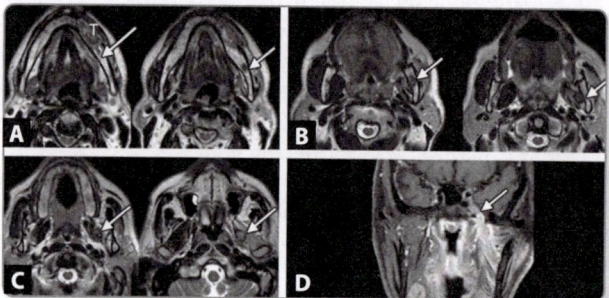

**Figures 7.11A to D** MRI imaging shows a lip carcinoma which had invaded deeply to involve the mandible (T). The arrows show perineural tumor spread along the inferior alveolar nerve in the mandible and then along the mandibular division of the trigeminal nerve in the masticator space. The coronal fat saturated postgadolinium enhanced image reveal tumor tracking back to the cavernous sinus

erosive changes. MRI is superior for assessment of central bone marrow involvement. Care must be taken in MRI as it may overestimate the extent of tumor invasion with false positive findings secondary to hemorrhage and inflammatory change.

## Floor of mouth carcinoma

The majority of SCCa's arise near the anterior midline floor of mouth. Floor of mouth carcinomas (**Figures 7.12A and B**) have a propensity for lateral spread with involvement of the adjacent mandible or submucosally to involve the ipsilateral or contralateral lingual neurovascular bundle in the sublingual compartment. Assessment as to whether tumor has crossed the midline lingual septum or involves the contralateral neurovascular bundles are factors that will influence whether a surgeon will attempt a hemiglossectomy or total glossectomy. Additional critical factors that may upstage a FOM cancer to a stage 4 include, bone involvement, extension to the base of tongue

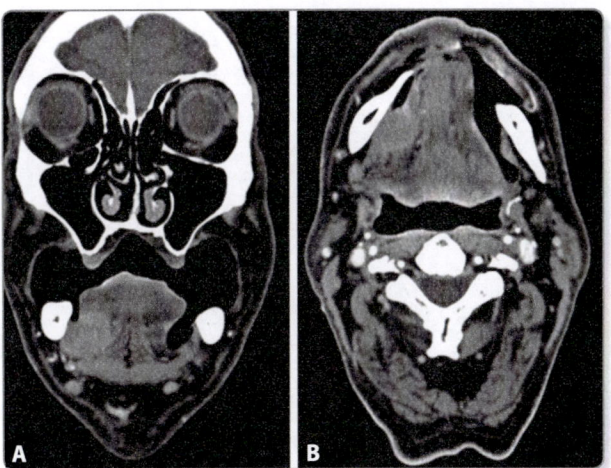

**Figures 7.12A and B** Contrast enhanced CT imaging with distension of the cheeks shows a hyperdense carcinoma involving the right floor of mouth mucosa. There is medial extension into the sublingual compartment. Bone algorithm images (not shown) did not reveal bone erosion

and beyond the posterior edge of the mylohyoid muscle into the neck. Other radiographic findings in FOM carcinoma may include secondary dilatation of the salivary ducts secondary to tumor obstruction (**Figures 7.13A and B**). Lymph node drainage pathways that need to be assessed include level IA, IB and internal jugular lymph nodes.

## Upper and lower alveolus and gingiva and buccal mucosa

Although tumors of the gingiva account for less than 10 percent of oral cavity carcinomas, the proximity of these tumors to bony cortical margins will increase the risk for potential bone and perineural extension (**Figures 7.14A and B**). Buccal carcinomas most commonly originate along the lateral margins. The most common routes of spread include lateral submucosal extension into the buccinator muscle and posteriorly towards the pterygomandibular raphe and subsequent bony involvement.

## Oral tongue

Approximately 16 to 22 percent of oral cavity SCCa arises in the tongue. Tumors present as a nonhealing ulcer or as a neck (nodal)

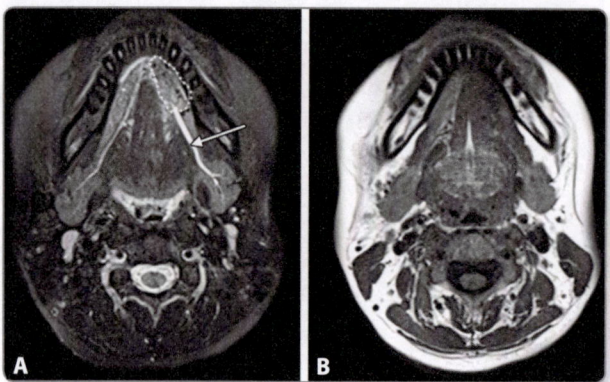

**Figures 7.13A and B** Dashed line outlines a mucoepidermoid carcinoma involving the left FOM. Note secondary dilatation (arrow) of the submandibular duct due to obstruction by the tumor

mass. Most oral tongue squamous cells carcinomas arise from the lateral undersurface of the tongue. Imaging should specifically assess whether there is extension across the midline raphe, invasion of the FOM, and the status of the adjacent mandible. Extension across midline may indicate the need for total glossectomy (**Figures 7.15 and 7.16**). Involvement of the tongue base is also important to

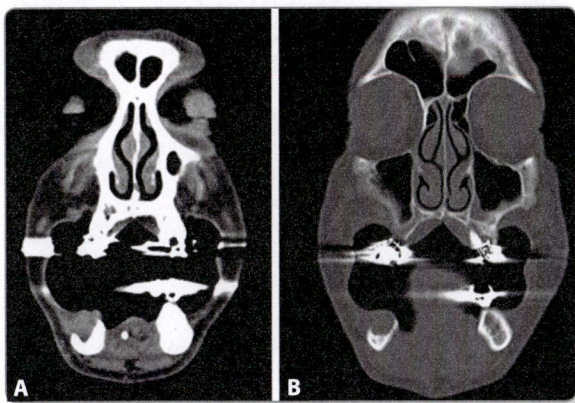

**Figures 7.14A and B** Coronal CT demonstrating a carcinoma involving the right mandibular alveolus

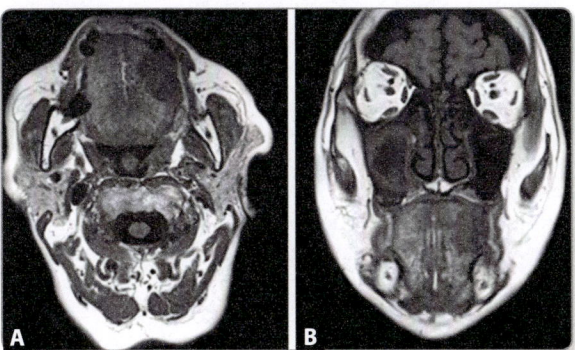

**Figures 7.15A and B** MRI of a left lateral oral tongue carcinoma. The lesion does not invade the tongue base or sublingual space and spares the midline

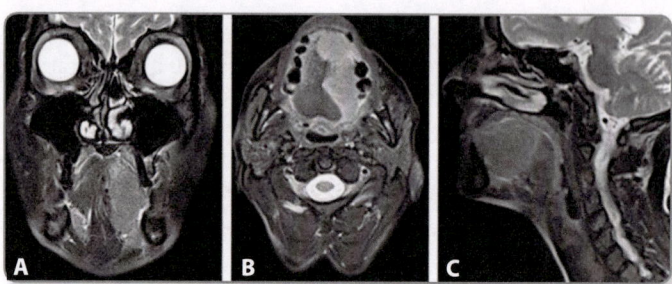

**Figures 7.16A to C** T2-weighted MRI shows a large carcinoma involving the entire left oral tongue. Coronal scan shows extension into the sublingual space. The tumor is also crossing the midline anteriorly

identify as there would be potential for disease extension across the glossotonsillar sulcus onto the oropharyngeal wall.

## Hard palate

Evaluation of hard palate SCCa requires careful assessment for bony palate destruction as well as for perineural tumor spread. While SCCa can also give rise to perineural tumor spread, adenoid cystic carcinomas can also arise in the palate. These tumors have a high propensity for perineural tumor spread. In the palate, such perineural disease can extend along the greater and lesser palatine nerves (**Figures 7.17 and 7.18**) and eventually into the pterygopalatine fossa. Once tumor has reached the pterygopalatine fossa there will be further routes for perineural tumor spread including along CN V2 into foramen rotundum or anteriorly along the infraorbital nerve. Tumor may also spread along the Vidian nerve in the Vidian canal. The Vidian nerve is a combination of the greater superficial petrosal nerve (GSPN) and deep petrosal nerve. All of these nerves serve as routes for potential perineural tumoral spread into skull base and cavernous sinus.

## Retromolar trigone

Retromolar trigone (RMT) tumors account for 7 percent of tumors affecting the oral cavity. The retromolar trigone is situated behind

Radiographic anatomy and pathology of the oral cavity 319

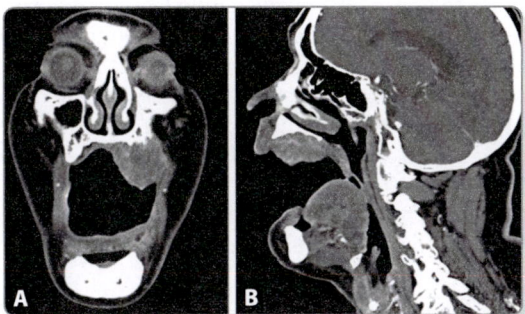

**Figures 7.17A and B** CT imaging shows a large lobulated carcinoma involving the lingual surface of the left hard palate. Even without the bone algorithm images, there is clear erosion of the left maxillary alveolus

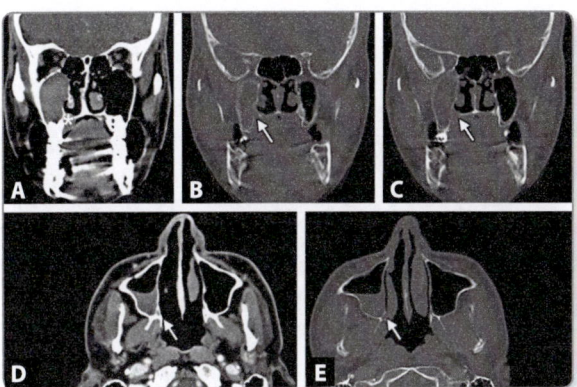

**Figures 7.18A to E** Another patient with an adenoid cystic carcinoma involving the right hard palate (*). Note the enlargement of the right greater palatine nerve canal and increased soft tissue density within it. Perineural tumor spread was confirmed at the time of surgery

the posterior molars and is the ridge of tissue posterior to the last mandibular molar that runs up along the ascending ramus. The RMT is a rather unique location as it is a junction point between the oral cavity, oropharynx, and nasopharynx. Muscles such as the buccinator and superior constrictor muscles insert into the retromolar trigone and can facilitate different routes of tumor growth. Beneath the mucosal surface of the retromolar trigone is the pterygomandibular raphe which attaches superiorly to the hook of the hamulus arising from the medial pterygoid plate and inferiorly to the posterior mylohyoid line of the mandible. This raphe allows tumor access to both the skull base and nasopharynx. Bony cortical involvement of the mandibular ramus must also be sought. Tumors involving the retromolar region can extend into the adjacent tonsillar fossa and masticator space (**Figures 7.19 and 7.20**).

## Mandible and maxilla

The maxilla and mandible can be affected by a diverse range of pathologic processes. In addition to tumor, many developmental, metabolic, inflammatory, and traumatic lesions or disorders which affect the skeleton can present in the jaws. Numerous benign and malignant soft tissue tumors as well as metastatic malignancies may present centrally within the maxilla or mandible. SCCa can arise primarily within the substance of the mandible or invade the mandible from adjacent gingival or buccal primaries.

Given the presence of teeth and associated structures, there are also a variety of pathologies which are unique to the jaws. The goal of imaging in this region is not only to determine the extent of disease,

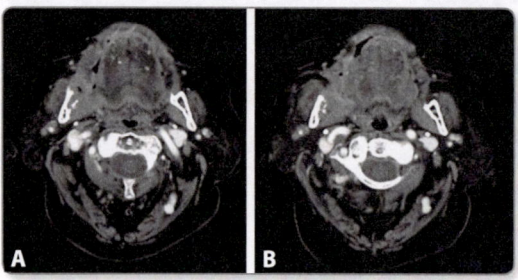

**Figures 7.19A and B** Infiltrative squamous carcinoma in the right retromolar trigone. There is asymmetric enlargement of the medial pterygoid muscle corresponding to masticator space involvement. Mandibular invasion is also evident

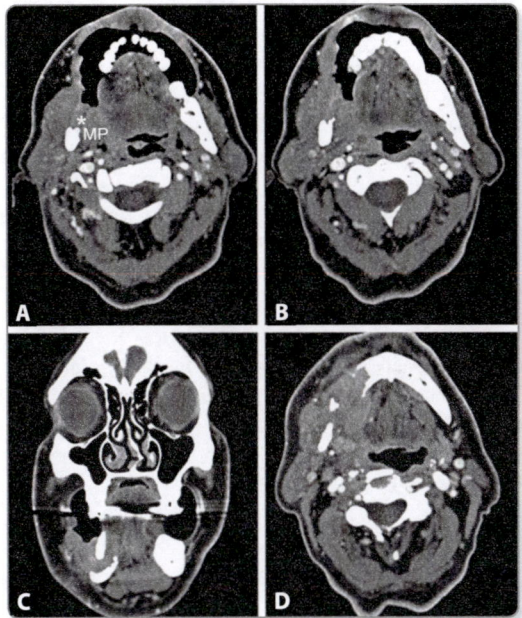

**Figures 7.20A to D** Large tumor mass centered in the right retromolar trigone (*). There is contiguous extension to involve the medial pterygoid (MP) and anteriorly along the buccal mucosa. Tumor is also noted to have extended across the lower buccoalveolar sulcus to invade the right body of the mandible

but also to characterize the radiographic features as an aid in differential diagnosis and treatment planning. Assessment of lesional shape, borders, internal architecture, relationship and effects on surrounding teeth, expansion or perforation of cortical plates, and extension to soft tissue are fundamental to radiographic analysis.

Three jaw lesions that have fairly characteristic imaging appearances are the odontogenic keratocyst, the ameloblastoma and the dentigerous cyst.

The odontogenic keratocyst accounts for 10 percent of all jaw cysts. It arises from the dental lamina. Most arise in the posterior body of the mandible. These cysts are usually unilocular and have a characteristic epicenter located above the inferior alveolar nerve canal. They are minimally expansile and tend to enlarge along the long axis of the mandible (**Figures 7.21A to F**).

An ameloblastoma is a locally aggressive neoplasm that originates from odontogenic epithelium. It is the most common odontogenic tumor. It has a characteristic expansile, multiloculated cystic appearance. MRI may reveal the presence of a mural nodule. It most commonly affects the posterior mandible (**Figures 7.22 and 7.23**).

A dentigerous cyst is the second most common jaw cyst, "with the periapical inflammatory cyst being most common". They have a characteristic location around the crown (pericoronal) of an unerupted tooth which is usually a posterior mandibular molar. The cyst will always insert at the cementoenamel junction of the tooth (**Figures 7.24A and B**). Dentigerous cysts can also arise in the maxilla. In these instances, the unerupted tooth and cyst can prolapse into the maxillary antrum (**Figures 7.25A and B**).

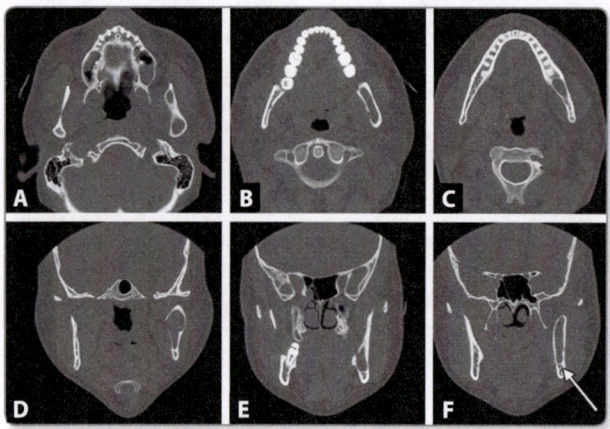

**Figures 7.21A to F** CT imaging of an odontogenic keratocyst. The lesion is mildly expansile and extends along the long axis of the mandible. The cyst epicenter is above the inferior alveolar nerve canal (arrow)

Radiographic anatomy and pathology of the oral cavity 323

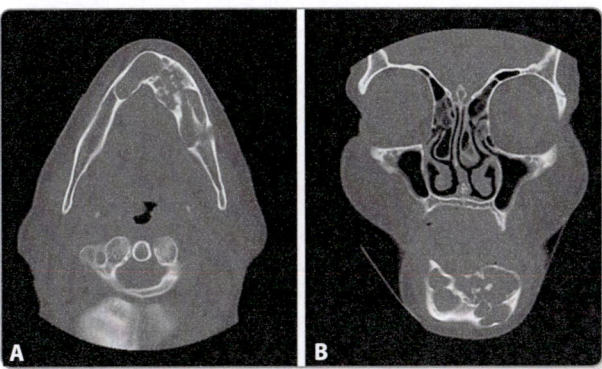

**Figures 7.22A and B** CT imaging of an ameloblastoma involving the mandibular symphysis and left body of the mandible. These tumors have a characteristic bubbly expansile appearance

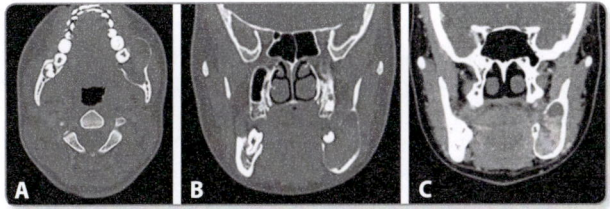

**Figures 7.23A to C** Another ameloblastoma. These are expansile lesions that can demonstrate internal scalloped margins and a central enhancing soft tissue component

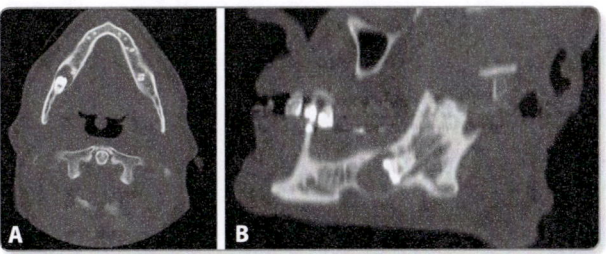

**Figures 7.24A and B** Dentigerous cyst located in the right posterior mandible. The cyst arises from the crown of an unerupted mandibular molar

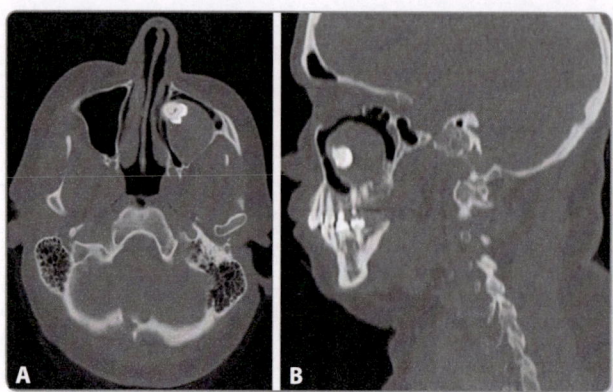

**Figures 7.25A and B** Another dentigerous cyst arising from the right maxilla. The cyst and it is associated unerupted tooth have extended into the right maxillary antrum.
*Courtesy*: Dr Eric Bartlett

Another type of growth that affects the jaws and palate are bony exostosis. These are bony hyperplasias of bone that can arise along the lingual aspect of the hard palate (torus palatinus) and along the lingual aspect of the mandible (torus mandibularis). On imaging, these appear as very dense lobulated bony protrusions (**Figures 7.26A and B**).

## AJCC staging

The American Joint Committee on Cancer (AJCC) has designated staging by TNM classification.

## TNM definitions

### Primary tumor (T)
- *TX*: Primary tumor cannot be assessed
- *T0*: No evidence of primary tumor
- *Tis*: Carcinoma *in situ*
- *T1*: Tumor no larger than 2 cm in greatest dimension

Radiographic anatomy and pathology of the oral cavity  325

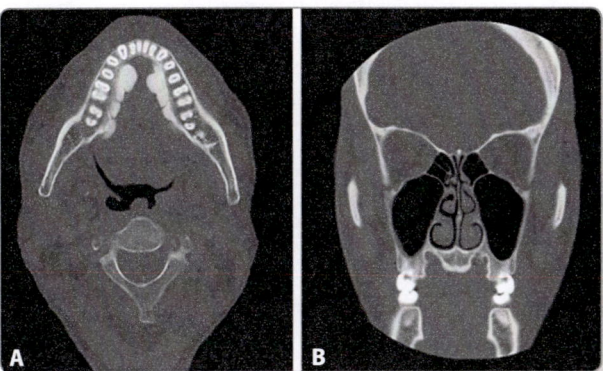

**Figures 7.26A and B** CT imaging in two different patients with tori involving the jaws. (A) Dense lobulated calcifed exostoses along the inner margin of the mandible–torus mandibularis. (B) The coronal CT shows a protruberant torus palatinus along the undersurface of the hard palate

- *T2*: Tumor larger than 2 cm but no larger than 4 cm in greatest dimension
- *T3*: Tumor larger than 4 cm in greatest dimension
- *T4*: (lip) Tumor invades through cortical bone, inferior alveolar nerve, floor of mouth, or skin of face, i.e. chin or nose:
  - *T4a*: (oral cavity) Tumor invades adjacent structures (e.g. through cortical bone, into deep [extrinsic] muscle of tongue [genioglossus, hyoglossus, palatoglossus, and styloglossus], maxillary sinus, and skin of face)
  - *T4b*: Tumor invades masticator space, pterygoid plates, or skull base and/or encases internal carotid artery.
  
  *[Note: Superficial erosion alone of bone/tooth socket by gingival primary is not sufficient to classify a tumor as T4]*

### Regional lymph nodes (N)
- *NX*: Regional lymph nodes cannot be assessed
- *N0*: No regional lymph node metastasis
- *N1*: Metastasis in a single ipsilateral lymph node, no larger than 3 cm in greatest dimension

- *N2*: Metastasis in a single ipsilateral lymph node, larger than 3 cm but no larger than 6 cm in greatest dimension; or in multiple ipsilateral lymph nodes, no larger than 6 cm in greatest dimension; or in bilateral or contralateral lymph nodes, no larger than 6 cm in greatest dimension
  - *N2a*: Metastasis in a single ipsilateral lymph node larger than 3 cm but no larger than 6 cm in dimension
  - *N2b*: Metastasis in multiple ipsilateral lymph nodes, no larger than 6 cm in greatest dimension
  - *N2c*: Metastasis in bilateral or contralateral lymph nodes, no larger than 6 cm in greatest dimension
- *N3*: Metastasis in a lymph node larger than 6 cm in greatest dimension.

In clinical evaluation, the actual size of the nodal mass should be measured and allowance should be made for intervening soft tissues. Most masses larger than 3 cm in diameter are not single nodes but are confluent nodes or tumors in soft tissues of the neck. The three stages of clinically positive nodes are: N1, N2, and N3. The use of subgroups a, b, and c is not required but is recommended. Midline nodes are considered homolateral nodes.

## Distant metastasis (M)
- *MX*: Distant metastasis cannot be assessed
- *M0*: No distant metastasis
- *M1*: Distant metastasis

## AJCC Stage Groupings

### Stage 0
- Tis, N0, M0

### Stage I
- T1, N0, M0

### Stage II
- T2, N0, M0

### Stage III
- T3, N0, M0
- T1, N1, M0
- T2, N1, M0
- T3, N1, M0

### Stage IVA
- T4a, N0, M0
- T4a, N1, M0
- T1, N2, M0
- T2, N2, M0
- T3, N2, M0
- T4a, N2, M0

### Stage IVB
- Any T, N3, M0
- T4b, any N, M0

### Stage IVC
- Any T, any N, M1

## Degenerative
Denervation atrophy of the hypoglossal nerve (CNXII) is a process that can mimic the presence of a tongue mass. Initially the denervated tongue may be more swollen and over time, fatty replacement of the tongue musculature will occur. This can make the affected side appear larger and raise suspicion for an underlying tumor (**Figures 7.27A and B**).

## Inflammatory
Inflammatory disorders of the oral cavity are multifold, and can include any of the inflammatory disease found elsewhere in the body. More specific inflammatory lesions of the oral cavity include herpetic gingiviostomatitis and also Behçet's syndrome that can results in multiple oral ulcers similar to aphthous stomatitis (known more commonly as canker sores), pemphigoid, or condyloma (venereally transmitted warts).

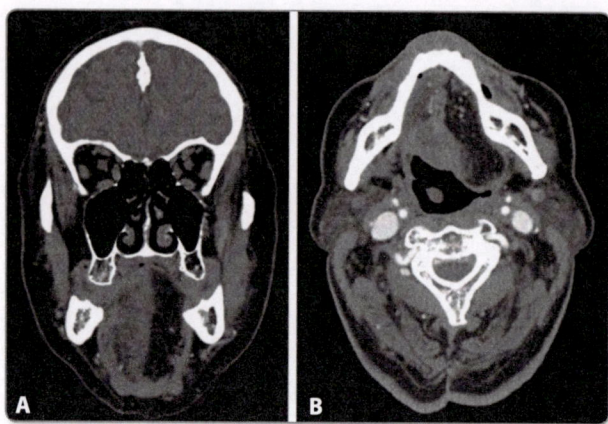

**Figures 7.27A and B** Example of tongue denervation. The affected left hemitongue demonstrates fatty atrophy. Axial imaging shows the tongue appears larger than the unaffected side. This could potentially give the impression of a left sided tumor mass

Patients who have undergone radiation therapy to the oral cavity or nearby regions can occasionally develop osteoradionecrosis of the jaws. This can arise decades after initial therapy and is most common in the mandible. Patients will present with soft tissue swelling and pain. Bony exposure can arise. Pathologic fracture can also occur. Imaging shows features very similar to osteomyelitis such as cortical erosion, mixed areas of permeative internal lucency and sclerosis. Sequestra may also be seen (**Figures 7.28A to D**). "Similar clinical and radiographic changes can be seen in antiresorptive agent-induced osteonecrosis of the jaws, with patients taking bisphosphonates or other antiresorptive medications."

Ranulas are mucous retention phenomena that arise in the floor of mouth. They arise secondary to local trauma to the sublingual, submandibular or minor salivary gland duct, resulting in spillage of mucous into the surrounding soft tissue. A simple ranula is confined in the sublingual space and is not a true cyst, as it lacks an epithelial lining. They appear as a well-defined fluid density mass (**Figure 7.29**).

Radiographic anatomy and pathology of the oral cavity

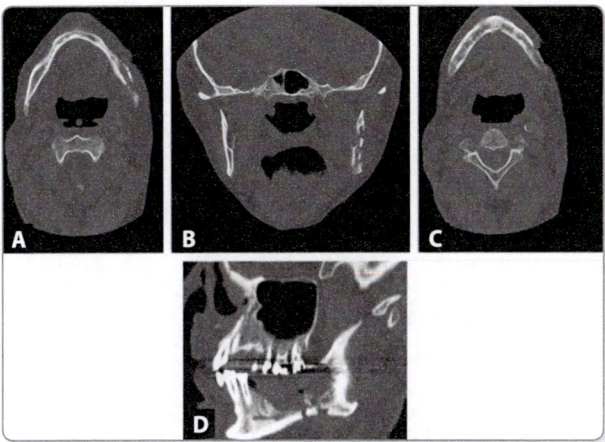

**Figures 7.28A to D** Radiation related osteoradionecrosis of the mandible in four different patients. Not the patchy erosive changes (A and B) involving the cortex and internal marrow space. (C) Loss of overlying soft tissue coverage. (D) Obliqued sagittal reconstructed shows the presence of a pathologic fracture

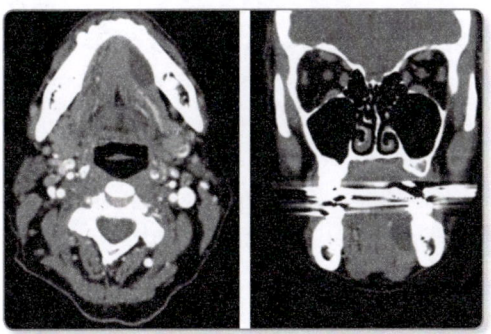

**Figure 7.29** Ranula of the left sublingual space. Imaging shows a well-defined fluid density mass

A diving or plunging ranula arises when extravasated mucous of a simple ranula dissects through the mylohyoid muscle and extends

**330** Introductory head and neck imaging

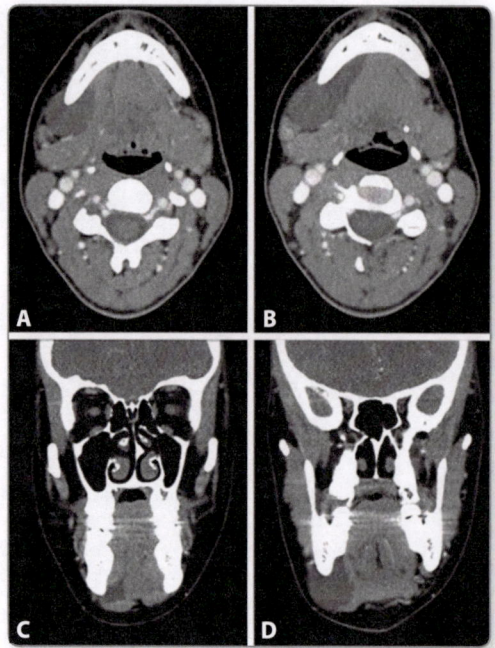

**Figures 7.30A to D** A diving ranula is a pseudocyst and appears as a fluid density mass that extends from the sublingual space into the submandibular compartment

into the submandibular space, but often still maintains a component in the sublingual region (**Figures 7.30A to D**).

### Congenital

Congenital and developmental lesions of the oral cavity include hemangiomas, lymphangiomas, lingual thyroid or thyroglossal duct cysts, teratomas and dermoid cysts.

Dermoid cysts are rare congenital epithelial inclusion cysts that contain both epithelial and dermal elements. Imaging can range from the presence of a low attenuation fluid density mass to a complex

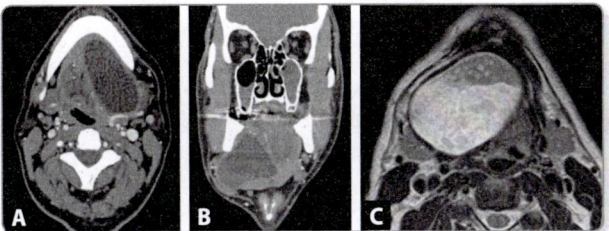

**Figures 7.31A to C** Imaging of dermoid cysts in three patients. Dermoids appear as cystic collections in the floor of mouth with internal foci of fatty attenuation. Some dermoids will show areas of internal calcification and may be trans-spatial with components spanning the sublingual and submandibular compartments

mass with internal foci of rounded calcification and/or fat. They can involve the sublingual and/or submandibular spaces (**Figures 7.31A to C**).

In addition specific disorders such as Gorlin-Goltz syndrome or basal cell nevus syndrome are associated with odontogenic keratocysts and epidermal cysts of the jaw, along with basal cell cancers, palmoplantar pits, calcified dura, and neoplasms including medulloblastoma, ovarian fibroma, lymphomesenteric cysts, fetal rhabdomyoma and bone anomalies include cleft lip and palate.

### Traumatic

Fractures of the oral cavity are easily imaged by CT and can involve the mandible. Fractures may involve the symphysis and parasymphyseal regions with disruption of the genioglossus and digastric attachments. This can lead to posterior displacement of the tongue secondary to the unopposed suprahyoid musculature and blockage of the airway.

## Conclusion

In summary, the anterior location and easy accessibility allow the unique anatomy of the oral cavity to be easily clinically inspected. However, lesions that extend below the submucosa including any of the various vascular, infectious, neoplastic, degenerative, inflammatory, congenital, allergic and traumatic pathologies presented here, may be better evaluated on cross-sectional imaging. CT as demonstrated here is excellent for bony detail and evaluation of odontogenic lesions. MRI allows for excellent evaluation of soft tissue detail, and both are often complementary.

# Bibliography

1. Brown B, Barnes L, Mazariegos J, Taylor F, Johnson J, Wagner RL. Prognostic factors in mobile tongue and floor of mouth carcinoma. Cancer 1989; 64:1195-1202.
2. Chong V. Oral cavity cancer. Cancer Imaging 2005; 5 Spec No A:S49-52.
3. Laine FJ, Smoker WR. Oral cavity: Anatomy and pathology. Semin Ultrasound CT MR 1995; 16: 527-45.
4. Mukherji SK, Pillsbury HR, Castillo M. Imaging squamous cell carcinomas of the upper aero digestive tract: what clinicians need to know. Radiology 1997; 205:629-46.
5. Rumboldt Z, Day TA, Michel M. Imaging of oral cavity cancer. Oral Oncol 2006; 42:854-65.
6. Smoker WR. The oral cavity. In: Som PM, Curtin HD, (Eds). Head and Neck Imaging, 4th edn. St. Louis, MO: Mosby 2003;1377-1464.
7. Stambuk HE, Karimi S, Lee N, Patel SG. Oral cavity and oropharynx tumors. Radiologic Clinics of North America: Elsevier 2007;1-20.
8. Tytor M, Olofsson J. Prognostic factors in oral cavity carcinomas. Acta Otolaryngol Suppl 1992;492:75-8.

# Oropharynx

chapter 8

Aditya Bharatha, Keng-Yeow Tay

**Abstract**

This chapter reviews the anatomy and normal radiological appearance of the oropharynx on CT and MRI. The most common pathologies of the oropharynx, including neoplasms, infectious and inflammatory pathologies, congenital lesions, trauma, and post-treatment change are described and illustrated.

**Keywords**

Oropharynx, CT, MRI.

## Radiologic anatomy

The oropharynx is the portion of the aerodigestive tract inferior to the nasopharynx, superior to the hypopharynx and larynx, and posterior to the oral cavity. The anterior border of the oropharynx is marginated by a ring of structures including the anterior tonsillar pillar, circumvallate papillae of the tongue, and junction of the hard and soft palate (**Figure 8.1**). The upper margin of the oropharynx is the level of the soft palate (**Figure 8.2**). The inferior margin is at the level of the base of the epiglottis and hyoid bone, marginated by the glossoepiglottic and pharyngoepiglottic folds which separate it from the larynx and hypopharynx at the level of the valleculae. The epiglottis itself is part of the supraglottic larynx.

Based on the definitions above, the oropharynx (**Figures 8.3A and B**) contains the base of tongue (the posterior third of the tongue posterior to the circumvallate papillae down to the valleculae), the anterior and posterior tonsillar pillars, and faucial (or palatine) tonsils, the (undersurface of the) soft palate and uvula, and the lateral and posterior oropharyngeal walls. The anterior tonsillar pillar is the mucosal fold overlying the palatoglossus muscle, while the posterior pillar is

## 334 Introductory head and neck imaging

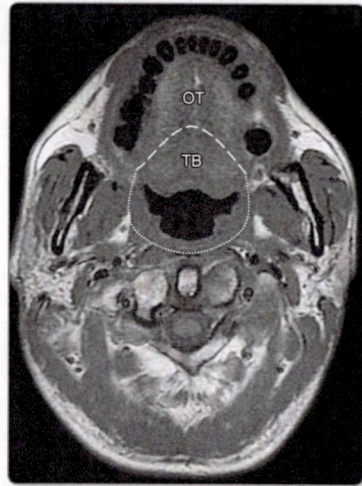

**Figure 8.1** Axial T1W MRI of the oropharynx. The dashed line represents the circumvallate papillae of the tongue, which separates the oral tongue (OT) from the tongue base (TB). The oropharynx is within the area bounded by the dashed line and dotted line

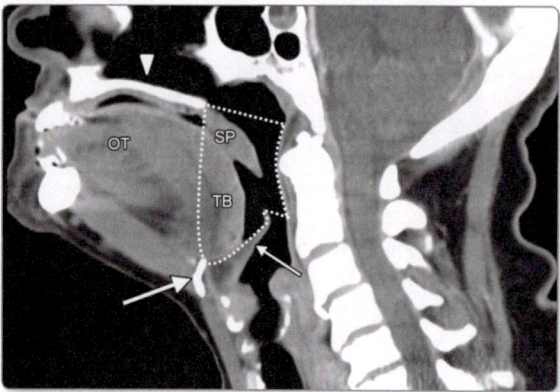

**Figure 8.2** Sagittal reformat of neck CT, the dotted line shows the boundaries of the oropharynx. Its superior border is formed by soft palate (SP) and the lower border by the hyoid bone (thick white arrow). The hard palate (white arrow head), oral tongue (OT), tongue base (TB) epiglottis (small white arrow) and hyoid bone (thick white arrow) have been labeled

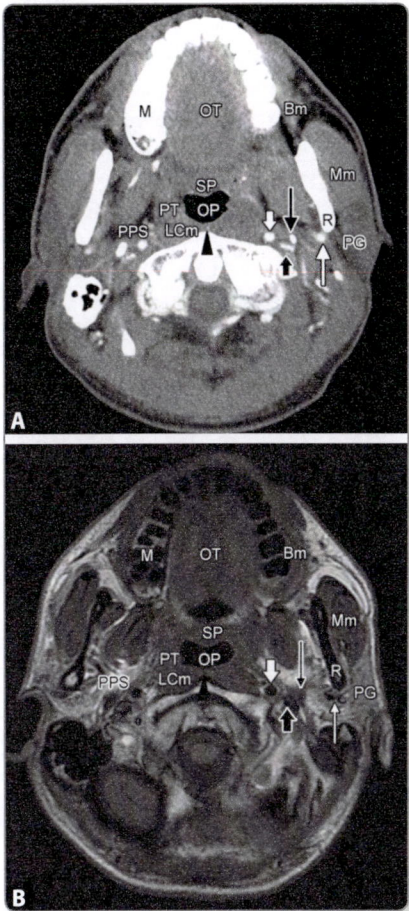

**Figures 8.3A and B** Axial CT of the oropharynx with IV contrast injection. Normal anatomical structures are labeled: M, maxillary alveolus with teeth; OT, oral tongue; Bm, buccinator muscle; Mm, masseter muscle; SP, soft palate; PT, palatine tonsil; OP, oropharynx; PPS, parapharyngeal space; LCm, Longus colli muscle; PG, parotid gland; Black arrowhead, posterior wall of the oropharynx; Thick white arrow, Internal carotid artery; Thin black arrow, styloid process; Thick black arrow, internal jugular vein; Thin white arrow, retromandibular vein

that overlying the palatopharyngeus. The glossotonsillar sulcus is the lateral mucosal fold where the palatine tonsils abut the tongue base, and serves as a potential pathway for tumor to spread between the tongue base and lateral oropharyngeal wall. The pterygomandibular raphe is a tendinous band of buccopharyngeal fascia attached to the hamulus of the medial pterygoid plate and to the mylohyoid line of the mandible. The superior pharyngeal constrictor muscle and the buccinator muscle attach to this raphe. It serves as an important conduit of disease from the oropharynx to the oral cavity.

The visceral layer of the deep cervical fascia surrounds the mucosa and musculature of the oropharynx and acts as a barrier to the spread of neoplasm and inflammatory disease. If this fascia is transgressed, tumor can spread posteriorly into the retropharyngeal space or into the prevertebral space, invading the longus muscles and/or the vertebrae. If tumor extends laterally, it can access the prestyloid or poststyloid (neurovascular) parapharyngeal space.

The main arterial supply to the oropharynx is derived from the ascending pharyngeal branch of the external carotid artery, the tonsillar branch of the facial artery and from a rich network of small arteries derived from the internal maxillary, lingual and facial arteries. Venous drainage is mainly via tonsillar veins which drain toward the facial venous system. Lymphatic drainage is toward level II and III cervical chain nodes, retropharyngeal nodes, and less often to level V or parotid nodes.

The palatine tonsils are one of the mucosa-associated lymphoid tissues that form a part of Waldeyer's ring (comprising the palatine, nasopharyngeal adenoid, tubal and lingual tonsils). These tissues form a ring of lymphoid tissue in the pharynx that serves as a key point of immune surveillance against pathogens that enter via the upper aerodigestive tract. There is marked variability in the size of the palatine tonsils between individuals. Also, the size of these lymphoid aggregates can increase greatly with upper respiratory tract infections, as well as other pathological states. In general terms, the palatine tonsils increase in size during childhood reaching a maximal size of around 2.5 (craniocaudally) cm x 1.5 (transversely) cm in adolescence. They then regress in size slowly during adulthood.

The lingual tonsils are lymphoid tissues at the base of the tongue. They are also quite variable in size. Lingual tonsillar tissue can extend inferiorly along the tongue base and anterior vallecular wall to the level of the base of the valleculae. "As" general guideline, lymphoid tissue here should not extend onto the floor or posterior wall of the vallecula. Tissue extending to such a degree should raise suspicion for neoplasm.

## Tumor

The majority of oropharyngeal tumors are squamous cell carcinomas (SCCa). Other malignant histopathological entities of the oropharynx include minor salivary tumors and hematologic malignancies. Risk factors for SCCa include tobacco use, alcohol abuse, and poor oral hygiene. Men are more commonly affected and the disease is more common in individuals over the age of 45 years. Infection with certain strains of human papilloma viruses (HPV) are also a risk factor for SCCa. The incidence of HPV associated carcinoma appears to be rising. Oropharyngeal SCCa often presents initially as a painless non-healing ulcer along the mucosa. With increasing size, the patient may experience pain, induration, or develop symptoms related to regional adenopathy. Sixty to seventy percent of patients have regional adenopathy at presentation; 15-30 percent of these are bilateral.

The current 7th edition of the American Joint Committee on Cancer (AJCC) TNM staging system for oropharyngeal SCCa is summarized in **Table 8.1**. It is worthwhile reviewing this table to ensure that the relevant information, notably size of the primary tumor, local extent of disease relevant to staging categories and nodal disease including size of largest nodes is reported.

The most common sites of involvement are the palatine tonsil, followed by the tongue base. Tumors in these locations are more prone to cause early symptoms including painful swallowing, referred otalgia, and speech difficulty. In advanced disease, there may be symptoms secondary to invasion of local structures; trismus can arise due to masticator space invasion, facial numbness due to inferior alveolar nerve involvement, or tongue atrophy/fasciculation due to sublingual space neurovascular involvement affecting the hypoglossal nerve.

| Primary tumor (T) | X | Primary tumor cannot be assessed |
|---|---|---|
| | 0 | No evidence of primary tumor |
| | is | Carcinoma *in situ* |
| | 1 | Tumor 2 cm or smaller in greatest dimension |
| | 2 | Tumor larger than 2 cm but 4 cm or smaller in greatest dimension |
| | 3 | Tumor larger than 4 cm in greatest dimension |
| | 4a | Tumor invades the larynx, deep/extrinsic muscle of tongue, medial pterygoid, hard palate, or mandible |
| | 4b | Tumor invades lateral pterygoid muscle, pterygoid plates, lateral nasopharynx, or skull base or encases carotid artery |
| Regional lymph nodes (N) | X | Regional lymph nodes cannot be assessed |
| | 0 | No regional lymph node metastasis |
| | 1 | Metastasis in a single ipsilateral lymph node, 3 cm or smaller in greatest dimension |
| | 2 | Metastasis in a single ipsilateral lymph node larger than 3 cm but 6 cm or smaller in greatest dimension |
| | 2a | Metastasis in multiple ipsilateral lymph nodes, 6 cm or smaller in greatest dimension |
| | 2b | Metastasis in bilateral or contralateral lymph nodes, 6 cm or smaller in greatest dimension |
| | 2c | Metastasis in bilateral or contralateral lymph nodes, 6 cm or smaller in greatest dimension |
| | 3 | Metastasis in a lymph node larger than 6 cm in greatest dimension |
| Distant metastasis (M) | X | Distant metastasis cannot be assessed |
| | 0 | No distant metastasis |
| | 1 | Distant metastasis |

**Table 8.1** AJCC staging for oropharyngeal carcinoma. *Adapted from:* AJCC Cancer Staging Manual, 7th edition, Springer-Verlag, New York 2010

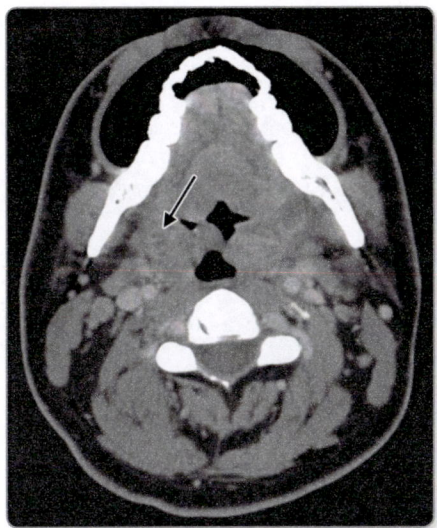

Figure 8.4 Axial CT of the oropharynx with IV contrast injection showing normal but prominent tonsillar crypts (black arrow)

Tumors arising in the tonsillar fossa likely arise from the mucosa lining the niche between the anterior and posterior pillars or from the palatine tonsil itself. Tumors there can arise from deep within the tonsillar crypts (**Figure 8.4**), presenting as clinically occult lesions with cervical nodal metastases. Lesions here may spread anteriorly or posteriorly to the adjacent tonsillar pillars, acquiring the potential spread pattern associated with these locations (see below), or may extend deep into the submucosal space, pharyngeal constrictor muscle, parapharyngeal space, neurovascular bundle, and along the pterygoid muscles to the skull base.

Tumors involving the anterior tonsillar pillar may spread superiorly to the palate and nasopharynx (**Figures 8.5 and 8.6**). From there tumor may extend into the upper parapharyngeal tissues along the tensor and levator veli palatini muscles to the skull base. They may also

## 340 Introductory head and neck imaging

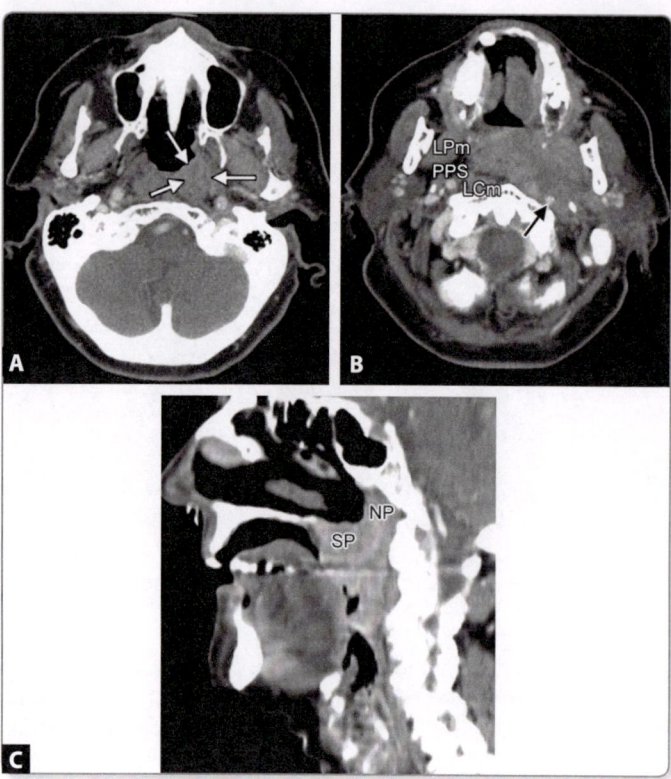

**Figures 8.5A to C** Spread of left tonsil squamous cell carcinoma; (A) Axial CT of the nasopharynx showing left nasopharyngeal (white arrows) involvement; (B) Axial CT of the oropharynx showing spread into the parapharyngeal space, lateral pterygoid muscle, longus colli muscle plus encasement of the internal carotid artery (black arrow). The normal right lateral pterygoid muscle (LPm), parapharyngeal space (PPS) and longus colli muscle (LCm) are labeled; (C) Sagittal reformat of neck CT showing spread of tumor into the soft palate (SP) and nasopharynx (NP)

Oropharynx 341

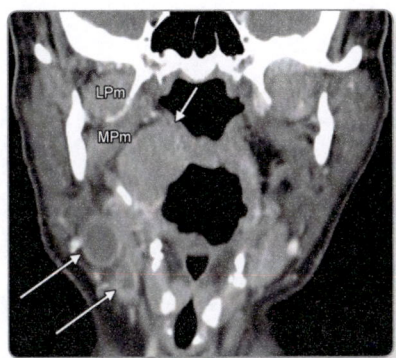

**Figure 8.6** Coronal reformat of neck CT demonstrating a patient with right tonsillar squamous cell carcinoma which has extended into the soft palate (small white arrow). The medial (MPm) and lateral (LPm) pterygoid muscles are not involved. Note the necrotic right sided lymph nodes (large white arrows)

spread anteriorly along the pterygomandibular raphe to the buccinator muscle and buccal space mimicking the appearance of tumor in the retromolar trigone. Inferiorly and anteriorly, tumor can extend to the glossotonsillar sulcus and then to the tongue base (**Figure 8.7**). Posteriorly, tumor may extend to the posterior tonsillar pillar, lateral and posterior oropharyngeal wall and may extend posteriorly to the retropharyngeal and prevertebral spaces, to involve the longus musculature or vertebrae. Inferiorly, tumor may extend along the posterior lateral pharyngeal wall to the hypopharynx or larynx.

Small SCCa arising in the base of tongue can be difficult to distinguish from lingual tonsillar tissue. Tongue base carcinomas are often clinically silent and are another common cause of "occult" malignancies in the head and neck. MR imaging, particularly non-enhanced T1-weighted images are particularly useful in imaging the full extent of these lesions, which can be underestimated on CT. These tumors can spread anteriorly to the sublingual space, oral tongue, or floor of mouth. Involvement of the neurovascular pedicle can include lingual artery, lingual nerve (V3), and cranial nerves 9 and 12 involvement

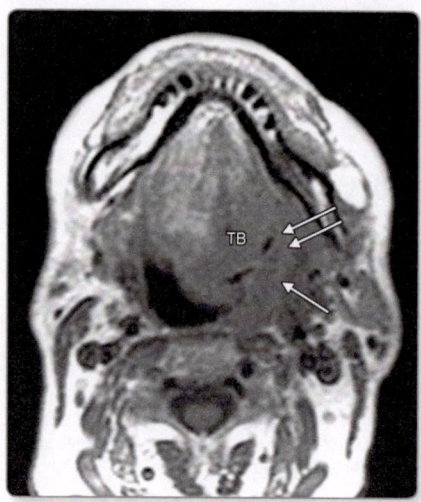

**Figure 8.7** Axial T1-weighted MRI showing a left tonsillar SCCa (single white arrow) which has extended across the glossotonsillar "sulcus" (double white arrows) and onto the adjacent left tongue base (TB)

(perineural disease). Tumor can extend posteriorly to the glossotonsillar sulcus (**Figure 8.8**), tonsillar pillars and pharyngeal wall, and submucosally under the valleculae to the supraglottic larynx. It is extremely important to evaluate the pre-epiglottic fat (**Figure 8.9**) for the presence of disease as this indicates laryngeal involvement. If surgery is being considered, the presence of laryngeal involvement implies the need for partial or total laryngectomy. The tongue base has a rich, bilateral lymphatic drainage system, bilateral nodal metastases are not uncommon.

While the majority of soft palate malignancies are also SCCa (**Figures 8.10A to C**), minor salivary tumors have their highest frequency in the posterior soft palate and hard palate. Although tumor extension of palate SCCa can occur in any direction, anterior spread toward the hard palate and inferior extension toward the tonsillar pillars usually occur first. Deep parapharyngeal invasion, nasopharyngeal involvement and spread to the skull base occur later. Tumor

## Oropharynx 343

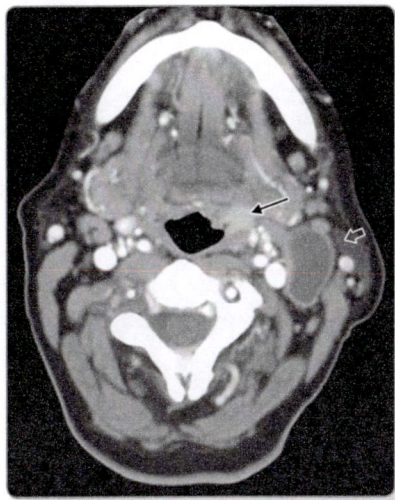

**Figure 8.8** Axial CT of the oropharynx with IV contrast injection showing a left glossotonsillar sulcus (black arrow) squamous cell carcinoma with a necrotic left level 2 lymph node (thick arrow)

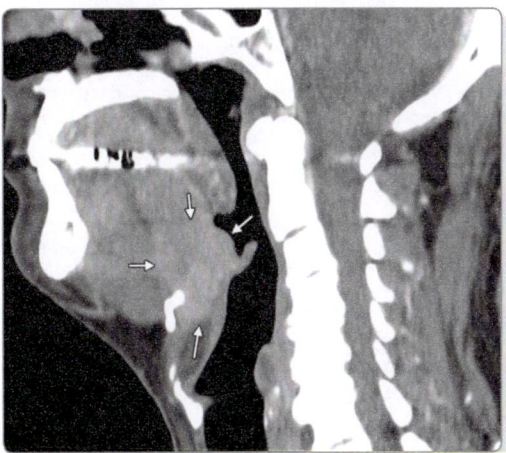

**Figure 8.9** Lateral reformat of neck CT showing infiltration of the pre-epiglottic space (long white arrow) by a tongue base squamous cell carcinoma (short white arrows)

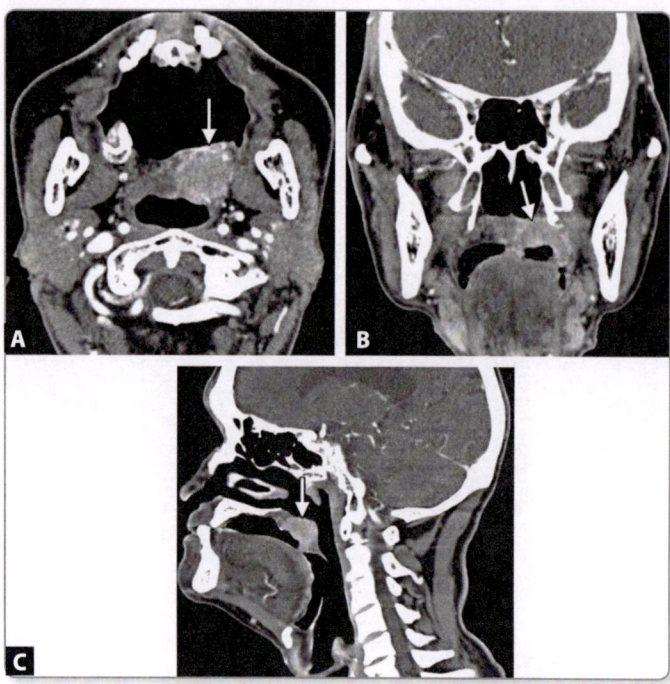

**Figures 8.10A to C** Axial CT (A) of the neck with IV contrast injection plus; (B) Coronal and; (C) Sagittal reformats of a patient with squamous cell carcinoma (white arrow) of the soft palate

can also arise primarily from other subsites, such as the posterior oropharyngeal wall (**Figures 8.11A and B**).

Treatment options for oropharyngeal SCCa include surgical excision, radical radiotherapy, and combined modality treatment. Soft tissue defects often require flap reconstruction. Neck dissection is commonly required because of high incidence of nodal metastases. **Table 8.2** summarizes the important anatomic features which should be reviewed in patients with oropharyngeal SCCa.

Oropharynx 345

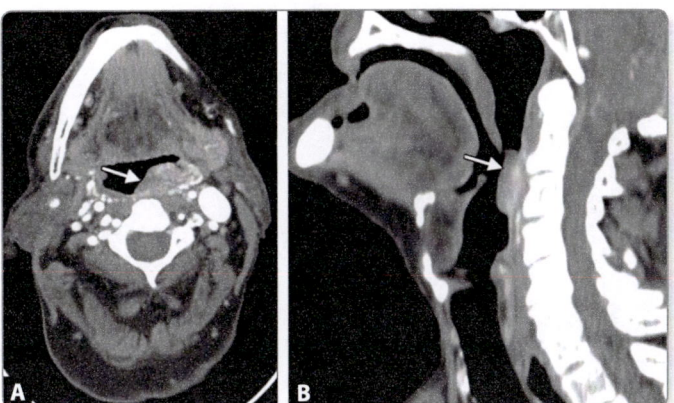

**Figures 8.11A and B** Squamous cell carcinoma of the posterior oropharyngeal wall. It has extended onto the left lateral oropharyngeal wall. There remains a clear separation from the vertebral body posteriorly

The most common lymphoproliferative disorder in the extracranial head and neck is lymphoma. Hodgkin's lymphoma (HD) is a hematopoietic malignancy primarily affecting young adults with a male predilection (2:1). HD typically presents with nodal disease, with extranodal disease in the head and neck being rare. Non-Hodgkin's lymphoma (NHL) is more commonly seen in older patients as well as immunodeficiency states including HIV. Males are more commonly affected than females. In contrast to HD, in which the vast majority of patients present with nodal disease, roughly 60 percent of NHL patients present with extranodal disease, of which 60 percent involve the head and neck. The extranodal sites commonly involved in NHL are the lymphoid tissues of Waldeyer's ring, the parotid gland, and the lacrimal gland (**Figures 8.12A to D**). However, other sites can also be affected. The imaging findings of head and neck lymphoma can mimic those of SCCa. However, the diagnosis can be suggested when there is a large homogenously enhancing nodal mass or masses, or a large homogenous mass involving the lymphoid tissues without the typical mucosal spread which may be expected with SCCa. However, locally

| | |
|---|---|
| Oropharyngeal mucosal involvement | |
| • | Tonsil |
| • | Posteriolateral oropharyngeal wall |
| • | Soft palate |
| • | Glossotonsillar sulcus |
| • | Tongue base |
| • | Extension across midline |
| Anterior | |
| • | Floor of mouth |
| • | Oral tongue, retromolar trigone, buccal mucosa |
| • | Sublingual space |
| • | Mandible |
| Lateral | |
| • | Parapharyngeal space |
| • | Neurovascular bundle |
| • | Carotid encasement |
| Posterior | |
| • | Prevertebral muscles |
| • | Vertebral erosions |
| Superior | |
| • | Nasopharynx |
| • | Upper parapharyngeal space |
| • | Skull base |
| Inferior | |
| • | Preepiglottic fat |
| • | Hypopharynx |
| • | Larynx |
| Nodes | |

**Table 8.2** List of imaging features to be evaluated in SCCa

extensive lymphomatous aggregates can infiltrate the deep spaces and mimic SCCa. Necrosis in the absence of treatment is uncommon but can be seen particularly in HIV-associated NHL.

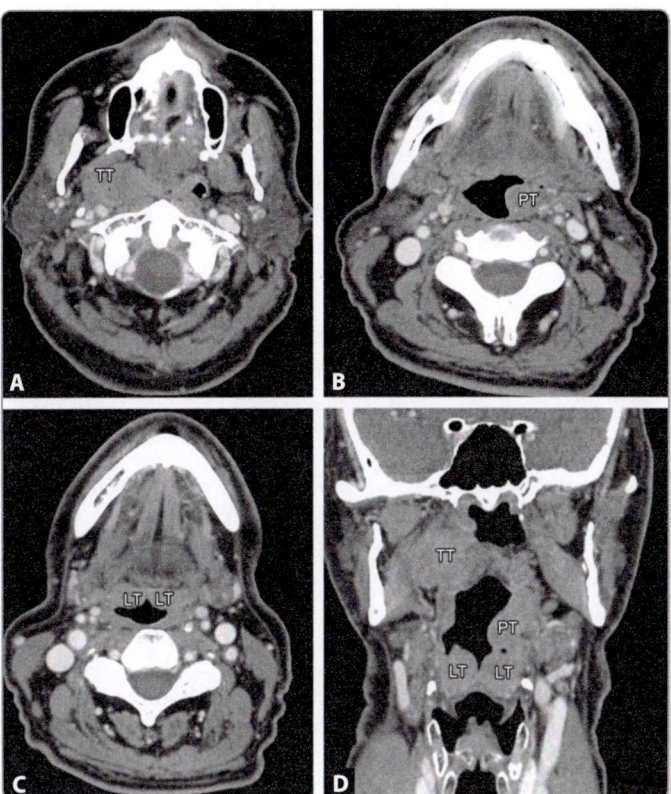

**Figures 8.12A to D** Mantle cell lymphoma, an uncommon form of non-Hodgkin's lymphoma with involvement of the tubal tonsil (TT), palatine tonsil (PT) and lingual tonsils (LT)

Minor salivary gland tissue is distributed throughout the mucosa of the upper aerodigestive tract, with the greatest concentration being located within the oral cavity and oropharynx. As a result tumors of salivary gland differentiation can also occur here. Minor salivary gland tumors account for 2-3 percent of all malignancies of the extracranial head and neck, most commonly in adults without gender predilection. The most common pathologies include histologies such as adenoid cystic carcinoma, mucoepidermoid carcinoma, adenocarcinoma, malignant mixed tumor, and acinic cell carcinoma; however, benign tumors such as pleomorphic adenoma can also occur. In the soft palate, which is the most common site of minor salivary tumors, their incidence approaches that of SCCa. The radiologic findings of these tumors tend to be nonspecific with the diagnosis tending to be based on tissue sampling. Pleomorphic adenomas can present as well circumscribed T2 hyperintense enhancing lesions similar to their appearance in the parotid gland or parapharyngeal space. The malignant minor salivary tumors have a variable appearance. Adenoid cystic carcinoma has a high predilection for perineural invasion, for which MR imaging with fat suppressed T1 postcontrast imaging is helpful.

Other tumors than can occasionally involve the oropharynx include neurogenic tumors, rhabdomyomas, rhabdomyosarcomas, granular cell tumors, and fibromatosis lesions. Hemangiomas may involve the oropharynx or face and have a similar appearance to those seen elsewhere in the body.

## Inflammatory

Acute tonsillopharyngitis is an infectious/inflammatory disease most commonly affecting adolescents and young adults. While viral pharyngitis is more common, bacterial (suppurative) tonsillopharyngitis (**Figure 8.13**) is associated with more severe symptoms and potential complications. The most common bacterial pathogens include beta-hemolytic *Streptococcus, Staphylococcus, Pneumococcus*, and *Haemophilus*. Untreated suppurative infection can go on to develop tonsillar (**Figure 8.14**) or peritonsillar abscess (quinsy). Peritonsillar abscesses (**Figures 8.15A to C**) can drain into the parapharyngeal, retropharyngeal, or submandibular space. Acute tonsillopharyngitis may present as nonspecific swelling and/or enhancement of the palatine tonsils and adjacent oropharyngeal mucosa. Abscess formation is characterized by a low attenuation necrotic abscess surrounded by

Oropharynx 349

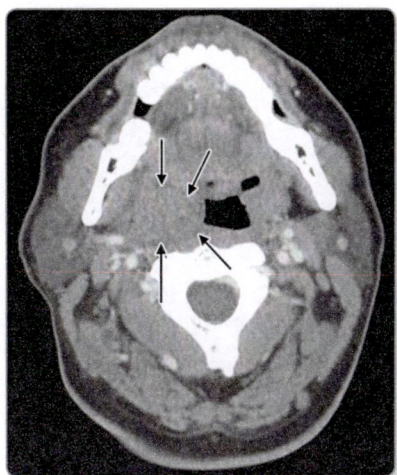

**Figure 8.13** Tonsillitis involving the right palatine tonsil (black arrows)

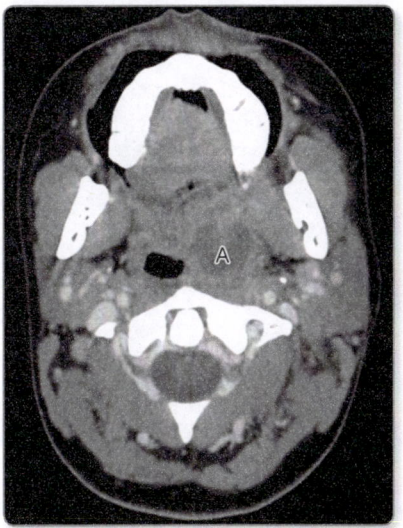

**Figure 8.14** Left tonsillitis complicated by tonsillar abscess (A)

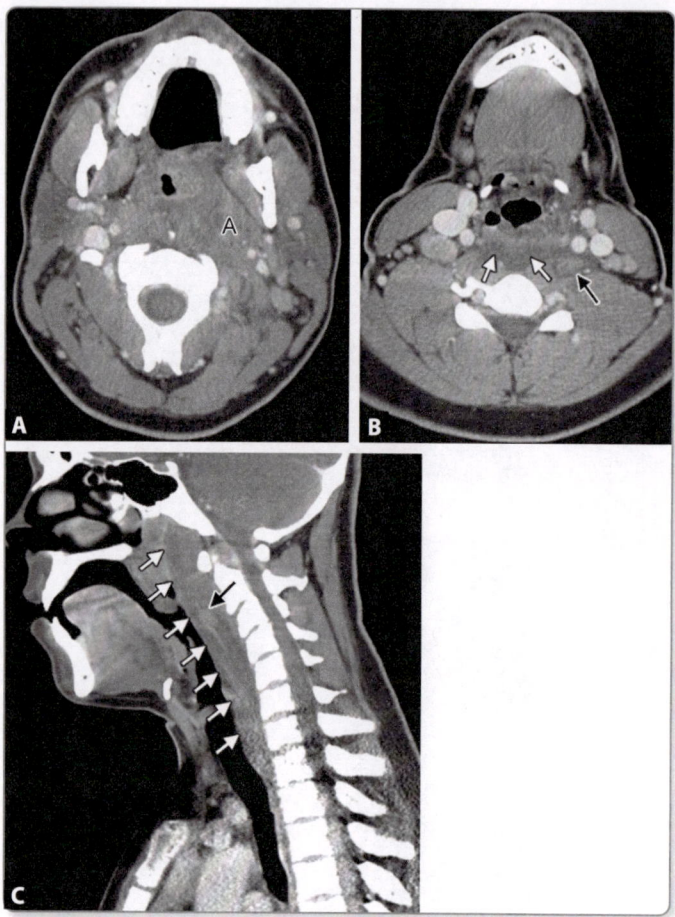

**Figures 8.15A to C** Left tonsillitis complicated by peritonsillar abscess (A). Note surrounding inflamed tissues and extension of inflammatory fluid into the retropharyngeal space (white arrows). Reactive left retropharyngeal lymph node enlargement is present (black arrows)

an enhancing rim. This should be distinguished from small 1-2 mm nonenhancing foci not uncommonly seen within the substance of tonsils likely representing normal tonsillar crypts.

## Congenital

Congenital lesions primarily involving the oropharynx are not particularly common. When a sinus or fistula is present in relation to a second branchial cleft anomaly, the internal orifice is in the region of the palatine tonsillar fossa. Although rare, thyroglossal duct cysts which are located proximally (near the foramen cecum) can involve the tongue base. Congenital lesions such as dermoids and venolymphatic malformations can involve the tissues of the oropharynx.

## Miscellaneous

Tortuosity of the internal carotid artery can result in a so-called retropharyngeal course of the ICA passing posteriorly to the oropharynx (**Figures 8.16A to C**) causing a pulsating submucosal impression visible to the endoscopist. Recognition of this variant is important in order to prevent inappropriate biopsy.

A retention cyst of a minor salivary gland is a small, superficial mucosal base cystic structure that can occur anywhere in the pharynx but is particularly common in the lateral nasopharynx and vallecula. When they occur in the vallecular fossa they are often referred to as vallecular cysts. Retention cysts can also occur secondarily in relation to tumor obstruction therefore clinical correlation of the mucosa adjacent to these cysts is advisable if there is any question of mucosal disease in the vicinity. Large vertebral osteophytes seen in degenerative disease and diffuse interstitial skeletal hyperostosis (DISH) can result in dysphagia.

Pharyngeal blunt trauma can result in mucosal or deep soft tissue hematoma. Iatrogenic trauma due to instrumentation, foreign body, or penetrating trauma can cause perforations of the oropharynx (**Figures 8.17A to C**). This can result in deep neck space infection, discussed elsewhere.

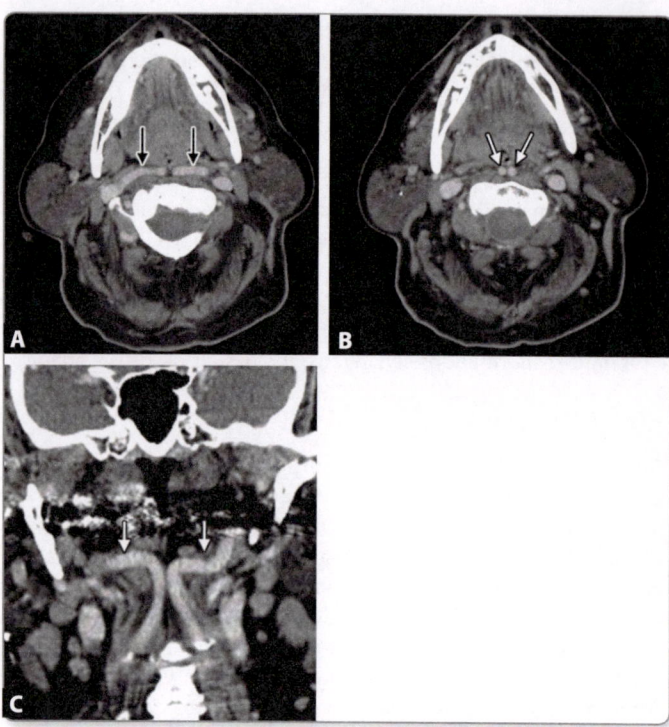

**Figures 8.16A to C** Retropharyngeal course of the internal carotid arteries bilaterally (arrows). Some call this appearance "Kissing carotids" when they meet in the midline

It is important to be aware of the spectrum of post-treatment change that can occur in the treated oropharynx. Following head and neck radiotherapy the pharynx often demonstrates increased enhancement of the mucosa which has been attributed to hyperemia and formation of telangiectatic vessels. The pharyngeal wall typically thickens and retropharyngeal edema may be present. Similar changes can be seen in patients with mucositis which can be a complication of

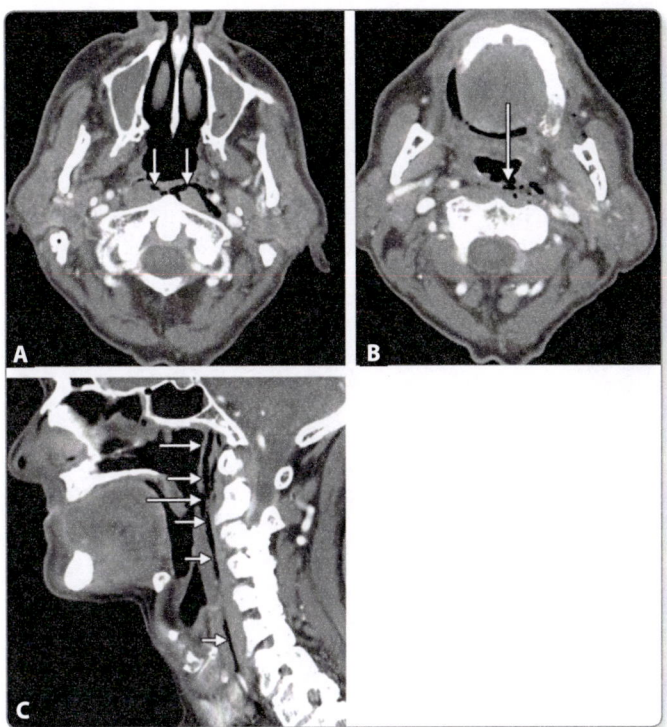

**Figures 8.17A to C** Traumatic perforation of the posterior pharyngeal wall resulting in interstitial emphysema (short white arrows). The site of perforation is very well demonstrated (long white arrow)

head and neck chemoradiation. Following surgical pharyngectomy there is significant variation in the appearance of the neopharynx depending on the type of surgical reconstruction and flaps that are used. A complete discussion of this topic is beyond the scope of this chapter, however, baseline postsurgical scanning done shortly postoperative can be extremely helpful in evaluating disease recurrence.

# Bibliography

1. Beil CM, Keberle M. Oral and oropharyngeal tumors. Eur J Radiol. 2008; 66(3):448-59.
2. Branstetter BF 4th, Weissman JL. Infection of the facial area, oral cavity, oropharynx, and retropharynx. Neuroimaging Clin N Am. 2003; 13(3):393-410.
3. Cohan DM, Popat S, Kaplan SE, Rigual N, Loree T, Hicks WL Jr. Oropharyngeal cancer: Current understanding and management.
4. Harnsberger HR. Handbook of Head and Neck Imaging 2nd edn. St Louis: Mosby 1995.
5. Som PM, Curtin HD. Head and Neck Imaging 4th edn. 2 vols. St. Louis: Mosby; 2003.
6. Stambuk HE, Karimi S, Lee N, Patel SG. Oral cavity and oropharynx tumors. Radiol Clin North Am. 2007; 45(1):1-20.
7. Tshering Vogel DW, Zbaeren P, Thoeny HC. Cancer of the oral cavity and oropharynx. Cancer Imaging. 2010;10:62-72. Curr Opin Otolaryngol Head Neck Surg. 2009;17(2):88-94.
8. Weber AL, Romo L, Hashmi S. Malignant tumors of the oral cavity and oropharynx: Clinical, pathologic, and radiologic evaluation. Neuroimaging Clin N Am 2003;13(3):443-64.
9. Wippold FJ 2nd. Imaging the treated oral cavity and oropharynx. Eur J Radiol. 2002;44(2):96-107.
10. Yousem DM, Gad K, Tufano RP. Respectability Issues with Head and Neck Cancer AJNR Am. J Neuroradiology. 2006;27:2024-36.

# Diseases of the parotid gland

chapter 9

Andrew Law, Andrew Thompson

**ABSTRACT**
Parotid gland anatomy and a review of the various imaging modalities available are reviewed. A discussion of normal anatomic variants, developmental, infectious and neoplastic entities is then presented.

**KEYWORDS**
Parotid, anatomy, neoplasm.

## Embryology

Development of the parotid glands commences in the sixth to eight week of gestation, derived from outpouchings of oral ectoderm into the surrounding mesenchyme. Epithelial thickening within the labiogingival sulcus progresses to form solid buds of tissue which branch repeatedly and eventually canalizes to form the parotid duct and ductules. Acinar cell proliferation at the ends of the ducts gives rise to the glandular component. As the parotid anlage grows and extends posteriorly, it envelops the extracranial facial nerve and its branches. The mesenchyme forms the capsule around the parotid gland and the fibrous septae between lobules but this only occurs late, after development of the lymphatic system, accounting for the presence of lymphoid tissue within the parotid gland. Development of the parotid gland is complete by the 3rd gestational month.

## Anatomy

The parotid gland is the largest salivary gland in the body and weighs approximately 14 to 28 grams. It extends from the external auditory canal and mastoid tip superiorly, over the mandibular ramus anteriorly, and below the mandibular angle inferiorly (parotid tail). Within the gland, from superficial to deep, are the extracranial facial nerve and branches; retromandibular vein; external carotid artery and its superficial temporal and mandibular artery terminal branches; and fibers of the auriculotemporal branch of the third division of the trigeminal nerve. There are 20 to 30 lymph nodes normally found within the parotid gland. The intraparotid group of lymph nodes are the primary drainage pathway from the external ear, external auditory canal, and skin of the forehead, temple, and lateral eyelids. Efferent lymphatic drainage from parotid nodes is received by the superior deep cervical lymph nodes along the internal jugular vein.

For surgical planning, the parotid gland is anatomically divided into superficial and deep lobes by the facial nerve. As the extracranial facial nerve is only visible in its proximal portion on MR, the retromandibular vein or stylomandibular tunnel is used to approximate the plane of the proximal intraparotid facial nerve and its ramifications. The "opening" or plane of the stylomandibular tunnel is a line drawn from the styloid process to the posterior margin of the mandibular ramus. The superficial and deep lobes are respectively located lateral and medial to these structures. The superficial lobe comprises around two-thirds of the parotid gland and the deep lobe extends into the lateral parapharyngeal space.

The parotid gland is composed almost entirely of serous acini. Parasympathetic secretomotor fibers arise from the inferior salivary nucleus within the lower pons and travel with the glossopharyngeal nerve (CN IX) and subsequently its tympanic nerve and lesser petrosal nerve branches. After synapsing within the otic ganglion, secretomotor fibers are carried by the auriculotemporal branch of CNV3 to the parotid gland. Sympathetic nerves to the parotid arise from the superior cervical ganglion, which travel with the external carotid artery. General sensation to the parotid gland and surrounding fascia is mediated via the auriculotemporal nerve and great auricular nerve respectively.

The parotid (Stensen's) duct is approximately 7 centimeters long and arises from the anterior margin of the parotid gland and passes superficially over the masseter muscle and inferior to the zygomatic arch. It turns medially to pierce the buccal fat and buccinator to open as a papilla on the mucous membrane adjacent to the 2nd maxillary molar.

# Imaging overview

## Plain radiographs

Plain radiographs are largely inadequate for the assessment of the salivary glands. Even for the detection of glandular or ductal calcification, ultrasound and CT are far more sensitive and have superseded plain radiographs as the initial examination of choice.

## Ultrasound

Ultrasound creates an image by using the varying reflective properties and sound-wave velocities in tissues to differentiate between tissue types. A linear, high-frequency transducer of around 7 to 10 MHz is generally used for parotid imaging, which gives high-resolution images at the expense of tissue penetration. The normal adult parotid gland is usually hyperechoic in relation to surrounding muscles, reflecting its higher fat content. The main intraparotid duct appears as paired hyperechoic streaks. The remaining intraparotid ducts are not usually visualized if normal in caliber. Ultrasound is useful for differentiating between solid and cystic lesions, but may be unable to completely image the deep lobe or provide full anatomic information for surgical planning and staging. It is the preferred modality for imaging-guided fine-needle aspiration or biopsy of a parotid gland lesion.

## Computed tomography

In children, the parotid gland is of soft tissue attenuation and resembles muscle. With age, the parotid gland gains fat as a normal process and the parenchyma is distributed within the fat in an interstitial pattern. The attenuation of the normal parotid gland in the adult approximates 15 to 25 Hounsfield units (HU) and is between that of fat and muscle. This provides good natural contrast for detecting tumors on unenhanced CT scanning. Rarely, particularly in younger patients, the administration of intravenous contrast may obscure

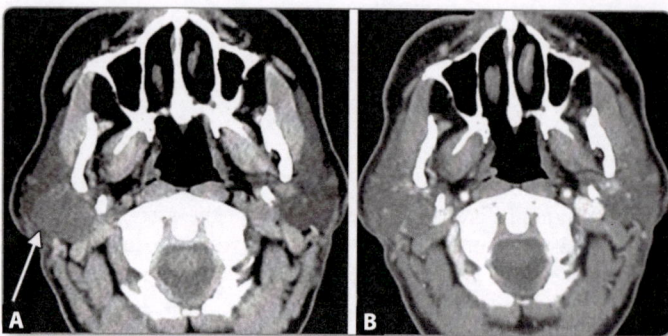

**Figures 9.1A and B** 55-year-old female. (A) Pre- and postcontrast CT (B), note the well circumscribed parotid mass (arrow) which following contrast administration becomes inconspicuous due to differential glandular and lesional enhancement characteristics. Enhanced imaging, in isolation, should be interpreted with caution if there is a clinically palpable mass

visualization of an intraglandular mass lesion (**Figures 9.1A and B**). Stensen's duct and the intraglandular ducts are not visualized on CT if they are of normal caliber.

At the musculotendinous attachment at the pinna, the parotid gland has a slightly higher attenuation compared to the rest of the gland, which should not be confused with a pathological lesion. CT is useful for detecting glandular calcification and for nodal staging. A well-defined, intraparotid soft tissue mass is a nonspecific CT finding and may be benign or malignant. Further evaluation with MRI as well as tissue sampling may be required.

## Magnetic resonance imaging

The normal parotid gland has a heterogenous appearance on MRI, with signal intensity between that of fat and muscle. It has predominantly intermediate to high signal on T1 reflecting the fat content with areas of low signal representing the parotid parenchyma. On T2-weighted imaging, the gland has intermediate to low signal.

MRI is particularly useful for assessing pericapsular tumor invasion and perineural spread, signs that point toward a malignant lesion.

Apparent diffusion coefficient (ADC) values have been proposed as a possible method of tissue characterization at a microscopic level, as malignancies tend to be more cellular than benign tumors and are therefore more likely to have a lower ADC value.

MR sialography is a method of imaging the ductal system without requiring ductal cannulation, reducing the number of unsuccessful investigations compared to conventional digital subtraction sialography. Several techniques have been described, all of which are based on T2-weighted sequences for contrast between high signal ductal contents and lower signal glandular fat and parenchyma. A secretagogue such as lemon juice may be given to assist in visualization of the intraparotid ducts.

## Digital subtraction sialography

Conventional sialography requires cannulating the opening of Stensen's duct and injection of approximately 1mL of radiopaque contrast media to avoid overfilling of the parotid acini as this can obscure ductal pathology. A secretagogue may be given to assist in excretory phase of the study, during which rapid and complete ductal emptying should be seen. Although employed less frequently due to advances in CT and MR imaging, DSS may be particularly useful for assessment of ductal complications of chronic inflammatory processes, including strictures and sialectasis. DSS has a higher spatial resolution and has a higher sensitivity for diagnosing subtle duct abnormalities compared to MR sialography.

## Nuclear medicine

Salivary gland scintigraphy is performed using Tc-99m pertechnetate, which accumulates normally within the salivary glands. It is most commonly used as an adjunctive study, especially in suspected Warthin's tumors or oncocytomas, which demonstrate marked focal increased uptake of 99m-Tc. In lesions with a negative Tc-99m study, subsequent F-18 Fluorodeoxyglucose Positron Emission Tomography (FDG PET) can assist in differentiating benign from malignant tumors as pleomorphic adenomas are not usually hot on PET imaging.

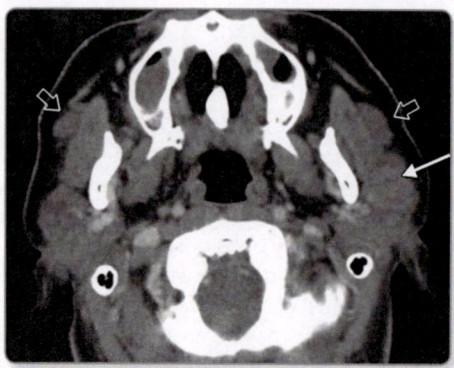

**Figure 9.2** Normal variant bilateral accessory parotid tissue (thick arrows). Note also benign mixed tumor left parotid gland in a young patient (arrow). The mildly enhancing tumor is of similar density to the parotid gland on postcontrast imaging

## Normal variants

### Accessory parotid tissue

Accessory parotid tissue is common, with a prevalence of 20 percent. It is most commonly located anterior to the main parotid gland and cranial to Stensen's duct as it passes over the masseter muscle (**Figure 9.2**). It has identical imaging characteristics as the main parotid gland and drainage into Stensen's duct is via a single main duct.

## Pathology

### Developmental

#### First branchial cleft cyst

The cystic remnant of the first branchial arch accounts for around 7 percent of all branchial cleft cysts. Two types of first branchial cleft cysts have been described, although overlap is not uncommonly seen. Associated sinus or fistulas may be present. Type I cysts are usually preauricular in location and can extend inferior and posterior to the pinna. They are usually only related to the membranous external auditory canal. Type 2 cysts are more common and are located at the mandibular angle. They can track superiorly and classically terminate at the junction of the bony and cartilaginous external auditory canal.

A noninfected cyst has a thin wall with a central area that is anechoic on ultrasound and of fluid attenuation on CT. On MR it follows fluid signal (low signal on T1-weighted imaging and high signal on T2-weighted imaging) with an isointense thin wall that shows no or slight-enhancement. Infection of the cyst results in a thickened, enhancing wall, with surrounding soft tissue stranding. There is an increase in attenuation and change in signal intensity of cyst contents, and these changes may persist after resolution of infection.

## Congenital absence or hypoplasia

Congenital absence of the parotid gland is a rare condition that usually affects multiple salivary glands. Due to hypertrophy and increased secretions from the remaining salivary glands, this condition may be asymptomatic. There are associations with facial developmental disorders, 1st branchial cleft abnormalities, and cleft palate. Ductal atresia is rare and more commonly affects the submandibular and sublingual ducts.

## Infective

### Sialolithiasis

Parotid calculi account for 19 percent of all cases of sialolithiasis compared to 80 percent from the submandibular gland. This is likely due in part to the serous composition of parotid secretions compared to the mucous secretion from the submandibular glands. Wharton's duct courses superiorly and has a narrower orifice compared to Stensen's duct. Obstruction can be either partial or complete and symptoms are often precipitated by food ingestion.

Computed tomography (CT) is the optimal modality for detecting parotid calculi. On ultrasound, calculi are echogenic and typically demonstrate posterior acoustic shadowing and may be accompanied by ductal dilation. Acute inflammation of the parotid gland is characterized by painful swelling with a heterogenous parenchymal

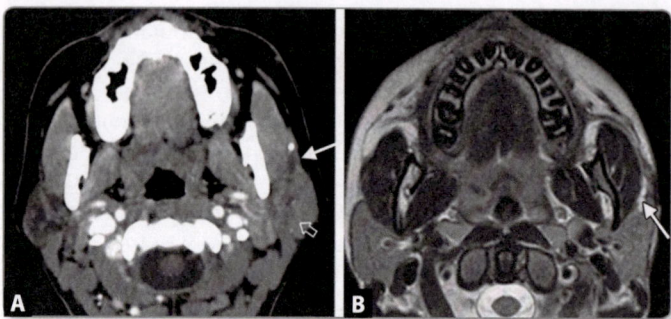

**Figures 9.3A and B** Enhanced axial CT. (A) Sialolith, sialectasis and parotitis. Note the dilated intraparotid duct (arrow) immediately posterior to the obstructing, hyperdense sialolith. The enlarged gland is hyperdense (thick arrow). (B) Right, axial T2 MR image, different patient with postinflammatory sialectasis, note T2 hyperintense dilated intraglandular duct (arrow)

echotexture. Small calculi of less than 2 mm can be difficult to detect sonographically as they do not usually demonstrate posterior shadowing. The acutely inflamed parotid gland usually has mildly increased attenuation on noncontrast CT, particularly if the premorbid gland was fatty, and increased T2 signal on MRI (**Figures 9.3A and B**). Stranding of the paraparotid fat is commonly seen and there is increased parenchymal enhancement following intravenous administration of contrast media. Patients with sialolithiasis have an increased risk of developing pyogenic sialadenitis and intraparotid abscesses.

Digital subtraction sialography (DSS) enables real-time assessment of calculus mobility, which can determine if endoscopic or surgical intervention is more appropriate. MR sialography is gaining favor as a noninvasive means of assessment and is also useful in patient with a documented severe allergy to contrast media, concurrent infective parotitis, and for investigating symptoms during pregnancy.

With recurrent sialolithiasis, the ducts become inflamed and scarred, resulting in dilatation and beaded-irregularity of Stensen's duct and the intraglandular ducts. This appearance is termed sialectasis and can be due to any cause of recurrent sialadenitis. Parenchy-

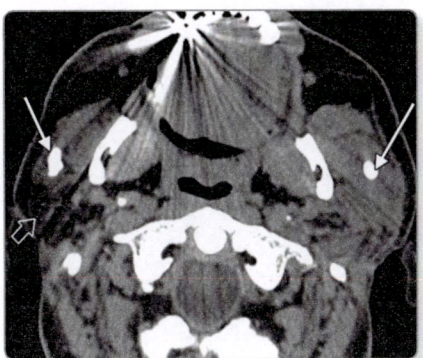

Figure 9.4 57-year-old male, bilateral parotid calculi (arrows). Note the postobstructive fatty atrophy of the right gland (thick arrow). *Courtesy:* Perth Radiological Clinic.

mal atrophy with reduced glandular function develops with chronic complete obstruction (**Figure 9.4**).

### Viral sialadenitis

Viral parotid infections are a disease of children and young adults. The diagnosis is made clinically and imaging is generally not required unless atypical features are present. Parvomyxovirus (mumps) is the most common viral infective organism. Other common organisms include cytomegalovirus; Epstein-Barr virus; and the Coxsackie viruses.

On ultrasound the gland is enlarged, hypoechoic and hypervascular with focal intraparotid areas of low echogenicity. Reactive lymphadenopathy within or around the parotid gland may be present. This nonspecific appearance is similar to other inflammatory diseases of the parotid gland. The parotid gland generally shows increased attenuation on CT with inflammatory stranding of the surrounding fat.

### Pyogenic sialadenitis

The majority of bacterial infection of the parotid glands is due to retrograde spread of oral flora secondary to a reduction in flow of saliva. This may be due to reduced saliva production, seen with Sjögren's

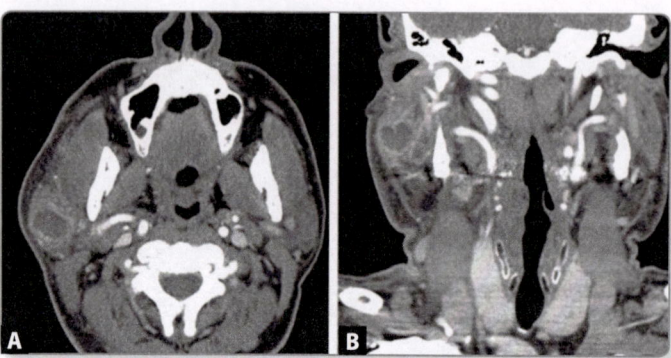

**Figures 9.5A and B** Peripherally enhancing right parotid abscess, *Streptococcus mitis* group isolated

syndrome; intraluminal ductal obstruction due to calculi, trauma, or strictures; or extraluminal ductal compression from a tumor. The most common infecting organisms are *Staphylococcus aureus*, *Streptococcus viridans*, *Hemophilus influenzae*, *Streptococcus pyogenes*, *Escherichia coli*, and *Streptococcus pneumoniae*.

The role of imaging in these cases is often to confirm or exclude the presence of a localized abscess as this may require more aggressive management in the form of drainage or surgery (**Figures 9.5A and B**).

# Autoimmune/inflammatory/infiltrative

## Sjögren's syndrome

Sjögren's syndrome is a disease in which autoantibodies are directed against exocrine glands such as the salivary glands and lacrimal glands causing chronic adenitis and ductal obstruction. This classically manifests as dry eyes and dry mouth but other body systems such as the skin can also be affected. It is nine times more common in females and usually presents around 40 years of age. It can develop alone (Primary Sjögren's syndrome) or in conjunction with other connective tissues diseases such as rheumatoid arthritis, systemic lupus erythematosus, or scleroderma (Secondary Sjögren's syndrome). Imaging characteristics of Sjögren's syndrome vary, depending on severity and chronicity of disease. In the primary form of disease, parotid involvement is slightly more common.

A definitive diagnosis usually involves a combination of positive sialographic findings, lymphocyte infiltration on minor salivary gland biopsy and the presence of antinuclear antibodies or antibodies to SS-A or SS-B. Lymphocyte-mediated destruction of ductal epithelial and acinar cells begin in the peripheral ducts. Ductal obstruction with focal ductal dilatation is best appreciated on MR or conventional sialography the size of which determines the stage of disease. They are seen as small cysts on ultrasound and cross-sectional imaging. Progression of acinar destruction causes formation of larger cysts of up to several centimeters in size.

Solid masses comprising of lymphocytic aggregates can develop at any stage but are more commonly seen in the late stages of disease.

Sonographically, in the early stages of disease the parotid gland has a granular heterogenous appearance and increased vascularity. As disease progresses, sialectasis is represented by hypoechoic foci. In addition echogenic foci may be seen which may represent mucous-filled ducts. On noncontrast enhanced computed tomography (NECT), the affected glands are initially enlarged and have increased attenuation and a heterogenous appearance. Punctate foci of calcification may be diffusely scattered throughout both glands. On magnetic resonance imaging (MRI), the gland has heterogenous signal with areas of high T1 signal represent foci of fat deposition, and low signal areas consistent with cysts. Cysts are seen as focal areas of T2 high signal (**Figures 9.6A and B**). There is heterogenous enhancement on both CT and MRI following administration of contrast media.

With ongoing inflammation and glandular destruction, there are large cystic areas, glandular atrophy and replacement of parenchyma with fat and fibrosis. Individuals with Sjögren's of the parotid have an increased risk of lymphoma, most commonly of the Non-Hodgkin's type. Serial imaging should be performed and biopsy is recommended of any dominant (>2 cm), rapidly growing, or invasive soft tissue mass (**Figure 9.6B**).

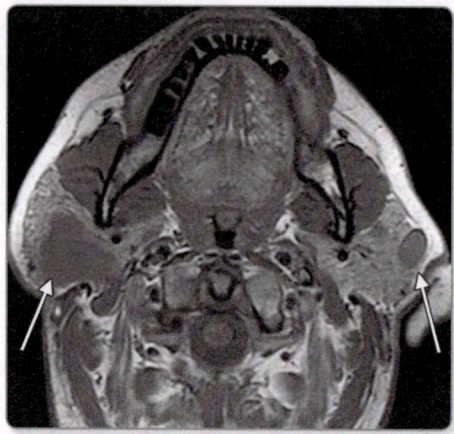

**Figure 9.6A** Axial T1 MR, bilateral fluid signal simple cysts, Sjögren's syndrome

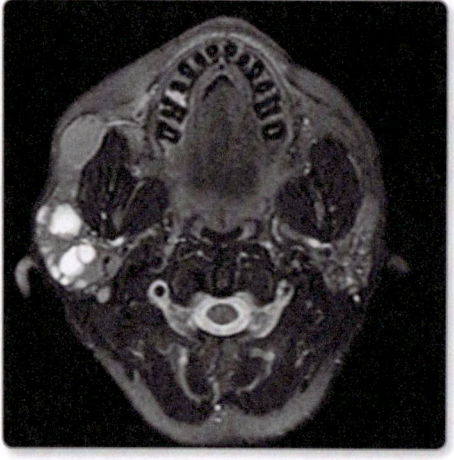

**Figure 9.6B** Another patient with Sjögren's syndrome. Note the large cysts in the right parotid. The patient also developed NHL as manifest by the mass located anteriorly in the region of the right accessory parotid tissue

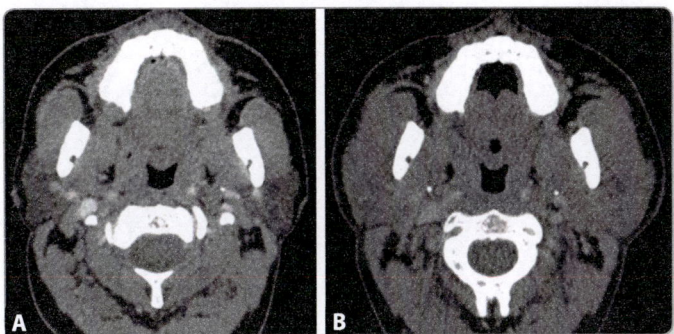

**Figures 9.7A and B** Nonspecific inflammatory sialadenitis, young adult male. Enhanced CT images prior to (A) and at presentation with purulent bilateral parotid discharge and gross submandibular and parotid sialadenitis. Bacterial and viral microbiological testing was negative, the symptoms resolved with steroid. Note enlarged and hyperdense parotid glands (B)

In certain instances, a noninfectious, inflammatory sialadenitis can arise. Imaging can be fairly nonspecific with increased CT attenuation and gland enlargement (**Figures 9.7A and B**).

## Sarcoidosis

Sarcoidosis is an idiopathic systemic disease characterized by the formation of noncaseating granulomas. It is more common in Africans and women. Up to 30 percent of patients with sarcoidosis have disease involving the parotid gland and of these patients 83 percent will have bilateral disease. Heerfordt syndrome refers to a clinical triad of patients with sarcoidosis, uveitis, and facial nerve palsy.

On cross-sectional imaging, granulomas within the parotid have a benign, noncavitating appearance. There are usually multiple and bilateral granulomas accompanied by cervical lymphadenopathy. In some cases, a solitary mass may be present, which is indistinguishable from other parotid tumors.

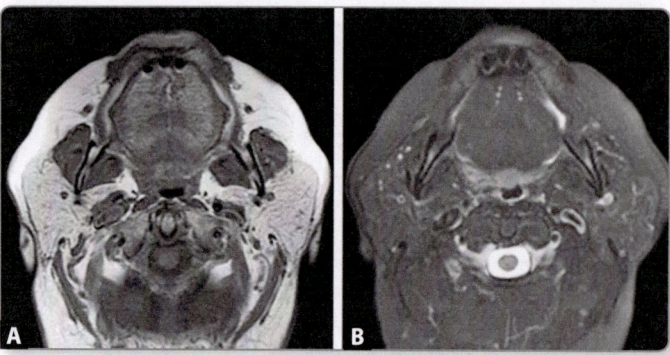

**Figures 9.8A and B** T1 (A) and enhanced T2 axial fat-saturated images (B), parotid sialosis in 58-year-old male with fatty deposition

## Sialosis

Sialosis, also known as sialadenosis is a benign non-inflammatory, non-neoplastic cause of bilateral and symmetric parotid swelling secondary to glandular hypertrophy, interstitial edema, and fat deposition. It is associated with several conditions including endocrine abnormalities such as diabetes mellitus and hypothyroidism, chronic alcoholism, hepatic cirrhosis and vitamin deficiencies, and certain medications including diuretics. Reversal may occur with treatment of the primary cause.

Attenuation of the parotid is reduced on CT and there is increased signal on T1- and T2-weighted MR imaging reflecting fatty deposition (**Figures 9.8A and B**).

## Radiation-induced sialadenitis

As with radiation-related changes elsewhere in the body, acute and chronic manifestations of disease have been described. Acute radiation-induced sialadenitis typically develops after a single dose of 10Gy or more and clinically presents as painful swelling with xerostomia that usually resolves within days. Chronic changes are characterized by parenchymal volume loss and fibrosis with increased

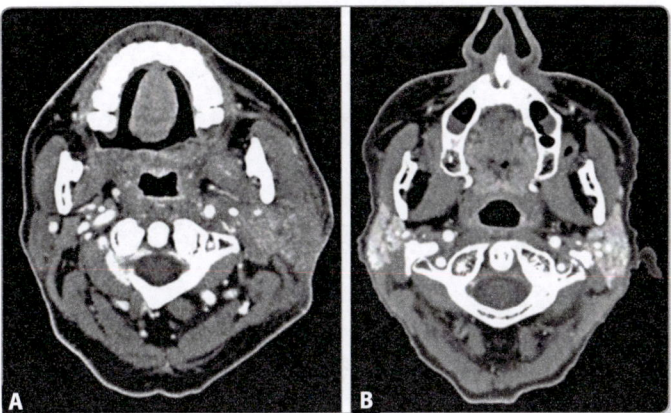

**Figures 9.9A and B** (A) Left image demonstrates left parotid enlargement and mild enhancement in patient undergoing radiation therapy. Note periparotid inflammatory changes. (B) Right image in another patient shows the chronic appearance of radiation related parotitis. The glands have atrophied and demonstrate marked enhancement

attenuation of CT (**Figures 9.9A and B**) and reduced signal on T1- and T2-weighed MR imaging.

## Trauma

### Parotid laceration, duct laceration and sialocele

Blunt trauma to the parotid gland can result in glandular contusions and intraglandular hemorrhage. Penetrating injury can cause laceration of the parotid gland or parotid duct. A sialocele is a cystic collection of saliva that develops secondary to duct rupture (**Figure 9.10**). Persisting communication with the main ducts may be seen on sialography with contrast filling the cyst.

## Benign neoplasms

The likelihood of a salivary gland tumor being malignant is inversely related to the size of the salivary gland. Approximately 80

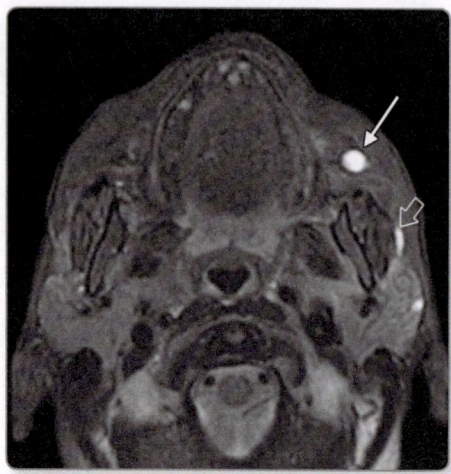

Figure 9.10 T2-weighted axial MRI, traumatic sialocele (arrow) of Stensen's duct following buccal space surgery. Note dilatation of the proximal duct (thick arrow)

percent of all parotid gland tumors are benign compared to a rate of 50 to 60 percent within the submandibular gland. In comparison, around 66 percent of all minor salivary gland tumors are malignant. Ultrasound guided fine needle aspiration (FNA) is often performed for cytological assessment of parotid masses prior to definitive excision. As a general rule, all parotid gland neoplasms are considered for excision as low grade malignant lesions may be well-circumscribed and have a 'benign appearance' on imaging.

## Pleomorphic adenoma (benign mixed tumor)

Pleomorphic adenomas are the most common tumor of the parotid gland and are named as they contain epithelial, myoepithelial, and stromal cellular elements. They account for 80 percent of all benign parotid masses and occur far more commonly in the parotid gland (85%) than in other salivary glands. Benign mixed tumor (BMT) is most prevalent in people over 40 years of age and is twice as common in females compared to males. The most common presentation is a slow-growing painless cheek or mandibular angle mass.

The majority (80%) of lesions are located within the superficial parotid lobe and less than 1 percent are multicentric. Margins are well circumscribed and the tumor has a lobulated appearance. Superficially located lesions tend to be smaller on presentation and lesions within the deep lobe can measure up to 8 cm at presentation. Smaller lesions have homogenous appearances on imaging and are hypoechoic on ultrasound and of low attenuation on noncontrast CT. The presence of dystrophic calcification on CT can help distinguish this lesion from a Warthin's tumor.

MR appearances vary with the degree of myxoid content but are usually hypointense on T1-weighted imaging and hyperintense on T2-weighted imaging (**Figures 9.11A to D**). A T2 low-signal capsule may be seen. Mild-moderate homogenous enhancement is present on CT and MRI following intravenous contrast administration. Necrosis and hemorrhage may be present in larger lesions (**Figure 9.12**). On angiography and dynamic contrast-enhanced CT and MRI, the hypovascular nature of pleomorphic adenomas is reflected by slow wash-in (**Figures 9.13A and B**) and increase in signal intensity with a plateau phase with slow washout of contrast. There is no uptake of fluoro-2-deoxy-D-glucose (FDG) on PET imaging. Occasionally, exophytic lesions arising from the deep lobe can project into the parapharyngeal space, and hence present clinically as a submucosal parapharyngeal space mass (**Figures 9.14A and B**).

All pleomorphic adenomas are surgically removed due to the risk of malignant transformation (carcinoma ex-pleomorphic adenoma), which increases over time. Special care is taken to prevent rupture of the fibrous capsule as this reduces the risk of recurrence through tumor cell seeding of the surgical site (**Figures 9.15A to D**).

## Warthin's tumor (adenolymphoma)

Warthin's tumor is also known as papillary cystadenoma lymphomatosum, adenolymphoma, or lymphomatous adenoma. It is the second most common salivary tumor and accounts for up to 10 percent of all parotid tumors. They arise from lymphoid tissue within the intra- or

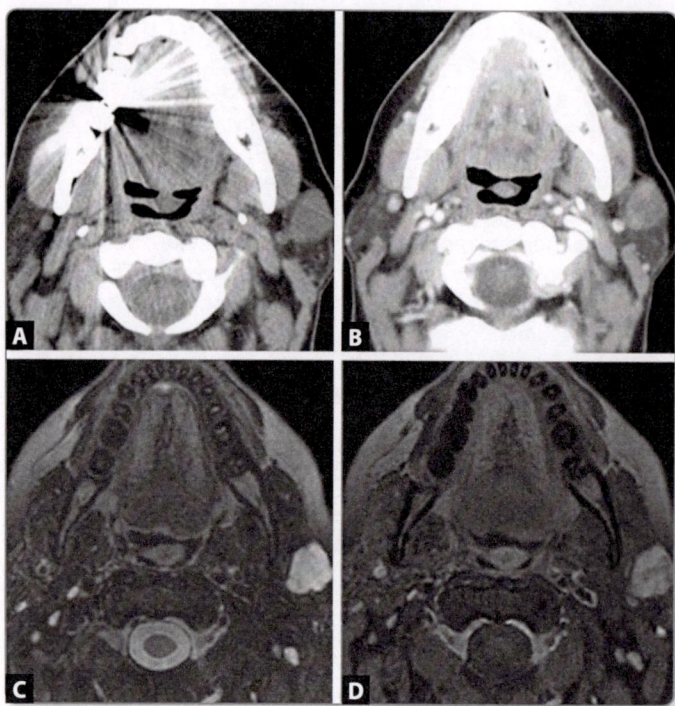

**Figures 9.11A to D** Pre- and postcontrast CT (A and B), T2 (C and D), enhanced T1 (D) MRI. Well circumscribed, T2 hyperintense, mildly enhancing tumor, pleomorphic adenoma. Benignity cannot be confirmed from imaging appearance and excisional biopsy is required

peri-parotid lymph nodes and contain both epithelial and lymphoid cellular elements. Most prevalent in males over 60 years of age, there is a strong link between Warthin's tumor and tobacco smoking. Smoking is associated with a relative risk of 40 of developing Warthin's tumor compared to nonsmokers, and 90 percent of patients with Warthin's tumor are smokers. Malignant transformation is extremely rare, occurring in less than 1 percent of cases.

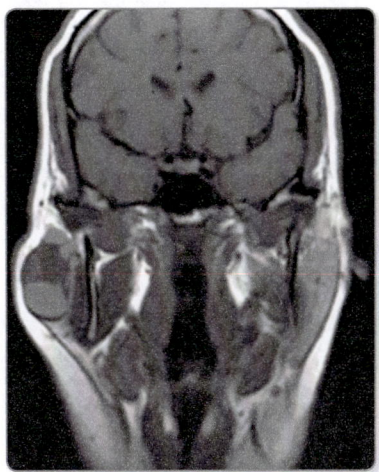

**Figure 9.12** Coronal T1-weighted image shows a pleomorphic adenoma with cystic change. High T1 signal is present compatible with the presence of hemorrhage

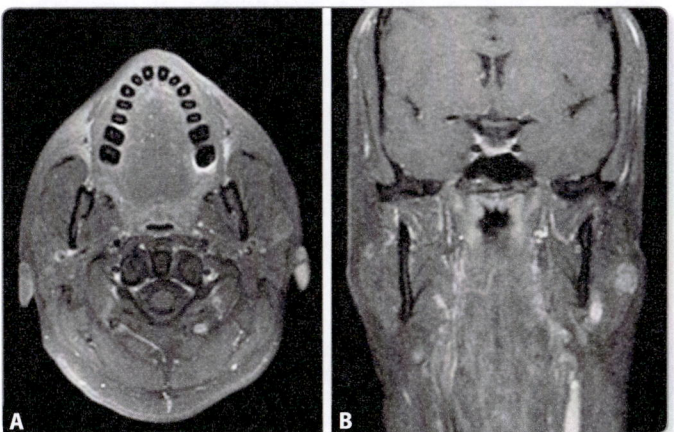

**Figures 9.13A and B** Axial and coronal gadolinium enhanced fat saturated imaging shows the delayed gradual enhancement of the pleomorphic adenoma in the left lobe of parotid. The coronal scan was performed approximately 5 minutes after the axial series

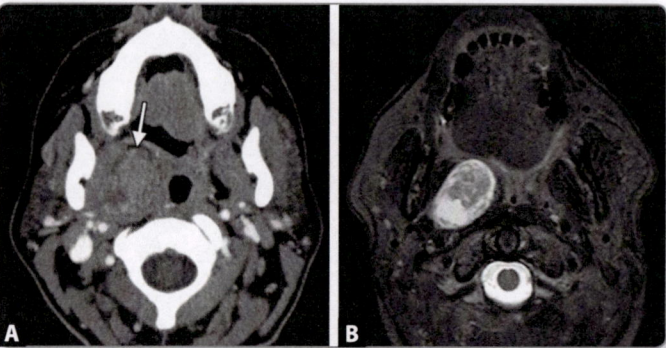

**Figures 9.14A and B** CT and T2-weighted MRI, benign mixed tumor in an elderly female arising from the deep lobe. Note the heterogenous nature of the lesion and displaced parapharyngeal fat (arrow), confirmation that the lesion is separate from the oropharynx

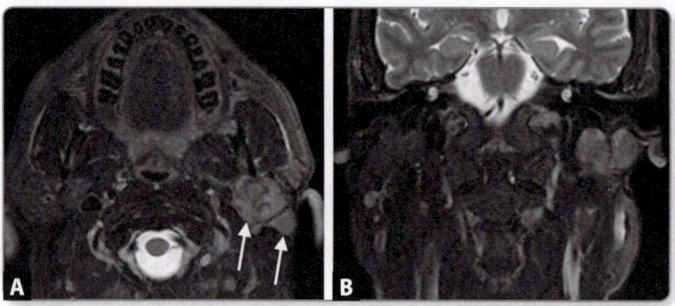

**Figures 9.15A and B** Multifocal BMT recurrence in the left parotid bed, 55-year-old male. Axial and coronal T2 imaging shows multiple, mildly hyperintense masses

These tumors are classically located within the parotid tail (posteroinferior aspect of the superficial parotid) and present as a painless mass at the mandibular angle. It is the most common lesion to be multicentric or bilateral, either synchronously or metachronously, in approximately 20 percent of cases. Warthin's tumors are typically well-circumscribed, smoothly marginated, heterogenous lesions and may

## Diseases of the parotid gland

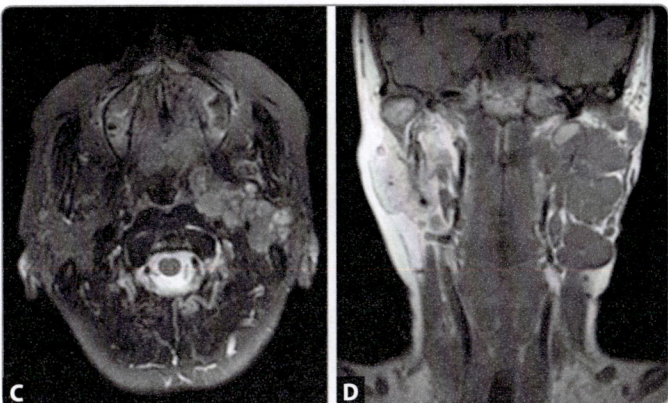

**Figures 9.15C and D** Multifocal BMT recurrence in the left parotid bed in another patient. Note the clustered appearance which is characteristic of recurrent disease

contain solid and cystic components. On ultrasound there are multiple irregular anechoic areas with posterior acoustic enhancement reflecting the cystic component. Hypervascularity is demonstrated with the application of color Doppler imaging.

On CT the cystic components may be reflected in fluid-attenuation Hounsfield values however if complicated by hemorrhage or infection, this may increase the attenuation to mimic that of soft tissue (**Figures 9.16A and B**). In contrast to pleomorphic adenomas, calcification is not present. Both the solid and cystic components are low signal on T1-weighted imaging compared to the remainder of the parotid gland. Hemorrhage and proteinaceous debris within cysts may have variable MRI signal depending on the stage of breakdown of blood products and the protein concentration. On T2-weighted imaging the simple cystic and solid components have high signal and intermediate-high signal respectively. There is mild enhancement of the solid component on CT and MRI following administration of intravenous contrast.

PET imaging can assist in the diagnosis of Warthin's tumors which show increased uptake of FDG, reflecting the large numbers of mitochondria within the columnar epithelial cells (oncocytes) in a

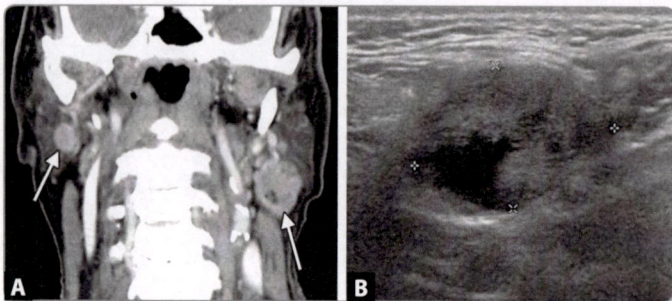

**Figures 9.16A and B** Bilateral Warthin's tumors in an 83-year-old male. Note the left parotid tail lesion heterogeneity on CT and ultrasound. *Courtesy:* Perth Radiological Clinic

Warthin's tumor. As malignant tumors also have increased FDG uptake, salivary gland scintigraphy demonstrating increased uptake of Tc-99m sodium pertechnetate with delayed washout after administration of a secretagogue can assist in differentiation.

## Benign lymphoepithelial lesions

Benign lymphoepithelial lesions are also known as AIDS-related parotid cysts but patients need only be infected with human immunodeficiency virus (HIV) to have this manifestation. These lesions arise from epithelial inclusions within intraparotid lymphoid tissue. It has been documented to occur in up to 5 percent of HIV-infected patients, although the incidence is decreasing with the introduction of combination antiretroviral agents. Clinically, this manifests as painless bilateral parotid gland swelling. There is a small risk of transformation into B-cell lymphoma.

There may be a range of imaging appearances from simple cysts to mixed, predominantly solid lesions, which vary from a few millimeters to several centimeters (**Figures 9.17A to D**). Mixed lesions have heterogenous and variable contrast enhancement of the solid component.

Benign lymphoepithelial cysts are associated with non-necrotic cervical lymphadenopathy and hypertrophy of the palatine, lingual,

Diseases of the parotid gland 377

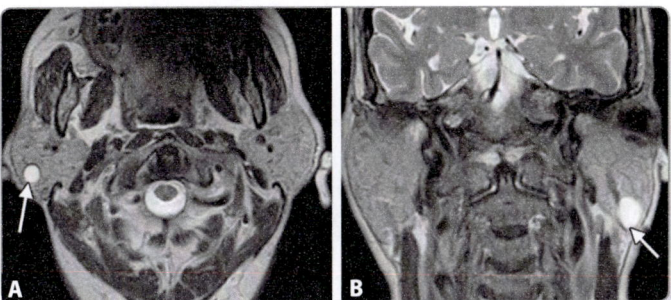

**Figures 9.17A and B** HIV associated simple lymphoepithelial cysts in a 48-year-old female, axial and coronal T2 MRI

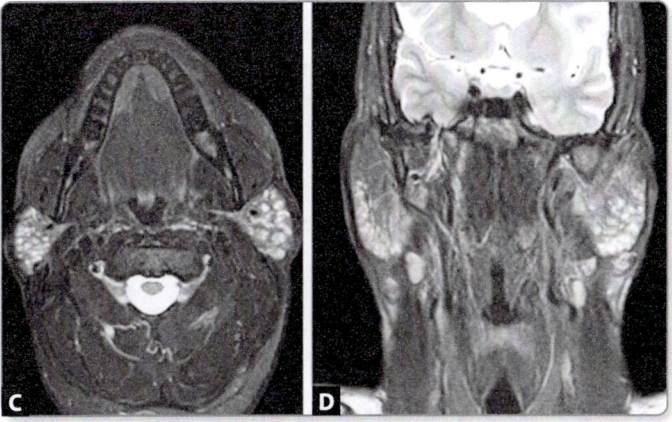

**Figures 9.17C and D** Multiple HIV associated simple lymphoepithelial cysts located bilaterally within both parotid glands

or adenoid tonsils, which can also help differentiate between benign lymphoepithelial lesions and Sjogren's disease on imaging.

## Oncocytic neoplasms

An oncocyte is a large cell that contains abundant mitochondria within its cytoplasm giving it an intensely eosinophilic histological appearance. This group of disorders is believed to be due to errors in mitochondrial DNA. The World Health Organization classifies oncocytic neoplasms into 3 entities. Oncocytosis is a benign condition with multifocal collections of oncocytes. Oncocytomas are rare lesions, accounting for less than 2 percent of all parotid tumors. Most present as a painless unilateral mass and around 20 percent have an associated history of radiation therapy. Approximately 7 percent are multicentric and bilateral on presentation (**Figures 9.18A and B**). They have a nonspecific benign imaging appearance with uptake of Tc-99m sodium pertechnetate on nuclear imaging scans. There is a small risk of malignant transformation into oncocytic carcinoma.

## Vascular malformations

Capillary hemangiomas are the most common head and neck tumor in infants, and account for 90 percent of parotid tumors in this age group. These nonencapsulated and lobulated tumors arise from endothelial cells and are histologically characterized by thin-walled capillary sized spaces separated by fibrous septae. Around 30 percent are clinically apparent at birth and may undergo a period of proliferation and rapid enlargement. Surgical treatment is usually avoided as most of these lesions spontaneously regress and there is no risk of malignant transformation.

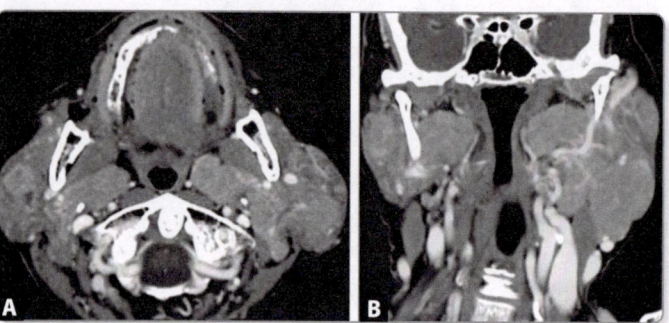

**Figures 9.18A and B** Enhanced axial and coronal CT, bilateral multifocal benign oncocytic tumors involving both deep and superficial lobes in an adult female.
*Courtesy:* Perth Radiological Clinic

Ultrasound demonstrates a vascular hypoechoic lesion. In the proliferative phase it has a similar appearance to muscle on noncontrast CT and T1-weighed MR imaging. On T2-weighted imaging it has a signal between muscle and fluid. Prominent flow voids may be seen in larger lesions. Calcifications are not associated with capillary hemangiomas and there is diffuse and intense contrast enhancement.

Venous vascular malformations are usually present at birth but do not become clinically apparent until late childhood or early adulthood. These well-circumscribed, multi-lobulated lesions are composed of variably sized vascular sinusoids and are characterized by the presence of phleboliths. In contrast to capillary hemangiomas, they do not tend to spontaneously regress. Vascular channels are visible on ultrasound and venous flow can be augmented with compression of the mass by the transducer.

On noncontrast CT the lesion has similar attenuation to that of muscle. Depending on the size of the vascular channels, they can appear isointense or hyperintense on T2-weighted imaging. Flow voids may be visible and phleboliths have T1 and T2 low signal (**Figures 9.19A and B**). Enhancement is usually present but variable with delayed and heterogenous, or early and homogenous patterns described. These lesions are classically angiographically occult, although a subtle blush may be present.

## Lymphatic malformations

Lymphatic malformations or lymphangiomas are most commonly diagnosed within the first 2 years of life, as this is the stage when lymphatic proliferation is the greatest. They are extremely uncommon in adults and may be secondary to trauma in this age group. Lymphangiomas are characterized by dilated lymphatic channels and classification of these lesions is dependent on vessel size. In the head and neck, cystic hygroma is the most common form of lymphangiomas and is associated with Turner's syndrome, Noonan's syndrome, and fetal alcohol syndrome. Lymphatic and venous malformations can occur within the same lesion and are referred to as venolymphatic malformations.

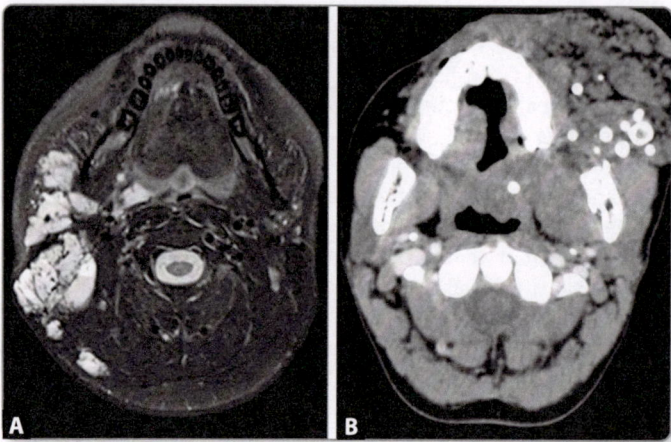

**Figures 9.19A and B** Axial fat saturated T2 (B) and contrast enhanced CT (A) in two different patients with venous vascular malformations. The first image shows lobulated T2 bright signal involving the right parotid and extending into the adjacent posterior cervical space. The CT shows characteristic phleboliths and lobulated soft tissue density in the left cheek and face

These lesions are most commonly located within the posterior cervical triangle and can infiltrate through fascial planes to involve the parotid gland. They are usually composed of multiple communicating locules although septation may be imperceptible on imaging. Normal fluid attenuation and signal is seen within the lesion unless there has been hemorrhage or previous infection. Pure lymphangiomas have no or minimal enhancement (**Figures 9.20A to C**).

## Nerve sheath tumors

Benign nerve sheath tumors include schwannomas and neurofibromas. They are the most common benign nonepithelial tumors after hemangiomas and lymphangiomas. Schwannomas are derived from Schwann cells, which are supporting cells for axons. There are peripherally located within the sheath, theoretically making nerve sparing

# Diseases of the parotid gland

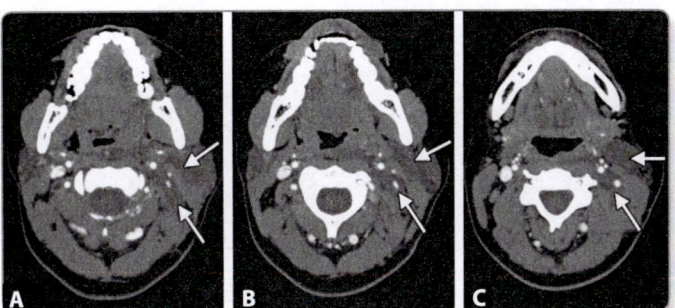

**Figures 9.20A to C** Lymphangioma. Contrast enhanced CT scan showing multifocal nonenhancing fluid density foci in the left parotid space and posterior cervical space (arrows)

surgery possible. In contrast, neurofibromas are derived from neuronal and perineural elements. They are surgically inseparable from axons as they infiltrate nerve fascicles and incorporate axons into the lesion. Plexiform neurofibromas are associated with neurofibromatosis type 1 (von Recklinghausen disease) and can undergo transformation into a malignant peripheral nerve sheath tumor.

Nerve sheath tumors within the parotid gland are usually ovoid and well-circumscribed tumors that arise from branches of the facial nerve. Cystic areas may be seen on both CT and MR. With MR imaging, schwannomas have a nonspecific appearance and are usually hypointense or isointense to muscle on T1-weighted imaging, hyperintense on T2-weighted imaging, and enhance avidly (**Figures 9.21A to D**). Review of the petrous, canalicular and cisternal portions of the facial nerve is mandatory to exclude neoplastic involvement. The elongated nature of these lesions and their extension along the course of a nerve are clues to the diagnosis. Fine needle aspiration of a nerve sheath tumor is usually extremely painful, a hint to the underlying histopathology.

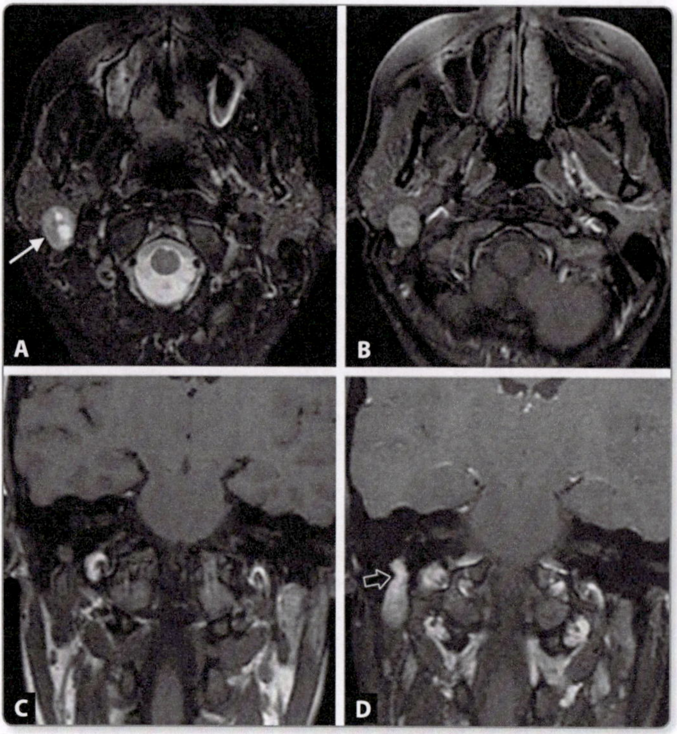

**Figures 9.21A to D** Axial and coronal MR, of intraparotid facial nerve schwannoma. Note heterogeneous T2 signal (arrow) and involving descending mastoid segment of the nerve (thick arrow), extending through stylomastoid foramen. *Courtesy:* Perth Radiological Clinic

# Malignant neoplasms

## Salivary gland epithelial malignancies (Tables 9.1 and 9.2)

### Mucoepidermoid carcinoma

Mucoepidermoid carcinoma is most common between the ages of 35 and 55 years. It accounts for 10 percent of all salivary gland tumors,

|  | TNM Stage | Description |
| --- | --- | --- |
| Primary tumor (T) | TX | Primary tumor cannot be assessed |
|  | T0 | No evidence of primary tumor |
|  | T1 | Tumor 2 cm or less in greatest dimension without extraparenchymal extension* |
|  | T2 | Tumor more than 2 cm but not more than 4 cm in greatest dimension without extraparenchymal extension* |
|  | T3 | Tumor more than 4 cm and/or tumor having extraparenchymal extension |
|  | T4a | Moderately advanced disease – tumor invades skin, mandible, ear canal and/or facial nerve |
|  | T4b | Very advanced disease – tumor invades skull base and/or pterygoid plates and/or encases carotid artery |
| Regional lymph nodes (N) | NX | Regional lymph nodes cannot be assessed |
|  | N0 | No regional lymph node metastasis |
|  | N1 | Metastasis in a single ipsilateral lymph node, 3 cm or less in greatest dimension |
|  | N2 | Metastasis in a single ipsilateral lymph node, more than 3 cm but not more than 6 cm in greatest dimension, or in bilateral or contralateral lymph nodes, none more than 6 cm in greatest dimension |
|  | N2a | Metastasis in a single ipsilateral lymph node, more than 3 cm but not more than 6 cm in greatest dimension |
|  | N2b | Metastasis in multiple ipsilateral lymph nodes none more than 6 cm in greatest dimension |
|  | N2c | Metastasis in bilateral or contralateral lymph nodes, none more than 6 cm in greatest dimension |
|  | N3 | Metastasis in a lymph node, more than 6 cm in greatest dimension |
| Metastases (M) | M0 | No distant metastasis (no pathologic M0; use clinical M to complete stage group) |
|  | M1 | Distant metastasis |

*Note: Extraparenchymal extension is clinical or macroscopic evidence of invasion of soft tissues. Microscopic evidence alone does not constitute extraparenchymal extension for classification purposes.

**Table 9.1** AJCC major salivary gland staging – 7th edition

| Stage I | T1 | N0 | M0 |
| --- | --- | --- | --- |
| Stage II | T2 | N0 | M0 |
| Stage III | T3<br>T1<br>T2<br>T3 | N0<br>N1<br>N1<br>N1 | M0<br>M0<br>M0<br>M0 |
| Stage IVA | T4a<br>T4a<br>T1<br>T2<br>T3<br>T4a | N0<br>N1<br>N2<br>N2<br>N2<br>N2 | M0<br>M0<br>M0<br>M0<br>M0<br>M0 |
| Stage IVB | T4b<br>Any T | Any N<br>N3 | M0<br>M0 |
| Stage IV C | Any T | Any N | M1 |

**Table 9.2** Anatomic stage/prognostic group

30 percent of salivary gland malignancies, and forms the majority (60%) of malignant parotid gland lesions. In contrast, adenoid cystic carcinoma is the most common malignancy in the submandibular gland. Mucoepidermoid carcinoma is also the most common salivary gland malignancy in children but only 3 percent of all such tumors occur in the pediatric population. On palpation, the lesion feels hard and manifestations of perineural spread to the facial and/or mandibular cranial nerves may be evident. Histologically, mucoepidermoid carcinomas are derived from ductal epithelium and are composed of both epidermoid and mucous components in varying amounts.

Mucoepidermoid carcinomas are more commonly found in the superficial parotid lobe and are usually 1 to 4 centimeters at presentation. Unenhanced T1-weighted imaging is the best sequence for delineating the margins or extent of tumor involvement due to inherent contrast with the normal intraparotid fat. Low-grade carcinomas are ovoid with well-defined margins and can resemble pleomorphic adenoma. There is a heterogenous appearance on CT and MRI with predominantly low signal on both T1- and T2-weighted imaging

Diseases of the parotid gland **385**

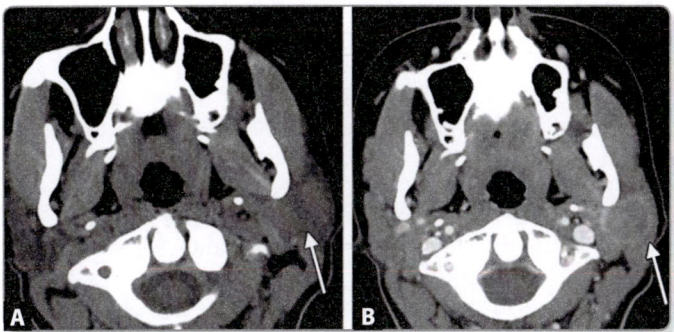

**Figures 9.22A and B** 26-year-old female, well-circumscribed, mildly enhancing left parotid mass, mucoepidermoid carcinoma. *Courtesy:* Perth Radiological Clinic

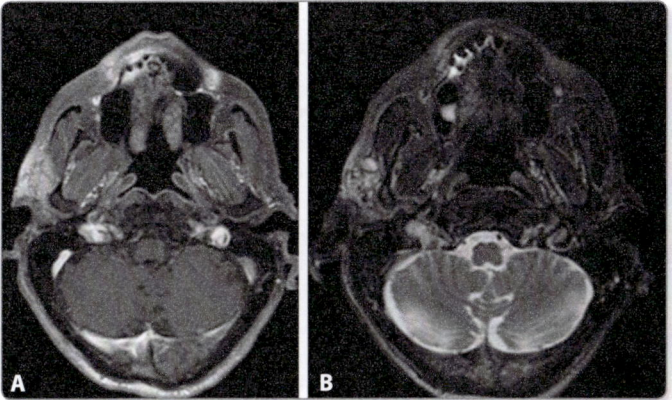

**Figures 9.23A and B** Mucoepidermoid carcinoma. Fat saturated postcontrast T1 (right) and T2-weighted MRI shows a enhancing mass in the superficial lobe of the right parotid. T2 imaging shows the lesion with predominantly high signal

(**Figures 9.22 and 9.23**). Cystic foci are commonly seen, and in rare instances calcification may be present.

High-grade mucoepidermoid carcinomas have soft tissue signal with ill-defined margins and an infiltrative and aggressive imaging appearance. The presence of enlarged and morphologically abnormal intraparotid and cervical lymph nodes strongly suggests a malignant process.

Recurrence and survival rates in mucoepidermoid carcinomas are dependent on histological grade. Due to the tendency of recurrence, clinical and imaging follow-up for at least 10 years is recommended.

## Adenoid cystic carcinoma

Adenoid cystic carcinoma is most common between 40 and 70 years of age and is slightly more common in females. It is the second most common major salivary gland malignancy and accounts for 2 to 6 percent of all parotid gland tumors. It is a slow-growing tumor that usually arises in the superficial parotid lobe, and is palpable as a hard and painful mass. Of all the salivary gland malignancies, adenoid cystic carcinoma has the highest tendency for perineural spread, with pain and facial nerve paralysis present in up to a third of cases.

Low-grade lesions appear well-defined and high-grade lesions are ill defined and infiltrative. High-grade tumors also tend to have lower signal on T2-weighted imaging, reflective of denser tumor cellularity. Metastatic disease to lung and bone is more common than nodal spread.

Although these lesions are slow growing, there is a high rate of local recurrence and remote perineural spread, which can occur up to 20 years after diagnosis, necessitating long-term follow-up.

There are numerous other recognized subtypes of epithelial parotid malignancy. Acinic cell carcinoma is a rare lesion, but occurs overall in younger population, has a 2:1 female predominance and is the second most common malignant lesion occurring in children. Imaging features are nonspecific (**Figures 9.24A and B**).

## Carcinoma ex-pleomorphic adenoma

The World Health Organization divides malignant derivatives of salivary gland pleomorphic adenomas into three separate clinicopathological entities: carcinoma ex-pleomorphic adenoma (malignant transformation of underlying pleomorphic adenoma), carcinosarcoma and metastasizing benign pleomorphic adenoma. Carcinoma

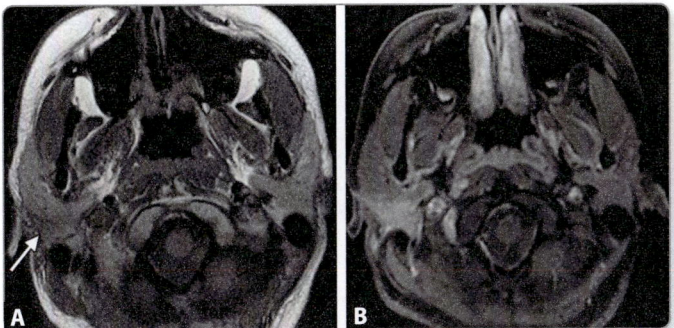

**Figures 9.24A and B** Acinic cell carcinoma, 14-year-old female. Note the ill-defined, relatively T1 hypointense (left, arrow) enhancing (right) tumor

ex-pleomorphic adenoma is by far the most common subtype. The rate of malignant degeneration of the epithelial elements of pleomorphic adenoma increases with time and is estimated at around 9.5 percent over a period of 15 years. These malignancies are usually high-grade adenocarcinomas and account for only around 5 percent of all parotid gland malignancies but have a high rate of recurrence and metastases. They typically occur in patients with a long-standing history of pleomorphic adenoma, most common between 50 to 70 years of age.

## Lymphoma

Primary lymphoma of the parotid gland is rare, and this diagnosis can only be made with histological confirmation of lymphoma within the parotid gland parenchyma without evidence of intraparotid lymph node involvement. These painless lesions are classified as MALT (mucosa-associated lymphoid tissue) lymphomas and clonal B cells can be demonstrated on PCR. The majority of primary lymphoma is indolent and therefore carries a good prognosis. Sjogren's syndrome increases the risk of developing MALT lymphoma with a relative risk of approximately 44 compared to the general population. Lymphoma in these patients is not merely confined to the exocrine glands and can involve lymph nodes and the spleen. Imaging appearances of primary lymphoma is nonspecific with a nodular, infiltrative lesion that can mimic chronic sialadenitis.

In the vast majority of parotid lymphoma, intraparotid lymphadenopathy is part of a systemic disease involving multiple nodal and extranodal sites. Salivary gland involvement occurs in 8 percent of systemic disease, most frequently (80%) involves the parotid gland and is most commonly seen in high-grade diffuse large cell lymphoma. The most common CT imaging appearance is of multiple, homogenous and benign-appearing intraparotid nodal masses. It can also present with diffuse glandular infiltration (**Figures 9.25A and B**). They demonstrate intermediate signal on both T1- and T2-weighted MR imaging with mild to moderate uniform contrast enhancement. Central necrosis is uncommon and the presence of extraglandular disease may assist with an imaging diagnosis.

## Metastatic disease to the parotid gland

Lymphangitic or hematogenous spread to the intraparotid or adjacent lymph nodes occurs most commonly in the setting of head and

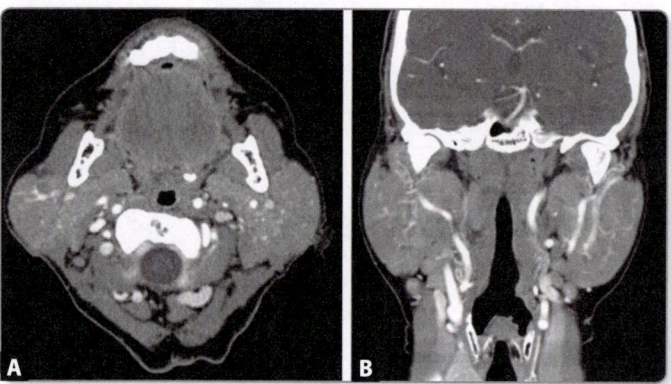

**Figures 9.25A and B** CT imaging of lymphoma that is diffusely infiltrating the parotid glands

neck squamous cell carcinoma or melanoma. In most cases there is a known primary and around 75 to 89 percent of primary tumors are located in the skin of the face, external ear, or scalp. Lung, kidney and breast are the most common systemic malignancies to metastasize to the parotid gland and can rarely affect both parotid glands. Peak incidence occurs in the 7th decade and is twice as common in males compared to females.

Typically, multifocal unilateral parotid necrotic metastases are demonstrated on imaging. Less commonly a solitary metastasis is present (**Figures 9.26A and B**), which mimics a primary high-grade parotid tumor. It is important to determine on imaging if there is tumor infiltration of the parotid parenchyma, which is characterized by ill-defined margins on imaging. This portends a poorer prognosis with a significantly higher rate of local recurrence.

## Perineural spread

Perineural spread into the skull base is best assessed on postcontrast MRI T1-Fat saturated imaging which demonstrates asymmetric thickening and enhancement of the facial (**Figures 9.27A and B**) or mandibular nerve. On CT, look for widening of the bony neural canal with obliteration of the fat surrounding the external canal orifice.

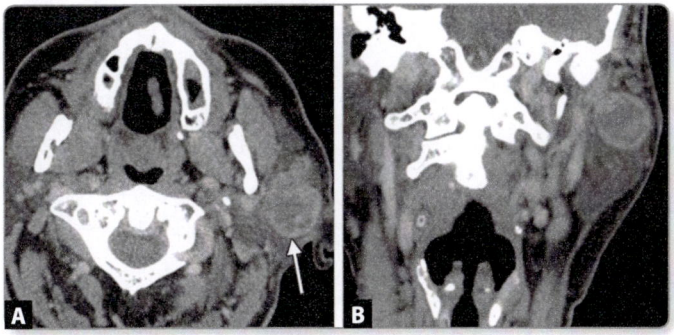

**Figures 9.26A and B** Solitary left parotid squamous cell carcinoma metastasis, primary cutaneous scalp lesion

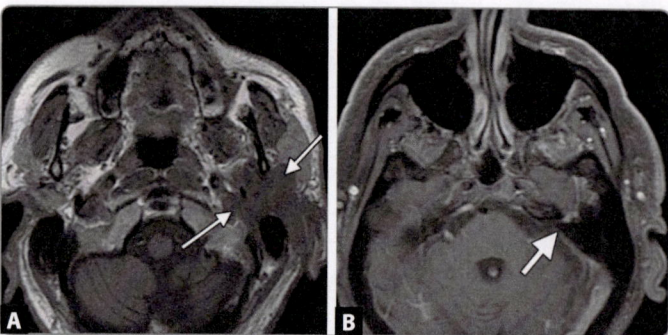

**Figures 9.27A and B** 68-year-old male, large cell carcinoma left parotid with facial nerve perineural spread. Note the large infiltrating tumor involving deep and superficial lobes (A). There was abnormal thickening and enhancement of the intratemporal facial nerve, depicted (B) at the labyrinthine canal and geniculate fossa (thick arrow) on axial T1 enhanced imaging

# Bibliography

1. Anacak Y, Miller R, Constantinou N, Mamusa A, Epelbaum R, Li Y, et al. Primary Mucosa-Associated Lymphoid Tissue Lymphoma of the Salivary Glands: A Multicenter Rare Cancer Network Study. Int J Radiat Oncol Biol Phys 2010 [Epub ahead of print].
2. Aro K, Leivo I, Maktie A. Management and Outcome of Patients With Mucoepidermoid Carcinoma of Major Salivary Gland Origin: A Single Institution's 30-Year Experience. Laryngoscope 2008;118:258-62.
3. Becker M, Marchal F, Becker C, Dulguerov P, Georgakopoulos G, Lehmann W, et al. Sialolithiasis and Salivary Ductal Stenosis: Diagnostic Accuracy of MR Sialography with a Three-dimensional Extended-Phase Conjugate Symmetry Rapid Spin-Echo Sequence. Radiology 2000;217:347-58.
4. Bialek EJ, Jakubowski W, Zajkowski P, Szopinski KT, Osmolski A. US of the Major Salivary Glands: Anatomy and Spatial Relationships, Pathologic Conditions, and Pitfalls. Radiographics. 2006;26:745-63.
5. Boahene D, Olsen K, Lewis J, Pinehiro D, Pankratz V, Bagniewski S. Mucoepidermoid Carcinoma of the Parotid Gland: The Mayo Clinic Experience. Arch Otolaryngol Head Neck Surg 2004;130:849-56.
6. Capone RB, Ha PK, Westra WH, et al. Oncocytic neoplasms of the parotid gland: A 16-year institutional review. Otolaryngol Head Neck Surg 2002;126:657-62.

7. Childers EL, Furlong MA, Fanburg-Smith JC. Hemangioma of the Salivary Gland: A Study of Ten Cases of a Rarely Biopsied /Excised Lesion. Ann Diagn Pathol 2002;6:339-44.
8. Choi SS, Zalzal GH. Branchial Anomalies: a review of 52 cases. Laryngoscope 1995;105:909-13.
9. Christoforidis GA, Spickler EM, Recio MV, Mehta BM. MR of CNS Sarcoidosis: Correlation of Imaging Features to Clinical Symptoms and Response to Treatment. AJNR 1999;20:655-69.
10. Donnelly LF, Adams DM, Bissett III GS. Vascular Malformations and Hemangiomas: A Practical Approach in a Multidisciplinary Clinic. AJR 2000;174:597-609.
11. Edge SB, Byrd DR, Compton CC, Fritz AG, Greene FL, Trotti A (Eds). American Joint Committee on Cancer: Cancer Staging Manual. 7th edn. New York: Springer; 2010.
12. Fiorella R, Di Nicola V, Fiorella ML, et al. Major salivary gland diseases. Multicentre study. Acta Otorhinolaryngol Ital 2005;25:182-190.
13. Goode R, Auclair P, Ellis G. Mucoepidermoid Carcinoma of the Major Salivary Glands: Clinical and Histopathological Analysis of 234 Cases with Evaluation of Grading Criteria. Cancer 1998;82:1217-24.
14. Gopinathan A, Tan TY. Kimura's Disease: Imaging Patterns on Computed Tomography. Clin Radiol 2009;6:994-9.
15. Gritzmann N, Rettenbacher T, Hollerweger A, Macheiner P, Hubner E. Sonography of the salivary glands. Eur Radiol 2003;13:964-75.
16. Harrison JD. Causes, Natural History, and Incidence of Salivary Stones and Obstructions. Otolaryngol Clin N Am 2009;42:927-47.
17. Hyde J, Takashima M, Dodson B, Said S. Bilateral multinodular oncocytoma of the parotid arising in a background of bilateral oncocytic nodular hyperplasia. Ear Nose Throat J 2008;87:51-4.
18. Ikeda K, Katoh T, Ha-Kawa SK, Yamashita T, Tanaka Y. The usefulness of MR in establishing the diagnosis of parotid pleomorphic adenoma. AJNR 1996;17:555-9.
19. Ikeda M, Motoori K, Hanazawa T, Nagai Y, Yamamoto S, Ueda T, et al. Warthin Tumor of the Parotid Gland: Diagnostic Value of MR Imaging with Histopathologic Correlation. AJNR 2004;25:1256-62.
20. Izumi M, Eguchi K, Uetani M, et al. MR Imaging of the Parotid Gland in Sjogren's Syndrome: A Proposal for New Diagnostic Criteria. AJR 1996;166:1483-87.
21. James DG, Sharma OP. Parotid Gland Sarcoidosis Vasc Diffuse Lung Dis 2000;17:27-32.
22. Kakimoto N, Gamoh S, Tamaki J, Kishino M, Murakami S, Furukawa S. CT and MR Images of Pleomorphic Adenoma in Major and Minor Salivary Glands. Eur J Radiol 2009;69:464-72.
23. Kalinowski M, Heverhagen JT, Rehberg E, Klose KJ, Wagner HJ. Comparative Study of MR Sialography and Digital Subtraction Sialography for Benign Salivary Gland Disorders. AJNR 2002;23:1485-92.
24. Kato H, Kanematsu M, Mizuta K, Ito Y, Hirose Y. Carcinoma Ex-pleomorphic Adenoma of the Parotid Gland: Radiologic-Pathologic Correlation with MR Imaging Including Diffusion-Weighted Imaging. AJNR 2008;29:865-67.

25. Khafif A, Anavi Y, Haviv J, Feinmesser R, Calderon S, Marshak G. Adenoid cystic carcinoma of the salivary glands: A 20-year review with long-term follow-up. Ear Nose Throat J 2005;84:664-7.
26. Kim KH, Sung MW, Chung PS, Rhee CS, Park CI, Kim WH. Adenoid Cystic Carcinoma of the Head and Neck. Arch Otolaryngol Head Neck Surg 1994;120:721-6.
27. Koch BL. Cystic Malformations of the Neck in Children. Pediatr Radiol 2005;35:463-77.
28. Liyanage SH, Spencer SP, Hogarth KM, Makdissi J. Imaging of salivary glands. Imaging. 2007;19:14-27.
29. Longo N, Ghaderi M. Primary Parotid Gland Sarcoidosis: Case Report and Discussion of Diagnosis and Treatment. Ear Nose Throat J 2010;89:E6-10.
30. Lowe LH, Stokes LS, Johnson JE, et al. Swelling at the Angle of the Mandible: Imaging of the Pediatric Parotid Gland and Periparotid Region. Radiographics 2001;21:1211-27.
31. McCormick JT, Newton ED, Geyer S, Caushaj PF. Sarcoidosis Presenting as a Solitary Parotid Mass. Ear Nose Throat J 2006;86:664-5.
32. Moonis G, Patel P, Koshkareva Y, Newman J, Loevner LA. Imaging Characteristics of Recurrent Pleomorphic Adenoma of the Parotid Gland. AJNR 2007;28:1532-6.
33. Oguz KK, Ozturk A, Cila A. Magnetic resonance imaging findings in Kimura's disease. Neuroradiology 2004;46:855-8.
34. Olsen KD, Lewis JE. Carcinoma ex-pleomorphic adenoma: a clinicopathologic review. Head Neck 2001;23:705-12
35. Rivera LK, Nelson BL. Juvenile Hemangioma of the Parotid Gland. Head Neck Pathol 2008;2:81-6.
36. Schroeder JW Jr, Mohyuddin N, Maddalozzo J. Branchial Anomalies in the Pediatric Population. Otolaryngol Head Neck Surg 2007;137:289-95.
37. Shah G. MR imaging of salivary glands. Magn Reson Imaging Clin N Am 2002;10:631-62.
38. Shellenberger TD, Williams MD, Clayman GL, Kumar AJ. Parotid Gland Oncocytosis: CT Findings with Histopathologic Correlation. AJNR 2008;29:734-6.
39. Som PM, Curtin HD. Head and Neck Imaging. 4th edn. St. Louis: Mosby; 2003.
40. STATdx. Salt Lake City, Utah: Amirsys.; c2005-2010 [cited 2010 September 15]. Available from: https://my.statdx.com/
41. Tagnon B, Theate I, Weynand B, Hamoir M, Coche E. Long-Standing Mucosa-Associated Lymphoid Tissue Lymphoma of the Parotid Gland: CT and MR Imaging Findings. AJR 2002;178:1563-5.
42. Takagi Y, Sumi M, Sumi T, Ichikawa Y, Nakamura T. MR Microscopy of the Parotid Glands in Patients with Sjogren's Syndrome: Quantitative MR Diagnostic Criteria. AJNR 2005; 26: 1207-14.
43. Tonami H, Ogawa Y, Matoba M, Kuginuki Y. et al. MR Sialography in Patients with Sjogren Syndrome. AJNR 1998;19:1199-1203.
44. Triglia JM, Nicollas R, Ducroz V, Koltai PJ, Garabedian EN. First Branchial Cleft Anomalies: a study of 39 cases and review of the literature. Arch Otolaryngol Head Neck Surg 1998;124:291-5.

## Diseases of the parotid gland 393

45. Uchida Y, Minoshima S, Kawata T, Motoori K, Nakano K, Kazama T, et al. Diagnostic Value of FDG PET and Salivary Gland Scintigraphy for Parotid Tumors. Clin Nucl Med 2005;30:170-76.
46. Veillon F, Ramos Taboada L, Abu Eid M, Riehm S, Debry C, Schultz P, et al. Pathology of the Facial nerve. Neuroimaging Clin N Am 2008;18:309-20.
47. Yabuuchi H, Matsuo Y, Kamitani T, et al. Parotid gland tumors: Can Addition of Diffusion-weighted MR Imaging to Dynamic Contrast-enhanced MR Imaging Improve Diagnostic Accuracy in Characterisation. Radiology 2008;249:909-16.
48. Yousem DM, Kraut MA, Chalian AA. Major Salivary Gland Imaging. Radiology. 2000; 216:19-29.
49. Zenk J, Iro H, Klintworth N, Lell M. Diagnostic Imaging in Sialadenitis. Oral Maxillofac Surg Clin North Am 2009;21:275-92.

# Perineural disease in the head and neck

chapter 10

Manas Sharma, Laurent Létourneau-Guillon

**ABSTRACT**
The common pathways of perineural tumor spread in head and neck oncology is reviewed.

**KEYWORDS**
Perineural tumor spread, trigeminal, facial nerve, pterygopalatine fossa.

## Introduction

Spread of tumor through the perineural lymphatics, perineurium or the endoneurium is known to occur in many of the malignancies affecting the head and neck region. This process, collectively termed perineural spread (PNS), remains a critical clinical problem as it may be clinically silent and its early detection relies mostly on modern CT and MR imaging techniques, although indirect signs have been described earlier on plain film imaging. It should be noted that perineural tumor spread differs from perineural invasion (PNI) as the latter refers to microscopic tumor cell infiltration around nerve branches which is a histologic process and not appreciated radiographically. PNS refers to macroscopic disease spreading along the course of a nerve. Knowledge of neural anatomy, awareness of the probability of PNS in relation to the primary tumor type, location, clinical presentation as well as knowledge of its imaging characteristics are extremely important for early detection of disease. The implications of PNS on patient management can be profound as it will often alter the course of therapy and prognosis. Failure to recognize perineural spread may lead to worsening of treatment outcome and increased risk of tumor recurrence.

## Types of tumors

Although many head and neck tumors may involve the cranial nerves, some primary tumors are more prone to perineural spread. Adenoid cystic carcinoma and desmoplastic melanoma are especially neurotropic but other minor salivary gland tumors, squamous cell carcinoma, as well as metastasis, lymphoma and even sarcomas may also invade and track along nerves (**Table 10.1**).

## Nerves most commonly involved

The 5th cranial nerve (trigeminal) and its branches and the 7th cranial nerve (facial) are the two most frequently involved by PNS in the head and neck. Interconnections between the two also facilitate spread from, one to the other. The branches of the superficial cervical plexus and the 12th cranial nerve (hypoglossal) are less frequently involved.

## Sites and routes

Virtually every head and neck malignancy may demonstrate PNS but it appears that tumors arising in certain primary sites have an increased predilection for this pattern of dissemination. Cutaneous malignancies, especially on the side of the nose and lower lip, areas supplied by the maxillary division of the 5th cranial nerve have a higher predilection. Tumor involving the palate can track along the palatine nerves and is a notorious site for perineural spread. Nasopharyngeal tumors can extend into the pterygopalatine fossa and thus involve the maxillary (V2) division of the 5th cranial nerve. They can

- Adenoid cystic carcinoma
- Squamous cell carcinoma (SCC)
- Mucoepidermoid carcinoma
- Cutaneous malignancy (including SCC, basal cell carcinoma, desmoplastic melanoma)
- Non-Hodgkin lymphoma
- Sarcomas (especially rhabdomyosarcoma)
- Metastasis

**Table 10.1** Head and neck malignancies associated with perineural spread

also extend laterally into masticator space and invade the mandibular (V3) division of the 5th cranial nerve. Any tumor extending into the parotid space can potentially result in perineural spread to the 7th cranial nerve or the auriculotemporal branch of the mandibular division of 5th cranial nerve. Thus, tumors located in the masticator space, the pterygopalatine fossa, cavernous sinuses and Meckel's cave, by virtue of their primary location, can have higher rates of perineural spread. Finally, it is important to the underscore the fact that PNS can be retrograde, as well as antegrade.

Surprisingly, tumors in certain regions of the head and neck, such as the submandibular glands, tongue, buccal mucosa, tonsil, larynx, pharynx and the floor of mouth, rarely show perineural spread. However, once they breach these local geographic margins and invade adjacent areas, they may disseminate perineurally.

Among those with increased predilection of PNS are salivary gland tumors, especially those arising in the parotid or the minor salivary glands of the palate. SCC of the mucosal lining of the head and neck cavities, particularly those arising from the retromolar triangle, soft palate or nasopharynx, also show an increased predilection. Finally, skin cancer may demonstrate spread, more often in the setting of cutaneous SCC or desmoplastic melanoma. **Table 10.2** summarizes the most frequent location of tumor associated with PNS and their pattern of perineural spread.

## Symptoms and signs

Forty percent of affected patients can be asymptomatic or have nonspecific symptoms. Pain, paresthesias, numbness, and fornication (feeling of tiny insects creeping subcutaneously) are common complaints. Motor weakness may be seen in the affected nerve distribution, for example, facial or masticator muscle weakness in cases of facial nerve or trigeminal involvement. Multiple cranial neuropathies are rarely reported. It is important to underscore the fact that symptoms related to perineural spread may be the initial presenting feature of a primary head and neck malignancy. This pattern of presentation appears to be most frequent with submucosal tumor arising from the soft palate, such as adenoid cystic carcinoma. Similarly, tumor recurrence may manifest only in the form of perineural spread.

| Tumor type | Location | Susceptible nerves |
|---|---|---|
| Mucosal primary neoplasm (SCC or minor salivary gland tumor, especially adenoid cystic) | Palate | Greater and lesser palatine nerves → PPF → V2 |
| | Nasopharynx | 1. PPF invasion → V2<br>2. Masticator space invasion → V3 → Meckel's cave |
| Major salivary gland tumor | Parotid (either primary parotid malignancy or metastatic skin cancer to the parotid gland) | 1. Facial nerve<br>2. Auriculotemporal branch → V3 |
| Cutaneous malignancy (SCC, desmoplastic melanoma) | Side of the nose, lower lip | Infraorbital nerve → V2 |
| Cutaneous or mucosal malignancy | Lower lip<br>Mandibular invasion | Inferior alveolar nerve → V3 |
| Any malignancy | PPF invasion | V2 |
| Any malignancy | Masticator space invasion | V3 |

*Abbreviations:* SCC: squamous cell carcinoma; PPF: pterygopalatine fossa; V2: maxillary division of the trigeminal nerve; V3: mandibular division of the trigeminal nerve.

**Table 10.2** Frequent sites and routes of perineural spread

## Clinical features of possible PNS

1. Neurologic deficits on initial presentation of a head and neck malignancy or after its treatment.
2. Patient with past tumor resection developing new cranial neuropathy, or deficits along nerve distribution.
3. *Patient presenting with cranial neuropathies*: Clinically silent primary tumor in one of the proximal locations needs to be suspected. Care should be taken to exclude PNS before assuming that the symptoms are related to Bell's palsy or trigeminal neuralgia.

Regardless, since perineural spread may be asymptomatic, systematic radiographic evaluation of this possibility must be an integral part of the imaging evaluation of head and neck malignancy.

## Anatomy

A thorough review of the minute neuroanatomy of the nerves primarily involved in perineural spread of malignancies in the head and neck is beyond the scope of this book. However, basic knowledge of the main branches and functions is important in understanding the patterns of perineural spread and clinical manifestations, and are highlighted here.

### Trigeminal/5th cranial nerve (CN V)

The trigeminal nerve is primarily responsible for sensation in the face, but is also responsible for the motor functions of mastication and partly deglutition. The nerve primarily connects to three sensory nuclei within the brainstem (mesencephalic nucleus, principal sensory nucleus and the spinal nucleus) and one motor nucleus. Anatomically, the nerve emerges from the mid-lateral surface of the pons as a larger sensory root and a smaller motor root, which together traverses the prepontine CSF space and enters into Meckel's cave (**Figure 10.1**).

Within the Meckel's cave this nerve gives off three divisions: ophthalmic (V1), maxillary (V2) and mandibular (V3).

The ophthalmic division (V1) provides pure sensory innervation to the eye, conjunctiva, the lacrimal gland, and some parts of nasal mucosa, skin of nose, eyelids, forehead and scalp. It emerges from the Gasserian ganglion in the Meckel's cave, courses through the cavernous sinus, entering the orbit through the superior orbital fissure and finally dividing into the nasociliary, lacrimal and frontal nerves. The frontal nerve will then divide into the supratrochlear and supraorbital branches. Perineural disease is reported along the supraorbital and supratrochlear nerves most commonly from cutaneous cancers. The lacrimal nerve innervates the lacrimal gland and it also receives a small branch from V2, while the nasociliary branches innervate the frontal dura and the nasoethmoid mucosa. Perineural spread of cancers in these nerves has been rarely seen.

The maxillary division (V2) provides sensory innervation to the skin of midface, sinonasal region, maxillary gingiva, teeth and the palatal mucosa. From the Meckel's cave/cavernous sinus, this nerve

Perineural disease in the head and neck 399

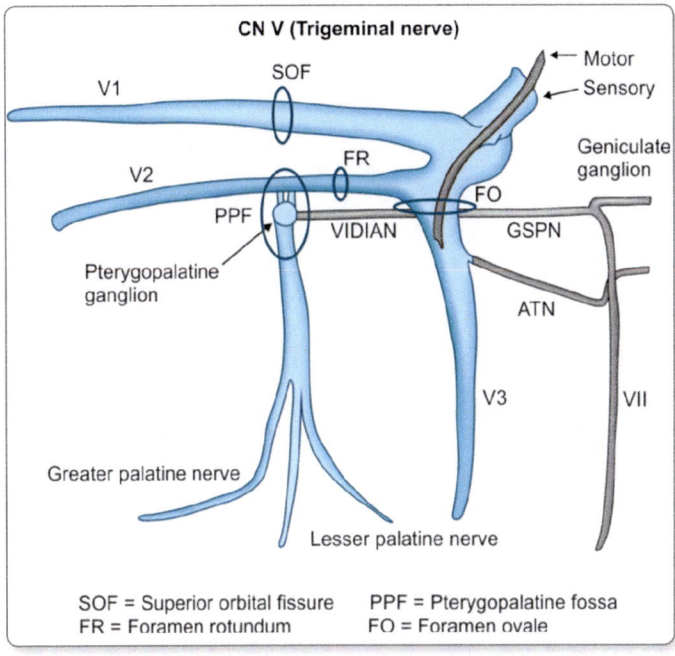

Figure 10.1 Anatomy of CN V (trigeminal nerve) and its relation to the CN VII (facial nerve)

travels through the foramen rotundum (**Figures 10.2 and 10.3**) and enters into the pterygopalatine fossa (PPF) and therein it gives rise to several palatine branches, the zygomatic nerve and the posterior superior alveolar nerve to the maxillary sinus. The palatine branches emerge through the greater and lesser palatine foramina while the zygomatic nerve enters the orbit through the inferior orbital fissure and runs along the lateral orbital wall dividing into the zygomaticotemporal and zygomaticofacial branches, which innervate the temporal and lateral skin of the cheek. The maxillary nerve then enters the infraorbital canal and gives off the anterior and middle superior alveolar nerves (which supply sensation to the maxillary teeth and

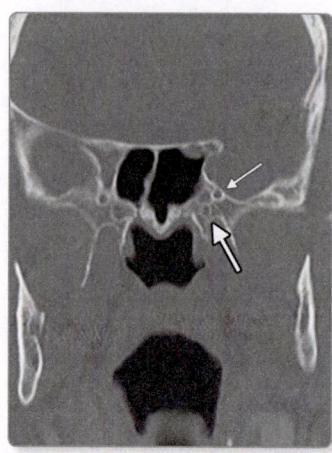

**Figure 10.2** Coronal CT section in bone window shows the foramen rotundum (thin arrow) and the vidian canal (thick arrow)

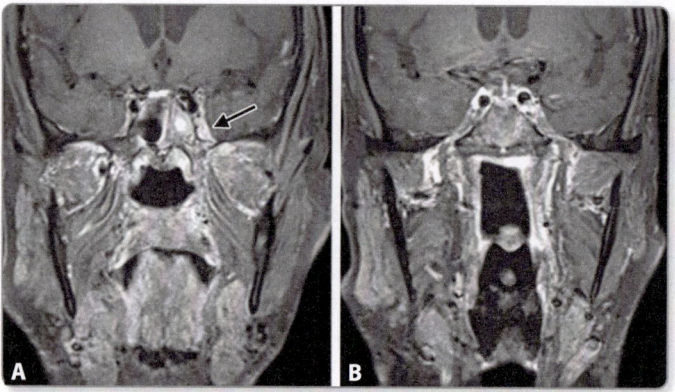

**Figures 10.3A and B** (A) Postgadolinium coronal T1-weighted image shows enhancement and widening at the left foramen rotundum seen with perineural spread of malignancy; (B) Postgadolinium coronal T1-weighted images are very important for assessment of the foramen ovale

gingiva) and then emerges as the infraorbital nerve which supplies sensation to the mid-facial and lateral nasal skin. Tumors arising in the cheek/upper lateral face/temporal region/palate/maxillary sinus are particularly prone to develop perineural spread along the infraorbital nerve.

The mandibular division (V3) is responsible for sensory innervation to the skin of the preauricular region and lower face, mandibular teeth, gingival mucosa, floor of mouth, anterior two-thirds of tongue and the buccal mucosa. It also provides motor innervation to the muscles of mastication (masseter, pterygoid and temporalis), the mylohyoid and the anterior belly of the digastric muscle. The V3 division exits the cranium through the foramen ovale (**Figures 10.4A and B**) and travels inferiorly into the masticator space and dividing there into the anterior and posterior trunks. The anterior trunk primarily gives off the motor branches, while the posterior trunk gives off auriculotemporal, inferior alveolar and lingual nerves. The first two of these, i.e. the auriculotemporal and the inferior alveolar nerves are more often associated with perineural spread.

The auriculotemporal nerve (also separately described below) provides cutaneous innervation over a broad area of the lateral and

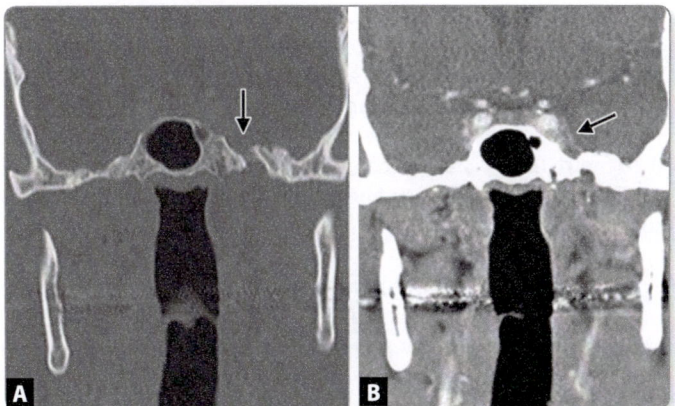

**Figures 10.4A and B** Coronal CT images with the arrows marking the foramen ovale in the bone window (A) and the cavernous sinus in the soft tissue window (B)

upper face and also gives of parotid branches. Thus parotid neoplasm can potentially give rise to auriculotemporal PNS. The inferior alveolar nerve enters the mandibular foramen and courses through the mandibular canal, providing sensory innervation to the mandibular gingiva and teeth, and exits out of the mental foramen as the mental nerve providing cutaneous innervation to the skin overlying the chin including lower lip. Tumors in these regions, such as skin malignancies, lateral facial and parotid tumors, can invade these nerve branches and give rise to PNS that can track in a retrograde fashion to ultimately reach the cavernous sinus and brain stem. Any tumor that extends into the masticator space can end up having PNS into the cranium through this route.

## Facial nerve/7th cranial nerve (CN VII)

The facial nerve exits the lateral aspect of the pontomedullary junction medial to the vestibulocochlear nerve. After traversing the internal auditory canal, the nerve then enters the petrous temporal bone. Its labyrinthine segment travels through the fallopian canal to reach the geniculate ganglion. It then travels posteriorly (the tympanic or horizontal segment) inferior to the lateral semicircular canal in the middle ear cavity. At the level of the sinus tympani, the nerve curves inferiorly to become the mastoid (vertical) segment and exits the temporal bone through the stylomastoid foramen. The nerve then enters the parotid gland, lateral to the retromandibular vein. The facial nerve acts as a boundary dividing the deep and superficial lobes of the parotid gland. Finally, the nerve divides into five branches which reach their motor units distally to control the muscles of facial expression.

There are three main branches of the facial nerve: the greater superficial petrosal nerve, the nerve to the stapedius and the chorda tympani.

i. The greater superficial petrosal nerve (GSPN) arises from the geniculate ganglion, passes through the hiatus for the GSPN (or facial hiatus), travelling anterior to the petrous apex, then inferior to Meckel's cave to reach the foramen lacerum. At this point it joins the deep petrosal nerve (arising from the sympathetic carotid plexus) to become the vidian nerve (see Vidian Nerve section below). The proximal GSPN may demonstrate physiological enhancement of its arteriovenous plexus after contrast administration.

ii. The nerve to the stapedius arises from the high mastoid segment opposite the pyramidal eminence and passes through a small canal in this eminence to reach the stapedius muscle.

iii. The chorda tympani arise from the distal mastoid segment of the facial nerve. After leaving the facial nerve, it runs superiorly in the mastoid to enter into the middle ear cavity and travels along the medial surface of the tympanic membrane, between the malleus and the incus. The nerve continues through the petrotympanic fissure and exits the temporal bone to reach the lingual branch of V3. The parasympathetic fibers for the submandibular and sublingual glands synapse in the submandibular ganglion. Special sensory (taste) fibers also extend from the chorda tympani to the anterior 2/3rds of the tongue via the lingual nerve. This is a potential route for perineural communication between the facial and trigeminal nerves but is seldom seen in radiologic practice.

The facial nerve has four main functions: motor, parasympathetic, general and special sensory. It controls the muscles of facial expression, is responsible for taste from the anterior two-thirds of the tongue, supplies somatosensory sensation from the concha skin and has parasympathetic function to the lacrimal glands as well as submandibular and sublingual glands.

The lesions that involve the facial nerve include primary or secondary parotid malignancies. Primary neoplasms arising in the parotid gland such as adenoid cystic carcinoma, acinic and mucoepidermoid carcinoma are the main source of perineural spread from a primary parotid malignancy. Secondary neoplastic processes invading into the parotid gland, such as cutaneous malignancies like SCC or desmoplastic melanoma may also give rise to perineural spread. These lesions will more often involve the mastoid segment of the facial nerve but may propagate in a retrograde fashion to reach the intracanalicular segment and possibly the brain stem.

## Hypoglossal nerve

The hypoglossal nerve (XII) exits the brainstem, courses through the perimedullary cistern and then enters the hypoglossal canal

(**Figures 10.5A and B**). The nerve leaves the skull base and enters the carotid sheath, close to cranial nerves IX to XI. At the angle of the mandible, the nerve passes inferior to the posterior belly of the

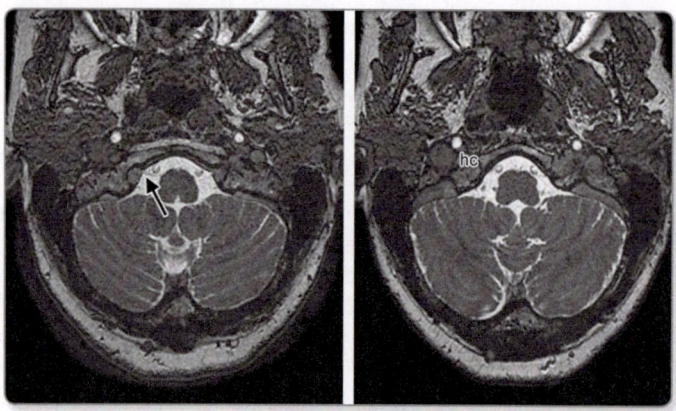

**Figure 10.5A** Axial FIESTA images show the right hypoglossal canal and nerve (arrow)

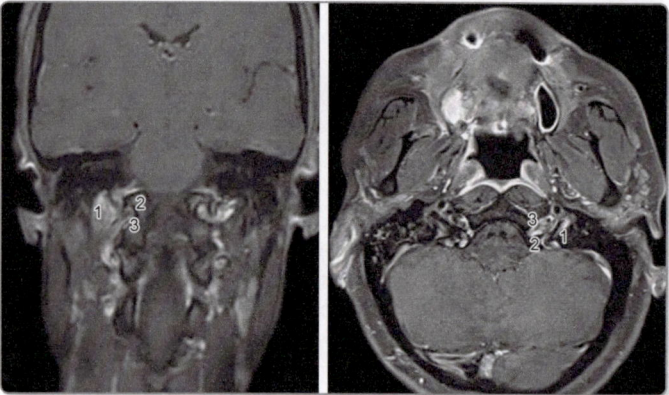

**Figure 10.5B** Coronal postgadolinium T1 fat-saturated image shows the close relation of hypoglossal canal and nerve to the jugular tubercle and foramen. (1) Marks the jugular bulb, (2) Jugular tubercle, (3) Hypoglossal canal with the nerve seen traversing within it

digastric muscle and hyoid bone. It then enters the sublingual space, runs along the surface of the hyoglossus muscle, above the mylohyoid muscle and reaches the tongue musculature. The hypoglossal nerve may be rarely involved by tumor arising from the tongue, such as minor salivary gland neoplasm.

## Spinal nerves

Branches of the superficial cervical plexus have cutaneous innervation to much of the neck and parts of the face. Branches such as the greater auricular, lesser occipital or transverse cutaneous nerves are mostly derived from the ventral divisions of the first four spinal nerves. Retrograde PNS from cutaneous malignancies are occasionally seen along these routes.

## Connections between the facial and trigeminal nerves

Connections exist between the facial and trigeminal nerves and may act as pathway for perineural spread (see **Figure 10.1**). As a result, neoplasms that arise from an area primarily innervated by the trigeminal nerve may also involve the facial nerve.

### Vidian nerve

Also called nerve of the pterygoid canal, the vidian nerve is formed by the greater superficial petrosal nerve (GSPN) a branch of the facial nerve, and deep petrosal nerve. This nerve connects the pterygopalatine ganglion and hence V2, and the facial nerve (**Table 10.3**). The vidian nerve passes forward through the pterygoid or vidian canal (see **Figure 10.2**) along with the artery of the pterygoid canal. It then enters the pterygopalatine fossa (PPF), with some branches going to the pterygopalatine (or sphenopalatine) ganglion; some fibers join the palatine nerves and others are directed toward the branches of V2, ultimately supplying the palate, nasal cavity, nasopharynx and lacrimal glands. This nerve provides parasympathetic innervation to the lacrimal glands, and sensory innervation of the mucous membrane lining the nasal cavity, palate as well as sphenoid, frontal and maxillary sinuses. Any tumor reaching the PPF can have potential PNS via the vidian nerve back to the GSPN, and then to the geniculate ganglion

| Nerves | Comments |
|---|---|
| Auriculotemporal nerve | • Facial and auriculotemporal nerves cross at a right angle within the parotid gland where they both are susceptible to PNS from parotid malignancy. Nerve fibers also directly connect the ATN and facial nerves near the posterior margin of the mandibular ramus. |
| Greater petrosal superficial nerve (GPSN) and vidian nerve | • The vidian nerve may be involved by lesions infiltrating the PPF. From there, the facial nerve may be involved through retrograde extension via the GPSN to the geniculate ganglion. The maxillary division of the trigeminal nerve (V2) is also vulnerable to PNS from malignancy involving the PPF.<br>• Direct extension to the GSPN from a lesion involving Meckel's cave may also occur. |

**Table 10.3** Important connections between CN V and CN VII in the setting of PNS

of the facial nerve. Also of note is that a tumor reaching the Meckel's cave can involve the GSPN and facial nerve in a retrograde manner by virtue of anatomic proximity to the origin of vidian nerve near the foramen lacerum.

### Auriculotemporal nerve (ATN)

Arising from the posterior division of V3 just below its emergence from foramen ovale, the auriculotemporal nerve traverses the stylomandibular tunnel before reaching the parotid gland. The nerve transmits somatosensory information from the lateral aspect of the cheek and scalp, including preauricular and external ear skin as well as from the temporomandibular joints (TMJ). It also conveys parasympathetic fibers from the glossopharyngeal nerve (IX) via the otic ganglion to the parotid gland. The auriculotemporal and facial nerve cross at a right angle in the parotid gland. Two connections usually exist between the auriculotemporal nerve and the facial nerve near the posterior margin of the mandible. Similar to the facial nerve, the auriculotemporal nerve is vulnerable to PNS from primary or secondary malignancy of the parotid gland. Concomitant involvement of the auriculotemporal and facial nerves may potentially arise.

## Pterygopalatine fossa

The pterygopalatine fossa (PPF) is a major cross-road for tumor invasion. The PPF is a small anatomical space located between the posterior walls of the maxillary sinus anteriorly and the sphenoid bone posteriorly. On imaging, it is predominantly a fat filled space (**Figures 10.6A to F**). Most of the medial boundary is made from the perpendicular plate of the ethmoid, whereas the lateral aspects communicate freely with the masticator space through the pterygomaxillary fissure. Several communications exist with other anatomical structures and are listed in **Table 10.4**. The PPF contains the maxillary division of the trigeminal nerve (V2), the pterygopalatine ganglion (receiving the vidian nerve), the vidian nerve and the terminal third of the maxillary artery.

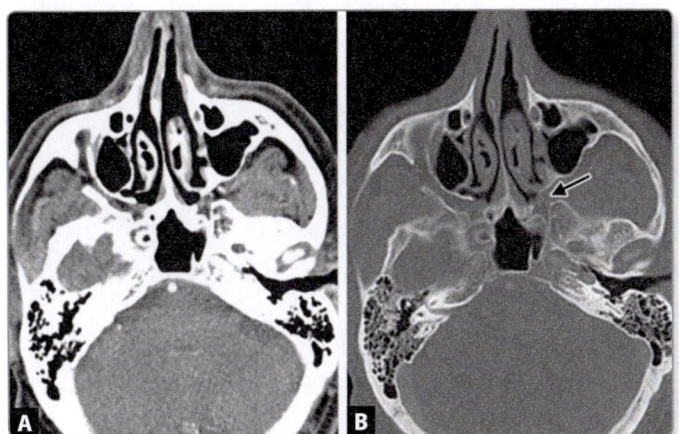

**Figures 10.6A and B** Axial CT (soft tissue and bone windows) shows normal fat-filled and bony-outlined pterygopalatine fossa

## 408 Introductory head and neck imaging

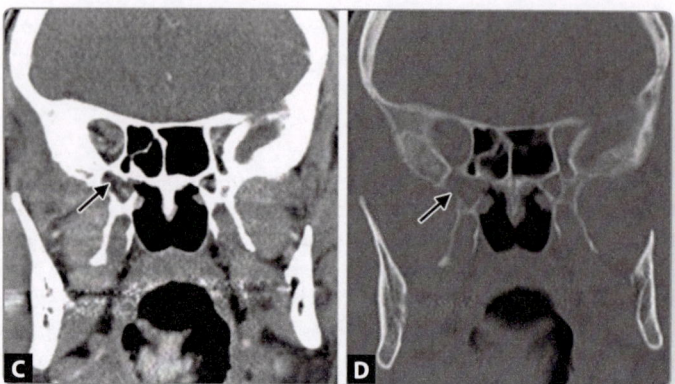

**Figures 10.6C and D** Pterygopalatine fossa on coronal CT (soft tissue and bone windows). Note fat-filled normal appearance

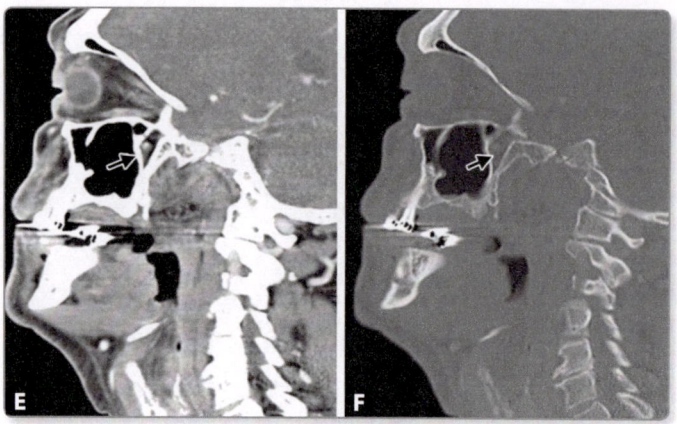

**Figures 10.6E and F** Pterygopalatine fossa on sagittal CT (soft tissue and bone windows)

| Foramen/Fissure | Connection |
|---|---|
| Foramen rotundum | Meckel's cave and cavernous sinus, middle cranial fossa |
| Vidian canal | Foramen lacerum, middle cranial fossa |
| Greater and lesser palatine foramina | Palate |
| Pharyngeal (palatovaginal) canal (*usually not depicted on imaging*) | Nasopharynx |
| Sphenopalatine foramen | Posterior nasal fossa (superior meatus) |
| Pterygomaxillary fissure | Masticator space |
| Inferior orbital fissure | Orbit |

**Table 10.4** Anatomical connections between the PPF and adjacent structures

## Imaging considerations: techniques and features

Computed tomography (CT) and MRI have complimentary roles in the diagnosis of perineural spread. CT is better at evaluation of the osseous component of neural foramina. The greater soft tissue resolution of MRI lends itself well to the detection of abnormal enhancement along the nerve course and the loss of normal fat planes in and around the neural foramina.

High resolution imaging technique is the key for detection of PNS. A small field of view (FOV; preferably 16–18 cm) and thin-slice imaging (3–5 mm) are important. At our institution, we incorporate an unenhanced T1-weighted series without fat suppression. Such sequences are less prone to artifacts and nicely delineate the normally visible hyperintense fat present in the PPF. Axial and coronal T1-weighted images also show the course of V3 in the masticator space and the course of the inferior alveolar nerve nicely. Lastly, unenhanced T1 images facilitate reference when comparing with postcontrast series in evaluation of abnormal nerve enhancements. We obtain postgadolinium T1-weighted images with fat suppression in order to highlight abnormal perineural enhancement. In addition to abnormal enhancement, asymmetric thickening of the nerve and widening of its foramen are other radiographic features of PNS. Having said this, it is important to be aware of normal enhancement that can be seen along some of the nerves: e.g. moderate enhancement along the geniculate, tympanic, and mastoid segments of the facial nerve due to presence of peri- and epineural venous plexuses.

Primary and secondary radiographic signs of perineural spread are listed in the **Table 10.5**. Nerves affected by PNS may appear discontinuous on imaging, i.e. — "skip" lesions. Thus, the entire course of the nerve needs to be assessed. Rarely, intracranial spread with enhancement of the cisternal segments of affected nerves may be observed. Perineural tumor spread image gallery as shown in **Figures 10.7–10.20**.

| Most frequent sites of anatomical involvement | – *V1*: Supraorbital foramen<br>– *V2*: Infraorbital foramen, PPF, Vidian canal, foramen rotundum, greater and lesser palatine foramina<br>– *V3*: Mandibular foramen for the inferior alveolar nerve, foramen ovale<br>– *Facial nerve*: Mastoid segment, stylomastoid foramen<br>– *Hypoglossal nerve*: Hypoglossal canal |
|---|---|
| Primary signs | – Widening or destruction of neural foramina/canals<br>– Loss of normal fat in neural foramina/canals<br>– Thickening, irregularity and/or nodularity of the nerve<br>– Abnormal enhancement in the neural foramina/canals<br>– Replacement of CSF by soft tissue mass in Meckel's cave<br>– Abnormal enhancement or mass effect in the cavernous sinus<br>– Rarely, enhancement of the cisternal segment of the affected nerve |
| Secondary signs | – Muscular denervation (Acute and subacute: Edema and enhancement, chronic: atrophy, fatty metaplasia) |

**Table 10.5** Main imaging features of perineural spread

Perineural disease in the head and neck 411

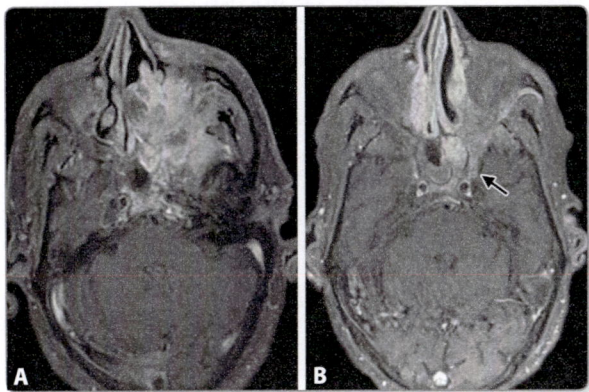

**Figures 10.7A and B** Cavernous sinus, pterygopalatine fossa. Postgadolinium T1 axial MR images in a 70-year-old male with adenoid cystic carcinoma of the left maxillary sinus, postradical radiation therapy. Large irregular enhancing left maxillary sinus mass extending to the retroantral region, left masticator space, left orbital apex. Note perineural spread along left trigeminal nerve to the cavernous sinus and Meckel's cave (*Courtesy:* Dr Makki Almuntashri)

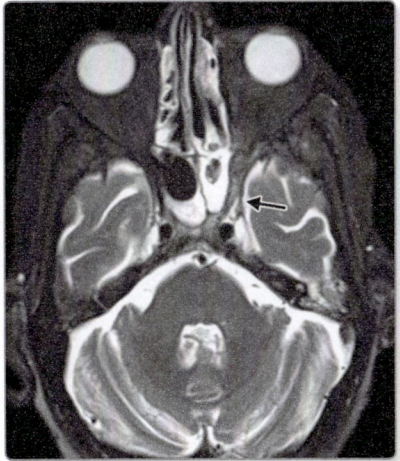

**Figure 10.8** Cavernous sinus. Axial T2-weighted image in the same patient as above, shows T2 hypointensity along the perineural extension of disease

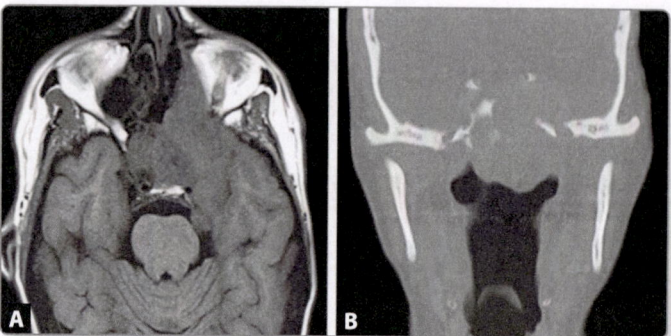

**Figures 10.9A and B** Cavernous sinus. Axial T1-weighted MR image reveals large lobulated infiltrative mass with an epicenter in the left nasopharynx in a 55-year-old female with recurrent adenoid cystic carcinoma. There is a large intracranial component in left middle cranial fossa with mass effect on left temporal lobe. Coronal CT image in bone window showing marked skull base bony destruction. Note widening of the left foramen ovale

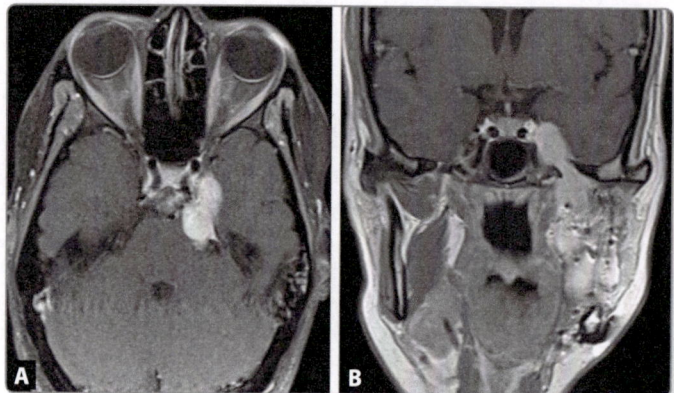

**Figures 10.10A and B** Mandibular division V3. Axial and coronal postgadolinium T1-weighted images reveal a fairly large lobulated enhancing mass centered in the region of left Meckel's cave and protruding into the prepontine area. This is perineural spread along V3 from a recurrent left mandibular angiosarcoma, well appreciated on the coronal image

Perineural disease in the head and neck **413**

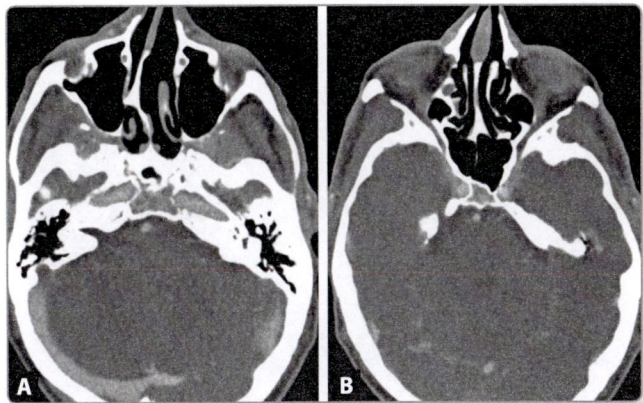

**Figures 10.11A and B** Pterygopalatine fossa. Perineural spread can be very subtle even to the trained eye. CT images show effacement of fat densities seen within the pterygopalatine fossae bilaterally in this case of lymphoma with bilateral diffuse adenopathy (not shown). Subtle soft tissue densities appear to extend to the cavernous sinus region bilaterally, more on the left. MRI may help better delineate these features

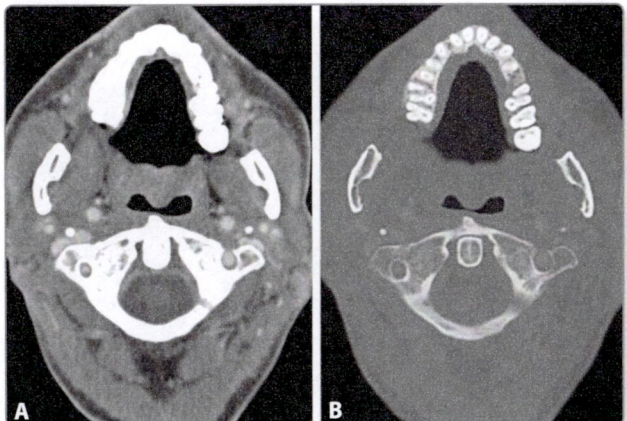

**Figures 10.12A and B** Inferior alveolar nerve canal. CT images (A) Soft tissue; (B) Bone window reveal radiographically suspicious widening of the inferior alveolar nerve canals bilaterally, which could also represent lymphomatous infiltration along the inferior alveolar nerves in this confirmed patient of lymphoma

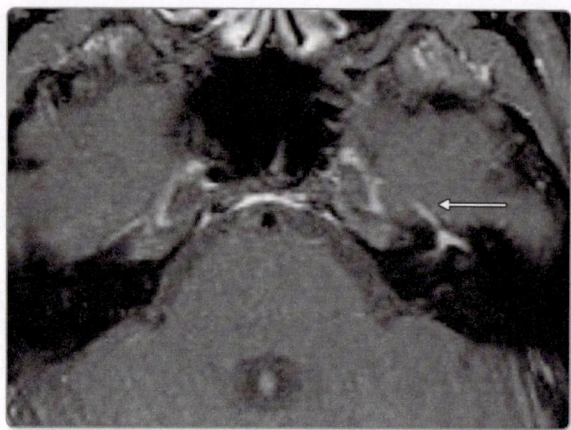

**Figure 10.13** Greater superficial petrosal nerve. Postgadolinium T1-weighted, fat-saturated image. In this patient with a presumed viral neuritis, the greater superficial petrosal nerve (GPNS) was seen exiting the facial hiatus and travelling toward the foramen lacerum. The geniculate ganglion and labyrinthine segment of the facial are avidly enhancing in a linear and uninterrupted fashion. No enhancement is seen on the normal contralateral side

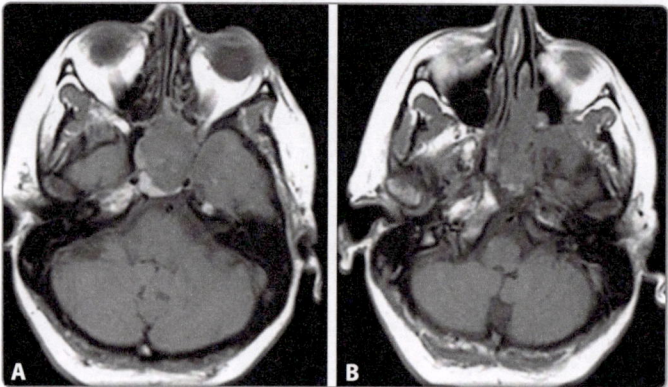

**Figures 10.14A and B** Pterygopalatine fossa. Axial T1-weighted images in this patient of adenocystic carcinoma reveal loss of fat plane within the left pterygopalatine fossa (PPF)

Perineural disease in the head and neck **415**

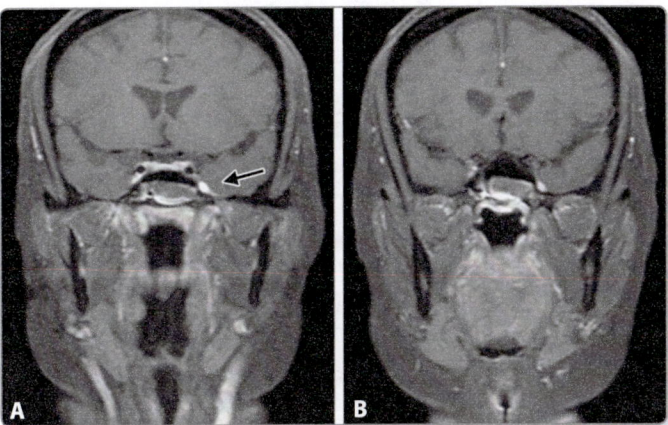

**Figures 10.15A and B** Foramen rotundum V2. Postgadolinium coronal T1-weighted fat-saturated images reveal thickening and enhancement in the left foramen rotundum in this patient with an adenoid cystic carcinoma

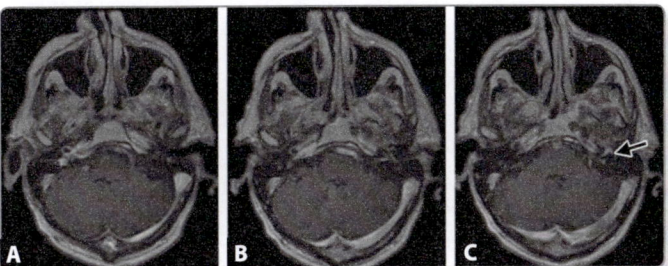

**Figures 10.16A to C** Facial nerve. There is abnormal enhancement and thickening seen along the left CN 7 in the distal canalicular, genicular, tympanic and mastoidal portions of the facial nerve in this patient with a squamous cell carcinoma in the left parotid gland. Note that enhancement without thickening in the tympanic and mastoidal segments of the facial nerve may be seen normally

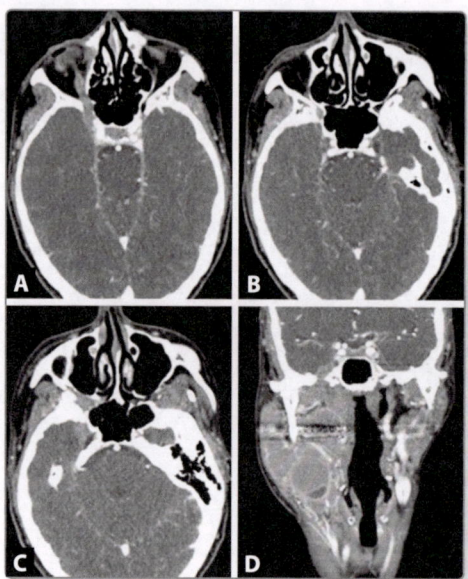

**Figures 10.17A to D** Pterygopalatine fossa, V2 and V3. Patient with lymphoma. Contrast-CT images reveal widened right PPF with effaced fat planes. This suggests involvement of the V2 and V3. On the coronal reformat note the widened foramen ovale

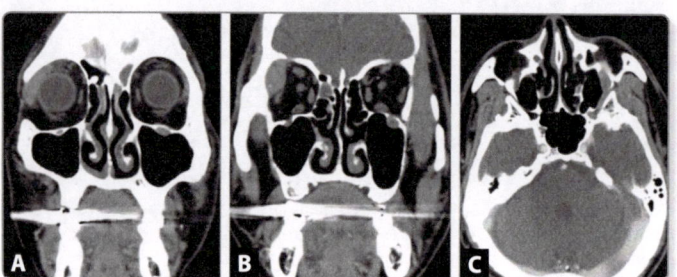

**Figures 10.18A to C** Infraorbital nerve. Contrast CT scan images in a patient with lymphoma shows thickening and enhancement along the left infraorbital nerve, suggestive of perineural involvement

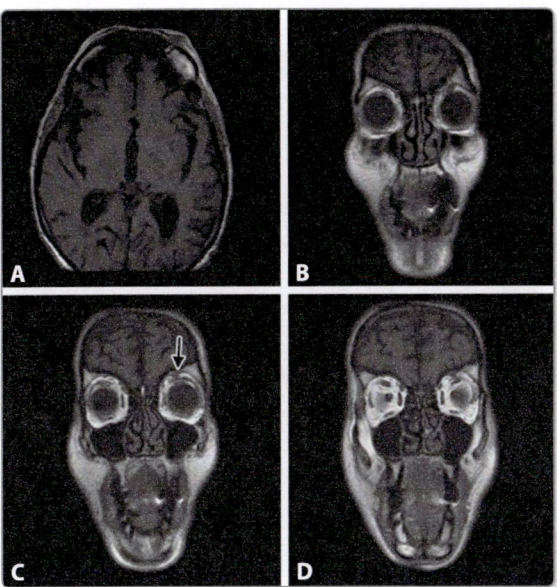

**Figures 10.19A to D** Ophthalmic division V1. Patient with skin SCC above left brow. T1-weighted axial and coronal images reveal thickened appearances of the V1 and branches on the left consistent with perineural spread of disease

A secondary imaging feature of PNS is muscular denervation. One such example can be seen when there is PNS affecting the mandibular division (V3) of the trigeminal nerve. This nerve supplies the muscles of mastication, the anterior belly of the digastric and mylohyoid muscles. The muscles of facial expression may also be involved secondary to PNS along the facial nerve. Hemiatrophy of the tongue may be seen in the setting of hypoglossal nerve infiltration (**Figures 10.21A to C**). In the acute (<1 month) and subacute stages (1–20 months), increased T2 signal and enhancement may be seen in the affected muscles. In the chronic stage (> 20 months), atrophy and fatty infiltration is noted.

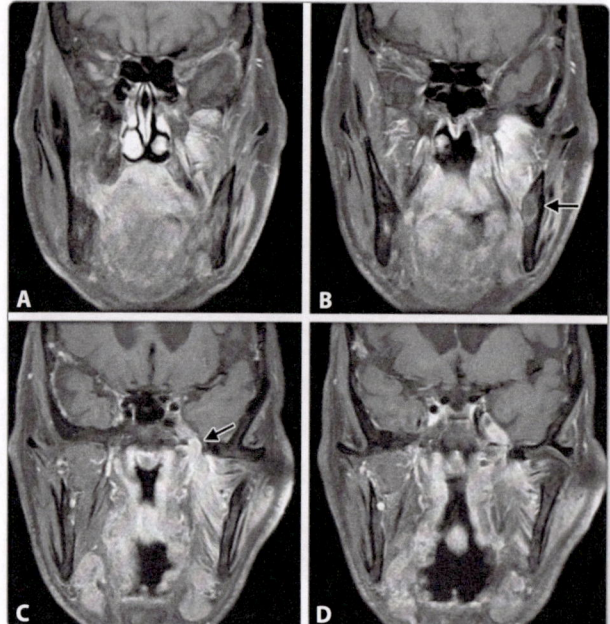

**Figures 10.20A to D** Inferior alveolar nerve to V3 and cavernous sinus. Coronal MR images in a patient of squamous cell carcinoma of the lip. Postgadolinium fat-saturated sequence images well highlight invasion of the left mandible, inferior alveolar canal going into the V3, foramen ovale and coming anterograde into the cavernous sinus

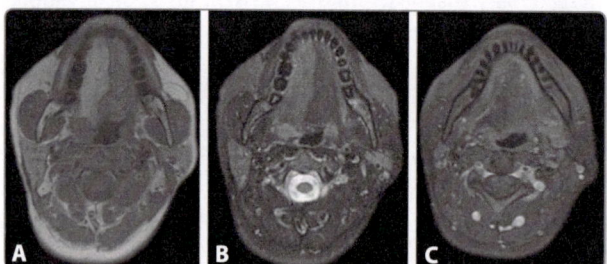

**Figures 10.21A to C** Axial T1, T2 and postgadolinium T1 fat-saturated images show right hemiatrophy and fatty change in the tongue, in a patient with hypoglossal nerve infiltration

| Infections | *Viral:* HSV I, CMV, VZ |
| --- | --- |
| | *Bacterial:* TB, Lyme disease |
| | *Fungal:* Rhinocerebral mucormycosis, Cryptococcus neoformans, Aspergillus |
| | *Parasitic:* Cranial neuro-schistosomiasis |
| **Postinfectious and demyelination disorders** | *e.g.* Bell's palsy, ophthalmoplegic migraine |
| **Granulomatosis** | *e.g.* sarcoidosis, idiopathic hypertrophic cranial pachymeningitis, Tolosa-Hunt syndrome |
| **Postradiation neuritis** | *Uncommon, usually delayed, complication of radiation therapy or radiosurgery* |
| **Tumors** | *e.g.* nerve sheath tumors, meningioma, hemangioma, etc. |

**Table 10.6** Some other causes of neural-perineural enhancement

# Normal variants and differential diagnosis

Emissary veins traversing neural foramina normally enhance after contrast administration. This finding is usually symmetrical which helps to distinguish it from PNS. As mentioned earlier, circumneural arteriovenous plexus surrounding the facial nerve at the geniculate ganglion, tympanic and mastoid segments also enhance normally and should not be confused for PNS. Nerve sheath tumors and meningiomas may cross foramina and resemble PNS. There are few reports of perineural spread secondary to rhinocerebral mucormycosis or Aspergillus infection as well as inflammatory involvement from sarcoidosis, and one should be wary of this in the appropriate clinical setting. Some of the common causes of neural-perineural enhancement on imaging are listed in **Table 10.6**.

# Bibliography

### Perineural spread of malignancy
1. Gandhi D, Gujar S, Mukherji SK. Magnetic resonance imaging of perineural spread of head and neck malignancies. Top Magn Reson Imaging. 2004;15(2):79-85.

2. Gandhi MR, Panizza B, Kennedy D. Detecting and defining the anatomic extent of large nerve perineural spread of malignancy: Comparing "targeted" MRI with the histologic findings following surgery. Head Neck. 2010. [Epub ahead of print]
3. Ginsberg LE. MR imaging of perineural tumor spread. Magn Reson Imaging Clin N Am. 2002;10(3):511-25, vi.
4. Ginsberg LE. MR imaging of perineural tumor spread. Neuroimaging Clin N Am. 2004;14(4):663-77.
5. Lee KJ, Abemayor E, Sayre J, Bhuta S, Kirsch C. Determination of perineural invasion preoperatively on radiographic images. Otolaryngol Head Neck Surg. 2008;139(2):275-80.
6. Liebig C, Ayala G, Wilks JA, Berger DH, Albo D. Perineural invasion in cancer: A review of the literature. Cancer. 2009;115(15):3379-91.
7. Maroldi R, Farina D, Borghesi A, Marconi A, Gatti E. Perineural tumor spread. Neuroimaging Clin N Am. 2008;18(2):413-29, xi.
8. Nemec SF, Herneth AM, Czerny C. Perineural tumor spread in malignant head and neck tumors. Top Magn Reson Imaging. 2007;18(6):467-71.

## Cranial nerve enhancements

9. Gebarsk SS, Telian SA, Niparko JK. Enhancement along the normal facial nerve in the facial canal: MR imaging and anatomic correlation. Radiology. 1992;183:391-4.
10. Ong CK, Chong VF. Cancer Imaging. Imaging of perineural spread in head and neck tumors. 2010;10 Spec no A:S92-8.
11. Williams LS, Schmalfuss IM, Sistrom CL, et al. MR imaging of the trigeminal ganglion, nerve, and the perineural vascular plexus: Normal appearance and variants with correlation to cadaver specimens. Am J Neuroradiol. 2003;24:1317-132.

## Trigeminal nerve

12. Becker M, Kohler R, Vargas MI, Viallon M, Delavelle J. Pathology of the trigeminal nerve. Neuroimaging Clin N Am. 2008;18(2):283-307.
13. Warden KF, Parmar H, Trobe JD. Perineural spread of cancer along the three trigeminal divisions. J Neuro Ophthalmol. 2009;29(4):300-7.

## Facial nerve

14. Raghavan P, Mukherjee S, Phillips CD. Imaging of the facial nerve. Neuroimaging Clin N Am. 2009;19(3):407-25.

## Auriculotemporal

15. Schmalfuss IM, Tart RP, Mukherji S, Mancuso AA. Perineural tumor spread along the auriculotemporal nerve. AJNR Am J Neuroradiol. 2002;23(2):303-11.

## Greater superficial petrosal nerve

16. Ginsberg LE, De Monte F, Gillenwater AM. Greater superficial petrosal nerve: Anatomy and MR findings in perineural tumor spread. AJNR Am J Neuroradiol. 1996;17(2):389-93.

# Imaging evaluation of cervical lymph nodes

## chapter 11

Reza Forghani, Hugh D Curtin

### Abstract

Evaluation of cervical lymph nodes is an integral part of head and neck imaging, enabling characterization of clinically suspected cervical lymphadenopathy as well identification of pathologic nodes in deeper regions of the neck that are not well-evaluated on physical examination. The imaging-based cervical lymph node classification system has received widespread acceptance and has been adopted by the American Joint Committee on Cancer (AJCC). The goals of this classification system are to optimize and enhance reproducibility across different institutions and to reduce inter-reader variability by providing consistent and readily identifiable imaging landmarks. This chapter provides an overview of the radiologic anatomy of cervical lymph nodes and characteristics of normal, reactive and inflammatory, and neoplastic/metastatic lymphadenopathy. The different imaging characteristics of pathologic lymph nodes, as well as their limitations, are discussed. This is followed by an overview of both common and uncommon infectious, inflammatory, and neoplastic nodal disease. The goal of this chapter is to provide an overview of the basics and fundamentals of radiologic anatomy and pathology of nodal disease as well as a relatively thorough but brief overview of various inflammatory and neoplastic nodal diseases typically encountered in clinical practice.

### Keywords

Cervical nodes, lymph nodes, cervical lymphadenopathy, imaging-based lymph nodes classification, computed tomography (CT), magnetic resonance imaging (MRI), ultrasound, positron emission tomography (PET), reactive nodes, metastatic nodes, node size, nodal necrosis, nodal calcification, node morphology, node size ratios, nodal grouping, internal nodal heterogeneity, nodal necrosis, node enhancement, extranodal tumor extension, extracapsular spread of tumor, viral lymphadenitis, human immunodeficiency virus (HIV), infectious mononucleosis, bacterial lymphadenitides, suppurative lymphadenitis, Lemierre's syndrome, cat-scratch disease, mycobacterial lymphadenitis, tuberculosis, Kimura's disease, Kikuchi-Fujimoto disease, sinus histiocytosis with massive lymphadenopathy, Rosai-Dorfman disease, sarcoidosis, angiofollicular lymph node hyperplasia (Castleman's disease), metastatic thyroid carcinoma, lymphoproliferative disorders, lymphoma, leukemia.

# Introduction

Evaluation of cervical lymph nodes is an integral part of head and neck imaging. While an expert clinician may palpate enlarged nodes, computed tomography (CT), magnetic resonance imaging (MRI), and ultrasound (US) are important adjunctive tools that can provide confirmation and further characterization of clinically suspected cervical lymphadenopathy and enable identification of pathologic nodes in deeper regions of the neck that are not well evaluated on physical examination. CT and MRI are now routinely used for characterization and determination of extent of lymphadenopathy in inflammatory and neoplastic diseases affecting the head and neck and to follow-up response after treatment. At the same time, more advanced imaging techniques such as positron emission tomography (PET) are used selectively for specialized applications, primarily in cancer staging. Notwithstanding the widespread utility of these powerful techniques, it is important to be aware of the strengths and weaknesses of each modality in the overall clinical assessment of each patient. CT and MRI are excellent techniques for localization and determination of anatomic extent of pathologically enlarged nodes, but frequently lack specificity. As is frequently the case in head and neck imaging, the clinical context is very important and should be used in conjunction with the imaging findings to provide an optimal and clinically relevant differential diagnosis. In certain cases, biopsy may be required for a pathologic diagnosis and imaging can be used to select the most appropriate site and to guide the biopsy. This chapter provides an overview of the current radiologic classifications used for description of cervical nodes, imaging criteria used for determination of pathologic nodes, and the major diseases associated with cervical lymphadenopathy.

# Physiology and radiologic anatomy of cervical nodes

## Basic organization and function of the lymphatic system

In the head and neck, the lymphatic system consists of lymph nodes and the Waldeyer's ring structures that are considered part of the mucosal associated lymphoid tissue (MALT). Peripherally, the lymphatic system consists of an extensive capillary lymphatic network that begins as blind ended channels draining interstitial fluid. Once fluid enters the lymphatic capillaries, it is called lymph, a transparent colorless or slightly yellowish fluid that is similar to, but more dilute than plasma. Approximately 10 percent of the interstitial fluid is estimated to enter the lymphatic system and passes from the lymphatic capillaries into larger lymphatic vessels that carry the lymph to lymph nodes. As lymphatic fluid travels centrally, it can pass through multiple nodal stations. Upon passage through lymph nodes, lymph becomes enriched with lymphocytes and its cellularity increases. The cellularity of central lymph varies widely, depending on the state of antigenic stimulation. After passage through central nodal stations, lymph eventually drains into the main lymphatic trunks consisting of the thoracic duct on the left side (the main lymphatic collecting channel, also called the left lymphatic duct) and the right lymphatic duct, and ultimately into the venous system.

Lymph nodes serve as filtration areas for foreign materials and their main function is lymphopoiesis and the creation of the immune response. In general, lymph nodes are organized into groups or chains that drain discrete anatomic regions. Lymph nodes are typically oval or bean shaped structures with a depression called the hilum where arterioles, venules, and efferent lymphatic vessels enter and exit. Lymph enters a node through multiple afferent lymphatic vessels that enter at the periphery of the node, away from the hilum. Lymph brings antigens to the node and carries out antibodies, T cells, macrophages, and activated B cells. Phagocytes within the lymph node sinuses also filter the lymph and retain foreign antigens and substances. As lymph passes from one chain of lymph nodes to the next, immunity is conveyed from peripheral to more central lymph nodes.

Blood enters lymph nodes via one or more arterioles at the nodal hilum. The majority of lymphocytes are brought to the lymph through blood rather than the afferent lymphatics. The blood vessels within a lymph node are for the most part morphologically identical to those in other organs, except for the high endothelial venules (HEV) which in addition to lymph nodes are also found in tonsillar tissue and in Peyer's patches in the gastrointestinal tract. Within lymph nodes, HEVs are generally found in the paracortical and interfollicular regions and occasionally in the medullary cords. HEVs contain specialized lymphocyte-homing receptors and mediate the trafficking of circulating lymphocytes into the lymph nodes through expression of specific combinations of cell adhesion molecules and chemokines, and occasionally may even provide a pathway for entry of tumor cells into the lymphatic system (discussed below).

As discussed earlier, approximately 10 percent of the interstitial fluid is estimated to enter the lymphatic system. This fluid can contain soluble as well as mobile solid material, including tumor cells. There are significant structural differences between the lymphatic capillaries and blood capillaries that facilitate metastatic spread of tumor cells. Lymphatic capillaries have loose cell junctions between endothelial cells, valve openings, and lack a basement membrane or surrounding pericytes. As a result, the dominant pathway for tumor cell entry into the lymphatic system is via passive intravasation. This is in contrast to the active process of intravasation of tumor cells into blood vessels. However, passive intravasation is not the only mechanism of entry of tumor cells into the lymphatics. There is also some evidence that tumor cells may occasionally enter a lymph node hematogenously, through interactions with specialized cell receptors on the HEVs, with experiments demonstrating preferential attachment of squamous cell carcinoma cells to HEVs.

## Radiologic anatomy and classification of cervical lymph nodes

### Historical overview and rationale for cervical lymph node classifications

Approximately 40 percent of the lymph nodes in the body are located in the head and neck. Over the past century, numerous classification systems have been proposed for description of cervical lymph nodes with the ultimate goal of producing a uniformly accepted and reproducible system for description of pathologic nodes and patient staging. Prior to routine use of cross-sectional imaging for evaluation of cervical soft-tissues in the 1980s, the landmarks used for nodal classification were based in large part on the palpable structures of the superficial triangles of the neck. The Rouvière classification described in 1938 was widely used for nearly 4 decades until in early 1980s it was suggested that the anatomic based classifications be replaced with a simpler "level" system. In the ensuing years, a number of classification systems were developed, eventually leading to 2 widely used classifications in the late 1990s consisting of the classification proposed by the American Joint Committee on Cancer (AJCC) and nomenclature proposed by the Committee for Head and Neck Surgery and Oncology of the American Academy of Otolaryngology — Head and Neck Surgery (AAO-HNS). However, some of the landmarks used in these classifications were only well seen at the time of surgery or were broadly defined anatomic structures that could not be always relied on for a reproducible classification on cross-sectional studies. Given that nearly all head and neck cancer patients (excluding those with skin cancer) are evaluated with CT, MRI, or PET/CT as part of their initial work-up and many head and neck cancer patients are no longer treated surgically, in 1999 Som et al. proposed an imaging based classification system that would allow radiologists and clinicians to use a single classification system that was reproducible regardless of the method of treatment. This system has been received enthusiastically and the imaging based system has now been adopted by the AJCC.

## Overview of classic anatomic and level based lymph node classifications

As alluded to earlier, a large number of lymph node classifications have been proposed over the years, sometimes with inconsistent use of terminology, leading to confusion in the literature. In the Rouvière system, the groups of cervical nodes at the top of the neck have been described as a "collar" of nodes composed of the occipital, mastoid, parotid, facial, retropharyngeal, submaxillary, submental, and sublingual lymph nodes (**Figures 11.1A and B**) (**Table 11.1**). Descending from this collar of nodes are the anterior and lateral cervical groups of lymph nodes which extend along the front and sides of the neck,

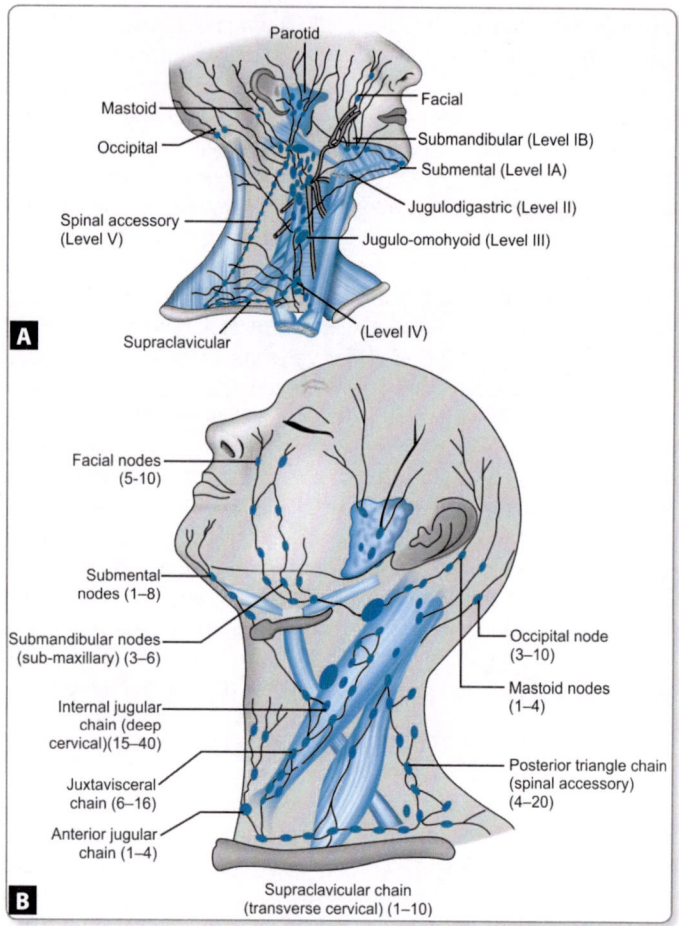

**Figures 11.1A and B** Major nodal chains in the neck. Drawing of the head and neck region as seen from the upper (A) and down (B) sides demonstrates the major nodal chains as described by Rouvière (A, B) with their corresponding nodal levels (A). For a detailed description of the nodal chains, please refer to the text (*Adapted from Som and Brandwein in Som and Curtin, Head and Neck Imaging, 5th Edition, Elsevier, 2011*)

| Nodes | Description | Region drained by nodes | Route of drainage of nodes |
|---|---|---|---|
| Occipital nodes | 3 to 10 nodes situated at the junction of the upper posterior portion of the neck and the lower lateral cranial vault. | Occipital region. | Spinal accessory chain of the lateral cervical nodes. |
| Mastoid nodes | 1 to 4 nodes that lie just behind the ear. | Parotid region, parietal scalp, and skin of the auricle. | Inferior parotid nodes and superior internal jugular chain of the lateral cervical nodes. |
| Parotid nodes | 7 to 19 nodes situated both superficial to the gland and within the gland and commonly referred to as either extraglandular or intraglandular. | An extensive and varied territory including the forehead and temporal scalp, portions of the mid and lateral parts of the face, the auricle and external auditory canal, the eustachian tube, portions of the posterior part of the cheek, buccal mucous membrane, gums, and the parotid gland itself. The most common area to drain into these nodes is the skin, and thus the most common tumors to metastasize to them are melanomas and squamous cell carcinomas. | A variety of local pathways leading to the internal jugular chain of the lateral cervical nodes. |

*Contd...*

*Contd...*

| Nodes | Description | Region drained by nodes | Route of drainage of nodes |
|---|---|---|---|
| Facial nodes | 5 to 10 nodes situated in the subcutaneous tissues of the face that, in general, follow the course of the external maxillary artery and the anterior facial vein. | Eyelids, cheek, mid portion of the face and, rarely, the gums and palate. | Submandibular nodes. |
| Retropharyngeal nodes | These are separated into medial and lateral groups. The medial group lies near the midline and is usually directly posterior to the upper pharynx near the level of the second cervical vertebra. These nodes can, however, occur as low as the level of the greater cornua of the hyoid bone. There usually are only 1 or 2 nodes in this inconstant group. The lateral group consists of 1 to 3 nodes situated near the lateral aspect of the posterior pharyngeal wall, overlying the longus capitus and longus coli muscles. These nodes can extend along the entire length of the pharynx and are often enlarged in newborn infants with a pharyngeal infection. The lateral retropharyngeal nodes lie medial to the carotid artery. | As a group, the retropharyngeal nodes primarily drain the nasopharynx and oropharynx. However, they also drain the palate, nasal fossae, paranasal sinuses, and middle ear. | Superior internal jugular chain of the lateral cervical nodes. |

*Contd...*

## Imaging evaluation of cervical lymph nodes

*Contd...*

| Nodes | Description | Region drained by nodes | Route of drainage of nodes |
|---|---|---|---|
| Submandibular (submaxillary) nodes | 3 to 6 nodes situated in the submandibular triangle of the neck, lateral to the anterior belly of the digastric muscle and near the submandibular gland. | These drain the lateral portion of the chin, the lower and upper lips, cheek, nose, anterior nasal fossae, most of the gums, teeth, palate, anterior portion of the tongue, medial portion of the eyelids, submandibular and sublingual glands, and the floor of the mouth. | Internal jugular chain of the lateral cervical nodes. |
| Submental nodes | 1 to 8 nodes that lie in the submental triangle of the neck, superficial to the mylohyoid muscle and between the anterior bellies of the digastric muscles. | Chin, lower lip, cheeks, anterior gingiva, floor of the mouth, and tip of the tongue. | Submandibular nodes and internal jugular chain of the lateral cervical nodes. |
| Sublingual nodes | Some dispute the existence of sublingual nodes. These are inconsistent nodes that are proposed to lie in a lateral group along the anterior lingual vessels and in a medial group between the genioglossus muscles. They probably should not be strictly | Tongue and floor of the mouth. | Submandibular and submental nodes and the internal jugular chain of the lateral cervical nodes. |

*Contd...*

Contd...

| Nodes | Description | Region drained by nodes | Route of drainage of nodes |
|---|---|---|---|
|  | grouped as lymph nodes, but rather as small lymph nodules located along the collecting lymphatic trunks of the tongue and sublingual glands. |  |  |
| Anterior cervical nodes | These lie in the infrahyoid portion of the neck, between the two carotid sheaths, and consist of 2 divisions. These are the anterior (superficial) jugular chain and the juxtavisceral chain. The anterior (superficial) jugular chain contains 1 to 4 small, inconstant nodes and follows the course of the anterior jugular vein, lying in the superficial fascia of the neck overlying the strap muscles. The juxtavisceral chain of the anterior cervical nodes lies in relationship to the larynx, thyroid gland, and tracheoesophageal grooves. One of the pretracheal nodes, the Delphian node, lies on the cricothyroid membrane. | The anterior (superficial) jugular chain: drain the skin and muscles of the anterior portion of the neck. The juxtavisceral chain: This nodal chain drains the supraglottic and infraglottic larynx, pyriform sinuses, thyroid gland, trachea, and esophagus. One of the pretracheal nodes, the Delphian node, lies on the cricothyroid membrane and receives lymph from the subglottic larynx. Thus, when this node is enlarged, subglottic disease is suspected. | The anterior (superficial) jugular and the juxtavisceral chains: Both chains drain into the thoracic duct or anterior mediastinal nodes on the left side and into the lowest internal jugular chain or highest intrathoracic node on the right side. |

Contd...

Contd...

## Imaging evaluation of cervical lymph nodes

| Nodes | Description | Region drained by nodes | Route of drainage of nodes |
|---|---|---|---|
| | The juxtavisceral nodes have been subdivided into prelaryngeal, prethyroid, pretracheal, and laterotracheal groups. There are 6 to 16 nodes in this category, with most (6–9 nodes) in the tracheoesophageal grooves. The highest nodes in the tracheoesophageal grooves may lie directly behind the posterior thyroid lobes. When in this location, these nodes may be confused on both CT and MR scans with either a thyroid nodule or parathyroid adenoma. | | |
| Lateral cervical nodes | These make up the primary nodes of clinical interest in the evaluation of head and neck malignancies, providing the major drainage route for all of the other nodal chains. These nodes have been grouped according to location. The superficial group contains 1 to 4 nodes and follows the course of the external | Internal jugular (deep cervical): Parotid, submandibular, submental, retropharyngeal, and some anterior cervical nodes. The nodes caudal to the level of the crossing of the omohyoid muscle also receive lymph from the arm and the superficial aspect of the thorax. The jugulodigastric (sentinel or tonsillar) | Internal jugular (deep cervical): The terminations of these chains differ slightly on each side. First, the respective chains form jugular lymphatic trunks. On the right side this trunk enters either the right lymphatic duct, the subclavian vein, or the internal jugular vein. On the left side the jugular |

Contd...

*Contd...*

| Nodes | Description | Region drained by nodes | Route of drainage of nodes |
|---|---|---|---|
| | jugular vein, lying superficial to the sternocleidomastoid muscle. The deep group is divided into 3 subgroups: the internal jugular (deep cervical), the spinal accessory (posterior triangle), and the transverse cervical (supraclavicular) chains. The internal jugular (deep cervical) chain lies close to the internal jugular vein. Just under the skull base, these nodes become inseparable from the highest lymph nodes of the posterior triangle chain. Most of the 15 to 40 nodes in the deep cervical chain are concentrated below the level where the posterior belly of the digastric muscle crosses the vein and above the level where the omohyoid muscle traverses the system. This latter muscle divides the nodal chain into 2 clinically important groups: the superior (upper) or supraomohyoid nodes and the infraomohyoid (inferior) | node receives lymph from the tonsils, neighboring mucous membranes, and the submandibular nodes. The jugulo-omohyoid node receives all of the lymph from the tongue. The nodes of Virchow (Trosier nodes) receive metastatic implants from tumors originating in the abdominal and thoracic cavities. The spinal accessory (posterior triangle) chain nodes: Occipital and mastoid nodes, the parietal and occipital regions of the scalp, the nape, lateral portions of the neck, and the shoulder. Transverse cervical (supraclavicular) nodes: These nodes primarily connect the distal posterior triangle chain with the internal jugular chain and the central neck veins. The transverse cervical nodes also receive lymph from the subclavicular nodes, the skin of the anterolateral portion of the neck, and the upper anterior chest wall. | lymphatic trunk terminates either in the arch of the thoracic duct or directly into the subclavian or internal jugular veins. The spinal accessory (posterior triangle) chain nodes: Their lymph drains primarily into the transverse cervical chain, but there are also communications with the internal jugular chain. Transverse cervical (supraclavicular) nodes: These nodes primarily connect the distal posterior triangle chain with the internal jugular chain and the central neck veins. They drain in a manner similar to the internal jugular nodes. |

*Contd...*

*Contd…*

| Nodes | Description | Region drained by nodes | Route of drainage of nodes |
|---|---|---|---|
| | nodes. The superior group of nodes lies anterolateral to the vein, while the infraomohyoid nodes may be either anterior, medial, or posterior to the vein. The deep cervical nodes are arranged either in a single series or in 2 or 3 roughly parallel, interconnecting rows that are side by side. A single node in the deep cervical chain, which is usually larger than the adjacent nodes, is situated near the junction of the posterior belly of the digastric muscle and the internal jugular vein. This is called the jugulodigastric, sentinel, or tonsillar node. Similarly, at the level where the omohyoid muscle crosses the internal jugular vein is the jugulo-omohyoid node, which is larger than the adjacent nodes. Among the most inferior nodes in the deep cervical chain are the nodes of Virchow (Trosier nodes). | | |

*Contd…*

*Contd...*

| Nodes | Description | Region drained by nodes | Route of drainage of nodes |
|---|---|---|---|
| | They may receive metastatic implants from tumors originating in the abdominal and thoracic cavities. The spinal accessory (posterior triangle) chain nodes consist of 4 to 20 nodes that follow the course of the spinal accessory nerve in the posterior triangle of the neck. The most superior nodes blend with the highest nodes of the internal jugular chain, but while the internal jugular nodes descend almost vertically in the neck, the posterior triangle nodes descend obliquely downward and posterolaterally in the neck. Transverse cervical (supraclavicular) nodes consist of 1 to 10 nodes that follow the course of the transverse cervical vessels. | | |

NB: Another group of nodes, not described by Rouvière, are the nuchal nodes. These consist of 1 to 3 nodes that lie under the origin of the trapezius muscle tendon and extend downward and parallel to the midline. These typically become palpable in patients with infectious mononucleosis.

**Table 11.1** The major drainage routes in the classic Rouvière classification of cervical nodes (*Source: Som PM, Radiology. 1987;165:593–600*)

respectively. The lateral group of cervical nodes is divided into superficial and deep groups with the deep subgroup consisting of the internal jugular chain, the spinal accessory (posterior triangle) chain, and the transverse cervical (supraclavicular) chain that are joined at their ends, forming a triangle (**Table 11.1**). The lateral cervical nodes make up the primary nodes of clinical and radiological interest in the evaluation of head and neck malignancies, since they provide the major route of drainage for all of the other nodal chains. It is important to be familiar with the Rouvière system since the terminology is still used, especially in describing superficial nodes, and it forms the basis of the classification systems developed later. **Table 11.1** provides a review of the nodal chains and drainage routes in this system.

Other early classifications proposed in the 1990s divided the head and neck nodes into 12 groups. These consisted of: (1) submental, (2) submandibular, (3) cranial jugular nodes, (4) medial jugular nodes, (5) caudal jugular nodes, (6) dorsal cervical nodes along the spinal accessory nerve, (7) supraclavicular nodes, (8) prelaryngeal and paratracheal nodes, (9) retropharyngeal nodes, (10) parotid nodes, (11) buccal nodes, and (12) retroauricular and occipital nodes. Yet others have proposed that with the exception of the tongue, the lymphatics of the head and neck can be thought of as being organized into two circles or cylinders: In this classification, the outer cylinder contains the superficial nodes, extending from the chin to the occiput, and consisting of the submental, submandibular, buccal, mandibular, preauricular, and occipital nodes. The inner cylinder surrounds the upper aerodigestive tract and includes the retropharyngeal, pretracheal, and paratracheal nodes. Lying vertically between the two cylinders and extending along the internal jugular veins are the deep cervical nodes (or the jugular chain). Virtually all of the lymph from both the inner and outer cylinders drains into the deep cervical or internal jugular lymph node chain, which is the primary drainage pathway of the head and neck. Two nodes in this chain are particularly important. One is the jugulodigastric (JD) node, also known as the sentinel node, located near the angle of the mandible. The JD node drains lymph from the tonsils, pharynx, mouth, and facial region. Given the extent of exposure to microorganisms and the frequency of infections in its drainage area, this node tends to be hyperplastic and larger than most other lymph nodes. The second node of special importance in the deep cervical chain is the jugulo-omohyoid (JO) node, located near the point at which the inferior belly of the omohyoid muscle crosses the internal jugular chain. The JO node drains lymph from the tongue, and if enlarged, may be the first sign of an otherwise clinically silent tongue malignancy.

With time, level based systems were proposed and became widely accepted. In the initial level based systems, cervical nodes were divided into levels I through VI, with further subdivisions into sublevels (**Table 11.2**). Briefly, these consisted of level IA (submental), IB (submandibular), IIA and IIB (upper jugular), III (middle jugular), IV (lower jugular), VA and VB (the posterior triangle group), and level VI (the anterior compartment group). Lymph nodes in regions not covered by these levels were referred to by the name of their specific nodal group, such as superior mediastinal, retropharyngeal, periparotid, the buccinator, postauricular, and suboccipital nodes. **Table 11.2** provides a detailed summary of the landmarks used in the determination of each level and sublevel in this classification system as well as the primary sites/regions with greatest propensity to metastasize to these levels.

## Imaging-based lymph node classification

### Overview and technique

The imaging based cervical lymph node classification system has received widespread acceptance and has now been adopted by the AJCC. The goals of this classification system are to optimize and enhance reproducibility across different institutions, regardless of the specific scanner used, and to reduce inter-reader variability by providing consistent and readily identifiable imaging landmarks. To accomplish these goals, the use of a consistent technique is encouraged, especially for CT where patient positioning and gantry angulation are more variable. The patient's head should be positioned in a comfortable neutral position with the hard palate perpendicular to the table top and the shoulders as far down as possible. The scanner gantry should be aligned along the inferior orbitomeatal plane.

## Imaging evaluation of cervical lymph nodes

| Level | General description | Sublevels | Common primary site(s) of metastasis |
|---|---|---|---|
| Level I | Divided into sublevels IA (submental) and IB (submandibular) lymph nodes. | Sublevel IA<br>Submental lymph nodes within the triangular boundary of the anterior belly of the digastric muscles and the hyoid bone. | These nodes are at greatest risk for harboring metastases from cancers arising from the floor of mouth, anterior oral tongue, anterior mandibular alveolar ridge and lower lip. |
| | | Sublevel IB<br>Submandibular lymph nodes within the boundaries of the anterior belly of the digastric muscle, the stylohyoid muscle, and the body of the mandible. It includes the preglandular and the postglandular nodes and the prevascular and postvascular nodes. The submandibular gland is included in the specimen when the lymph nodes within the triangle are removed. | These nodes are at greatest risk for harboring metastases from cancers arising from the oral cavity, anterior nasal cavity, and soft tissue structures of the midface, and submandibular gland. |
| Level II | Upper jugular (includes sublevels IIA and IIB) lymph nodes located around the upper third of the internal jugular vein and adjacent spinal accessory nerve extending from the level of the skull base (above) to the level of the inferior border of the hyoid bone (below). The anterior (medial) boundary is the stylohyoid muscle (the radiologic correlate is the vertical plane defined by the posterior surface of the submandibular gland) and the posterior (lateral) boundary is the posterior border of the sternocleidomastoid muscle. | Sublevel IIA<br>These nodes are located anterior (medial) to the vertical plane defined by the spinal accessory nerve. | The upper jugular nodes are at greatest risk for harboring metastases from cancers arising from the oral cavity, nasal cavity, nasopharynx, oropharynx, hypopharynx, larynx, and parotid gland. |
| | | Sublevel IIB<br>These nodes are located posterior (lateral) to the vertical plane defined by the spinal accessory nerve. | |

*Contd...*

*Contd...*

| | | | |
|---|---|---|---|
| Level III | Middle jugular lymph nodes located around the middle third of the internal jugular vein extending from the inferior border of the hyoid bone (above) to the inferior border of the cricoid cartilage (below). The anterior (medial) boundary is the lateral border of the sternohyoid muscle, and the posterior (lateral) boundary is the posterior border of the sternocleidomastoid muscle. | No sublevels. | These nodes are at greatest risk for harboring metastases from cancers arising from the oral cavity, nasopharynx, oropharynx, hypopharynx, and larynx. |
| Level IV | Lower jugular lymph nodes located around the lower third of the internal jugular vein extending from the inferior border of the cricoid cartilage (above) to the clavicle below. The anterior (medial) boundary is the lateral border of the sternohyoid muscle and the posterior (lateral) boundary is the posterior border of the sternocleidomastoid muscle. | No sublevels. | These nodes are at greatest risk for harboring metastases from cancers arising from the hypopharynx, thyroid, cervical esophagus, and larynx. |

*Contd...*

Contd...

| | | | |
|---|---|---|---|
| Level V | Posterior triangle group (includes sublevels VA and VB). This group is composed predominantly of the lymph nodes located along the lower half of the spinal accessory nerve and the transverse cervical artery. The supraclavicular nodes are also included in posterior triangle group. The superior boundary is the apex formed by convergence of the sternocleidomastoid and trapezius muscles, the inferior boundary is the clavicle, the anterior (medial) boundary is the posterior border of the sternocleidomastoid muscle, and the posterior (lateral) boundary is the anterior border of the trapezius muscle. | Sublevel VA is separated from sublevel VB by a horizontal plane marking the inferior border of the anterior cricoid arch. Thus, sublevel VA includes the spinal accessory nodes, whereas sublevel VB includes the nodes following the transverse cervical vessels and the supraclavicular nodes with the exception of the Virchow node, which is located in level IV. | The posterior triangle nodes are at greatest risk for harboring metastases from cancers arising from the nasopharynx, oropharynx, and cutaneous structures of the posterior scalp and neck. |
| Level VI | Anterior compartment group of lymph nodes include the pretracheal and paratracheal nodes, precricoid (Delphian) node, and the perithyroidal nodes including the lymph nodes along the recurrent laryngeal nerves. The superior boundary is the hyoid bone, the inferior boundary is the suprasternal notch, and the lateral boundaries are the common carotid arteries. | No sublevels. | These nodes are at greatest risk for harboring metastases from cancers arising from the thyroid gland, glottic and subglottic larynx, apex of the piriform sinus, and cervical esophagus. |

**Table 11.2** Classic 6 level cervical lymph node classification and associated primary sites of metastases *(Source: Robbins et al., Neck Dissection Classification Update, Arch Otolaryngol Head Neck Surg. 2002;128:751-8).*

In addition, the occlusal plane should be perpendicular to the table top in order to minimize artifact. To improve distinction of nodes from adjacent soft tissue structures and vessels, intravenous contrast should be administered unless contraindicated. The recommended field of view is 16 to 18 cm. The scan should start above the skull base and extend caudally to the level of the manubrium and be reconstructed as contiguous 1.5 mm to 2.5 mm slices when using a multidetector CT. When performing a MRI, the scan should include axial images with a slice thickness of 3 to 4 mm with either a 1 mm interslice gap or no interslice gap.

In patients with a history of thyroid cancer, cancer of the cervical esophagus, or subglottic laryngeal cancer, the caudal margin of the study (typically CT) should be extended down to the level of the carina in order to provide coverage of the superior mediastinum. Using these techniques, all of the nodal chains as well as the most likely potential primary sites along Waldeyer's ring are visualized. Slight variations from the techniques described do not appear to significantly alter interpretation and assignment of nodal levels.

### Nodal chain classification, landmarks, and approach to interpretation

The ultimate goal of the imaging based classification is to provide a consistent and reproducible system that is acceptable to both treating physicians and radiologists, building on the early major nodal classifications. In the imaging based classification, the cervical nodal chains are divided into 7 levels (**Table 11.3; Figures 11.2A and B**). Level I consists of submental (IA) and submandibular (IB) nodes (**Figures 11.3A and B; Table 11.3**). Levels II to IV are comprised of internal jugular nodes (**Figures 11.4A to D; Table 11.3**). Level II nodes extend from the skull base to the level of the lower body of the hyoid bone and are subclassified into IIA and IIB. Level IIA includes nodes which lie anterior, lateral, or medial to the internal jugular vein or those that lie posterior to it but are inseparable from the vein. Level IIB includes level II nodes which lie posterior to the internal jugular vein and have a fat plane separating the node from the vein. These nodes are located in the fat deep to the sternocleidomastoid muscle. Level III

| Level I | All of the nodes below the mylohyoid muscles, anterior to a transverse line drawn through the posterior edge of the submandibular gland in the axial plane, and above the bottom of the body of the hyoid bone. These include previously classified submental and submandibular nodes. Level I nodes can be subclassified into levels IA and IB.<br>*Level IA*<br>Nodes that lie between the medial margins of the anterior bellies of the digastric muscles, above the bottom of the body of the hyoid bone and below the mylohyoid muscle (previously classified as submental nodes).<br>*Level IB*<br>Nodes that lie posterior and lateral to the medial edge of the anterior belly of the digastric muscle (previously classified as submandibular nodes) |
|---|---|
| Level II | Nodes around the internal jugular vein extending from the lower bony margin of the jugular fossa at the skull base to the level of the lower body of the hyoid bone. These nodes lie anterior to a transverse line drawn on each axial image through the posterior edge of the sternocleidomastoid muscle and lie posterior to a transverse line drawn on each axial scan through the posterior edge of the submandibular gland. In the area within 2–3 cm of the skull base, a node located anterior, lateral, or posterior to the internal carotid artery is classified as a level II node. However, if the node lies medial to the internal carotid artery, it is classified as a retropharyngeal node. More caudally, level II nodes include those located anterior, lateral, medial, or posterior to the internal jugular vein. Level II nodes can be subclassified into levels IIA and IIB.<br>*Level IIA*<br>Nodes that lie anterior, lateral, or medial to the internal jugular vein (previously classified as upper internal jugular nodes) as well as nodes that lie posterior to the internal jugular vein and are inseparable from the vein.<br>*Level IIB*<br>Nodes that lie posterior to the internal jugular vein and are separated from the vein by a fat plane (previously classified as upper spinal accessory nodes). These nodes are located in the fat deep to the sternocleidomastoid muscle. |
| Level III | Nodes around the internal jugular vein between the level of the lower body of the hyoid bone and the level of the lower margin of the cricoid cartilage arch. These nodes lie anterior to a transverse line drawn on each axial image through the posterior edge of the sternocleidomastoid muscle. Level III nodes also lie lateral to the medial margin of either the common carotid artery or the internal carotid artery. On each side of the neck, the medial margin of carotid arteries separates level III nodes (located laterally) from level VI nodes (located medially). Level III nodes were previously known as mid-jugular nodes. |

*Contd...*

Contd...

| | |
|---|---|
| Level IV | Nodes around the internal jugular vein between the level of the lower margin of the cricoid cartilage arch and the level of the top of the manubrium. These nodes lie anterior and medial to an oblique line drawn through the posterior edge of the sternocleidomastoid muscle and the lateral posterior edge of the anterior scalene muscle. The medial margin of the common carotid artery is the landmark that separates level IV nodes (located laterally) from level VI nodes (located medially). Level IV nodes were previously known as the low jugular nodes (including the prescalene nodes). |
| Level V | Nodes extending from the skull base, at the posterior border of the attachment of the sternocleidomastoid muscle, to the level of the clavicle, as seen on each axial scan. All these nodes lie anterior to a transverse line through the anterior edge of the trapezius muscle in the axial plane. From the skull base to the bottom of the cricoid arch, these nodes are located posterior to a transverse line through the posterior edge of the sternocleidomastoid muscle in the axial plane. More caudally, between the level of the bottom of the cricoid arch and top of the manubrium, they lie posterior and lateral to an oblique line through the posterior edge of the sternocleidomastoid muscle and the lateral posterior edge of the anterior scalene muscle. Level V nodes can be subdivided into VA and VB nodes.<br><br>*Level VA*<br>Nodes between the skull base and the level of the lower margin of the cricoid cartilage arch, behind the posterior edge of the sternocleidomastoid muscle.<br><br>*Level VB*<br>Nodes between the lower margin of the cricoid cartilage arch and the level of the clavicle, as seen on each axial scan. They are behind an oblique line through the posterior edge of the sternocleidomastoid muscle and the lateral posterior edge of the anterior scalene muscle. |
| Level VI | Nodes located between the medial margins of the left and right common carotid or internal carotid arteries, extending from the level of the lower body of the hyoid bone to the level superior to the top of the manubrium. These are the visceral nodes. |
| Level VII | Nodes in the substernal region extending from the level of the top of the manubrium to the level of the innominate vein, between the medial margins of the left and right common carotid arteries. |

Note: The facial, parotid, retropharyngeal, occipital, and other nodes are referred to by their respective names in all classifications.

**Table 11.3** Current imaging based classification of cervical lymph nodes (*Source: Som et al, Arch Otololaryngol Head Neck Surg 1999;125:388-96*)

Imaging evaluation of cervical lymph nodes **443**

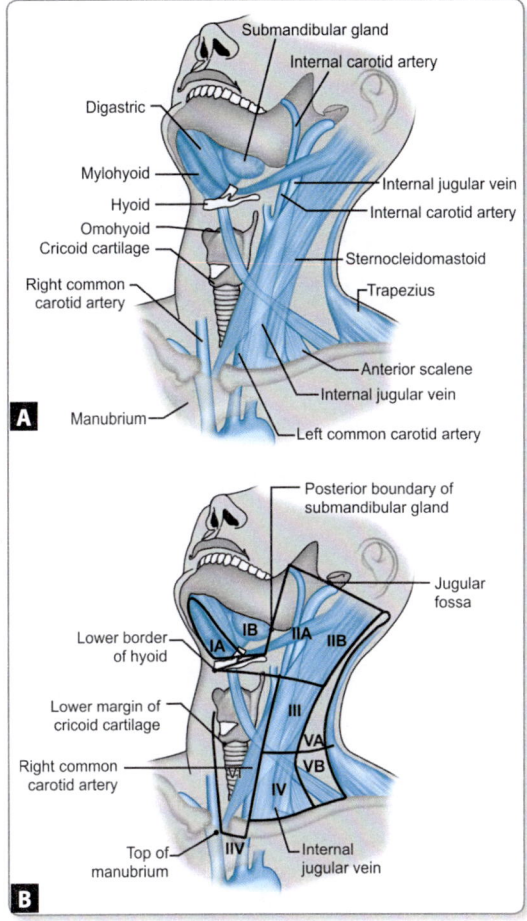

**Figures 11.2A and B** Imaging based nodal classification. Schematic diagram of the head and neck viewed from the left anterior oblique projection (A) demonstrates the major anatomic landmarks used in the imaging-based nodal classification. In (B), broad lines are used to outline the boundaries of the nodal levels I through VII using the imaging-based nodal classification (*Adapted from Som and Brandwein in Som and Curtin, Head and Neck Imaging, 5th Edition, Elsevier, 2011*)

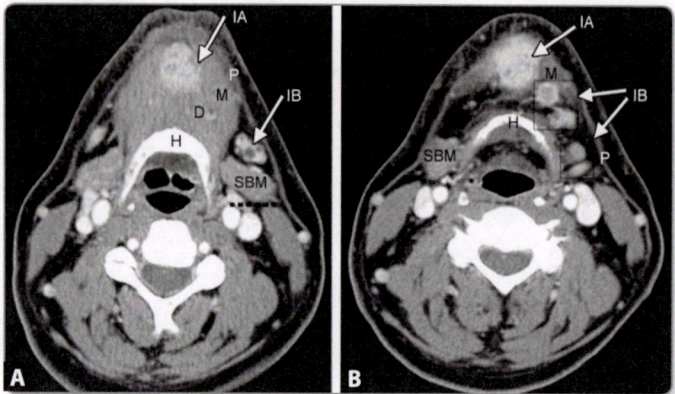

**Figures 11.3A and B** Imaging based nodal classification: Level I nodes. Axial images from a contrast enhanced CT scan demonstrate examples of level IA and IB nodes. (A) There are pathologic level IA (Between the medial margins of the anterior bellies of the digastric muscles) and IB nodes. The dashed line indicates an imaginary line drawn beyond the posterior margin of the submandibular gland (SBM) and used to separate level I from level II nodes. (B) Image caudal to that shown in A again demonstrates the large pathologic level IA node as well as multiple left level IB nodes (Box-Arrows), some clearly pathologic. The ipsilateral left submandibular gland is no longer seen although the contralateral submandibular is still visible. Note that all level I nodes are superior to the level of the bottom of the hyoid bone (H). *Abbreviations*: D – anterior belly of digastric muscle; H – hyoid bone; M – mylohyoid; P – platysma; SBM – submandibular gland

nodes consist of nodes around the internal jugular vein between the level of the lower body of the hyoid bone and the level of the lower margin of the cricoid cartilage arch, and level IV nodes extend from the level of the lower margin of the cricoid cartilage arch to the level of the top of the manubrium.

Level V nodes are subdivided into VA and VB and lie posterior to the sternocleidomastoid muscle in the upper neck (VA) or posterolateral to an oblique line drawn from the posterior edge of the sternocleidomastoid muscle and the lateral posterior edge of the anterior scalene muscle (VB) in the lower neck. Both groups are anterior to a line drawn on each axial scan through the anterior

Imaging evaluation of cervical lymph nodes **445**

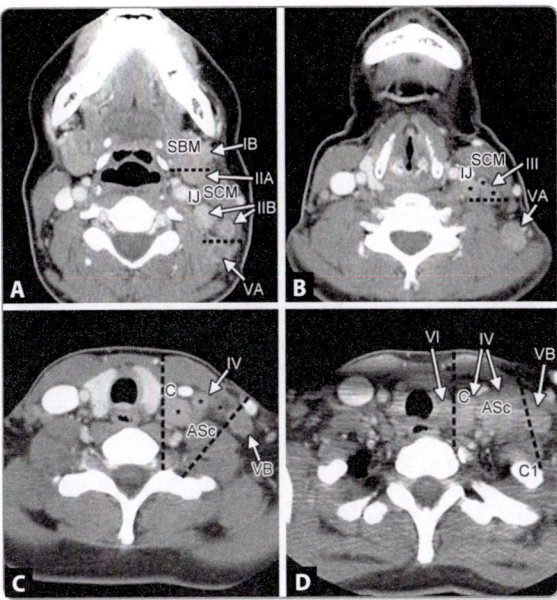

**Figures 11.4A to D** Imaging based nodal classification: Levels II – VI. Axial images from a contrast enhanced CT scan demonstrate examples of nodes at various levels, many pathologic (see Table 11.3 for a detailed description of landmarks used for nodal level designation). Dashed lines designate imaginary lines used to distinguish different levels. (A). The left level IIA node is anterior to the IJ but mostly (more than 50%) posterior to a line drawn along the posterior margin of the SBM, distinguishing it from the more anteriorly located level IB node. The level IIB nodes are posterior to the IJ and separated from it with a fat plane. A line drawn along the posterior margin of the SCM is used to separate level IIB from VA nodes. (B) This section is below the hyoid bone but above the lower margin of the cricoid arch and demonstrates left level III (individually marked by asterisks) and VA nodes. (C) This section is below the lower margin of the cricoid arch but above the manubrium. Left level IV (individually marked by asterisks) and VB nodes are shown. There are also right level IV nodes. (D) More caudally, this section demonstrates multiple and conglomerate left level IV lymphadenopathy as well as level VB and VI nodes. *Abbreviations*: ASc – anterior scalene muscle; C – carotid artery; Cl – Clavicle; IJ – internal jugular vein; SBM – submandibular gland; SCM – sternocleidomastoid muscle

edge of the trapezius muscle. Level VA consists of the upper nodes, extending between the skull base and the level of the lower margin of the cricoid cartilage arch. On axial scans, these lie behind the posterior edge of the sternocleidomastoid muscle. Level VB are the lower level V nodes, extending between the level of the lower margin of the cricoid cartilage arch and the level of the clavicle, as seen on each axial scan. On axial images, these lie behind an oblique line drawn from the posterior edge of the sternocleidomastoid muscle and the lateral posterior edge of the anterior scalene muscle. Level VI nodes are the visceral nodes that lie between the medial margins of the left and right common carotid arteries or the internal carotid arteries, extending from the level of the lower body of the hyoid bone to the level of the top of the manubrium. Lastly, level VII nodes are those that lie caudal to the top of the manubrium in the substernal region between the medial margins of the left and right common carotid arteries (**Figures 11.4A to D; Table 11.3**). These nodes extend caudally to the level of the innominate vein. The landmarks used for classification of nodes into levels I through VII are further described in **Table 11.3**. To maintain consistency with prior classifications, the following nodal groups, as well as other superficial nodes of the neck, are referred to by their anatomical names, including supraclavicular, retropharyngeal, parotid (periparotid and intraparotid), buccinator (facial), suboccipital, and preauricular nodes.

When interpreting scans, axial images are used for determination of a nodal station and it is recommended that each side of the

| | |
|---|---|
| • | Axial images are used for assignment of nodal stations |
| • | Each side of the neck should be evaluated separately |
| • | When appropriate, use an imaginary line to define the boundaries of the levels, using the landmarks described in Table 11.3. These should be "drawn" separately for each side of the neck |
| • | When a lymph node is transected by a line separating two levels or sublevels, the side of the line on which the majority of the nodal cross-sectional area lies is the level to which the lymph node should be assigned. |

**Table 11.4** Approach for interpretation and assignment of nodal stations using the imaging classification

neck be evaluated separately. Imaginary "lines" are used to define the boundaries of the levels, and these should be "drawn" separately for each side of the neck (**Figures 11.3 and 11.4; Tables 11.3 and 11.4**). When a lymph node is transected by a line separating two levels or sublevels, the side of the line on which the majority of the nodal cross-sectional area lies is the level to which the lymph node should be assigned. The supraclavicular fossa is a triangular region caudal to a plane defined by the upper medial (sternal) end of the clavicle, upper lateral end of the clavicle, and where the posterior neck meets the shoulder. This triangular region is difficult to precisely identify in the axial plane given that it is oblique to that plane and not seen in its entirety on a single slice. This area is most accurately identified clinically but can be approximated on axial images whenever any portion of the clavicle is identified on one side of the neck, provided the patient's shoulders are as low as possible. Note that this would include the caudal portions of the level IV and VB nodes. If a node is located below the level of the clavicle and lateral to the ribs, it is considered a deep axillary node.

# Pathology

## Overview

Most nodal pathology is either inflammatory, including those secondary to a regional infection or the wide spectrum of less common nonspecific reactive lymphadenopathies, or neoplastic. Evaluation of nodal disease requires a multidisciplinary approach including clinical physical examination, imaging, and biopsy. The clinician can detect palpable lymphadenopathy, and imaging can confirm and characterize abnormalities identified on physical exam and detect nonpalpable disease in the deep spaces of the neck. Histopathology is considered the gold standard in the evaluation of a pathologic lymph node, enabling the identification of a specific pathogen or neoplasm as well as identification of micrometastases not detectable on physical exam or by conventional anatomic imaging. However, even histopathologic analysis is not free of potential error. It is estimated that 1 billion malignant cells are required to create a mass of only 1 mm$^3$, and it has been shown that a significant percentage of micrometastases may be missed if a lymph node is simply bisected sagittally, as opposed to when a more thorough evaluation with serial sectioning is performed. These issues highlight the challenges faced by the clinical team in evaluation of lymphadenopathy, particularly when staging metastatic carcinoma.

Cross-sectional imaging with CT or MRI are powerful methods for detection of the anatomic extent of lymphadenopathy and characterization of pathologic lymph nodes. They are routinely performed as part of the standard work-up and staging of most head and neck cancers, with the exception of skin cancer. Ultrasound (US) can also be used for characterization of cervical lymphadenopathy. However, given that US is operator dependent and not all nodal levels can be thoroughly evaluated, it is not as widely and routinely used for staging of head and neck cancer and will not be discussed further in this chapter. Lastly, PET combined with anatomic imaging with CT or MRI can enhance the accuracy of nodal staging and may be used as an adjunctive tool for staging of cancer patients.

It is important to be aware of limitations of imaging in detection and characterization of pathologic lymph nodes. Determination of a pathologic node on imaging relies in large part, although not entirely, on nodal enlargement and therefore micrometastases are frequently not detectable by CT or MRI alone. Another limitation of nodal imaging is that the imaging appearance of pathologic nodes is frequently nonspecific and does not enable identification of the specific pathologic agent without additional clinical information and/or information from biopsy. This highlights the importance of considering all information, including the clinical context, in order to provide a clinically relevant differential diagnosis. In the following sections, we will review and discuss the imaging characteristics of pathologic lymph nodes with emphasis on CT and MRI. We will begin with a discussion of the various imaging characteristics of pathologic lymph nodes, followed by an overview of the major inflammatory and neoplastic etiologies presenting as cervical lymphadenopathy.

# Imaging criteria for characterization of pathologic lymph nodes

## Normal nodes

Normal "non-challenged" cervical nodes are small structures embedded in the normal fat within the neck (**Figures 11.5 and 11.6**). These measure no more than a few millimeters in their greatest dimension and are frequently difficult to identify and separate from adjacent soft tissue structures on imaging or even at the time of surgery or autopsy. On imaging, normal lymph nodes have well defined borders and are usually oval. In addition, normal lymph nodes have a fatty hilum that can frequently be seen on CT and MRI. Before administration of IV contrast, normal nodes are isodense to muscle on CT. On MRI, normal nodes are isointense to muscle on T1 and variably hyperintense to muscle on T2 weighted images. After administration of IV contrast, normal nodes enhance slightly more than muscle on both CT and MRI. On imaging, normal lymph nodes and mildly reactive nodes (see below) cannot be definitively distinguished but the distinction is not relevant clinically and therefore these are simply referred to as normal nodes.

## Reactive or inflammatory nodes

When a lymph node is challenged by an infection, there is an increase in the number and size of its germinal centers, pathologically referred to as reactive follicular hyperplasia. This results in enlargement of the lymph node and the reaction to inflammation is referred to as reactive lymphadenopathy. In nodal stations draining sites of frequent inflammation and infection, lymph nodes are frequently challenged over many years. In the head neck, these are exemplified by the jugulodigastric and submandibular nodes which are the primary drainage sites for common inflammations associated with teething, tonsillitis, pharyngitis, sinusitis, and skin infections. As a result, these "chronically challenged" nodes tend to be larger than other cervical nodes (**Figures 11.5A and B**).

On imaging, nodes are characterized based on their size, internal architecture, and morphology. Reactive nodes are typically

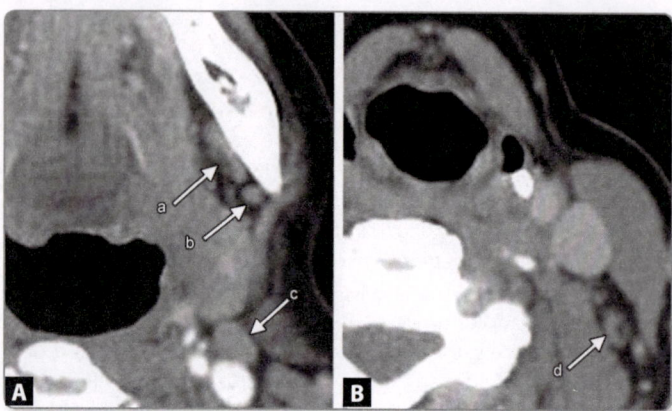

**Figures 11.5A and B** Normal and reactive nodes. Axial images from a contrast enhanced CT scan demonstrate the different appearances of normal and/or reactive nodes. Normal nodes have smooth margins and a fatty hilum and are oval and lima-bean shaped (a, d). However, small normal nodes can also have a rounded appearance, either because of variations in shape or the plane of the section (b). Occasionally, nodes can be slightly prominent, like the level IIA node shown here (c). This is most commonly encountered at levels IIA and IB because these are primary drainage sites of common inflammations and these nodes are chronically challenged. As a response to chronic inflammation, some nodes develop fatty hilar metaplasia (d), with a U-shape or lima bean configuration and a low-attenuation central region that extends to the peripheral surface of the node. If large enough, the central low-attenuation region can be characterized as fat on imaging, allowing a clear distinction from central nodal necrosis

homogeneous, have smooth and noninfiltrating margins, and typically retain their fatty hilum (**Figures 11.7, 11.8 and 11.12**). On CT, reactive nodes usually have an attenuation similar to or slightly less than that of muscle. On MRI, these nodes typically have homogeneous low to intermediate signal intensity on T1 and fairly high signal on T2-weighted images. Reactive nodes demonstrate variable enhancement after administration of IV contrast.

Size is a major criterion used for characterization of pathologic lymph nodes. It is important both for the radiologist and the surgeon to understand the limitations of nodal size assessment. Because of

Imaging evaluation of cervical lymph nodes 451

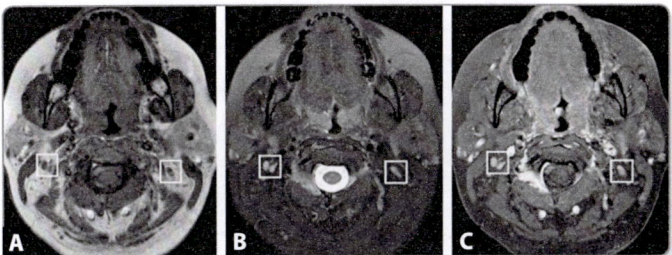

**Figures 11.6A to C** Normal nodes. Axial images from a contrast enhanced MRI scan are shown including (A) T1, (B) fat saturated T2, and (C) contrast enhanced fat-saturated T1-weighted images. Representative examples of small normal nodes are shown in white boxes. Normal nodes have smooth margins and are oval/lima-bean shaped. They are of intermediate signal on T1, variably hyperintense on T2, and can enhance after administration of contrast

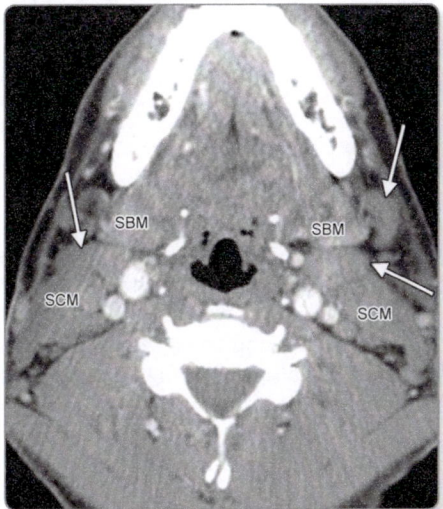

**Figure 11.7** Reactive nodes in a HIV positive patient. Axial contrast enhanced CT image demonstrates multiple enlarged but sharply defined and homogenous lymph nodes in a HIV positive patient (arrows). The appearance of these nodes is nonspecific and may be seen in other reactive lymphadenopathies or even lymphoma. *Abbreviations*: SBM – submandibular gland; SCM – sternocleidomastoid muscle

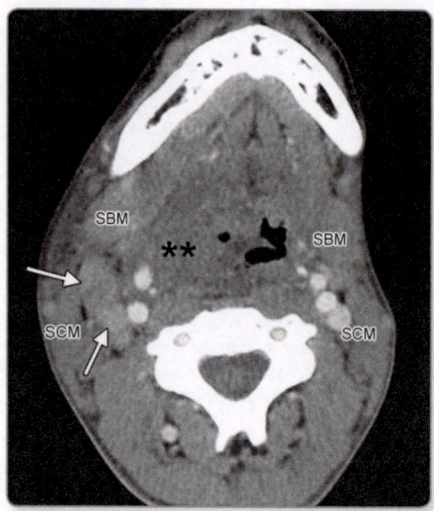

**Figure 11.8** Reactive nodes in a patient with severe pharyngitis. Axial contrast enhanced CT image demonstrates two adjacent reactive nodes (arrows) in a patient with severe pharyngitis (center marked by double asterisks) extending to multiple adjacent spaces with inflammation of the ipsilateral subcutaneous tissues. *Abbreviations*: SBM – submandibular gland; SCM – sternocleidomastoid muscle

considerable variability and overlap between the size of normal or reactive nodes and metastatic nodes, there is always a tradeoff between sensitivity and specificity when evaluating nodes based on size. Typically, studies evaluating nodal size have sought to establish criteria to distinguish malignant (metastatic) lymphadenopathy from reactive lymphadenopathy, given the obvious implications for patient diagnosis and management. Although a variety of size parameters have been proposed and none is perfect, many authors use the minimal axial dimension for distinguishing reactive from metastatic lymphadenopathy. Most authors consider nodes reactive if their minimal axial diameter does not exceed 11 mm in the jugulodigastric region and 10 mm at all other cervical nodal levels, with the exception of the retropharyngeal region. Retropharyngeal nodes are considered reactive if they do not exceed 5 mm in their minimal axial (transverse) diameter (or 8 mm in their maximal axial diameter) although no measurement is perfect and these are not absolute. The different size criteria and their limitations are discussed in greater detail below in the section on nodal metastases, as well as in **Table 11.5**. *It is important to note that all the proposed size criteria apply to homogenous, sharply delineated nodes.*

Notwithstanding the typical imaging characteristics and size criteria described above for reactive lymph nodes, if an otherwise healthy young patient presents with a large focus of inflammation or abscess, the nodes, even if markedly enlarged or heterogenous, are likely to be inflammatory. Therefore, evaluation of lymphadenopathy is best performed by taking into account the clinical context and patient's risk profile rather than isolated interpretation based solely on the appearance of the lymph nodes.

| Minimum axial diameter: |
| --- |
| Jugulodigastric nodes: 11 mm or less are normal, >11 mm are abnormal<br>All other nodes: 10 mm or less are normal, >10 mm are abnormal<br>Retropharyngeal nodes: 5 mm or less are normal, >5 mm are abnormal |
| Maximal longitudinal diameter: |
| Jugulodigastric and submandibular nodes: 15 mm or less are normal, >15 mm are abnormal<br>All other nodes except retropharyngeal nodes: 10 mm or less are normal, >10 mm are abnormal<br>Retropharyngeal nodes: 8 mm or less are normal, >8 mm are abnormal |
| Other proposed criteria for minimum axial diameter for nodes other than the jugulodigastric and retropharyngeal nodes: |
| 8 mm or less are normal, >8 mm are abnormal (compared to a cut-off of 10 mm, this results in increased sensitivity but decreased specificity). |
| Regardless of the size criterion used, the overall error rates for false-positive and false-negative diagnoses are in the range of approximately 15 and 20%, reflecting the limitations of the use of size criteria for determination of metastatic lymphadenopathy. |

**Table 11.5** Generally accepted size criteria for determination of pathologic lymphadenopathy and distinction from benign reactive lymphadenopathy for single homogenous sharply delineated nodes

## Neoplastic nodal pathology

### Imaging criteria for assessment of metastatic nodes

*Overview*

Imaging plays an essential role in staging of head and neck cancer, and correct staging of nodal disease has important implications both for patient management and prognosis. It is therefore not surprising that a large number of investigations have sought to establish criteria to help distinguish metastatic nodes from reactive lymph nodes. The parameters used in imaging evaluation of lymphadenopathy include size, shape, internal nodal architecture, and nodal grouping, with nodal size and change in internal architecture (central inhomogeneity) constituting the most important criteria. Central inhomogeneity is frequently simply referred to as central necrosis although histologically this simplification is not always accurate, as discussed below. Other features that need to be evaluated include node enhancement, calcification, extension of disease outside the node capsule, and relationship to vital structures. The criteria discussed are to a large extent based on studies performed using CT scans although they are meant to apply to CT, MRI, or US. CT and MRI are the main modalities currently used for staging of head and neck cancer, and some have suggested that CT performs slightly better than MRI when all interpretive criteria are taken into account, especially when both size and internal architecture are considered.

*Node size*

As alluded to earlier, nodal size criteria are not perfect. It has long been recognized that there is considerable variability in the size of "normal" (nonmetastatic) lymph nodes, and a variety of size criteria have been proposed over the past decades for determination of metastatic cervical lymphadenopathy. The challenge has been to select a size that has sufficient sensitivity yet a reasonable specificity, a trade-off that is well demonstrated in different studies looking at the sensitivity and specificity of nodal size for determination of metastatic cervical lymphadenopathy. As a smaller size is selected, there is increased sensitivity for detection of metastatic nodes but decreased specificity (resulting in an unacceptable number of false positives) and vice versa. Over the years, criteria have been proposed based on all 3 nodal dimensions, namely the maximal longitudinal, the minimal short axis, and maximal short axis dimensions. Given that none of these criteria is perfect, their use to some extent depends on individual preference, although some are more widely accepted and more practical for routine implementation. It is important to note that all the proposed size criteria apply to homogenous, sharply delineated nodes.

Some have advocated that in patients suspected of having a head and neck carcinoma, nodes should be considered pathologic if they have a maximum diameter greater than 1.5 cm in the jugulodigastric region and submandibular triangles, or a maximal diameter greater than 1 cm elsewhere in the neck. The advantage of using the greatest nodal dimension is that it corresponds to the size used for assessment of cervical lymphadenopathy clinically. However, these criteria alone are inaccurate in 20 to 28 percent of cases, either underestimating or overestimating the presence of tumor. Furthermore, assessment of nodal size in the craniocaudal plane in not as practical on imaging and given that no advantage has been demonstrated for the use of the longest nodal dimension as a criterion, the most widely used criteria are those based on measurements in the axial plane (**Tables 11.5 and 11.6**). Some investigators have suggested that the minimal axial dimension is more reliable for determination of metastatic lymph nodes. One set of commonly used size criteria for determination of a metastatic node based on the minimal short axis diameter is: nodes are considered pathologic (metastatic) if they measure: (1) greater than 11 mm in the jugulodigastric region or (2) greater than 10 mm at all other cervical nodal levels, with the exception of the retropharyngeal region. Retropharyngeal nodes are considered pathologic if they measure greater than 5 mm in their minimal axial dimension (**Table 11.5**). Others have proposed using a minimal axial diameter of 8 mm as the upper limits of normal for nodes other than the jugulodigastric and retropharyngeal nodes. This increases sensitivity but it comes at the expense of specificity. Interestingly, regardless of the size criterion used, the overall error

| | |
|---|---|
| For a group of three or more nodes in the drainage area of the tumor, suspect metastases if: | |
| • | The maximal longitudinal diameter is greater than 8 to 15 mm |
| • | The minimum axial diameters are greater than 9 to 10 mm in level II or greater than 8 to 9 mm in the remaining neck |

**Table 11.6** Proposed size criteria for groups of homogenous sharply delineated nodes for distinction from benign reactive lymphadenopathy from metastatic lymphadenopathy

rates for false-positive and false-negative diagnoses are in the range of approximately 15 and 20 percent, reflecting the limitations of the use of size criteria for determination of metastatic lymphadenopathy.

*Node morphology and size ratios*

The shape of a node has also been used to evaluate for metastases. While hyperplastic nodes tend to be elliptical or "lima-bean" shaped, metastatic nodes tend to be rounded spherical structures. The pitfalls of this approach are that there are variations in nodal shape depending on their location in the neck and it may be difficult to apply these criteria to smaller nodes. As a result, in general, this is frequently not a reliable criterion. In addition to a qualitative evaluation of node shape, some investigators have proposed using the ratio of the maximum longitudinal nodal length to the maximum axial nodal length (L/T). In one study, this criterion was used to evaluate nodes measuring greater than 8 mm in size in any plane. The authors found that normal and reactive hyperplastic nodes typically have a L/T ratio greater than 2, whereas nodes harboring metastases have a L/T ratio of less than 2 with a high accuracy of 97 percent (**Table 11.7**). By default, the use of this criterion requires assessment of node size in the axial as well as the craniocaudal planes.

*Nodal grouping and size*

The presence of groups of borderline enlarged nodes has also been proposed as a criterion for the presence of nodal metastases, *provided that the nodes are in the drainage area of the primary tumor site* (*see* **Table 11.6**). Therefore, the presence of three or more lymph nodes

| Criterion | Pitfalls |
|---|---|
| Heterogenous internal architecture or central inhomogeneity (frequently simply referred to as central necrosis although histologically this is not always accurate — see text): When present, this is considered one of the most reliable signs of pathologic lymphadenopathy. | May be indistinguishable from the normal fatty hilum, particularly in small nodes. Intranodal abscess can have an identical appearance but frequently is distinguishable based on clinical context and patient demographics. Fatty hilar metaplasia. Other cystic neck lesions including branchial cleft cyst and soft tissue abscess. |
| L/T Ratio (Longitudinal length/Transaxial width) < 2 is suggestive of metastasis (round node vs. lima bean-shaped node). | The criteria provided are based on nodes measuring greater than 8 mm; not reliable for smaller nodes. Normal variations in node shape. Overall not a very specific or reliable criterion. |
| Node enhancement is frequently seen in acute infections but can also be seen with metastases (although less commonly seen with squamous cell carcinoma). | Non-specific finding that can be seen in both reactive and metastatic nodes. |
| Nodal calcifications: Relatively rare finding in cervical nodes. Can be seen in both inflammatory (particularly TB or healed abscessed nodes) and neoplastic nodes (most commonly papillary thyroid cancer or less commonly treated lymphoma) (see text for other rare causes of nodal calcification). | Not specific for distinction of inflammatory and neoplastic processes but may be useful when used in conjunction with other clinical information and imaging findings. |
| Irregular nodal contour and extracapsular spread of tumor. Nodal contour irregularity and infiltration of adjacent tissues is abnormal. Macroscopic extranodal tumor spread can present as a thickened enhancing rim with infiltration of the adjacent fat planes or other soft tissue structures. This is associated increased risk of recurrence and a poorer prognosis. | Can be seen with neoplastic and inflammatory nodal pathology as well as after treatment such as radiation or surgical manipulation. |

**Table 11.7** Other criteria used for determination of pathologic lymphadenopathy and distinction from benign reactive lymphadenopathy

with minimum axial dimensions of 9 to 10 mm at level II or minimum axial dimensions of 8 to 9 mm elsewhere in the neck are suggestive of metastatic lymphadenopathy. Similar to absolute size criteria, these criteria apply to homogenous, sharply delineated nodes.

*Internal nodal architecture and homogeneity*

The spread of tumor to a lymph node can result in a mixture of cells within the node center consisting of tumor cells, residual lymph node tissues, and areas of necrosis. On imaging, this can result in areas of relatively low, water attenuation (CT) or signal (MRI). For a long time, it was common practice to simply refer to such lymph nodes as being necrotic or having central nodal necrosis. However, pathologically, not all low attenuation foci within a metastatic node correspond to necrosis per se. As tumor proliferates and invades the lymph node medulla, some areas contain a mix of tumor cells and interstitial fluid and even though not necrotic, have lower attenuation than the soft tissue attenuation of a normal node. This may explain why at least some studies have found that foci of "central necrosis" tend to appear larger on CT than on MRI, where truly necrotic areas have signal intensities similar to water. Therefore, some prefer to refer to this as internal nodal heterogeneity, central inhomogeneity, internal nodal abnormality, or heterogenous internal architecture, rather than necrosis.

When greater than 3 mm in size, internal nodal heterogeneity ("central necrosis") can be frequently identified on CT and MRI and represents the most reliable imaging finding of metastatic disease. On contrast-enhanced CT, necrotic nodes have a central region of low water attenuation measuring approximately 10 to 25 HU with a variably thick rim of tissue demonstrating variable enhancement (**Figures 11.9 to 11.11**). On MRI, foci of internal nodal heterogeneity appear hypointense on T1 and hyperintense on T2-weighted images, similar to water (**Figures 11.9 and 11.11**). On T2-weighted images, metastatic nodes have both areas of high signal, presumably corresponding to foci of true liquefaction and necrosis, and foci of intermediate signal, corresponding to tumor cells and residual infiltrated lymphoid tissues. Therefore, as discussed earlier, the truly necrotic hyperintense foci on T2-weighted images frequently (but not

Imaging evaluation of cervical lymph nodes 459

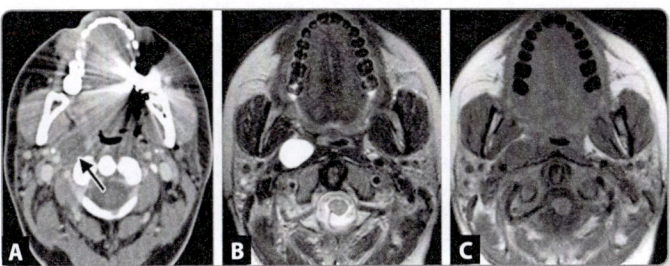

**Figures 11.9A to C** Internal nodal heterogeneity (central necrosis) from recurrent papillary thyroid carcinoma. Axial (A) contrast enhanced CT, (B) T2W MRI, and (C) T1W MRI images demonstrate an enlarged node with central water attenuation on CT (A; arrow) and fluid signal on MRI. Incidentally, the small calcification lateral to the node seen on CT (A) corresponded to the styloid process and stylohyoid ligament and not nodal calcification

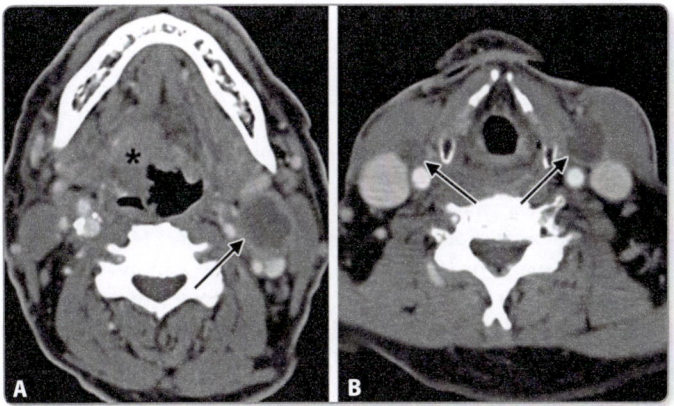

**Figures 11.10A and B** Internal nodal heterogeneity (central necrosis) from metastatic base of tongue squamous cell carcinoma. Axial contrast enhanced CT images demonstrate an infiltrative base of tongue mass (A; *) with bilateral metastatic nodes with central water attenuation and rim enhancement (arrows). In a cancer patient without an active infection, these findings are essentially pathognomonic for metastatic lymphadenopathy

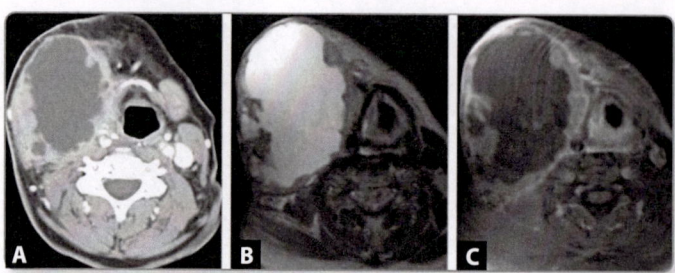

**Figures 11.11A to C** Massive node enlargement and internal heterogeneity ("central necrosis") as a first presentation of a metastatic squamous cell carcinoma of the tongue. Massive necrotic cervical lymphadenopathy as a first presentation of a squamous cell carcinoma (SCC) of the tongue. Axial (A) contrast enhanced CT, (B) T2W MRI, and (C) gadolinium-enhanced fat-saturated T1W MRI images demonstrate a large heterogeneously enhancing mass with central cystic/necrotic change and irregular and nodular margins. Further investigation revealed a SCC of the tongue (not shown) (*Adapted from Forghani, Smoker, and Curtin in Som and Curtin, Head and Neck Imaging, 5th Edition, Elsevier, 2011*)

necessarily all the time) tend to be smaller than the central region of low attenuation seen on CT. Unenhanced T1-weighted images are not as reliable for evaluation of central nodal necrosis but postcontrast fat saturated images are useful for demonstrating the central nonenhancing region, similar to the appearance on contrast enhanced CT. These sequences should be part of the routine neck MRI evaluation.

The primary imaging differential diagnoses of internal nodal heterogeneity or "central necrosis" are the normal fatty hilum of the node (*see* **Figures 11.5A and B**), fatty hilar metaplasia, or an intranodal abscess (**Figures 11.12 and 11.13**), although other rare cystic lesions in the neck should also be considered (**Figures 11.14 and 11.15**). Fatty hilar metaplasia represents a response to chronic inflammation. In cases of fatty hilar metaplasia, there can be a pronounced U-shape or lima bean configuration with a low-attenuation central region that extends to the peripheral surface of the node. If large enough, the central low attenuation region can be characterized as fat on imaging, allowing a clear distinction from central nodal necrosis

# Imaging evaluation of cervical lymph nodes 461

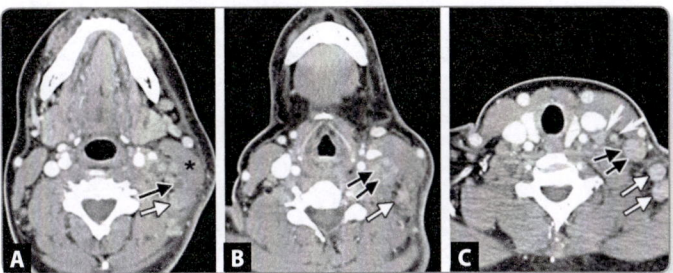

**Figures 11.12A to C** Internal nodal heterogeneity (central necrosis) secondary to an intranodal abscess and reactive nodes in a patient with bacterial adenitis. Axial contrast enhanced CT images demonstrate a left level IIB node with internal low-attenuation (A; black arrow). Metastasis from squamous cell carcinoma can have an identical appearance, highlighting the importance of considering the clinical context and patient demographics in interpretation of pathologic appearing lymph nodes on imaging. There is also subtle internal heterogeneity of a left level IIB-III and a left level V node (B, C; double black arrows), although this is less pronounced than the more cranially located node shown in A. There are scattered enhancing and/or enlarged reactive nodes (white arrows) and asymmetric enlargement of the left sternocleidomastoid muscle secondary to inflammation (A; *). All the abnormalities resolved after antimicrobial therapy (not shown)

(**Figure 11.5B**). Unfortunately, in very small nodes or in cases where the hilar metaplasia is very small and/or located centrally within the node it may be impossible to differentiate fatty metaplasia from central heterogeneity. The other differential consideration is an intranodal abscess in patients with acute infections and suppurative lymphadenitis (see **Figures 11.12 and 11.13**). Intranodal abscesses cannot be distinguished from central nodal heterogeneity secondary to metastases based on the imaging appearance of the nodes in isolation. However, these cases are frequently evident based on the clinical presentation and many may have imaging findings demonstrating a primary site of infection such as cellulitis or a dental infection.

In addition to central low-attenuation, heterogeneity and foci of low attenuation may occasionally be seen in the subcapsular region of a metastatic lymph node on CT. This is because the majority of tumor

## 462 Introductory head and neck imaging

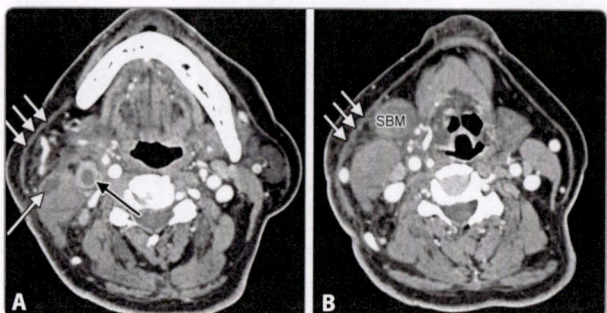

**Figures 11.13A and B** Internal nodal heterogeneity (central necrosis) secondary to an intranodal abscess and reactive nodes in a patient with group A *Streptococcus* bacterial adenitis with spread of infection to soft tissues of the neck and a small intramuscular abscess. Axial contrast enhanced CT images demonstrate a right level IIA node with internal low-attenuation (A; black arrow). There are extensive inflammatory changes in the soft tissues of the neck on the right with fat stranding, thickening of the right platysma (triple small white arrows), enlargement of the submandibular gland (B; *SBM*) and sternocleidomastoid muscle, and a small abscess in the sternocleidomastoid muscle (A; large white arrow). The patient responded to conservative management with intravenous and oral antimicrobial therapy

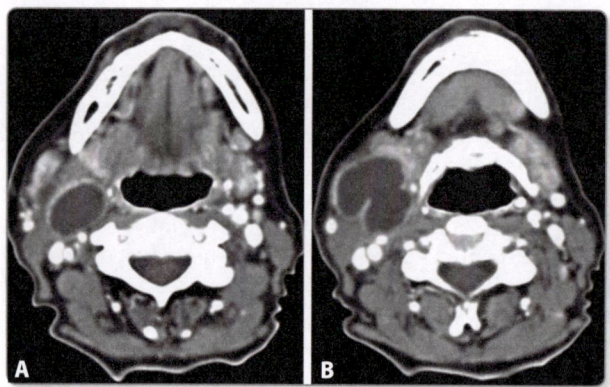

**Figures 11.14A and B** Differential diagnosis of large node with internal heterogeneity (central necrosis): Branchial cleft cyst. Axial contrast enhanced CT images demonstrate a pathologically proven right branchial cleft cyst

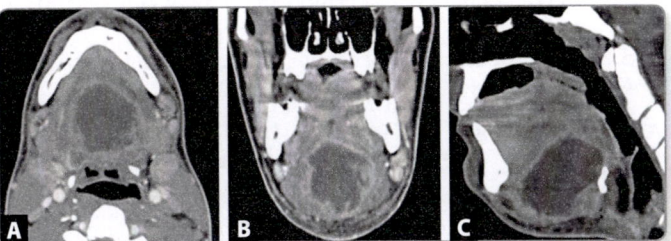

**Figures 11.15A to C** Differential diagnosis of large node with internal heterogeneity (central necrosis): Floor of mouth abscess. (A) Axial, (B) coronal reformatted, and (C) sagittal reformatted images from a 19-year-old man with recent infectious mononucleosis demonstrate a large rim enhancing low-attenuation collection involving the floor of the mouth bilaterally, contained inferiorly by the mylohyoid muscle. This was surgically drained and confirmed to represent an abscess (*Adapted from Forghani, Smoker, and Curtin in Som and Curtin, Head and Neck Imaging, 5th Edition, Elsevier, 2011*)

cells enters a lymph node via the afferent lymphatics and tumor cells first start to proliferate in the subcapsular regions. When present, this can be considered an additional sign suggestive of nodal metastasis.

### Nodal enhancement

Despite early assertions, nodal enhancement is a nonspecific finding reflecting increased vascularity of the node that can be seen with a variety of pathologies. The most common etiologies for increased node enhancement are acute infections (**Figure 11.12; Table 11.7**). These nodes are typically mildly enlarged, homogeneous, and have variable enhancement. Occasionally, aggressive acute infections such as *Staphylococcus* can further result in nodal necrosis and simulate a necrotic metastatic lymph node (**Figure 11.13**). In addition to acute infections, TB and HIV can result in nodal enhancement. Metastases from a variety of neoplasms can also result in nodal enhancement. Nodes involved by lymphoma, papillary and medullary thyroid carcinomas, renal cell carcinoma, and Kaposi's sarcoma, among others, all can enhance. Although not typical, occasionally nodes harboring metastatic squamous cell carcinoma may also enhance. Lastly, rare diseases such as angiofollicular lymphoid hyperplasia (Castleman's disease), angioimmunoblastic lymphadenopathy with dysproteinemia, angiolymphoid hyperplasia with eosinophilia, Kimura's disease, and Kikuchi's disease can have enhancing lymph nodes (discussed in greater detail below).

*Nodal calcifications*

Cervical nodal calcifications are uncommon, occurring in about 1 percent of cases (**Table 11.7**). Even now, many of these are seen in patients with tuberculosis (**Figures 11.16A to C**). These may also be seen in healed necrotic and abscessed nodes. Uncommon causes of nodal calcification include amyloidosis and rarely, sarcoidosis. Among primary head and neck cancers, nodal calcifications are most commonly seen with metastatic papillary thyroid carcinomas (**Figures 11.17A and B**). Although nodal calcifications can be seen with lymphomas, this is usually seen after radiation and/or chemotherapy. Rarely, nodal calcifications may be seen with metastases from primary tumors outside the neck, especially mucinous adenocarcinomas such as breast and colon cancer.

*Nodal margin irregularity, extranodal tumor extension and arterial invasion*

Normal nodes have smooth well defined margins and irregularity of the nodal contour is suggestive of pathology. Extranodal extension of

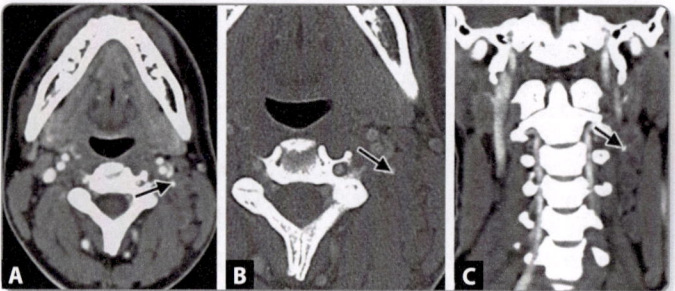

**Figures 11.16A to C** Nodal calcification in tuberculosis (scrofula). Axial contrast enhanced CT images (A, B) and a coronal reformatted image (C) from a 17-year-old with tuberculous lymphadenopathy (scrofula) demonstrate internally heterogenous (necrotic) nodes, one containing a small focus of calcification (black arrow)

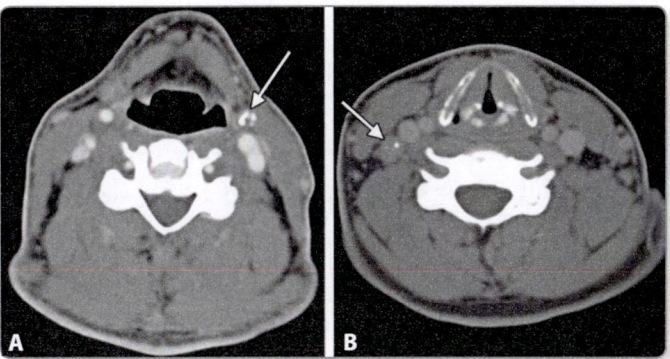

**Figures 11.17A and B** Nodal calcifications in papillary thyroid cancer metastases. Axial contrast enhanced CT images from 2 different patients demonstrate different appearances of nodal calcifications (arrow) in two cases of recurrent papillary thyroid cancer

tumor, also known as extracapsular or transcapsular spread of tumor refers to penetration of the node capsule by tumor and extension into the adjacent soft tissues (**Figures 11.18 to 11.20**). The presence of extracapsular tumor spread has important prognostic and management implications and is associated with an increased risk of recurrence and a decrease in patient survival. In histopathologic analyses, extranodal tumor extension has been seen both in normal sized and enlarged nodes, although the incidence of extracapsular tumor spread increases with an increase in node size. On CT, macroscopic extranodal tumor spread can present as a thickened enhancing rim with infiltration of the adjacent fat planes or other soft tissue structures (**Figures 11.18 to 11.20**). However, the imaging findings are not specific and a number of other nodal pathologies and treatment changes can mimic this appearance. Essentially, any process resulting in inflammation of the node capsule can result in this appearance, including recent nodal infection, recent irradiation, or surgical manipulation. This again highlights the importance of clinical information and context in interpretation of head and neck images. In the absence

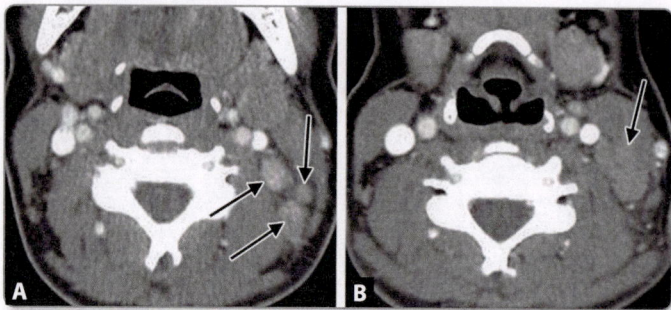

**Figures 11.18A and B** Nodal contour irregularity and extracapsular spread of tumor. Axial contrast enhanced CT images demonstrate "fuzzy" irregular margins of multiple level IIB and VA nodes (A; arrows) with infiltration of adjacent fat. In (B), there is loss of fat plane with focal infiltration of the adjacent sternocleidomastoid muscle (arrow). However, these findings are not specific for tumor and may be seen with acute infection or after treatment such as radiation or surgical manipulation

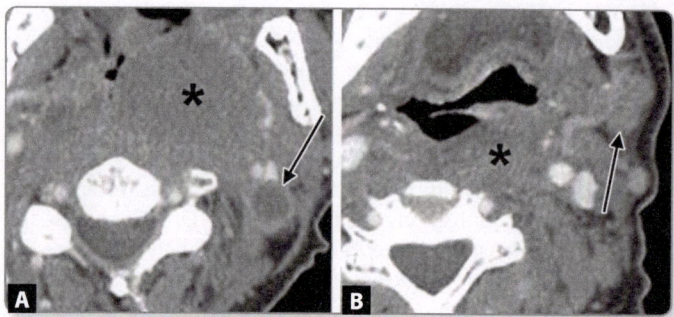

**Figures 11.19A and B** Nodal contour irregularity and extracapsular spread of tumor. Axial contrast enhanced CT images demonstrate caudal extension of an advanced invasive undifferentiated nasopharyngeal carcinoma (*) and multifocal lymphadenopathy with at least one node with internal heterogeneity (central necrosis). Note the "fuzzy" irregular and infiltrative of margins of some of the nodes with extension into adjacent soft tissue structures (arrows)

Imaging evaluation of cervical lymph nodes 467

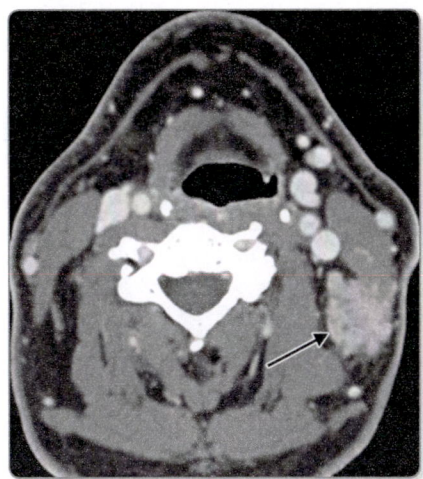

**Figure 11.20** Nodal metastasis from melanoma with macroscopic extracapsular spread of tumor. Axial contrast enhanced CT image demonstrates an enlarged hyperenhancing node/nodal conglomerate (arrow). The mass has irregular margins laterally with extracapsular spread and infiltration of the adjacent sternocleidomastoid muscle

of signs and symptoms of infection or recent treatment, these radiologic findings can be used to suggest extranodal tumor extension.

Computed tomography (CT) can demonstrate extranodal tumor extension well and some head and neck radiologists feel that extranodal spread tends to be less reliably identified on MRI, although this is debatable. When extranodal tumor spread is seen, it is important to identify the vascular, soft tissue, or osseous structures involved to enable appropriate treatment planning by the surgical team. While it is important to identify invasion of any major structure by nodal tumor, tumor extension to the internal carotid artery is of particular importance and a grave prognostic finding. The salvage rate for these patients is small and the prognosis invariably poor, but in select cases the involved artery segment can be resected and replaced with a graft.

From an oncologic management point of view, invasion of the arterial adventitia is as important as greater degrees of arterial invasion, such as invasion of the muscularis and intima. Since CT and MRI cannot reliably identify microscopic tumor infiltration of the arterial wall, invasion of the internal carotid artery is either determined by gross infiltration and invasion of that structure or suggested based on the extent of circumference that is potentially involved by tumor. The latter determination is made based on the presence of gross tumor abutting the arterial wall as well as more subtle obliteration of the normal fat plane surrounding the artery. This approach is not foolproof but it is generally believed that if 270° or more of the circumference of the artery is involved, there is a high likelihood that the artery wall has been invaded.

### Advanced nodal imaging and future prospects

A discussion of nodal imaging and staging is not complete without discussing PET-CT imaging. Currently, 2 [18F] fluoro-deoxy-D-glucose (FDG) is the agent of choice for evaluation of nodes with PET-CT. After intravenous administration, FDG accumulates within cells in direct proportion to the glycolytic rate. The basis of FDG-PET studies is that cancer cells have increased metabolic needs compared to normal cells and their increased glycolytic activity results in a preferential accumulation of FDG within active tumors cells. This does occur and the addition of PET to anatomic imaging such as CT or MRI has been shown to increase accuracy for identification of metastatic lymphadenopathy (**Figures 11.21A and B**). However, FDG-PET is not without problems. First, to be detectable, there has to be a sufficient number of live tumor cells within a lymph node. This can be particularly problematic in cases of necrotic nodes in which there may be insufficient metabolically active tumor cells to be detectable by PET. The second major problem is that increased metabolic activity is not specific for metastasis, and reactive and inflammatory lymph nodes also have increased glycolytic activity. Nonetheless, the addition of FDG-PET-CT has been shown to increase accuracy and its judicious use is an integral part of cancer imaging.

In addition to PET, advanced MRI imaging techniques and novel contrast agents have shown promise as additional noninvasive tools for evaluation of lymphadenopathy. Some investigators have

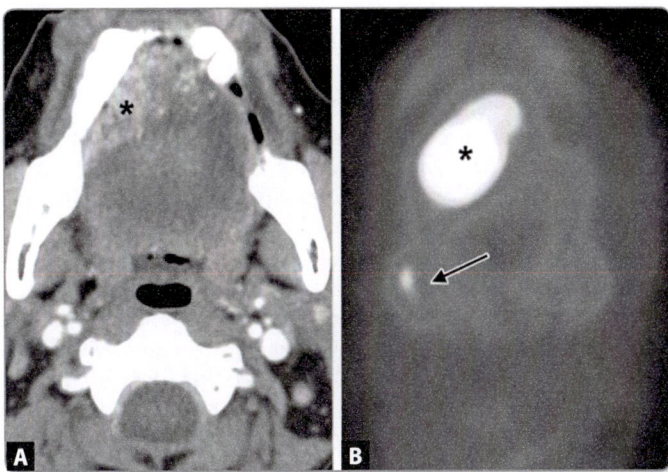

**Figures 11.21A and B** Metastatic node on PET. (A) Conventional axial contrast enhanced CT demonstrates an infiltrative lesion of the lateral right oral tongue and right floor of the mouth corresponding to a pathologically confirmed squamous cell carcinoma (black *). (B) PET component of a PET-CT performed subsequently demonstrates a highly FDG avid lesion corresponding to the invasive right tongue and floor of the mouth lesion. There is also increased asymmetric FDG uptake (short black arrow) that corresponded to a 6 mm, size-insignificant node on the nonenhanced fusion CT (*Adapted from Forghani, Smoker, and Curtin in Som and Curtin, Head and Neck Imaging, 5th Edition, Elsevier, 2011*) (*for color version of Figure 11.21B see Plate 17*)

evaluated the utility of diffusion weighted imaging (DWI) for evaluation of cervical lymphadenopathy. DWI is a technique based on diffusion of water molecules in tissues. A discussion of physics of DWI is beyond the scope of this chapter but in tissues with high and dense cellularity there are more barriers to free motion of water and therefore, those tissues tend to have relatively diminished (restricted) diffusion with lower apparent diffusion coefficient (ADC) values. Areas of cavitation or necrosis, on the other hand, represent relatively little barriers to free motion of water and therefore have elevated diffusion with increased ADC values (unless, of course, they contain viscous content such as pus in an abscess). Some studies have shown that nodes harboring lymphomas and metastases from undifferentiated nasopharyngeal carcinoma have lower ADC values than metastases from squamous cell carcinoma. Pitfalls of DWI evaluation of nodes include overlap between the measured ADC values and the presence of necrosis which can falsely elevate the measured ADC value. A definite role for DWI in evaluation of cervical lymphadenopathy has not yet been established.

Another MR based technique that has shown promise is the use of the ultra small iron oxide particles (USPIO). After intravenous administration, USPIOs pass through the vascular endothelium into the interstitium and are eventually taken up by normally functioning and inflamed lymph nodes. These are then phagocytosed by the cells of the reticuloendothelial system. Accumulation of iron within tissue has a T2 shortening effect and on USPIO enhanced MRI, normal lymph nodes show a decrease in signal on T2-weighted and T2* MR sequences because of accumulation of iron within normal lymphoid tissue. Metastatic lymph nodes, on the other hand, have replacement of their normal components with metastatic cells with loss of phagocytosis and therefore do not accumulate iron. As a result, they do not demonstrate a similar drop in signal as normal nodes. Therefore, on USPIO imaging, lymph nodes with a homogeneous signal decrease are considered normal whereas those without any signal decrease on USPIO enhanced images are considered pathologic. Lymph nodes with partial signal drop on USPIO enhanced images are considered to harbor partial metastatic infiltration. Although promising, USPIO imaging is not in widespread use at this time.

## Etiologies and clinical syndromes presenting as cervical lymphadenopathy

### Infectious and noninfectious inflammatory/reactive lymphadenopathies

#### General

Lymphadenitis refers to inflammation of lymph nodes secondary to an infectious process and suppurative adenitis indicates an infected lymph node that has undergone liquefactive necrosis. As discussed earlier, the imaging findings of lymphadenopathy frequently do not enable a specific diagnosis of the underlying pathology or distinction of an inflammatory from a malignant etiology. The clinical context and patient demographics are crucial elements that will help narrow down the differential diagnosis and as in other areas of medicine a close collaboration between the radiologist and ENT surgeon will yield the best result.

## Viral lymphadenitis

Viral infections are a frequent cause of lymph node enlargement, particularly in the pediatric population, where upper respiratory tract infections are the most common cause of enlarged lymph nodes. A large variety of viruses may cause acute or chronic lymphadenitis. Sometimes, the causative virus can be isolated from a lymph node. Other times, their presence is presumed on clinical grounds. On imaging, viral lymphadenitis can have a variable appearance but there is typically bilateral nodal involvement with an increase in number and prominence of nodes (*see* **Figure 11.7**). Most nodes have either a normal size or are mildly enlarged, are homogeneous, and typically there is little or no inflammatory change adjacent to the nodes. They are usually slightly hypoattenuating to muscle on CT, and have low to intermediate signal on T1-weighted images and high signal on T2-weighted MR images. After administration of IV contrast, these nodes enhance mildly on CT and MRI. Occipital nodes are frequently affected in this group of diseases. Many of the nonspecific viral lymphadenitis either do not come to medical attention or do not require evaluation by imaging. However, it is important to be aware of their appearance so as to not misinterpret them when encountered on imaging performed for other indications. Even though the majority of viral lymphadenitis do not have a specific imaging appearance, a few merit a separate discussion.

## Human immunodeficiency virus (HIV) infection

Human immunodeficiency virus type 1 (HIV-1) is a retrovirus and a member of the lentiviruses. Primary HIV infection may be entirely asymptomatic, but approximately 50 to 70 percent of individuals may present with a range of symptoms including fever, malaise, myalgias, diarrhea, pharyngitis, macular erythematous rash, lymphadenopathy, splenomegaly, and weight loss approximately 3 to 6 weeks after primary infection with virus, referred to as the acute HIV syndrome. The acute illness may last for up to 2 weeks, although milder symptoms may persist for months. In most patients, primary infection with or without the acute syndrome is followed by a prolonged period of clinical latency with variable duration with a median of approximately 10 years in untreated patients. However, there is active virus replication during the asymptomatic period. While symptoms of HIV may appear at any time during the disease, the more severe and life-threatening complications of HIV infection appear in patients with a CD4+ count of less than 200 cells/µL. A diagnosis of AIDS is made in anyone with HIV infection and a CD4+ count less than 200 cells/µL or a number of AIDS defining illnesses.

A high percentage of AIDS cases initially come to medical attention because of symptoms related to the head and neck, especially oral complaints. These include oropharyngeal symptoms such as candida oropharyngitis or HSV infections, cervical lymphadenopathy, and Kaposi's sarcoma (KS), discussed later in the section on tumors. Persistent generalized adenopathy (PGA) can also be commonly seen with AIDS and may be the presenting symptom of an otherwise undiagnosed HIV infection. Although many of the findings are not specific, there is a strong association between the presence of diffuse lymphadenitis (lymphadenopathy) and multiple benign-appearing parotid cysts (lymphoepithelial cysts) and HIV infection (**Figures 11.22A to C**). Therefore, when encountered, the radiologist should alert the clinician to the possibility of unrecognized HIV infection. In a significant percentage of these cases, there also is considerable enlargement of the adenoids (**Figures 11.22A to C**). Benign (nonmalignant) lymphadenopathy typically has homogenous CT density and MR signal intensity, in contradistinction to lymphadenopathy from KS or squamous cell carcinoma which frequently can have low density foci and nodal heterogeneity.

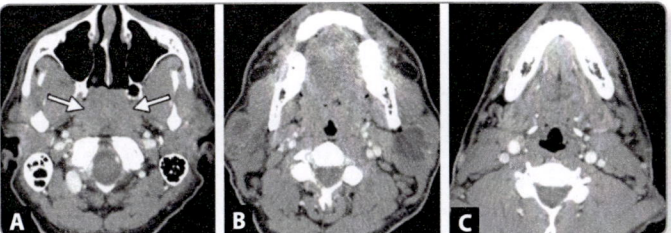

**Figures 11.22A to C** HIV related lymphadenopathy, lymphoepithelial cysts, and adenoid hypertrophy. Axial contrast enhanced CT images of a patient referred for bilateral "parotid masses" demonstrate enlargement of the lymphoid tissues of the Waldeyer's ring including marked adenoidal hypertrophy (A; arrows), multiple parotid lymphoepithelial cysts, and increased reactive lymph nodes. The constellation of findings is highly suggestive of HIV infection and the radiologist may be the first to suggest the diagnosis. Patient was subsequently diagnosed with HIV

## Infectious mononucleosis

Infectious mononucleosis (IM) is caused by the Epstein-Barr virus (EBV), a double-stranded DNA virus of the herpes virus family. This is a ubiquitous virus and over 95 percent of adults worldwide are infected with EBV based on seroepidemiologic surveys. Infection with EBV results in a lifelong infection in humans and the overwhelming majority of cases of IM occur during primary EBV infection, although infectious mononucleosis syndromes have been reported in chronically infected persons after T-lymphocyte depletion with monoclonal antibodies against CD3. Primary EBV infections are rare in the first year of life, presumably secondary to passive transfer of immunity from maternal antibodies. In developing countries and lower socioeconomic groups, most EBV infections occur in early childhood. On the other hand, in industrialized countries and higher socioeconomic groups, approximately half the population develops a primary EBV infection between 1 and 5 years of age, with another large percentage becoming infected later in the second decade of life. The latter demographic is changing with time and as less children develop a primary infection in early childhood secondary to improvements in sanitary conditions, a larger percentage of adolescents are at risk of developing a primary infection. There is a significant difference in susceptibility to developing IM after infection with EBV in these 2 demographics. Whereas primary infections in young children are often manifested as nonspecific illnesses and rarely develop into IM, IM develops in approximately 30 to 50 percent of the older patients developing a primary EBV infection.

Typically, patients with acute IM present with cervical adenopathy, pharyngitis, abdominal pain, and fever, after a nonspecific prodromal period of approximately 3 to 5 days. There is generalized lymphadenopathy, including lymphadenopathy in the posterior cervical chain, as well as hepatosplenomegaly. In the majority of patients, IM is a self-limited disease without any long-term sequelae. Typically, most clinical and laboratory findings resolve by 1 month although cervical adenopathy and fatigue may resolve more slowly. Most patients resume usual activities within 2 to 3 months although persistent fatigue and functional impairment lasting 6 months or longer has been described. IM can have associated acute complications including a variety of hematologic complications, neurologic complications such as Guillain–Barré syndrome, facial nerve palsy, meningoencephalitis, aseptic meningitis, transverse myelitis, peripheral neuritis, cerebellitis, and optic neuritis, and rarely life-threatening complications such as splenic rupture and upper airway obstruction due to lymphoid hyperplasia and mucosal edema. In most otherwise healthy adolescents, a diagnosis of infectious mononucleosis can be made on the basis of the clinical presentation, the presence of atypical lymphocytes on a peripheral-blood smear, and a positive heterophile antibody test. However, certain patient populations such as pregnant patients or those at risk for HIV infection require confirmation and a more extensive diagnostic work-up given the potential clinical impact of other mimicking infections to the patient and/or the fetus. When required, a definitive diagnosis of EBV infection can be made by testing for specific IgM and IgG antibodies against viral capsid antigens, early antigens, and EBV nuclear antigen proteins. Imaging of cervical adenopathy is not routinely performed in IM except in cases of uncertainty or when there is clinical suspicion for a complication.

## Other viral infections

A variety of other viral infections, usually of the upper respiratory tract or rarely disseminated infections may result in cervical lymphadenopathy. These include cytomegalovirus, varicella-zoster, adenovirus, rhinovirus, enterovirus, herpes simplex, measles, rubella, and vaccinia, among others. Regional lymphadenitis, most often cervical, axillary, and inguinal, may also develop within a few days to 2 weeks after vaccination with vaccines prepared from live, attenuated strains. A detailed discussion of these infections is beyond the scope of this chapter. However, many of these are diagnosed based on clinical grounds and laboratory analysis, and when imaged, there are usually no specific imaging findings that would enable a pathologic diagnosis of the specific etiologic agent.

## Bacterial lymphadenitides

Like viral infections, bacterial infections can result in enlarged enhancing nodes, although these tend to be more localized and present unilaterally on the side of the inciting primary infectious process (**Figures 11.12, 11.13 and 11.23**). In addition, compared to viral lymphadenitis, bacterial infections tend to result in larger nodes, have a greater propensity for central nodal necrosis, and more likely to have inflammation in the adjacent fat or cellulitis (**Figures 11.12, 11.13, and 11.23**). Some of these features can mimic metastases from carcinoma such as squamous cell carcinoma. The clinical context is extremely important and may help distinguish infectious necrotic lymphadenopathy from metastases. Imaging can help delineate the anatomic extent of lymphadenopathy (and the primary infection), identify complications such as abscess formation (**Figures 11.13, and 11.23**), guide aspiration and biopsy when necessary, or follow-up the progression of disease if warranted. Below we will review the imaging characteristics of select bacterial lymphadenitis.

## Routine suppurative lymphadenitis

Suppurative lymphadenitis refers to the process when there is invasion of lymph nodes by neutrophils with edema and rapid enlargement leading to capsular distention and ultimately necrosis

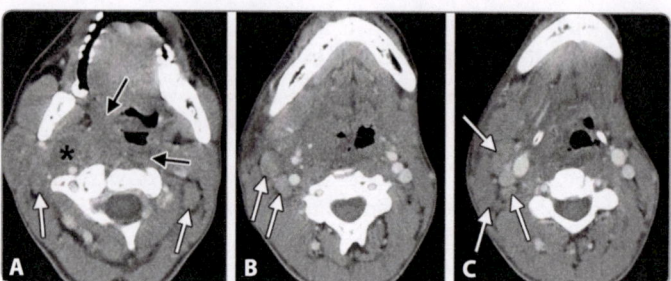

**Figures 11.23A to C** Reactive and heterogenous lymph nodes in complicated bacterial pharyngitis. Axial contrast enhanced CT images in a patient with complicated bacterial pharyngitis demonstrate marked swelling and inflammation of the right pharyngeal mucosal space with anterior extension to the glossotonsillar region and posterior extension to the retropharyngeal space (A; black arrows). Deep to the area of pharyngitis, there is an organizing collection (A; *) with generalized inflammatory changes of the soft tissues of the neck on the right. There are multiple scattered reactive nodes (the more prominent ones are marked by white arrows) that are mostly ipsilateral to the site of inflammation

and liquefaction. Although a variety of organisms can result in nodal necrosis, suppurative lymphadenitis typically refers to acute localized infections secondary to pyogenic bacteria such as *Staphylococcus aureus* and *Streptococcus pyogenes*. On imaging, there can be abscess or sinus formation with complete obliteration of the normal nodal architecture (see **Figures 11.12 and 11.13**) and clinically the involved nodes tend to be soft, enlarged, and tender with inflammatory change in the adjacent soft tissues. Other less common causes of acute lymphadenitis include yersinia, listeria, cat-scratch disease (discussed below), rarely gonorrhea, and even fungal infections. With widespread use of antibiotics, suppurative lymphadenitis is much less frequently encountered in developed countries.

### Lemierre's syndrome

Lemierre's syndrome is an uncommon complication of acute pharyngotonsillitis. In these patients, infection with anaerobic organisms results in septic thrombophlebitis of the ipsilateral internal jugular vein leading to septicemia and septic emboli, most often to the lungs and large joints. There is usually associated regional reactive (homogenous) lymphadenopathy on imaging. There are also case reports of an associated soft tissue abscess in the neck.

## Cat-scratch disease and bacillary angiomatosis

Cat-scratch disease (CSD) can result in a necrotizing granulomatous regional lymphadenitis secondary to infection by rochalimaea henselae. The organisms are typically introduced at a skin site by a scratch, splinter, or thorn and children and young adults are most commonly affected. Clinically, there is initially an erythematous lesion at the site of injury that typically resolves spontaneously within 1 to 3 weeks and often not brought to medical attention. However, within weeks of the primary lesion, there is painful enlargement of the regional lymph nodes prompting patients to seek medical attention. This may be accompanied by fever, headache, and myalgias. Thereafter, a typical erythema nodosum-type rash may follow although other forms of rash may also occur, including erythema annulare, erythema multiforme, or thrombocytopenic purpura. The disease typically has a self-limiting course lasting 2 to 4 months although a small percentage of patients may progress to severe systemic infections with multi-organ involvement. Antibiotics are not indicated in most cases, except for severe cases or cases of systemic dissemination. There are relatively few reports of imaging findings in the neck in CSD. CSD can result in both homogenous reactive lymph nodes and nodes with internal heterogeneity (central necrosis) with inflammatory changes in surrounding soft tissues. Cervical lymphadenopathy in CSD is commonly associated with axillary and upper extremity (particularly epitrochlear) lymphadenopathy. On histology, there may only be nonspecific reactive changes in early CSD lymphadenitis. The finding of coalescent epithelioid granulomata forming stellate necrotizing microabscesses suggests the diagnosis but bacilli are rarely present within the granulomata and in practice the bacilli are usually difficult to identify.

Bacillary angiomatosis (BA) is a rochalimaea infection that can affect AIDS patients and is related to CSD. Similar to CSD, patients affected by BA have a history of exposure to cats. Clinically, BA presents as a solitary or multiple red or violaceous, friable, cutaneous papules or nodules affecting the face, extremities, and scrotum that may resemble Kaposi's sarcoma. BA is responsive to antibiotics, with erythromycin-type drugs constituting the treatment of choice.

## Mycobacterial lymphadenitis

Both tuberculosis (TB) and atypical mycobacteria can result in variable appearing cervical lymphadenopathy. There has been a resurgence of tuberculosis in North America secondary to immigration from endemic countries, as well as from reactivation of disease in the elderly population and AIDS. Nonetheless, head and neck involvement in TB, known as scrofula, is rare. TB lymphadenitis can present as an increased number of nodes including homogenous enhancing nodes as well as internally heterogenous (necrotic) nodes (**Figures 11.16 and 11.24**). Sometimes, a localized abscessed node can develop, also known as a cold abscess. Typically, head and neck experts believe that there is little infiltration of surrounding fat although there are case reports describing irregular and infiltrative margins. There may be nodal calcification. Four general imaging patterns for TB lymphadenopathy have been described: (1) homogenous hyperplastic nodes with well-defined margins, (2) nodes with central low-attenuation and well-defined thick irregular peripheral enhancement, (3) a multilocular complex of nodes with central low-attenuation and peripheral rim enhancement, believed by some to represent the most specific appearance, and (4) a confluent area of low-attenuation with peripheral enhancement (**Figures 11.16 and 11.24**). There is a tendency for involvement of Level V nodes but some reports describe greater involvement of the internal jugular chain nodes. The lymphadenopathy is usually unilateral, but diffuse lymphadenopathy can also occur. Since the imaging appearance is not specific, other causes for lymphadenopathy have to be considered, including metastatic squamous cell carcinoma and lymphoma. However, known pulmonary disease as well as the patient's age and demographic group may help narrow the differential. Other head and neck manifestations of TB include gingivitis, otitis, nasopharyngeal,

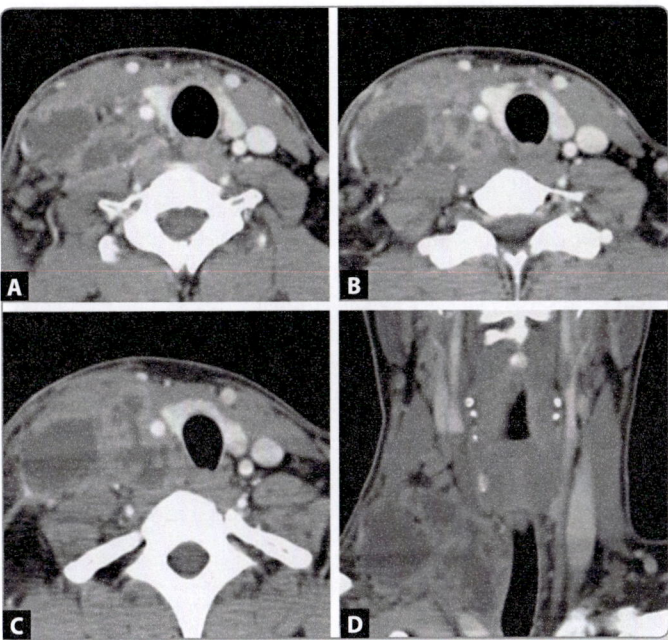

**Figures 11.24A to D** Tuberculous cervical lymphadenitis (scrofula). Axial contrast enhanced CT images (A, B, C) and a coronal reformatted image (D) from a 28-year-old patient demonstrate a multilocular complex of nodes with central low-attenuation and peripheral rim enhancement

sinonasal, or laryngeal disease. Primary nasopharyngeal infection can also occur and may mimic Wegener's granulomatosis clinically and histologically or nasopharyngeal carcinoma clinically.

In addition to tuberculous mycobacteria, a variety of atypical/non-tuberculous mycobacteria can result in cervical lymphadenitis. These organisms can be found in water, milk (especially unpasteurized milk), dust, soil, and birds. Cervical lymphadenitis is a common presentation of atypical mycobacteria in immunocompetent patients, most commonly secondary to infection with *Mycobacterium scrofulaceum*, *Mycobacterium kansasii*, and *Mycobacterium avium-intracellulare*.

These patients present with enlarged, erythematous lymph nodes, mostly in the upper cervical region, but are generally afebrile. Less commonly, there can be involvement of submental, preauricular, middle, or lower cervical nodes. On imaging, there is usually asymmetric adenopathy with low-attenuation ring enhancing or multichambered masses and variable inflammatory infiltration of adjacent soft tissues, subcutaneous fat, and skin. In a small percentage of patients, the nodes may be calcified. One theory is that atypical mycobacteria enter the lymphatics through a mucosal break in the tonsils. In these patients, lymph nodes may spontaneously fistualize to the skin. The treatment of choice for cervical lymphadenitis secondary to atypical mycobacteria is surgical excision and not incision and drainage. These organisms are not susceptible to standard anti-TB therapeutic agents and therefore antibiotic therapy is not indicated. Distinction of scrofula secondary to *Mycobacterium tuberculosis* from atypical mycobacteria requires special cultures and hybridization techniques, and is required to guide proper management. It is generally believed that human-to-human transmission of atypical mycobacteria does not occur.

### Fungal and protozoan lymphadenitis

Fungal infections are typically superficial, affecting mucocutaneous tissues, except in immunocompromised patients where they can occasionally result in pulmonary infection or disseminated systemic infections. Lymphadenitis may occur in the context of cryptococcosis, histoplasmosis or coccidioidomycosis, among others. In general, the imaging findings are nonspecific, often resulting in enlarged and hyperplastic nodes. Protozoal lymphadenitis may occur after infection with toxomplasma gondii. Normal hosts are commonly asymptomatic but uncommonly can develop cervical lymphadenopathy along with symptoms of fever, myalgia, anorexia, headache, sore throat, and rash. Rarely, a more severe necrotizing systemic infection may occur.

### Other causes of reactive lymphadenopathy

Reactive lymphoid hyperplasia may develop secondary to a variety of causes. In addition to bacterial and viral infections, exposure to chemicals, environmental pollutants, drugs, or foreign antigens may result in lymphoid hyperplasia. These may develop in the form of an acute inflammatory response or a chronic immune response. Their imaging appearance is nonspecific, similar to findings described for viral lymphadenitis, consisting of typically normal or slightly enlarged, variably enhancing, and homogenous lymph nodes with smooth margins.

## Clinical syndromes associated with cervical lymphadenopathy

A number of syndromes may be associated with cervical lymphadenopathy and can either be primarily localized to cervical lymph nodes or have more a generalized manifestation. Two general imaging patterns are seen in these syndromes. One pattern consists of enlarged, internally heterogenous or "necrotic" Kikuchi disease and enhancing nodes, typically affecting regional nodes, as seen in patients with Kimura's and Kikuchi-Fujimoto disease. These can have associated soft-tissue infiltration, frequently involving the parotid or submandibular glands. In the second group, there tends to be homogenous hyperplastic enlarged lymph nodes, similar to that seen with lymphomatous disorders. Disorders that can present in this manner include sinus histiocytosis with massive lymphadenopathy, sarcoidosis, dermatopathic lymphadenopathy, angiofollicular lymph node hyperplasia, and tumor-reactive lymphadenopathy.

## Kimura's disease

Kimura's disease (KD) typically affects young adults age 27 to 40 years and is endemic to Asia. It is characterized by eosinophilic infiltrates and vascular proliferation with plump reactive endothelium with involvement of the lymph nodes and deep subcutaneous tissues. KD should be distinguished from angiolymphoid hyperplasia with eosinophilia which is primarily restricted to the dermis but not the deeper tissues as in KD. Clinically, KD has an insidious onset and presents with enlarging subcutaneous nodules and nodes mainly affecting the head and neck. There is also frequently involvement of the parotid gland and periauricular soft tissues, with less common involvement of other regions such as the oral cavity or structures outside the head and neck including the axilla, groin, and limbs. Although the disease is primarily regional, there can be systemic involvement with development of allergic asthma, myocarditis, and focal segmental glomerulosclerosis as a result of the eosinophilia. On imaging, nodal disease in KD can present as diffusely enhancing nodes or nodes with rim enhancement. Overall, the disease usually has a benign course and surgery is the treatment of choice.

## Kikuchi-Fujimoto disease

Kikuchi-Fujimoto lymphadenopathy (KFL) or Kikuchi's disease is a necrotizing lymphadenopathy common in Japan and sporadically seen in Western countries. The disease typically affects young females with a mean age of 30 years. Its etiology is not known, but is thought to represent the sequela of an autoimmune disorder. Patients typically present with unilateral or less commonly bilateral cervical lymphadenopathy. The lymph nodes can be tender and there may be associated systemic symptoms such as fever, chills, myalgia, sore throat, skin rash, localized pain, leukopenia, or leukocytosis. Less commonly, there can be more severe systemic signs and symptoms including weight loss, nausea, vomiting, night sweats, arthralgias, and hepatosplenomegaly. Rarely, there may also be skin and bone marrow involvement. On imaging, KD lymphadenopathy can present either as homogenously enhancing lymph nodes or internally heterogenous "necrotic" nodes (**Figures 11.25A to D**). The disease typically has a self-limiting course and resolves spontaneously within a few weeks or months.

## Sinus histiocytosis with massive lymphadenopathy

Sinus histiocytosis with massive lymphadenopathy (SHML) is also known as Rosai-Dorfman disease. It usually affects children and teenagers although it has a wide age of presentation including the elderly group, with no racial or geographical predisposition. The disease consists of proliferation of histiocytes within distended sinuses in lymph nodes with histiocytes containing ingested lymphocytes, referred to as emperipolesis. There can also be infiltration of soft-tissues. Patients can present with lymphadenopathy and as well can have infiltration of extranodal soft tissues including the ear, upper respiratory tract, gastrointestinal tract, and meninges, among others. The lymphadenopathy is generally painless and although enlarged

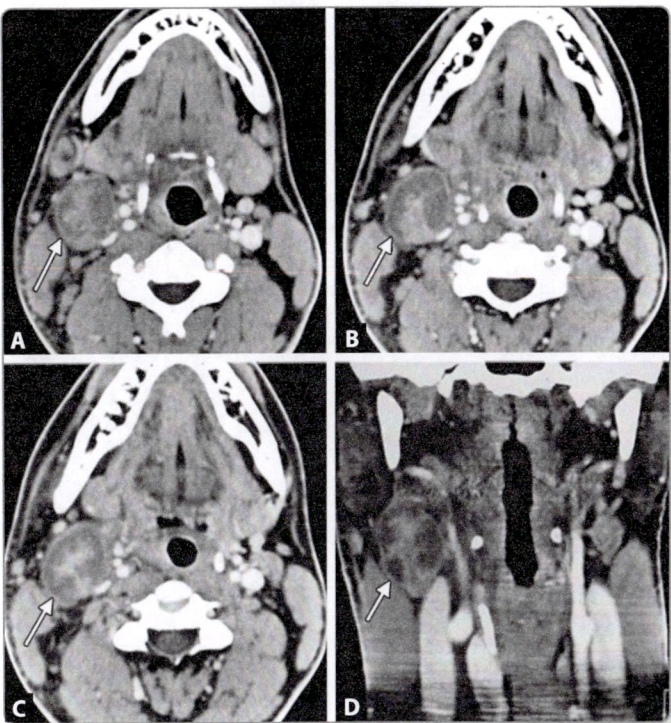

**Figures 11.25A to D** Kikuchi's disease. Axial contrast enhanced CT images (A, B, C) and a coronal reformatted image (D) from a 19-year-old man demonstrate a large internally heterogeneous (necrotic) node (arrow) with mixed areas of low-attenuation and enhancement in this patient with pathologically proven Kikuchi-Fujimoto lymphadenopathy, a necrotizing lymphadenopathy

lymph nodes can persist for several years, the disease is usually self-limited. Only rarely is there more severe disease with that can result in involvement of vital organs which can cause significant morbidity and mortality. On imaging, the typical appearance is that of massive nonspecific homogenous cervical lymphadenopathy that can measure up to 6 cm (**Figure 11.26**). There is no effective treatment.

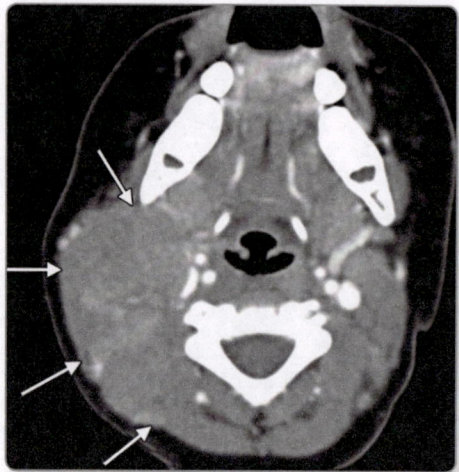

**Figure 11.26** Rosai-Dorfman disease (sinus histiocytosis with massive lymphadenopathy). Axial contrast enhanced CT image demonstrates a large enhancing nodal mass with an otherwise nonspecific appearance (arrows). Biopsy confirmed Rosai-Dorfman disease

## Sarcoidosis

Sarcoidosis is a systemic granulomatous disease of unknown etiology that can affect multiple organ systems, including lymph nodes. In the head and neck, sarcoid may involve the anterior or posterior cervical lymph node chains or present as extranodal disease. On imaging, sarcoidosis usually manifests as multiple reactive-appearing lymph nodes or enlarged nodes similar to those of lymphoma. Typically, there is no imaging evidence of extracapsular disease. When a patient has cervical lymphadenopathy and multiple parotid lymph nodes, the most likely diagnosis is either sarcoidosis or lymphoma.

## Dermatopathic lymphadenopathy

Dermatopathic lymphadenopathy is a disorder in which there is reactive lymph node hyperplasia in association with chronic inflammatory skin disease. Axillary, inguinal, and regional nodes are most commonly involved but cervical or facial lymph nodes can be involved when the dermatopathy affects the face. There are no specific imaging features to identify this uncommon disorder but it should be included as a possible differential in patients suffering from a chronic inflammatory skin disorder.

## Angiofollicular lymph node hyperplasia (Castleman's disease)

Angiofollicular lymph node hyperplasia, also known as Castleman's disease (CD), is a disease consisting of germinal center hyperplasia with interfollicular sheets of plasma cells and can be either unicentric, presenting as a solitary mass, or multicentric and systemic, presenting with widespread lymphadenopathy. The most common subtype is the hyaline vascular subtype, which can affect a wide age group but typically affects young patients. Patients present with single, asymptomatic masses of either cervical or mediastinal lymph nodes although there can be involvement of periparotid or intraparotid lymph nodes as well as extranodal soft tissues. Surgery is curative. The other subtype is the plasma cell subtype which tends to affect older patients. Unlike the hyaline vascular subtype, the plasma cell subtype is more likely to present and multicentric masses and often has systemic manifestations including the POEMS syndrome (polyneuropathy, organomegaly, endocrinopathy, monoclonal gammopathy, and skin abnormalities). It also follows a different clinical course from the hyaline vascular type with relapses or occasionally even progression to malignant lymphoma.

Involvement of the neck by CD is relatively uncommon. Typically, these present as a single neck mass although there are case reports of multicentric neck involvement (**Figures 11.27 and 11.28**). The imaging appearance is nonspecific and variable but there is typically marked enhancement (**Figures 11.27 and 11.28**). The nodes in KD can also have a heterogenous appearance and some have described a linear or stellate central low-attenuation area corresponding to a dense fibrous stroma forming a central scar.

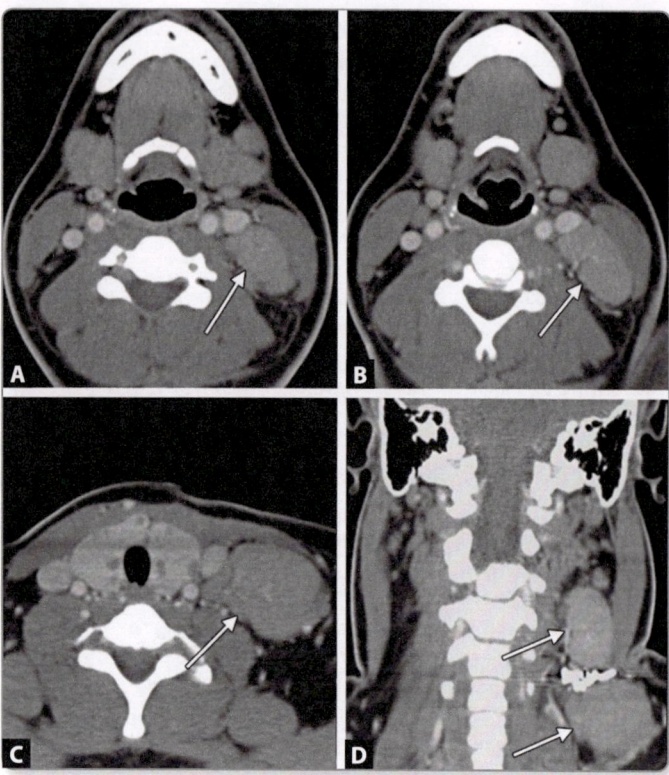

**Figures 11.27A to D** Angiofollicular lymph node hyperplasia (Castleman's disease). Axial contrast enhanced CT images (A, B, C) and a coronal reformatted image (D) from a 38-year-old patient demonstrate 2 large enhancing nodal masses (arrows). The surgical clips are from a prior biopsy. Incidentally, there is an enlarged thyroid gland with multiple small nodules. Although cervical lymphadenopathy in Castleman's frequently presents as a solitary mass, occasionally it can be multifocal as in this case

Imaging evaluation of cervical lymph nodes 487

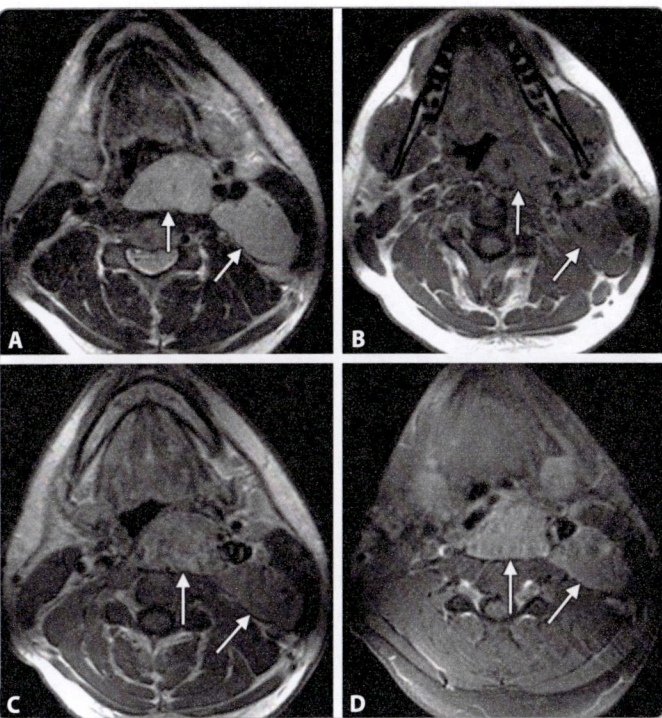

**Figures 11.28A to D** Angiofollicular lymph node hyperplasia (Castleman's disease). Axial T2 (A), T1 (B), postcontrast T1 (C) and fat-saturated postcontrast T1-weighted images are shown from a 15-year-old patient presenting with a neck mass. The images demonstrate large multifocal enhancing nodal masses. Biopsy demonstrated Castleman's disease

## Kawasaki's syndrome

Kawasaki's syndrome is also known as mucocutaneous lymph node syndrome. This is a systemic disorder of unknown etiology and manifests in infants or during early childhood. A variety of organ systems can be affected and these patients can present with fever, skin rash, aseptic meningitis, conjunctivitis, uveitis, strawberry tongue, and diffuse lymphadenopathy. The disease can also result in an acute necrotizing coronary arteritis leading to aneurysm formation, which may be fatal, and a small percentage of cases may have neurologic complications. On imaging, there can be unilateral nonspecific reactive appearing cervical lymphadenopathy.

### Tumor-reactive lymphadenopathy

Lymph nodes in the vicinity of a neoplasm are frequently enlarged, even though they may not harbor metastatic foci. On histology, there is typically reactive hyperplasia or occasionally the presence of sarcoid-type granulomas.

## Other miscellaneous causes of cervical lymphadenopathy on imaging

### Vascular-related lymphadenopathies

These are nonspecific entities thought to result from obstruction of nodal blood flow secondary to compression by tumor, vascular embolization and thrombosis, surgery or, rarely needle biopsy. Typically, the imaging findings are those of nonspecific reactive lymph nodes. The importance of vascular lymphadenopathies is the potential for confusion with vascular neoplasms in lymph nodes. Rarely, lymph nodes may infarct, most commonly secondary to involvement by either lymphoma or metastatic carcinoma.

### Foreign body lymphadenopathies

The presence of various endogenous or exogenous substances within tissues including but not limited to agents used for lymphangiography, silicone, Teflon, and gold may elicit a reactive adenopathy in the region of tissue drainage. If the inciting agent is radiodense, radiodensities may be seen within the reactive lymph nodes.

### Lymph node inclusions

Lymph nodes may harbor benign cellular inclusions including salivary gland inclusions, nevus cell inclusions, and thyroid follicles. The inclusions are typically microscopic and not identifiable on imaging. However, these may be seen within enlarged nodes on pathology and are important to recognize in order not to be confused as metastatic foci.

## Neoplastic causes of cervical lymphadenopathy

### Metastatic lymph nodes

*Overview of cervical lymph node staging*

The most widely accepted and clinically useful cancer staging system is the TNM (tumor, node, and metastasis) system. Metastases to lymph nodes carry a poor prognosis and determination of the extent of nodal metastasis is essential for proper patient staging and treatment planning. Essentially, any metastatic tumor may involve cervical nodes, either from a head and neck primary or a primary outside the head and neck. This includes head and neck squamous cell and other carcinomas (**Figures 11.10, 11.11, 11.19, 11.29 to 11.31, 11.36**), thyroid cancer (**Figures 11.9, 11.17, 11.32 to 11.34**), breast carcinoma, melanoma (**Figure 11.20**), renal cell carcinoma (**Figures 11.35A to C**), lung cancer (**Figure 11.37**), gastrointestinal tumors, and small round blue cell tumors (small cell carcinoma of lung, neuroblastoma, Ewing's sarcoma, alveolar rhabdomyosarcoma), among others. The imaging characteristics of cervical node metastases have already been described in detail in the section. *Imaging criteria for assessment of metastatic nodes.* The goal of nodal staging is to relate the overall number, size, and location of the affected nodes to the prognosis and to guide patient management. It should be noted that metastasis to any lymph node other than a regional node is considered distant metastasis. Furthermore, an increase in greatest nodal dimension above 3 cm and 6 cm, respectively, result in an increase in N stage (**Table 11.8**). It is noteworthy most nodal masses greater than 6 cm in diameter are not single nodes, but are either confluent conglomerate of nodes and/or tumor in the adjacent soft tissues.

There is a uniform N classification for cervical lymph node metastasis (**Table 11.8**) from all sites except for those arising from the nasopharynx, thyroid, and skin cancers (**Tables 11.9 to 11.13**). The reason is that tumors from the latter sites have sufficiently different behavior and prognosis that the AJCC has recognized the need for a separate nodal classification for these tumors. In addition, in the most recent 2010 AJCC manual, there has been a revision of the chapters describing nonmelanoma skin cancers. All nonmelanoma skin cancers

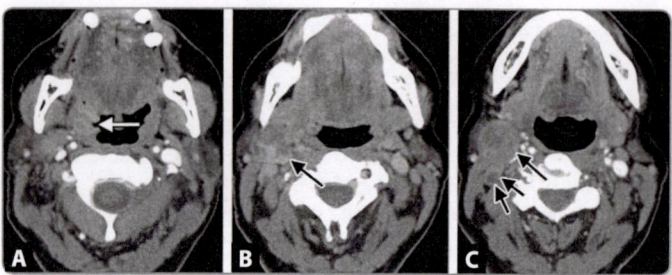

**Figures 11.29A to C** Pathologic nodes with internal heterogeneity (central necrosis) from tonsillar carcinoma. Axial contrast enhanced CT images demonstrate a mass centered in the right palatine tonsil (A; white arrow) with large and small right level II pathologic nodes with internal heterogeneity (frequently referred to as central necrosis) (B, C; black arrows). In a patient with a primary head and neck cancer, internal nodal heterogeneity is one of the most specific signs of a metastatic node, regardless of node size

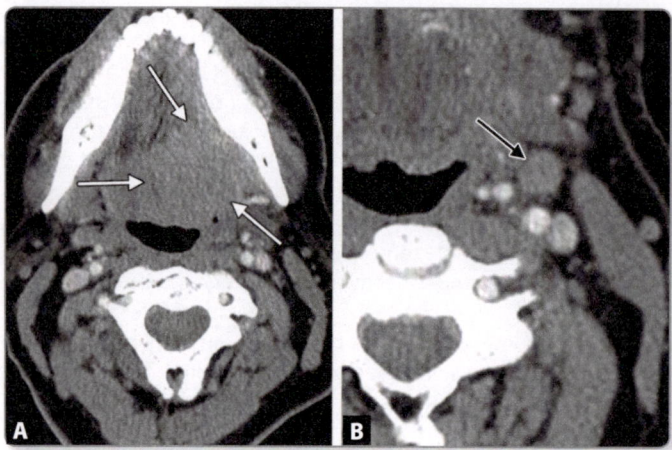

**Figures 11.30A and B** Pathologic node in a patient with squamous cell carcinoma of the tongue. Axial contrast enhanced CT images demonstrate a mass involving the posterior left oral tongue and base of tongue corresponding to a squamous cell carcinoma (A; white arrows). There is a rounded left level II node with fuzzy irregular margins (B; black arrow). Although not enlarged by size criteria, in the primary region of nodal drainage of a carcinoma, this appearance is highly suggestive of a nodal metastasis

Imaging evaluation of cervical lymph nodes **491**

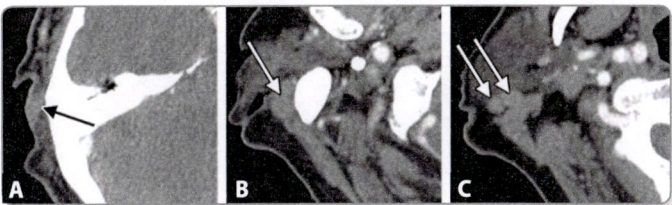

**Figures 11.31A to C** Metastatic nodes from Merkel cell skin carcinoma. Axial contrast enhanced CT images demonstrate focal skin thickening in the right periauricular area corresponding to a pathologically proven Merkel cell carcinoma (A; black arrow). There is a right postauricular node with subtle internal heterogeneity suspicious for a metastatic node (B; white arrow). There are also 2 small periparotid nodes with a rounded appearance and fuzzy margins (C; white arrows). While not definitive, these are also suspicious and were demonstrated to represent metastases on pathology. In cases of uncertainty, additional options for work-up of nodes include correlation with PET-CT or biopsy/resection

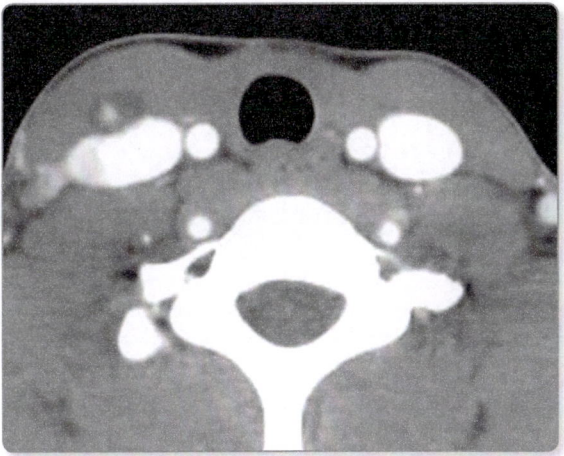

**Figure 11.32** Nodal metastasis from papillary thyroid cancer. Axial contrast enhanced CT image demonstrates a cystic right level IV node with a focus of nodular internal enhancement

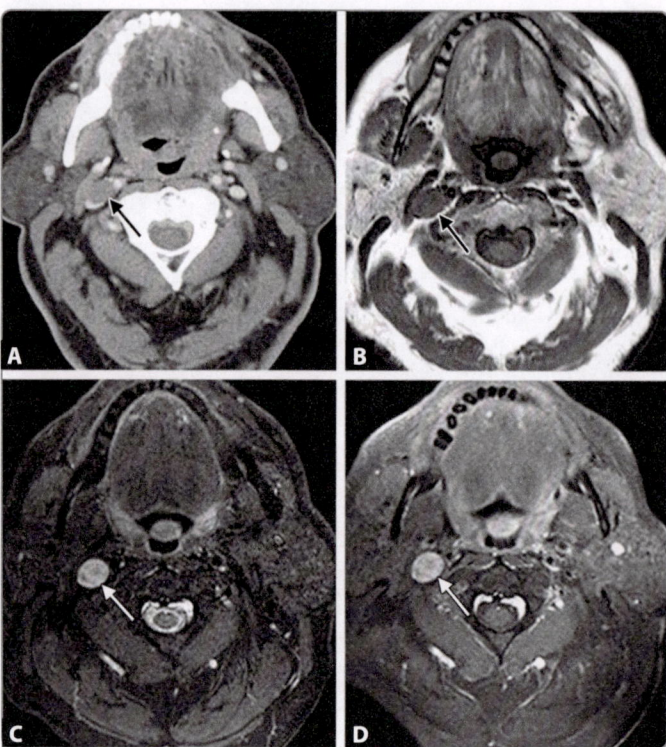

**Figures 11.33A to D** Nodal metastasis from papillary thyroid cancer. Axial (A) contrast enhanced CT, (B) T1W MRI, (C) STIR, and (D) postcontrast T1-SPIR MRI images are shown. On the CT scan, there is a right level IIA node (arrow) that is not significant by size but atypical because it exerts mass effect on the adjacent internal jugular vein. The MRI performed subsequently demonstrated growth of the node as well as mild internal heterogeneity (arrow)

other than Merkel cell carcinoma are staged according to the cutaneous squamous cell carcinoma staging system (**Table 11.11**). There is also a new separate chapter for Merkel cell carcinoma including a separate N classification system (**Table 11.12**). The melanoma N classification is described in **Table 11.13**.

Imaging evaluation of cervical lymph nodes  **493**

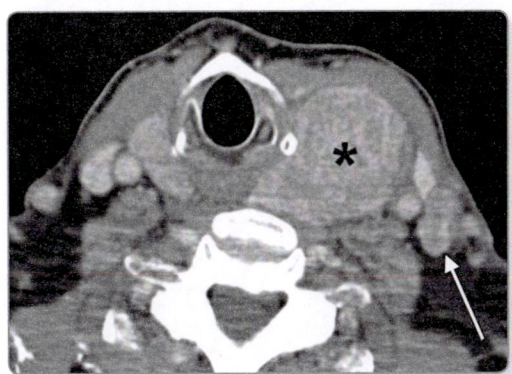

**Figure 11.34** Nodal metastasis from medullary thyroid cancer. Axial contrast enhanced CT image demonstrates a left thyroid mass (*) and an enlarged enhancing slightly heterogenous left level III node

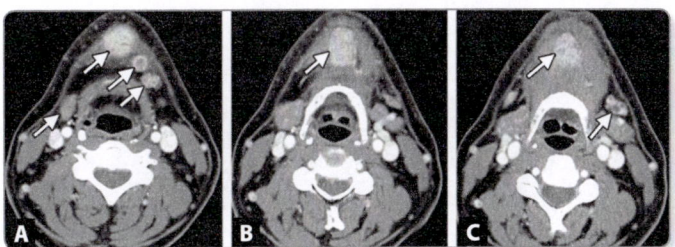

**Figures 11.35A to C** Nodal metastases from renal cell carcinoma. Axial contrast enhanced CT images demonstrate multiple avidly enhancing hypervascular level I nodes (arrows), some with internal heterogeneity (same case as in Figure 11.3)

## Specific neoplastic nodal pathologies

### Metastatic thyroid carcinoma

Although cervical node metastases can be seen with all histological subtypes of thyroid cancer, they are most commonly seen secondary to metastasis from papillary and follicular types. Metastatic nodes can have a variety of appearances and can present as either small

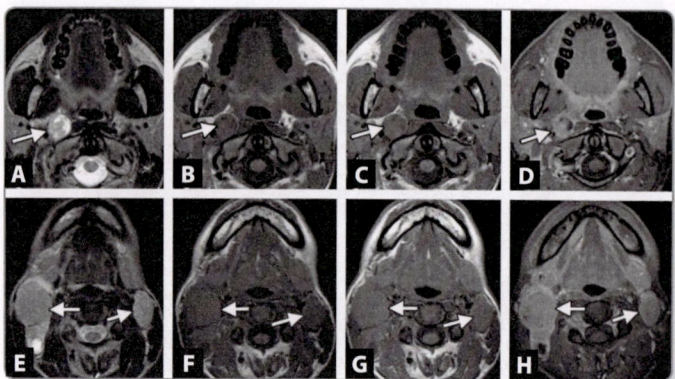

**Figures 11.36A to H** Nodal metastases from EBV related nasopharyngeal carcinoma. Axial (A, E) T2W, (B, F) T1W, (C, G) postgadolinium T1W, and (D, H) postgadolinium fat-saturated T1W MRI images demonstrate multiple pathologic nodes (arrows), some with internal heterogeneity (central necrosis). Note that the internal nodal heterogeneity and nodal contour irregularity with infiltration of the adjacent soft tissues (A – D) is most conspicuous on the fat-saturated contrast enhanced images (D, H)

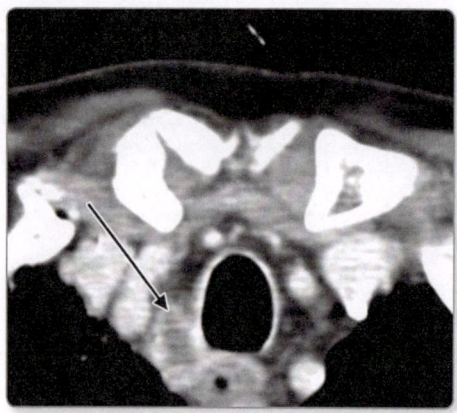

**Figure 11.37** Nodal metastasis from adenocarcinoma of the lung. Axial contrast enhanced CT image demonstrates a heterogeneously enhancing node in the right tracheoesophageal groove (arrow). Patient had vocal cord paralysis

| NX | Regional lymph nodes cannot be assessed |
|---|---|
| N0 | No regional lymph node metastasis |
| N1* | Metastasis in a single ipsilateral lymph node, 3 cm or less in greatest dimension |
| N2* | Metastasis in a single ipsilateral lymph node, more than 3 cm but not more than 6 cm in greatest dimension; or in multiple ipsilateral lymph nodes, none more than 6 cm in greatest dimension; or in bilateral or contralateral lymph nodes, none more than 6 cm in greatest dimension |
| N2a* | Metastasis in a single ipsilateral lymph node more than 3 cm but not more than 6 cm in greatest dimension |
| N2b* | Metastasis in multiple ipsilateral lymph nodes, none more than 6 cm in greatest dimension |
| N2c* | Metastasis in bilateral or contralateral lymph nodes, none more than 6 cm in greatest dimension |
| N3* | Metastasis in a lymph node more than 6 cm in greatest dimension |

*A designation of "U" or "L" may be used for any N stage to indicate metastasis above the lower border of the cricoid arch "U" or below this level "L". Similarly, clinical/radiological ECS (extracapsular spread) should be recorded as E− or E+, and histopathologic ECS should be designated En (not present), Em (microscopic), or Eg (gross).

**Table 11.8** The AJCC general nodal (N) staging system for head and neck cancers (from the AJCC Cancer Staging Manual, 7th Edn. Springer, 2010)

or hyperplastic nodes with variable enhancement (**Figures 11.9, 11.17, 11.32 to 11.34**). Nodes may harbor small foci of dystrophic calcification (although it should be noted that true psammomatous calcifications are only seen microscopically) (*see* **Figures 11.17A and B**). Lastly, thyroid nodal metastases can be completely cavitated or cystic, mimicking the appearance of a benign cyst which if encountered should alert the radiologist to the presence of a possible thyroid primary (*see* **Figures 11.9 and 11.32**). Hemorrhage may rarely be seen in thyroid nodal metastases (as well as other hypervascular tumors such as metastases from renal cell carcinoma). On MRI, metastatic thyroid cancer nodes typically have low to intermediate signal on T1- and high signal on T2-weighted images (*see* **Figures 11.9 and 11.33**)

| NX | Regional lymph nodes cannot be assessed |
|----|---|
| N0 | No regional lymph node metastasis |
| N1 | Unilateral metastasis in cervical lymph nodes (s), 6 cm or less in greatest dimension, above the supraclavicular fossa, and/or unilateral or bilateral, retropharyngeal lymph nodes, 6 cm or less, in greatest dimension* |
| N2 | Bilateral metastasis in cervical lymph nodes (s), 6 cm or less in greatest dimension, above the supraclavicular fossa* |
| N3 | Metastasis in lymph node (s)* > 6 cm and/or to supraclavicular fossa |
| N3a | Greater than 6 cm in greatest dimension |
| N3b | Extension to the supraclavicular fossa** |
| \* Midline nodes are considered ipsilateral nodes<br>\*\* Supraclavicular zone or fossa is the triangular region originally defined by Ho (see text). | |

**Table 11.9** The AJCC general nodal (N) staging system for nasopharyngeal carcinoma (from the AJCC Cancer Staging Manual, 7th Edn. Springer, 2010)

| NX | Regional lymph nodes cannot be assessed |
|----|---|
| N0 | No regional lymph node metastasis |
| N1 | Regional lymph node metastasis |
| N1a | Metastasis to level VI (pretracheal, paratracheal, and prelaryngeal/Delphian lymph nodes) |
| N1b | Metastasis to unilateral, bilateral, or contralateral cervical (Levels I, II, III, IV, or V) or retropharyngeal or superior mediastinal lymph nodes (level VII) |

**Table 11.10** The AJCC general nodal (N) staging system for thyroid carcinomas (from the AJCC Cancer Staging Manual, 7th Edn. Springer, 2010)

but occasionally the nodes may have high signal on both T1- and T2-weighted images, particularly with papillary thyroid carcinoma. This is believed to be secondary to high intranodal concentrations thyroglobulin or in rare cases secondary to intranodal hemorrhage.

## Imaging evaluation of cervical lymph nodes

| NX | Regional lymph nodes cannot be assessed |
|---|---|
| N0 | No regional lymph node metastasis |
| N1 | Metastasis in a single ipsilateral lymph node, 3 cm or less in greatest dimension |
| N2 | Metastasis in a single ipsilateral lymph node, more than 3 cm but not more than 6 cm in greatest dimension; or in multiple ipsilateral lymph nodes, none more than 6 cm in greatest dimension; or in bilateral or contralateral lymph nodes, none more than 6 cm in greatest dimension |
| N2a | Metastasis in a single ipsilateral lymph node more than 3 cm but not more than 6 cm in greatest dimension |
| N2b | Metastasis in multiple ipsilateral lymph nodes, none more than 6 cm in greatest dimension |
| N2c | Metastasis in bilateral or contralateral lymph nodes, none more than 6 cm in greatest dimension |
| N3 | Metastasis in a lymph node more than 6 cm in greatest dimension |

**Table 11.11** The AJCC nodal (N) staging system for cutaneous squamous cell carcinoma and other nonmelanoma skin cancers, except Merkel cell carcinoma (from the AJCC Cancer Staging Manual, 7th Edn. Springer, 2010)

| NX | Regional lymph nodes cannot be assessed |
|---|---|
| N0 | No regional lymph node metastasis |
| cN0 | Nodes negative by clinical exam* (no pathologic node exam performed) |
| pN0 | Nodes negative by pathologic exam |
| N1 | Metastasis in regional lymph node (s) |
| N1a | Micrometastasis** |
| N1b | Macrometastasis*** |
| N2 | In transit metastasis**** |

\* Clinical detection of nodal disease may be via inspection, palpation, and/or imaging
\*\* Micrometastases are diagnosed after sentinel or elective lymphadenectomy
\*\*\* Macrometastases are defined as clinically detectable nodal metastases confirmed by therapeutic lymphadenectomy or needle biopsy
\*\*\*\* In transit metastasis: A tumor distinct from the primary lesion located either (1) between the primary lesion and the draining regional lymph nodes or (2) distal to the primary lesion.

**Table 11.12** The AJCC nodal (N) staging system for Merkel cell carcinoma (from the AJCC Cancer Staging Manual, 7th Edn. Springer, 2010)

| NX | Patients in whom the regional lymph nodes cannot be assessed (e.g. previously removed for another reason) |
|---|---|
| N0 | No regional metastases detected |
| N1-3 | Regional metastases based upon the number of metastatic nodes and presence or absence of intralymphatic metastases (in transit or satellite metastases) |

*N1-3 and a-c subcategory assignment:*

| N classification | No. of metastatic nodes | Nodal metastatic mass |
|---|---|---|
| N1 | 1 node | a: Micrometastasis* <br> b: Macrometastasis** |
| N2 | 2–3 nodes | a: Micrometastasis* <br> b: Macrometastasis** <br> c: In transit met (s)/satellite (s) without metastatic nodes |
| N3 | 4 or more metastatic nodes, or matted nodes, or in transit met (s)/satellite (s) with metastatic node (s) | |

\* Micrometastases are diagnosed after sentinel lymph node biopsy and completion lymphadenectomy (if performed).
\*\* Macrometastases are defined as clinically detectable nodal metastases confirmed by therapeutic lymphadenectomy or when nodal metastasis exhibits gross extracapsular extension.

**Table 11.13** The AJCC nodal (N) staging system for melanoma (from the AJCC Cancer Staging Manual, 7th Edn. Springer, 2010)

## Lymphoproliferative disorders

Both lymphomas and leukemias consist of abnormal neoplastic proliferation of the cells of the immune system. Lymphomas are solid neoplasms consisting of proliferation of malignant cells within tissues, primarily the lymph nodes. Leukemia, on the other hand, is a neoplastic proliferation of either myelocytic or lymphocytic precursor cells, resulting in increased numbers of cells within the circulating blood compartment which may or may not have a discernible associated soft tissue infiltrative component. Classification of nodal regions is different for the lymphomas than for other metastatic cancers. In the currently accepted classifications of core nodal regions each entire side of the neck (including cervical, supraclavicular, occipital, and pre-auricular lymph nodes) is considered a core nodal region. Therefore, a single pathologic node on one side of the neck contaminates the entire side of the neck.

On imaging, nodes involved by lymphoma and leukemia have a similar appearance. Lymphomatous nodes can appear as normal-sized or enlarged lymph nodes with variable enhancement (**Figures 11.38 to 11.40**). The most common appearances are: (1) slightly enlarged, homogeneous nodes, similar to reactive lymphadenopathies, (2) enlarged, "foamy"-appearing nodes, (3) enlarged lymph nodes with a thin nodal capsule and central low-attenuation, or (4) a cluster of nodes with variable enhancement, some of which may have central low-attenuation. Usually, lymphomatous nodes are described as having relatively little extracapsular extension and infiltration of the adjacent fat planes and soft tissues, although the enlarged nodes will result in effacement of adjacent fat planes. While internal low-attenuation and heterogeneity "necrosis" can be seen in lymphoma, it is not as frequently seen as in comparably sized nodes from metastatic squamous carcinoma. As discussed earlier, if there is evidence of cervical lymphadenopathy and multiple parotid lymph nodes, the most likely differential considerations are lymphoma and sarcoidosis.

Another related and important group of disorders are the post-transplantation lymphoproliferative disorders (PTLD). These consist of lymphoid or plasmacytic proliferations that develop in the setting of solid organ or marrow transplantation and although uncommon, represent a significant cause of morbidity and mortality in that patient population. PTLD has variable pathology ranging from lymphoid hyperplasia to lymphoma. The major risk factors for development of PTLD are EBV-positive serology prior to transplantation, the type of organ transplanted, and the intensity and chronicity of the immunosuppressive regimen used after transplantation. On imaging, good immunosuppression after transplantation results in little if any adenoidal or palatine soft tissue fullness, even in young children. There are also typically fewer than normal small and reactive lymph

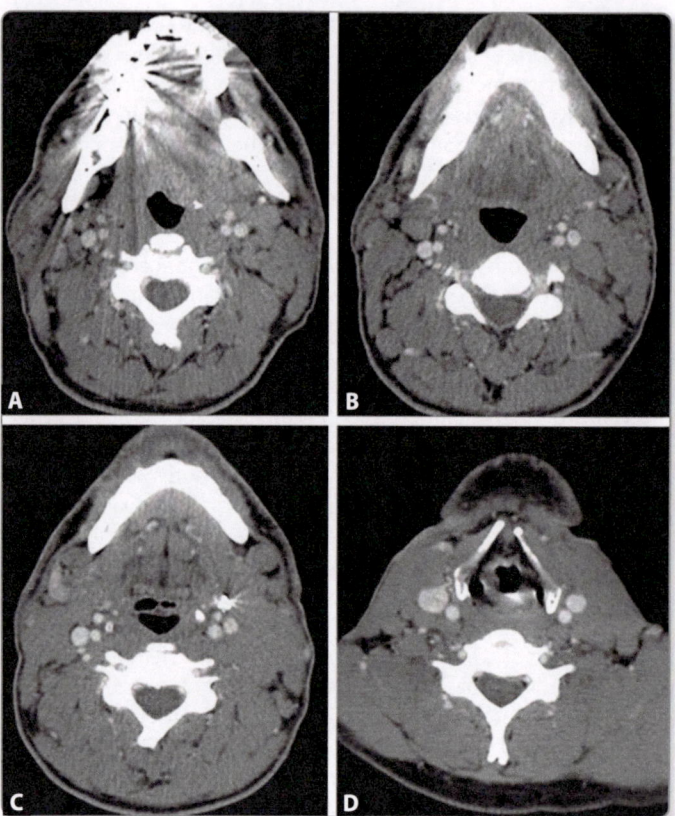

**Figures 11.38A to D** Non-Hodgkin's lymphoma. Axial contrast enhanced CT images demonstrate numerous homogenous nodes bilaterally. The surgical clips are from an excisional biopsy

nodes in the neck. Development of PTLD results in an increase in the size and number of cervical lymph nodes and thickness of lymphoid tissue of the Waldeyer's ring structures, with the adenoidal fullness being a more reliable sign than increases in the size of the palatine or lingual tonsils. In the setting of a transplant and immunosuppression,

Imaging evaluation of cervical lymph nodes  501

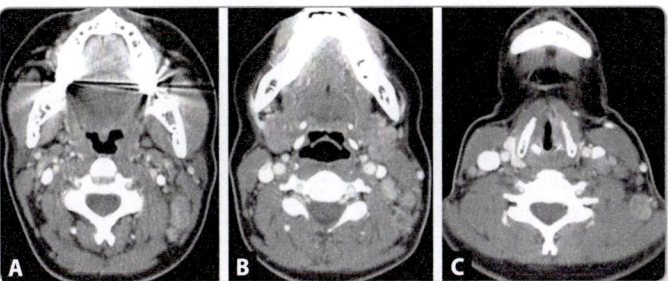

**Figures 11.39A to C** Non-Hodgkin's lymphoma. Axial contrast enhanced CT images demonstrate the variable appearance of lymph nodes in lymphoma, including internally heterogeneous nodes

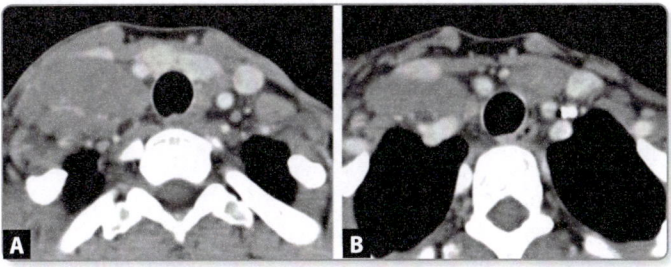

**Figures 11.40A and B** Hodgkin's lymphoma. Axial contrast enhanced CT images demonstrate variably enlarged nodes with a unilateral predominance

a serial increase in the adenoidal soft tissues or the size and number of cervical lymph nodes should raise suspicion for the presence of PTLD.

## Proliferative histiocytic disorders

Proliferative histiocytic disorders consist of a broad group of disorders of monocyte-macrophage and dendritic cell proliferation that are difficult to classify. A detailed discussion of these disorders is beyond the scope of this chapter, but they include, among others, entities such as true histiocytic lymphoma, hemophagocytic lymphohistiocytosis, Rosai-Dorfman disease (discussed earlier), and Langerhan's cell histiocytosis (LCH). LCH is the term applied to a group of childhood disorders of unknown etiology characterized by a polymorphous cellular infiltrate of mononuclear or multinucleated histiocytes (Langerhan's cells) mixed with eosinophils, granulocytes, and lymphocytes. Three forms of LCH are commonly described in the literature and include eosinophilic granuloma (EG), Hand-Schuller Christian disease, and Letterer-Siwe disease. EG is a localized manifestation of LCH, frequently presenting as a solitary bone lesion, whereas Hand-Schuller Christian disease and Letterer-Siwe disease present with multifocal disease, including involvement of lymph nodes. The head and neck is frequently involved in LCG including facial rash, cervical lymphadenopathy, and involvement of the skull and mandible with otitis media or destructive lesions of the temporal bone. Other disorders of the mononuclear phagocytic system include malignant histiocytosis (MH) and true histiocytic lymphoma (THL) with a somewhat arbitrary distinction between the two entities. MH usually presents with systemic symptoms, pancytopenia, adenopathy, and hepatosplenomegaly, whereas THL presents as a localized mass derived from the tissue histiocytes that may or may not disseminate.

### Other nodal neoplasms

Kaposi's sarcoma is a vascular neoplasm that among other organs can affect lymph nodes. KS can have a wide range of presentations including small raised reddish-purple skin nodules, involvement of various mucosal sites in the head and neck including the oral region and upper airway, enlarged lymph nodes, and occasionally fulminant disease with extensive cutaneous and visceral involvement. On imaging, KS nodes are typically enlarged, enhance, and often have a heterogenous internal morphology. Rarely primary spindle cell tumors and inflammatory nodal pseudotumors may arise in lymph nodes but a detailed discussion of these disorders is beyond the scope of this chapter.

## Conclusion

Evaluation of cervical lymphadenopathy is an essential part of head and neck imaging. Imaging can confirm and further characterize lymphadenopathy suspected on physical exam and identify nodes not palpable on physical examination. In addition, imaging can identify complications of nodal disease, enable follow-up, and in the setting of primary head and neck pathologies characterize the primary inciting disease. In staging of cancer, the radiologist and clinical team need to understand both the advantages and limitations of current anatomic criteria for identification of metastatic lymph nodes and use more advanced imaging techniques such as PET when warranted. Despite their limitations, cross-sectional imaging modalities such as CT and MRI are essential tool in work-up and staging of cancer patients. In the future, the use of iron oxide particles or advanced MRI sequences may further increase accuracy of imaging for staging of cancer and enable better distinction from non-neoplastic reactive lymph nodes.

## Acknowledgments

The authors would like to thank Ms Veronika Glyudza for assistance with the preparation of figures for this manuscript.

## Bibliography

1. Curtin HD, Ishwaran H, Mancuso AA, Dalley RW, Caudry DJ, McNeil BJ. Comparison of CT and MR imaging in staging of neck metastases. Radiology. 1998;207:123-30.
2. Don DM, Anzai Y, Lufkin RB, Fu YS, Calcaterra TC. Evaluation of cervical lymph node metastases in squamous cell carcinoma of the head and neck. Laryngoscope. 1995;105:669-74.
3. Edge SB. American Joint Committee on Cancer. AJCC cancer staging manual. New York: Springer; 2010.
4. Feinmesser R, Freeman JL, Noyek AM, Birt BD. Metastatic neck disease. A clinical/radiographic/pathologic correlative study. Arch Otolaryngol Head Neck Surg. 1987;113:1307-10.
5. Flint PW, Cummings CW. Cummings otolaryngology—head and neck surgery. Philadelphia, PA: Mosby/Elsevier; 2010.
6. Friedman M, Shelton VK, Mafee M, Bellity P, Grybauskas V, Skolnik E. Metastatic neck disease. Evaluation by computed tomography. Arch Otolaryngol. 1984;110:443-7.
7. Hayasaka H, Taniguchi K, Fukai S, Miyasaka M. Neogenesis and development of the high endothelial venules that mediate lymphocyte trafficking. Cancer Sci. 2010;101:2302-8.
8. Hopkins KL, Simoneaux SF, Patrick LE, Wyly JB, Dalton MJ, Snitzer JA. Imaging manifestations of cat-scratch disease. AJR Am J Roentgenol. 1996;166:435-8.

9. Kaji AV, Mohuchy T, Swartz JD. Imaging of cervical lymphadenopathy. Semin Ultrasound CT MR. 1997;18:220-49.
10. Mancuso AA, Harnsberger HR, Muraki AS, Stevens MH. Computed tomography of cervical and retropharyngeal lymph nodes: Normal anatomy, variants of normal, and applications in staging head and neck cancer. Part II: pathology. Radiology. 1983;148:715-23.
11. Nadel DM, Bilaniuk L, Handler SD. Imaging of granulomatous neck masses in children. Int J Pediatr Otorhinolaryngol. 1996;37:151-62.
12. Robbins KT, Clayman G, Levine PA, et al. Neck dissection classification update: revisions proposed by the American Head and Neck Society and the American Academy of Otolaryngology-Head and Neck Surgery. Arch Otolaryngol Head Neck Surg. 2002;128:751-58.
13. Robson CD, Hazra R, Barnes PD, Robertson RL, Jones D, Husson RN. Nontuberculous mycobacterial infection of the head and neck in immunocompetent children: CT and MR findings. AJNR Am J Neuroradiol. 1999;20:1829-35.
14. Som PM, Brandwein MS. Lymph Nodes. In: Som PM, Curtin HD (Eds). Head and neck imaging. 5th edn. St. Louis, Mo.: Mosby; 2011.
15. Som PM, Curtin HD, Mancuso AA. An imaging-based classification for the cervical nodes designed as an adjunct to recent clinically based nodal classifications. Arch Otolaryngol Head Neck Surg. 1999;125:388-96.
16. Som PM. Lymph nodes of the neck. Radiology. 1987;165:593-600.
17. Steinkamp HJ, Hosten N, Richter C, Schedel H, Felix R. Enlarged cervical lymph nodes at helical CT. Radiology. 1994;191:795-8.
18. Tohya K, Umemoto E, Miyasaka M. Microanatomy of lymphocyte-endothelial interactions at the high endothelial venules of lymph nodes. Histol Histopathol. 2010;25:781-94.
19. van den Brekel MW, Stel HV, Castelijns JA, et al. Cervical lymph node metastasis: Assessment of radiologic criteria. Radiology. 1990;177:379-84.
20. Vargiami EG, Farmaki E, Tasiopoulou D, et al. A patient with Lemierre syndrome. Eur J Pediatr. 2010;169:491-3.

# The larynx and the hypopharynx

**chapter 12**

**Eric S Bartlett**

### Abstract
The larynx and the hypopharynx occupy the mid-portion of the aerodigestive tract. Although the larynx and the hypopharynx have completely separate functions, they are essentially duplexed structures since they share a common wall. This close anatomic relationship has important implications in the setting of disease. This chapter discusses the anatomy, function and the imaging of the normal and diseased larynx and hypopharynx.

### Keywords
Larynx, supraglottic, glottic, subglottic, pharynx, hypopharynx, cricoid cartilage, arytenoid cartilage, thyroid cartilage, aryepiglottic folds, squamous cell carcinoma, laryngocele, vocal cord paralysis, Wegener's granulomatosis, laryngeal papillomatosis, chondrosarcoma.

## Introduction

The larynx and the hypopharynx occupy the mid-portion of the aerodigestive tract, extending from the level of the hyoid bone through to the level of the inferior cricoid cartilage. Although the larynx and the hypopharynx have completely separate functions, they are essentially duplexed structures since they share a common wall. Thus, any discussion of the larynx should always consider the hypopharynx and vice versa.

There are three main functions of the larynx:
1. Maintenance of the airway.
2. Protection against aspiration.
3. Phonation.

The larynx contains the only complete cartilaginous ring within the airway, the cricoid cartilage. The cricoid cartilage therefore plays a very important role in maintaining a patent airway as well as creating a foundation for the remaining structures of the larynx. Along the posterior wall of the larynx, the cricoid cartilage supports the arytenoid cartilages as well as many of the intrinsic muscles of the true vocal cords that function to protect the airway against aspiration and to create speech.

The hypopharynx is the lower portion of the pharynx. The primary function of the hypopharynx is less eloquent than that of the larynx, serving as a conduit from the oropharynx to the upper cervical esophagus. The tongue provides the major force that propels the food through the hypopharynx. The pharyngeal constrictor muscles also help to provide local peristalsis above a food bolus and receptive relaxation below the bolus to aid in its passage through the hypo-pharynx. The pyriform sinuses, the lateral pouches along the anterior wall of the upper hypopharynx, may have an additional minor function, serving as small acoustic chambers in the high frequency speech spectra. However, within the emergency medical setting, the pyriform sinuses have a more common and obvious function—the trapping of foreign bodies, such as coins and toys in children, and fish/chicken bones in adults. The pyriform sinuses are therefore prone to injury, including risk of perforation.

The larynx develops from two distinct embryologic components that are separated at the level of the laryngeal ventricle—the structure separates the supraglottic and glottic portions of the larynx. The upper and largest portion of the larynx, the supraglottic larynx, develops from the primitive buccopharyngeal anlage. The lower portions of the larynx, the glottis (level of the true vocal cords) and the subglottic larynx develop from the tracheobronchial buds within the tracheobronchial diverticulum. The clinical importance of this separation occurs within a pathologic setting such as infection or cancer. The embryologic origin of the supraglottic larynx is associated with a lush lymphatic system. The embryologic origin of the glottic and subglottic larynx is associated with a sparse lymphatic system. Therefore, a pathologic condition within the supraglottic larynx has a much higher likelihood to be associated with reactive or metastatic lymphadenopathy.

The hypopharynx forms from the 4th and 6th pharyngeal arch during embryologic development, with the 5th pharyngeal arch being quickly resorbed. Despite its origin from two separate pharyngeal arches, there is no corresponding clinical importance of this separation.

## The role of imaging

The endolaryngeal mucosa is readily visualized by the clinician, either indirectly with a mirror, or directly with an endoscope. If the visual examination of the mucosa is inconclusive, a more direct examination can be performed under anesthesia for a more complete visualization of the mucosa and the ability to biopsy any areas that appear suspicious for malignancy.

Laryngeal pathology is often identified relatively early in its development since even very small pathologic abnormalities can result in obvious changes to the functioning of the larynx. Common signs/symptoms of laryngeal pathology include: Changes in phonation (hoarseness), breathing difficulty (stridor, dyspnea), aspiration, hemoptysis, and referred otalgia (irritation of the vagus nerve—cranial nerve X).

Since the presence of laryngeal pathology is often clinically obvious, medical imaging has a minimal role in the initial detection of a laryngeal abnormality. Approximately, 95 percent of all malignancies of the larynx are squamous cell carcinomas (SCCa). Thus, SCCa is one of the most common indications for medical imaging. The role of the radiologist in this situation is to define the submucosal and deep soft tissue extension of the disease. Specifically, the radiologist plays an important role in defining cartilaginous tumor involvement and identifying extralaryngeal extension of tumor. Additionally, the radiologist plays an important role in staging the neck for nodal metastasis.

In contrast, since the function of the hypopharynx is primarily to act as a conduit to the upper esophagus, hypopharyngeal pathology is often asymptomatic until reaching an advanced stage, especially in the case of cancer. Thus, the majority of hypopharynx tumors present at highly advanced stages and typically have the worst prognosis among all cases of SCCa within the head and neck. These tumors also have a high rate of local and distant nodal metastases at the time of initial presentation.

Since hypopharyngeal pathology is often asymptomatic, medical imaging has a greater role in providing the initial diagnosis of disease. The radiologist is also essential in defining the local tumor extent around the hypopharynx, including potential involvement of the larynx anteriorly, the prevertebral soft tissues posteriorly and the internal/common carotid arteries lateral to hypopharynx.

Injury to the hypopharynx due to ingestion of foreign bodies is an obvious exception in the typical delayed timeline in hypopharyngeal pathology. This is especially true in cases of hypopharyngeal perforation that can be associated with ingestion of a fish bone or chicken bone. The perforation is often in the region of the pyriform sinus. In a case of hypopharyngeal perforation, computed tomographic (CT) imaging would typically show free air along the soft tissue and fascial planes of the neck around the hypopharynx. If the perforation involves the retropharyngeal space, there is a risk of developing a retropharyngeal abscess if not appropriately treated following injury. This can lead to a medical emergency if the retropharyngeal abscess extends inferiorly to involve the mediastinum.

Computed tomography is the primary imaging modality for both the larynx and the hypopharynx due to its fast speed of imaging, relatively high resolution and its availability within most communities. The use of IV contrast is preferred and is often performed using a 2-stage bolus. The first injection stage provides time for the contrast to reach the mucosa. The second injection stage insures that there is contrast present within the neck arteries. The neck should be imaged from vertex or near-vertex, through the level of the clavicular heads (**Figures 12.1A and B**). If the indication for imaging is due to vocal cord paralysis, the imaging should extend inferiorly through the level of the tracheal carina and the aortic arch to evaluate for potential upper mediastinal masses that may involve the recurrent laryngeal nerves. All axial images should be viewed in 2 mm increments. Reformats along the plane of the glottis should be performed in 1 mm increments with a smaller field of view (**Figures 12.2A to D**), extending from the hyoid bone through the cricoid cartilage. All cases should have 2 mm reformats in the coronal and sagittal planes (**Figures 12.3A and B**).

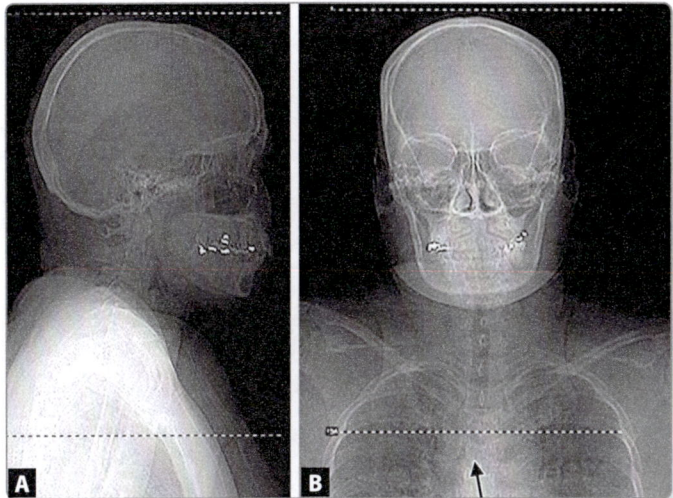

**Figures 12.1A and B** Computed tomography (CT) scout images showing the superior and inferior margins at the vertex and below the level of the clavicular heads, respectively. The solid black arrow is pointing to the carina

There is a limited application for magnetic resonance imaging (MRI) of the larynx and hypopharynx. Beyond having a lower image resolution than CT, MR imaging of the neck below the level of the hyoid bone is often of poor quality due to patient motion associated with breathing and swallowing. Tumor within the larynx and/or hypopharynx may also interefere with the patient's ability to lay supine within the MRI scanner for the duration of the exam (approximately 45 minutes). Patient discomfort, along with impaired respiration and difficulty with managing secretions, precludes MR imaging in some patients with advanced disease.

# Imaging anatomy—larynx

## Laryngeal cartilages

The laryngeal cartilages create the framework that protects the endolaryngeal structures and supports its functions of airway

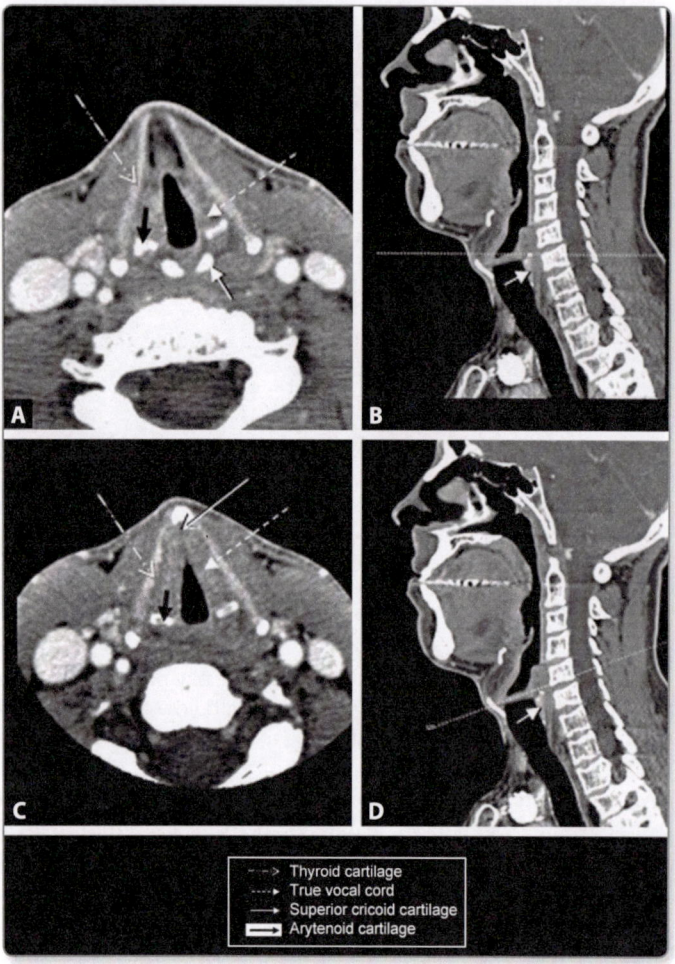

**Figures 12.2A to D** (A and B) Axial images through the posterior aspect of the true vocal cord: Sagittal showing the angle of imaging through the neck in a standard head and neck CT. This angle is not parallel to the true vocal cords; (C and D) Axial reformatted images through the true vocal cords: Sagittal showing the plane of the axial reformatted image that is parallel to the true vocal cords

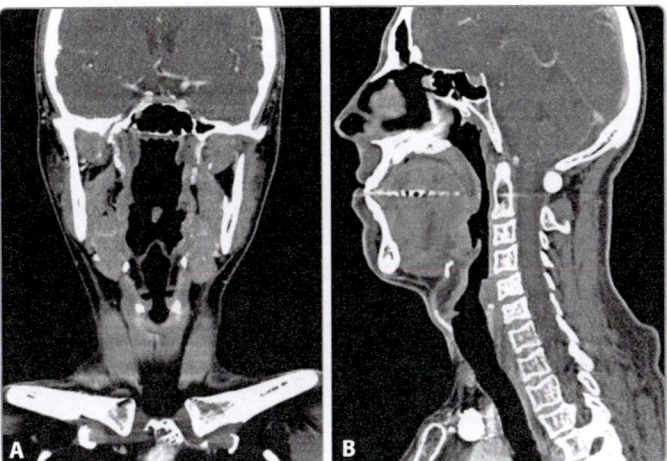

**Figures 12.3A and B** CT reformats in the coronal and sagittal planes (left and right, respectively). The reformats are created at 2 mm intervals

management and phonation. The largest and most superficial cartilage is the thyroid cartilage. The thyroid cartilage acts as a shield to protect the anterior larynx.

There are bilateral cornua along the superior and inferior margins of the posterior thyroid cartilage. The superior cornua of the thyroid cartilage are along the posterior margin of the thyrohyoid ligament that extends from the hyoid bone superiorly, to the top of the thyroid cartilage lamina. The inferior cornua of the thyroid cartilage extend inferiorly from the lower margins of the thyroid cartilage lamina to articulate with the medical aspects of the cricoid cartilage.

Along the anterior aspect of the thyroid cartilage, the midline thyroepiglottic ligament attaches at the inferior aspect of the epiglottic cartilage to the anterior thyroid cartilage (**Figure 12.4**). The endolaryngeal mucosa overlying this attachment helps to define the anterior aspect of the laryngeal ventricle. This is superior to another important anterior attachment to the anterior thyroid cartilage, the anterior attachment of the true vocal cords, called the anterior commissure (**Figure 12.4**). These structures are easily identified on the midline sagittal image through the larynx.

As previously mentioned, the cricoid cartilage is the only complete cartilaginous ring within the airway, and thus provides significant structural integrity to the airway and the larynx. The cricoid cartilage has a "signet" ring shape, with the anterior arch of the cricoid resembling the ring's "band", and the larger posterior lamina resembling the ring's "signet". The inferior border of the cricoid cartilage is the junction of the larynx and trachea.

The arytenoid cartilages are paired, pyramidal-shaped cartilages that sit along the superior aspect of the posterior cricoid cartilage lamina. The vertical height of the arytenoid cartilages spans the height of the laryngeal ventricle, thus the majority of the arytenoid cartilages are within the inferior aspect of the supraglottic larynx. The vocal and muscular processes at the base of the arytenoid cartilages provide

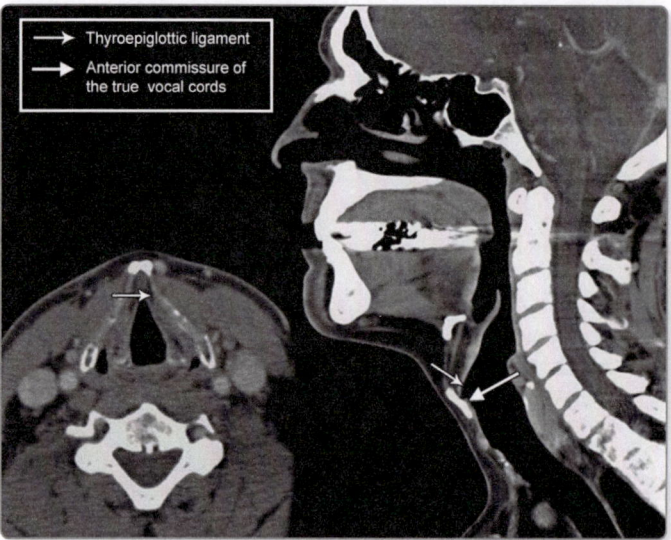

**Figure 12.4** Axial at the level of the thyroepiglottic ligament. Sagittal at midline

1. **Muscles varying the rima glottidis**
   **Transverse arytenoid**: Approximates the arytenoid cartilages and closes the rima glottidis posteriorly, decreasing the posterior commissure; causes adduction of the vocal cords; breath holds
   **Lateral cricoarytenoid**: Rotates the arytenoids medially to close the rima glottidis; adduction of the vocal cords; breath holds, helps to protect the airway against aspiration
   **Posterior cricoarytenoid**: Opposes the lateral cricoarytenoids; opens the rima glottidis by rotating the arytenoids laterally; abduction of the vocal cords; quiet respiration, relaxed state

2. **Muscles regulating tension in the vocal ligaments**
   **Cricothyroids**: Elongates and tenses the vocal cords by tilting the cricoid cartilage posteriorly and inferiorly in relation to the thyroid cartilage; important for phonation, especially higher pitch phonation
   **Posterior cricoarytenoids**: Elongates the vocal cords by medially rotating the muscular process of the arytenoids, thus laterally rotating the vocal process and opening the rima glottidis
   **Thyroarytenoid and vocalis**: Relaxes and shortens the vocal cords by pulling the arytenoid cartilages forward towards the thyroid cartilage

3. **Muscles modifying the laryngeal inlet**
   **Oblique arytenoid and aryepiglottic**: Narrows the rima glottidis during a cough or swallow to protect the airway
   **Thyroepiglottic**: Opens the rima glottidis; opposes the oblique arytenoid and aryepiglottic muscles

**Table 12.1** Three functional groups of the intrinsic laryngeal muscles.

the muscular attachments for the thyroarytenoid and cricoarytenoid muscles, respectively, and are at the level of the glottis.

## Intrinsic laryngeal musculature

There are three functional groups to the intrinsic laryngeal musculature: (1) muscles that vary the opening between the vocal cords and the arytenoid cartilages (the rima glottidis), (2) muscles that regulate the tension within the vocal ligaments, and (3) muscles that modify the size of the laryngeal inlet (**Table 12.1**).

## Mucosal surfaces of the endolarynx

There are three distinct regions within endolarynx: (1) the supraglottic, (2) glottic, and (3) the subglottic larynx (**Figure 12.5**).

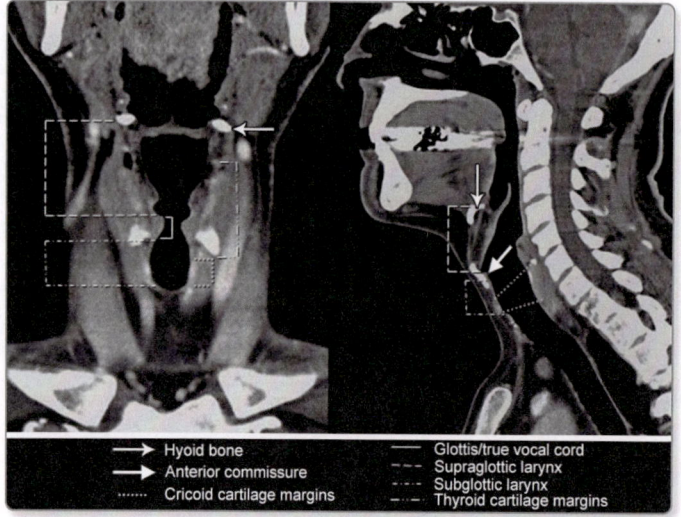

**Figure 12.5** Coronal image from the inferior mandible through the clavicular heads showing the three parts of the larynx. Sagittal and midline through the larynx

The supraglottic larynx extends from the level of the hyoid bone through the false vocal folds and the laryngeal ventricle, inferiorly. Anteriorly, the supraglottic larynx includes the pre-epiglottic fat and the paraglottic fat along the aryepiglottic folds. The medial or inner-mucosal surface of the aryepiglottic folds belongs to the mucosal surfaces of the supraglottic larynx (**Figures 12.6A to C**).

The glottis includes only the true vocal cords. The muscles of the true vocal cord include the larger thyroarytenoid muscle that attaches to the thyroid cartilage anteriorly to define the anterior commissure, and attaches to the vocal process of the arytenoid cartilage posteriorly. The vocalis muscle is the small medial muscle that is along the leading edge of the true vocal cord, deep to the vocal ligament. There is a thin paraglottic fat stripe between the thyroid cartilage and the thyroarytenoid muscle. When there is a glottic tumor, the preservation of this fat stripe proves that the tumor has not extended to or

The larynx and the hypopharynx 515

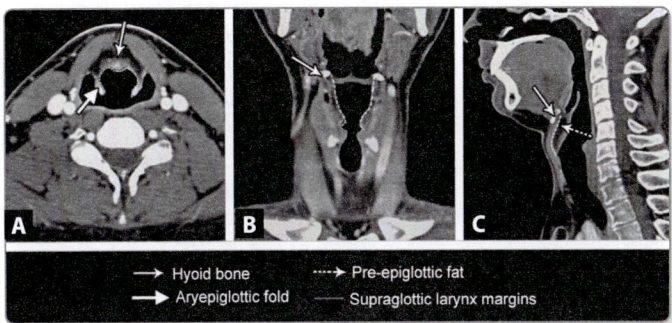

**Figures 12.6A to C** Axial, coronal and sagittal images through the supraglottic larynx

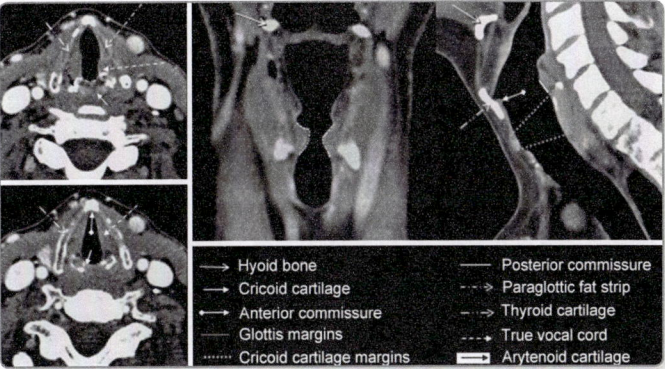

**Figure 12.7** Axial, coronal and sagittal images through the glottis. The axial images are not parallel to the true vocal cords; the superior image is through the posterior true vocal cords; the inferior image is 2 mm lower, showing the anterior commissure

through the overlying thyroid cartilage at the glottic level. The anterior commissure is easily visualized on the midline sagittal image through the larynx, appearing as a small triangular soft tissue along the endoluminal aspect of the thyroid cartilage, below the attachment of the thyroepiglottic ligament (**Figure 12.7**). On routine axial imaging through the glottis, the glottis is usually oblique to the axial imaging plane with the posterior glottis appearing in a more superior image in comparison to the anterior commissure. On these routine images, the posterior glottis will be on the first axial image where both the arytenoid cartilages and the posterior cricoid cartilage are present (**Figure 12.7**).

The subglottic larynx is below the level of the true vocal cords and extends inferiorly through the inferior aspect of the cricoid cartilage (**Figures 12.8A to C**). The superior trachea is inferior to the cricoid cartilage.

# Imaging anatomy—hypopharynx

The hypopharynx also extends from the level of the hyoid bone through the level of the inferior cricoid cartilage, connecting the oropharynx to the cervical esophagus. There are three main regions of the hypopharynx: (1) the posterior wall, (2) pyriform sinus, and (3) postcricoid hypopharynx (**Figures 12.9 and 12.10**).

The posterior wall is a flat mucosal layer that creates the posterior margin of the hypopharynx. The posterior hypopharyngeal wall is continuous with the posterior wall of the oropharynx (**Figures 12.9 and 12.10**).

The anterior wall of the hypopharynx is composed of the remaining two regions of the hypopharynx—the pyriform sinus and the postcricoid hypopharynx. The pyriform sinuses are paired anterolateral

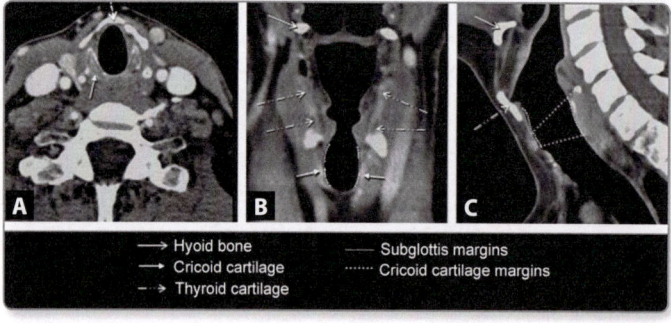

→ Hyoid bone
→ Cricoid cartilage
--→ Thyroid cartilage
— Subglottis margins
⋯ Cricoid cartilage margins

**Figures 12.8A to C** Axial, coronal and sagittal images through the subglottic larynx

The larynx and the hypopharynx 517

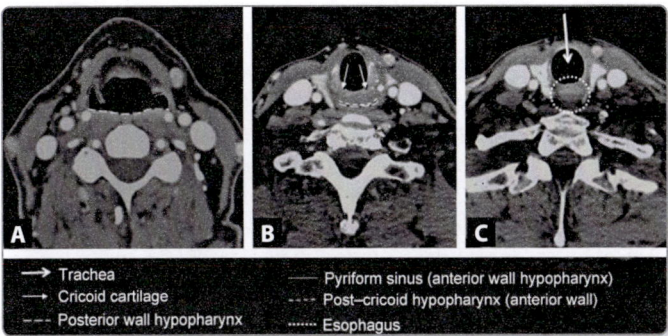

- → Trachea
- → Cricoid cartilage
- --- Posterior wall hypopharynx
- ⎯ Pyriform sinus (anterior wall hypopharynx)
- ---- Post–cricoid hypopharynx (anterior wall)
- ······ Esophagus

**Figures 12.9A to C** (A) Axial through the upper hypopharynx; (B) Axial through the lower hypopharynx (C) Axial inferior to the hypopharynx, showing the trachea and esophagus

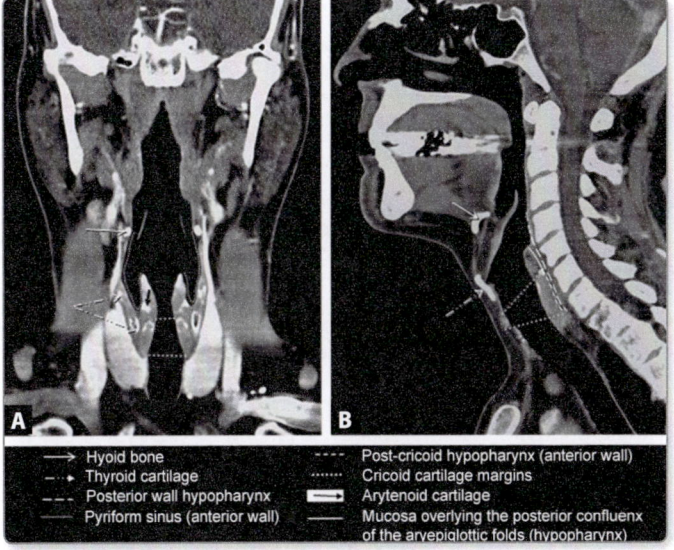

- → Hyoid bone
- --→ Thyroid cartilage
- --- Posterior wall hypopharynx
- ⎯ Pyriform sinus (anterior wall)
- ---- Post-cricoid hypopharynx (anterior wall)
- ······ Cricoid cartilage margins
- ⇨ Arytenoid cartilage
- ⎯ Mucosa overlying the posterior confluenx of the aryepiglottic folds (hypopharynx)

**Figures 12.10A and B** Coronal and sagittal images through the hypopharynx

recesses of the upper hypopharynx that have an inverted pyramid shape with the apex of the pyramid at the level of the true vocal cord (**Figures 12.9 and 12.10**). The anterior mucosal boundaries of the pyriform sinuses are defined by the lateral, outer-margins of the aryepiglottic folds (**Figures 12.9A and C**). The postcricoid hypopharynx is primarily defined by the mucosa overlying the posterior aspect of the cricoid cartilage, extending from the level of the cricoarytenoid joints through the inferior margin of the cricoid cartilage. There is a small focal area of mucosa that is superior to the postcricoid hypopharynx and medial to the bilateral pyriform sinuses. This mucosa belongs to the hypopharynx and is best described as the posterior confluence of the aryepiglottic folds, since the mucosa overlies the posterior margins of the transverse and oblique arytenoid muscles that are superior to the posterior cricoid cartilage lamina. The anterior wall of the hypopharynx is shared with the posterior wall of the larynx, creating a "bulkhead" of tissue that acts as an important interface between the larynx and the hypopharynx (**Figures 12.10A and B**).

# Anatomic details

## Innervation of the larynx and hypopharynx

Innervation of the larynx is via branches of the vagus nerve (cranial nerve X) specifically the paired superior laryngeal nerves and the recurrent laryngeal nerves. There are two branches to each of the superior laryngeal nerves, the external branch and the internal branch. The external branch of the superior laryngeal nerve supplies the extrinsic laryngeal musculature and the cricothyroid muscle. The internal branch of the superior laryngeal nerve provides sensation to the laryngeal mucosa.

The paired recurrent laryngeal nerves course between the thyroid cartilage and the cricoid cartilage and extend superiorly to the larynx within the groove of their respective tracheoesophageal junctions. The right recurrent laryngeal nerve loops around the subclavian artery. The left recurrent laryngeal nerve loops around the aortic arch. The recurrent laryngeal nerves innervate all of the intrinsic muscles of the larynx. When investigating the etiology of a vocal cord paralysis by CT, it is important to image inferiorly through the level of the aortic

| Nodal level | Larynx | Hypopharynx |
| --- | --- | --- |
| II | Supraglottic | All |
| III | Supraglottic, subglottic | All, except postcricoid |
| IV | Subglottic | Postcricoid |
| V | None | All, except postcricoid |
| VI | Subglottic | Postcricoid |
| Retropharyngeal | None | Posterior wall |
| Delphian (pre-laryngeal) | Rare: Glottic, subglottic | None |

**Table 12.2** Simplified nodal classification

arch to rule out the possibility that a mediastinal mass has interfered with the recurrent laryngeal nerves. Innervation of the hypopharynx is via the pharyngeal branches of the glossopharyngeal (cranial nerve IX) and the vagus nerves, which comprise the pharyngeal plexus. The pharyngeal plexus provides all motor and most sensory innervation of the pharynx, including the hypopharynx.

## Lymph node drainage

There is a relatively predictable pattern of lymph node drainage to the aerodigestive tract within the native neck (lymphatic drainage that is unaltered by surgery or radiation therapy). Within the larynx, nodal drainage can involve nodal levels II, III, IV and VI. Within the hypopharynx, nodal drainage can involve nodal levels II, III, IV, V, VI and the retropharyngeal nodes (**Table 12.2**).

# Pathology

## Squamous cell carcinoma

The larynx and hypopharynx are essentially two parallel tubes that share a common wall and are both lined by squamous cells. The first task of describing any tumor within the aerodigestive tract is to define the site of the tumor's origin—typically the center of the mass.

Squamous cell carcinoma (SCCa) can be predominantly exophytic or submucosal, however, the most common pattern of growth is along the mucosal (squamous cell lined) surfaces of the involved structure.

Therefore, when describing the extent of SCCa, it is important to know how the mucosal surfaces relate to each other so that you can accurately define the extent of the tumor.

Smoking and excessive alcohol are major risk factors for the development of SCCa within the aerodigestive tract. Several varieties of the human papilloma virus (HPV) are also risk factors to developing SCCa within the upper aerodigestive tract, specifically involving the oral cavity and oropharynx. HPV-related SCCa of the larynx and hypopharynx is rare.

In the evaluation of SCCa within the larynx and/or hypopharynx, there are several areas that can act as pitfalls in the diagnosis and/or description of the tumor. Some of these pitfalls include cartilaginous tumor involvement, extralaryngeal or extrahypopharyngeal spread of tumor, and involvement of the thyroarytenoid and/or cricothyroid tunnels (**Figures 12.11 and 12.12**).

## Laryngocele

A laryngocele can develop when there is an abnormal dilatation of the anterior appendage of the laryngeal ventricles (the small elliptical recess located between the false vocal cords and the true vocal cords below). A laryngocele can be filled with air, fluid, or a combination of both air and fluid. When a laryngocele gets infected, it is called a laryngopyocele. As the laryngocele gets larger, if it remains medial to the thyrohyoid membrane, it is termed an "internal" laryngocele. If the laryngocele extends laterally to the thyrohyoid membrane, then it is an "external" laryngocele. Combination internal/external laryngoceles can also be present. A minority of laryngoceles are due to a mass obstructing the appendage of the laryngeal ventricle (**Figure 12.13**).

## Vocal cord paralysis

The most common etiology for vocal cord paralysis is iatrogenic. Tumor, directly or indirectly, accounts for less than half of all cases of vocal cord paralysis. Paralysis can be secondary to dysfunction of either the superior or the recurrent laryngeal nerves; with both being branches of the vagus nerve (cranial nerve X). In the case of a superior laryngeal nerve dysfunction, there are typically no abnormal findings

The larynx and the hypopharynx 521

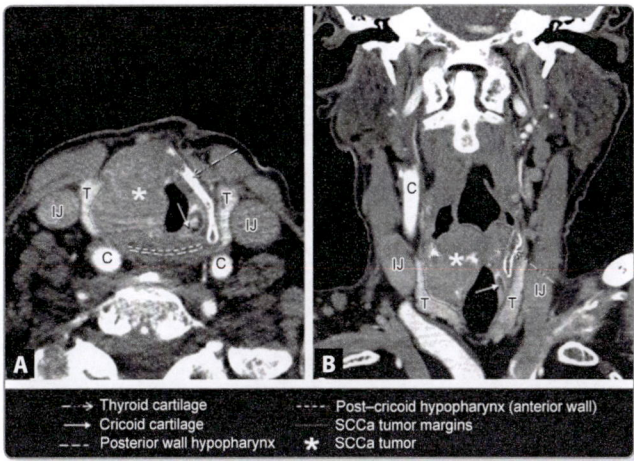

- - -> Thyroid cartilage
⟶ Cricoid cartilage
- - - Posterior wall hypopharynx
- - - - Post–cricoid hypopharynx (anterior wall)
▬▬ SCCa tumor margins
★ SCCa tumor

**Figures 12.11A and B** Squamous cell carcinoma (SCCa) involving the right transglottic larynx with extralaryngeal tumor extension. *Abbreviations*: T – Thyroid; IJ – Internal jugular vein; C – Common carotid artery

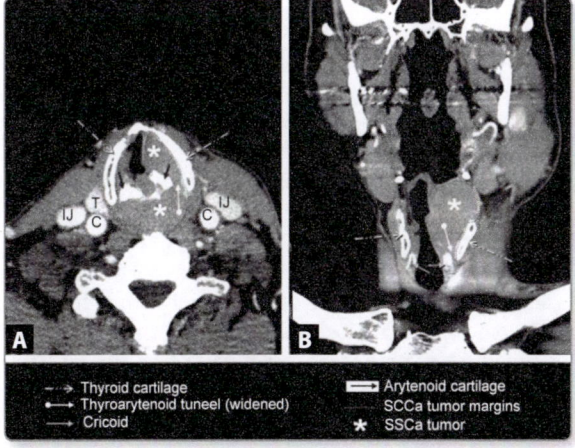

- - -> Thyroid cartilage
⟷ Thyroarytenoid tuneel (widened)
⟶ Cricoid
▬▬ Arytenoid cartilage
▬▬ SCCa tumor margins
★ SSCa tumor

**Figures 12.12A and B** Left transglottic squamous cell carcinoma (SCCa) with extension through a widened left thyroarytenoid tunnel to involve the postcricoid hypopharynx and pyriform sinus. *Abbreviations*: T – Thyroid; IJ – Internal jugular vein; C – Common carotid artery

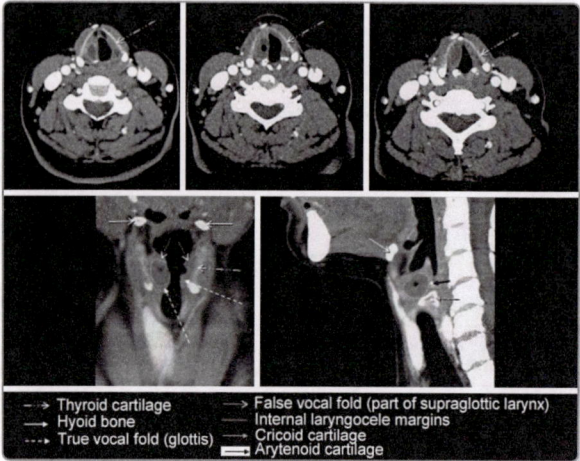

**Figure 12.13** Internal laryngocele primarily filled with fluid, however with a small focus of air

at the level of the cord to signify a superior laryngeal nerve etiology. When dysfunction of the recurrent laryngeal nerves is suspected, it is important to image the entire course of these nerves from the larynx through the upper mediastinum with the left recurrent nerve passing under the aortic arch and the right recurrent nerve passing under the aortic arch and the right subclavian artery. Within the lower neck, the recurrent laryngeal nerves run along the tracheoesophageal junction.

The classic findings of a vocal cord paralysis include dilatation of the vallecula, the ipsilateral pyriform sinus and ipsilateral laryngeal ventricle. Additionally, there is typically a medial rotation of the cricoarytenoid joint and adduction of the ipsilateral true vocal cord. There may be a medical location of the ipsilateral true vocal cord. If the vocal cord paralysis is chronic, there is often thinning of the thyroarytenoid muscle within the involved true vocal cord due to denervation atrophy (**Figure 12.14**).

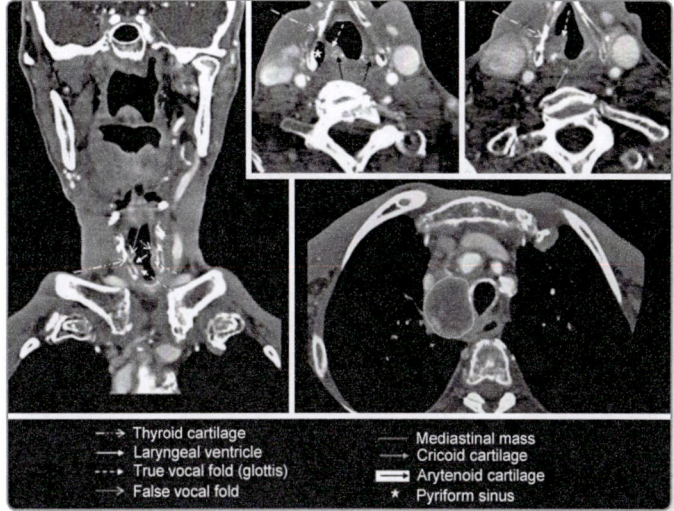

**Figure 12.14** Vocal cord paralysis involving the right vocal cord secondary to a metastatic mass in the right peritracheal region of the upper mediastinum

## Medialization thyroplasty

Thyroplasty is a subgroup of laryngoplasty that involves alteration or modification of the thyroid cartilage. The goals of medialization thyroplasty are to improve voice quality and to help protect the airway from aspiration in patients with a unilateral vocal cord paralysis (approximately 30 percent of patients with vocal cord paralysis routinely aspirate). Patients with bilateral vocal cord paralysis are not considered for medialization thyroplasty (not even a unilateral procedure) since a medialization procedure may cause significant compromise to the patient's airway. Bilateral vocal cord paresis, however, may be an indication for a unilateral medialization thyroplasty as long as there is adequate abduction of the contralateral vocal fold. Contraindications for medialization thyroplasty include malignant disease and poor abduction of the contralateral vocal fold.

Suboptimal results from a medialization thyroplasty result in an unsatisfactory improvement in the voice quality and persistent aspiration. Such results are often due to malpositioning of the implant superiorly (leading cause for revision) or anteriorly which can lead to under-medialization of the true vocal cord and/or a persistent posterior glottic gap. Potential complications from medialization thyroplasty include implant extrusion and airway obstruction. Implant extrusion is rare, but when it occurs, the implant typically extrudes into the airway. The risk for airway obstruction is greater when there is adduction of the arytenoid (**Figures 12.15A and B**).

## Subglottic stenosis due to Wegener's granulomatosis

Wegener's granulomatosis is a systemic disease, often controlled via steroids and cyclophosphamide. The head and neck manifestations of Wegener's granulomatosis include glottic/subglottic stenosis, nasal septal erosion, sinusitis, mastoiditis and occular disease. Forty percent of patients with Wegener's granulomatosis involving the head and neck will have occular disease, which can include optic neuropathy, conjunctivitis, scleritis, uveitis, and orbital granulomas (**Figure 12.16**).

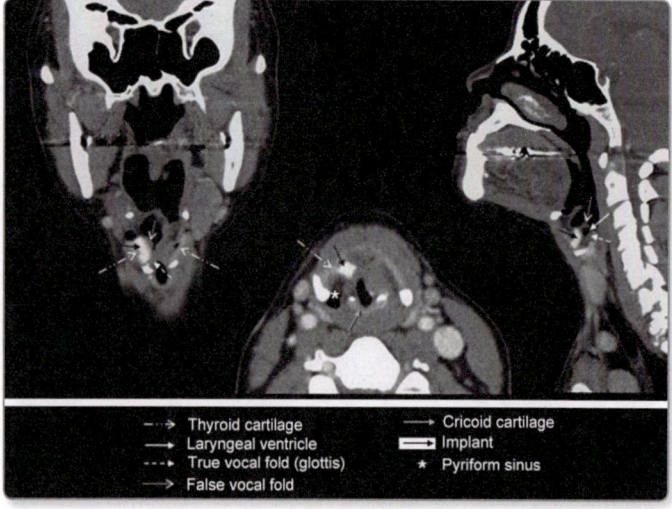

**Figure 12.15A** Patient with history of right vocal cord paralysis, following medialization thyroplasty with under-medialization of the vocal folds, before revision thyroplasty

The larynx and the hypopharynx 525

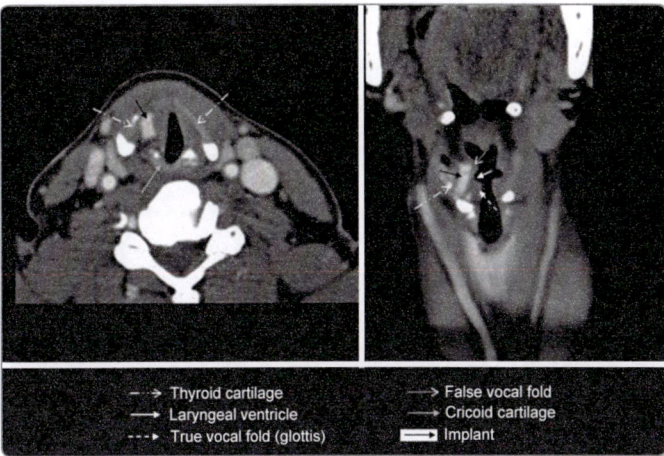

- - -> Thyroid cartilage
——> Laryngeal ventricle
- - -> True vocal fold (glottis)
——> False vocal fold
——> Cricoid cartilage
▬▬▶ Implant

**Figure 12.15B** Same patient with right vocal cord paralysis, following revision medialization thyroplasty with satisfactory medialization of the vocal folds

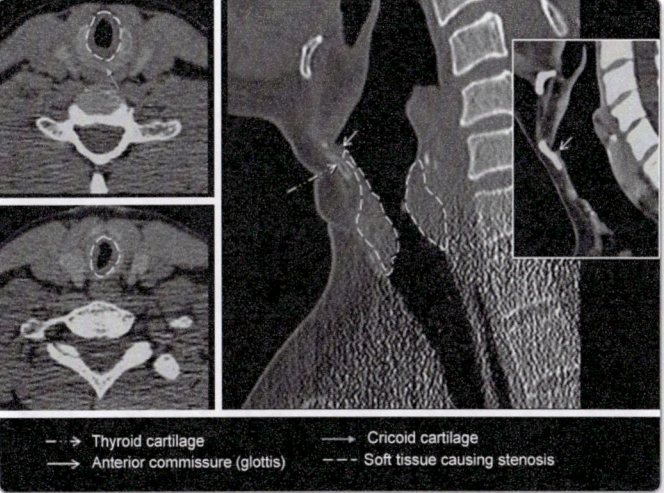

- - -> Thyroid cartilage
——> Anterior commissure (glottis)
——> Cricoid cartilage
- - -> Soft tissue causing stenosis

**Figure 12.16** Subglottic stenosis in a 40-year-old female with Wegener's granulomatosis that was diagnosed 4 years after first developing a stridor. Inlay: normal sagittal larynx with arrow on the normal appearance of the anterior commissure

## Tracheal enchondroma due to Maffucci syndrome

Maffucci syndrome is a rare disorder that is characterized by multiple enchondromas and angiomas. Lesions usually present in early childhood around age 4 to 5, and can involve the arms and legs asymmetrically. Sarcomatous degeneration has been reported in up to 30 percent of cases (**Figures 12.17A and B**).

## Laryngeal papillomatosis

Laryngeal papillomatosis, also known as recurrent respiratory papillomatosis, is a rare disorder that is caused by infection with the human papilloma virus (HPV). HPV types 6 and 11 are the most common. The larynx is the most common site of involvement. Lung nodules and cavitary lesions are usually present with pulmonary involvement (**Figures 12.18A to C**).

## Chondrosarcoma of the larynx

Chondrosarcomas of the head and neck are rare, with most occurring within the maxilla. The majority of laryngeal chondrosarcomas involve

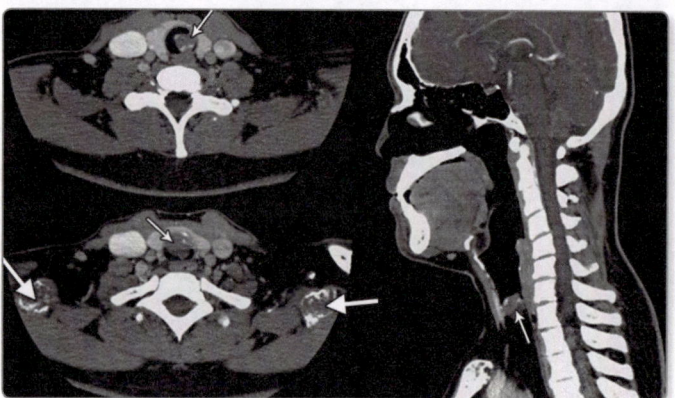

**Figure 12.17A** Tracheal enchondroma in a patient with Maffucci syndrome. Enchondromas are present within the bilateral humeral heads (Thin arrows). There is an endotracheal enchondroma (Thick arrows) that is significantly narrowing the tracheal airway

The larynx and the hypopharynx 527

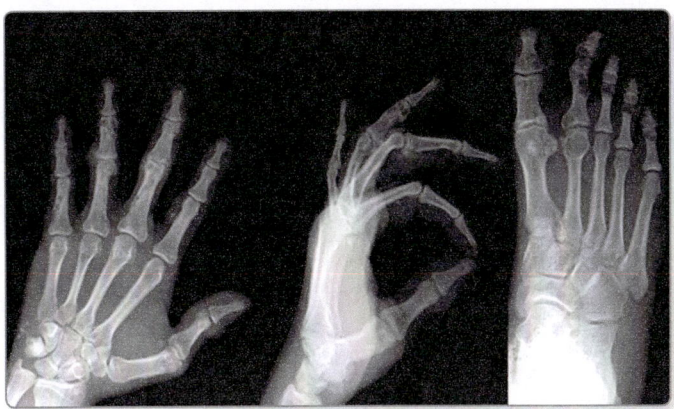

**Figure 12.17B** Multiple enchondromas (multiple lytic foci) in a patient with Maffucci syndrome

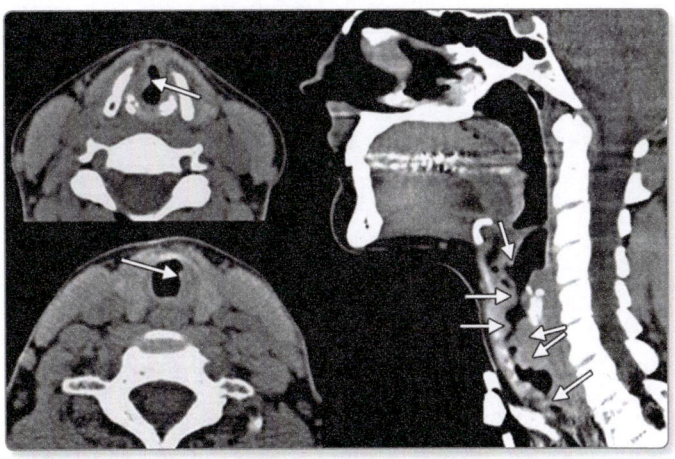

**Figure 12.18A** Laryngeal papillomatosis. Multiple papillomas within the larynx and trachea (arrows)

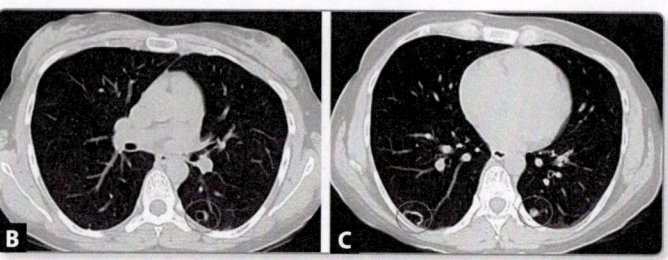

**Figures 12.18B and C** Laryngeal papillomatosis with several nodules and areas of cavitation within the lungs

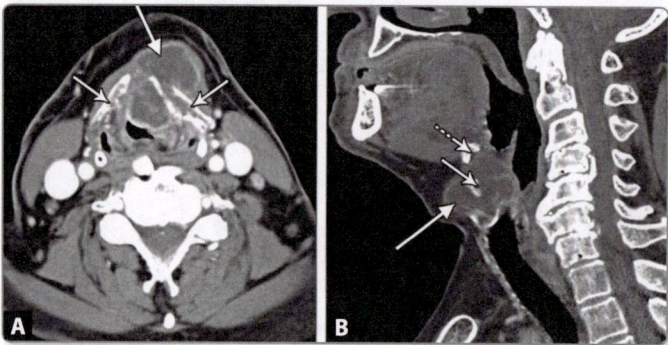

**Figures 12.19A and B** Chondrosarcoma of the larynx (long closed white arrows), centered at the left thyroid cartilage (open white arrow); hyoid bone (dashed arrow)

the cricoid cartilage, usually along the posterior or posterior-lateral aspects of the cricoid. The second most common laryngeal location for a chondrosarcoma is along the inferolateral thyroid cartilage. The chondrosarcoma mass tends to be hypodense to muscle tissue on CT imaging, with "ring and arcs" type of calcifications (however, not all will have associated calcifications). Cartilage and bony destruction is typical with local soft tissue invasion occurring in aggressive tumors. The mass often causes airway narrowing (**Figures 12.19A and B**).

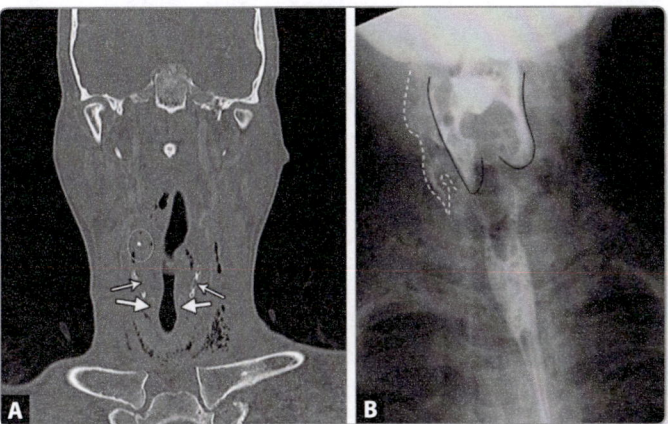

**Figures 12.20A and B** (A) Pyriform sinus perforation from an ingested chicken bone (white circle). Note the extraluminal free air within the neck on the coronal CT shown in bone algorithm. (B) upper GI contrast swallow exam shows extravasation of contrast (white dashed line) through the perforation at the right pyriform sinus (black solid line shows normal pyriform sinus contours). Thyroid cartilage = white open arrows. Cricoid cartilage = white closed arrows

## Pyriform sinus perforation

The dead-ended pouches of the pyriform sinus occasionally will collect ingested foreign bodies such as coins in children and bones from fish or chicken in adults. These foreign bodies, especially fish and chicken bones, can cause pyriform sinus perforation that can lead to further complications such as subcutaneous and mediastinal empysema, retropharyngeal and mediastinal abscess, and esophageal fistula and/or stricture (**Figures 12.20A to C**).

## Conclusion

Imaging of the larynx and hypopharynx can be challenging due to their anatomic complexity. The high resolution and fast imaging associated with CT, makes CT the preferred imaging modality for both the larynx and hypopharynx. Although their functions are completely

## 530 Introductory head and neck imaging

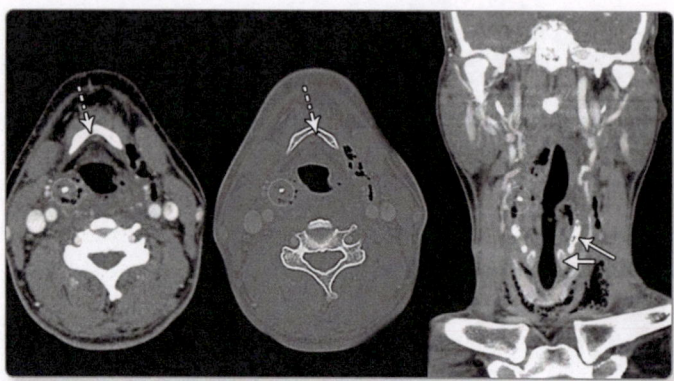

**Figure 12.20C** Pyriform sinus perforation from an ingested chicken bone (white circle). Note the extraluminal free air within the neck on the axia and coronal CT images. Thyroid cartilage = White open arrow, Cricoid cartilage = White closed arrow. Hyoid bone = Dashed open arrows

different, it is important to remember that the larynx and hypopharynx are duplexed structures that share a common wall, and therefore, may share a common pathology.

## Bibliography

1. Becker M. Larynx and hypopharynx. Radiol Clin North Am. 1998;36(5):891-920, vi.
2. Becker M, Burkhardt K, Dulguerov P, Allal A. Imaging of the larynx and hypopharynx. Eur J Radiol. 2008;66(3):460-79.
3. Castelijns JA, van den Brekel MW, Herman R. Imaging of the larynx. Semin Roentgenol. 2000;35(1):31-41.
4. Curtin HD. The Larynx. In: Som PM, Curtin HD (Eds). Head and Neck Imaging. St Louis: Mosby, 2003;1595-1699.
5. Herman R. Staging of laryngeal and hypopharyngeal cancer: Value of imaging studies. Eur Radiol. 2006;16(11):2386-400.
6. Mukherji SK. Pharynx. In Som PM, curtin HD (Eds). Head and Neck Imaging. St Louis: Mosby, 2003. pp. 1465-1520.
7. Pameijer FA, Mukherji SK, Balm AJ, van der laan BF. Imaging of squamous cell carcinoma of the hypopharynx. Semin Ultrasound CT MR. 1998;19(6):476-91.
8. Wycliffe ND, Grover RS, Kim PD, Simental A Jr. Hypopharyngeal cancer. Top Magn Reson Imaging. 2007;18(4):243-58.

# Carotid, prevertebral, and perivertebral spaces

chapter 13

Daniel M Mandell

**Abstract**
Radiographic anatomy, common infectious, inflammatory and neoplastic processes involving the carotid, prevertebral and perivertebral regions are discussed.

**Keywords**
Carotid, prevertebral, perivertebral space, anatomy.

## Carotid space

## Anatomy

The carotid space extends craniocaudally from the skull base to the level of the aortic arch. The space is bounded laterally by the carotid space, anteriorly by the prestyloid parapharyngeal space, anteromedially by the visceral space, posteromedially by the retropharyngeal space, and posteriorly by the prevertebral space. In the surgical literature, the carotid space is more commonly referred to as the post-styloid component of the parapharyngeal space. Accordingly, carotid space masses displace the styloid process anteriorly, narrowing the stylomandibular notch (space between the styloid process and the mandible). The carotid space is more formally defined by its fascial boundaries, with facial contributions from all 3 layers of the deep cervical facia: The carotid space is bounded laterally by the superficial layer of the deep cervical fascia, anteromedially by the middle layer of deep cervical fascia (around the aerodigestive tract), and posteromedially by the deep layer of deep cervical fascia (around the vertebral column and perivertebral musculature). One may categorize the craniocaudal extent of the carotid space into nasopharyngeal, oropharyngeal, cervical, and mediastinal segments. Lesions of the carotid space at the level of the nasopharynx are nonpalpable, whereas lesions at the level of the oropharynx or lower neck are palpable.

The carotid space contains the carotid artery, internal jugular vein, cranial nerves, sympathetic nervous plexus, paraganglion tissue, and lymph nodes. Cranial nerves 9 to 11 (glossopharyngeal nerve, vagus nerve, and spinal accessory nerve, respectively) exit the posterior fossa via the jugular foramen, and cranial nerve 12 (hypoglossal nerve) exits through the hypoglossal canal. Cranial nerves 9 to 12 all descend in the carotid space, with cranial nerves 9 to 11 exiting the carotid space at the level of the soft palate, and cranial nerve 12 descending within the entire length of the carotid space. The fascial "carotid sheath" is strong, so masses within the carotid space may compress structures such as the internal jugular vein.

## Pseudolesions

### Retropharyngeal carotid artery

One or both carotid arteries may deviate medially into the retropharyngeal region, either bowing the retropharyngeal space or truly penetrating into the retropharyngeal space (**Figure 13.1**). This tortuous course of the carotid arteries is more common in the elderly, and attributed to atherosclerotic changes. It is typically the distal common carotid artery and proximal portion of the internal carotid artery that are displaced. When bilateral, approximation of the carotid arteries has been called "kissing carotids". It is extremely important to convey this information to the referring physician as a medially displaced carotid artery may mimic a submucosal pharyngeal mass on clinical exam, and biopsy must be avoided.

### Asymmetric size of internal jugular veins

Commonly, one internal jugular vein is much larger than the other. This is considered a normal variation with no known clinical significance.

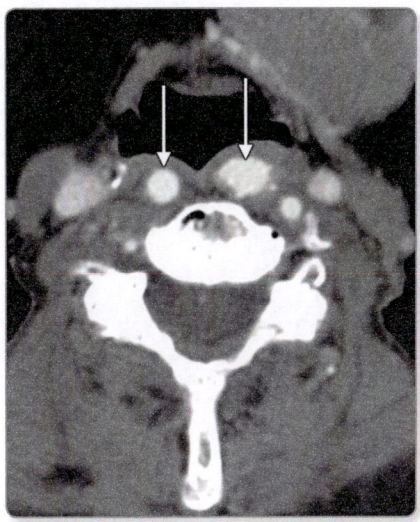

**Figure 13.1** Retropharyngeal carotid arteries in a 90-year-old women. Contrast-enhanced axial CT image demonstrates medial displacement of both internal carotid arteries (arrows). The arteries bulge into the posterior wall of the hypopharynx, potentially mimicking submucosal pharyngeal masses

## Vascular diseases

### Large artery vasculitis

Takayasu's arteritis is a chronic large artery vasculitis that primarily involves the aorta and its main branches, including the common carotid arteries. Giant cell (temporal arteritis) also involves large arteries, but more commonly the cavernous internal carotid artery than the cervical carotid artery.

### Idiopathic carotiditis

Idiopathic carotiditis is a disorder characterized by carotid artery wall and periarterial inflammation, with unilateral pain and tenderness in the region of the common carotid artery bifurcation and pain

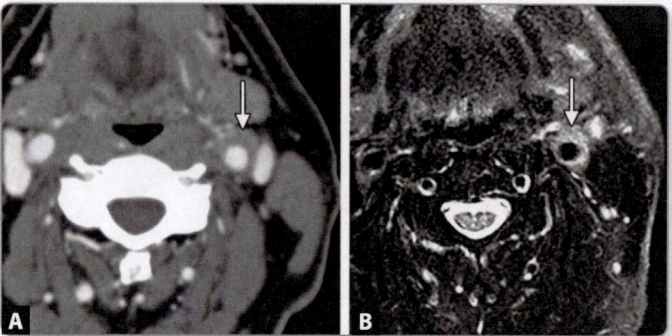

**Figures 13.2A and B** Idiopathic carotiditis. A fifty-two-year-old man presented to a hospital emergency department with pain and fullness in the left neck. Contrast-enhanced CT image (A) demonstrates a thick intermediate attenuation rim (arrow) surrounding the left common carotid artery, immediately proximal to the carotid bifurcation. T2-weighted fat-suppressed MR image and (B) shows a corresponding rim of hyperintensity (arrow)

radiating into the face. The disorder is self-limited, resolving within a few weeks. The term carotidynia ("dynia" = pain) is used more commonly than *idiopathic carotiditis* but the former is less specific, and might be used for cases of pain related to carotid artery dissection, aneurysm, lymphadenitis and a variety of other disorders. On imaging (**Figures 13.2A and B**), idiopathic carotiditis demonstrates carotid artery wall thickening, possibly wall enhancement, and surrounding inflammatory changes within the carotid space. Treatment is supportive and may include nonsteroidal anti-inflammatory drugs.

## Carotid artery dissection

Arterial dissection is characterized by sudden disruption of the intima, with penetration of circulating blood into the arterial wall. Dissecting blood then propagates longitudinally within the artery wall and or ruptures through the adventitia to form a pseudoaneurysm. Causes of carotid artery dissection include trauma, pre-existing arteriopathy (such as fibromuscular dysplasia, Marfan syndrome, osteogenesis imperfecta, and autosomal dominant polycystic kidney disease), and some cases are idiopathic. The typical clinical presentation is ipsilateral head or neck pain, sometimes a Horner's syndrome (ptosis, miosis, anhidrosis), and sometimes associated cerebral or retinal ischemic symptoms. The Horner's syndrome is only partial (lacking anhidrosis) if the dissection is distal to the carotid bifurcation as the sympathetic fibers supplying the iris and eyelid travel along the internal carotid artery, but fibers responsible for sweating traveling along the external carotid artery.

Either CTA or MRI/MRA is a reasonable first investigation for suspected carotid artery dissection. Dissection of the cervical carotid artery typically originates distal to the carotid bifurcation, and most commonly ends extracranially. The arterial wall is eccentrically thickened due to intramural hematoma (**Figures 13.3 and 13.4**). This thickening may be hyper-attenuating on nonenhanced CT in acute

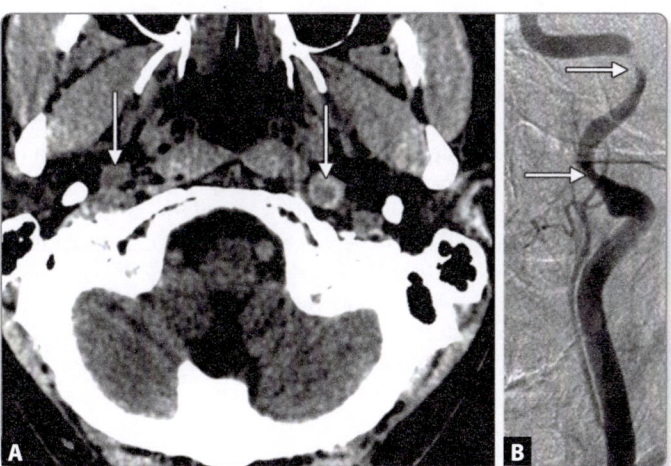

**Figures 13.3A and B** Left internal carotid artery (ICA) dissection. Non-enhanced CT brain (A) demonstrates an eccentric rim of hyperattenuation (arrow) around the left ICA just below the skull base, consistent with acute intramural blood. The right ICA (arrow) does not demonstrate intramural hematoma. (B) Catheter angiography (right) shows narrowing of the extracranial left ICA (arrow) and severe narrowing in the posterior bend of the petrosal segment of the ICA (arrow)

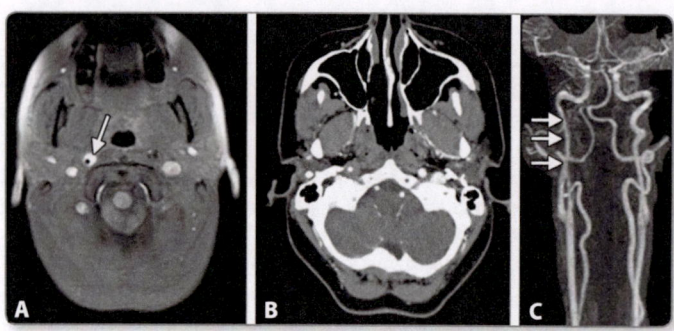

**Figures 13.4A to C** Right internal carotid artery dissection. Fat saturated T1 image (A) shows the presence of hyperintense mural hematoma (arrow). (B) shows the corresponding appearance on CTA. The lumen is narrowed as a result of the dissection. (C) is a contrast MRA showing subtle narrowing and irregularity of a large segment of the cervical ICA (arrows)

dissection, and hyperintense on fat suppressed T1-weighted MRI in the subacute phase (about 1 week to 2 months old). Dissection is typically isointense in the acute and chronic phases on T1-weighted MRI. CTA/MRA typically demonstrates narrowing (due to intramural hematoma) at the origin of the dissection, and segments of fusiform dilatation (due to outward bulging of the adventitia). An intimal flap or double lumen on CTA or MRA are pathognomonic, but not necessarily present.

Most carotid artery dissections resolve spontaneously. Treatment is anticoagulation unless there is a contraindication (such as recent major trauma). Endovascular treatment is generally reserved for patients who are refractory to medical therapy.

## Fibromuscular dysplasia

Fibromuscular dysplasia (FMD) is an idiopathic disorder characterized by slowly progressive overgrowth of smooth muscle and fibrous tissue in medium size arteries. The disorder is most common in young to middle-aged women. The disease is often asymptomatic, but clinically important as arterial stenosis may be hemodynamically significant, and there are associations with spontaneous arterial dissection and intracranial aneurysms. Carotid arteries are involved more commonly than vertebral arteries, and the disease tends to affect the middle and distal portions of these vessels. Fibromuscular dysplasia is classified into several subtypes. Medial fibroplasia (classic fibromuscular dysplasia) is the most common subtype, and is characterized by alternating segments of arterial constriction and dilatation, resulting in a string-of-beads appearance on angiography. Intimal fibroplasia, another subtype, is characterized by a long segment of smooth narrowing. The natural history of fibromuscular dysplasia is not well-known. If there is a history of an ischemic event, antiplatelet therapy may be used. Balloon angioplasty-stenting may be considered if there is evidence of hemodynamic impairment or ongoing ischemic events despite medical therapy.

## Internal jugular vein thrombosis

Internal jugular vein (IJV) thrombosis is most commonly secondary to an IJV central line, head and neck malignancy, prior surgery or radiation therapy, or drug abuse with intravenous access by IJV. Acute IJV thrombosis presents clinically as erythema, swelling, tenderness, and fever. The referring clinician may query neck abscess. On imaging, there is an enlarged vein with nonenhancing tubular filling defect, and inflammatory changes surrounding the vein (**Figure 13.5**). The disorder is self-limiting. Patients are not typically anticoagulated as consequential pulmonary thromboembolism is uncommon. An exception may be patients with intracranial extension of venous thrombosis. Patients develop collateral venous bypass of the occluded vein. A chronic IVJ thrombosis pattern emerges over weeks. On imaging, there remains a filling defect in the vein, but the inflammatory changes surrounding the vein have resolved, and venous collateral vessels may be apparent. The differential diagnosis of IJV thrombosis includes rim-enhancing neck abscess or necrotic mass, and IJV filling defect due to slow or turbulent blood flow.

Lemierre's syndrome refers to oropharyngeal infection (streptococcal or other), resulting in internal jugular thrombophlebitis, *Fusobacterium necrophorum* septicemia, and septic emboli (**Figures 13.6A to C**). The typical history is several days of sore throat and fever, then onset of more severe symptoms.

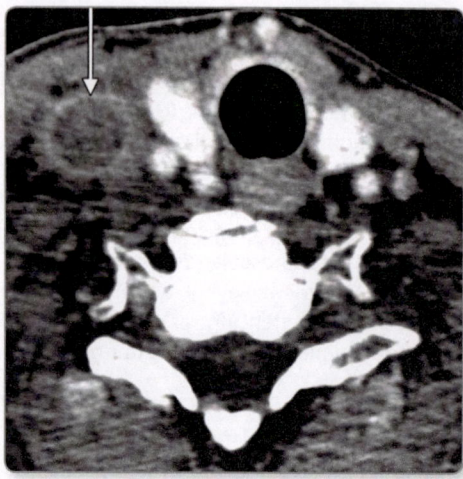

**Figure 13.5** Acute internal jugular vein thrombosis. The right internal jugular vein (arrow) is enlarged, with a filling defect occluding the lumen, enhancement of the venous wall, and perivenous inflammatory changes

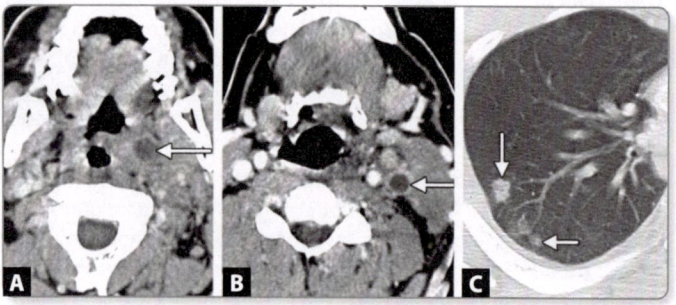

**Figures 13.6A to C** Lemierre's syndrome. Twenty-eight-year-old presented with sore throat, dysphagia, and fever. (A) Contrast-enhanced axial CT images demonstrated a left peritonsillar abscess; (B) Acute left IJV thrombosis, (C) CT chest demonstrated multiple parenchymal opacities that arise at the ends of pulmonary arteries (feeding vessel sign), consistent with pulmonary septic emboli. Blood culture grew *Fusobacterium necrophorum*. Constellation of findings is consistent with Lemierre's syndrome

# Neoplastic

## Paragangliomas

The paraganglia are small groups of neuroendocrine cells associated with the cervical carotid artery and vagus nerve in the carotid space. Paraganglioma is a neoplasm of these cells. Paragangliomas are usually benign, with metastatic spread in 5 to 10 percent. These tumors are highly vascular. Given their rich internal network of branching arteries, they are also called "glomus" (*L. ball* of thread) tumors. Most paragangliomas of the head and neck are hormonally inactive, and present clinically as a painless, slowly growing, and sometimes pulsatile neck mass. There may be a cranial neuropathy from mass effect. Head and neck paragangliomas are multiple in 5 to 10 percent of patients, and even more often multiple (20–30%) when they occur in an autosomal dominant familial form. Treatment of carotid space paragangliomas is typically surgical resection, sometimes with preoperative embolization.

On imaging, the classic appearance of a carotid space paraganglioma is a well-defined mass with a "salt and pepper" appearance on T2-weighted images. Hyperintense foci (salt) represent tumor, hemorrhage, and slow flow in vessels, and hypointense foci (pepper) represent vascular flow voids within the lesion. Paragangliomas at the skull base have an aggressive pattern of bone destruction, in contrast with the smooth bone remodeling typical of schwannomas and neurofibromas. Paragangliomas are strongly enhancing, typically homogeneously for smaller lesions, and more heterogeneously for larger lesions due to necrosis and hemorrhage. There is rapid wash-in and wash-out of contrast material due to arterial-venous shunting. The main differential diagnosis for a strongly enhancing carotid space mass is a vascular metastasis such as renal cell carcinoma or thyroid carcinoma.

There are 3 types of paragangliomas in the carotid space:

## Carotid body tumor (Figures 13.7 and 13.8)

The carotid bodies are paraganglia located at the level of the common carotid artery bifurcation bilaterally, either within or outside the

## 540 Introductory head and neck imaging

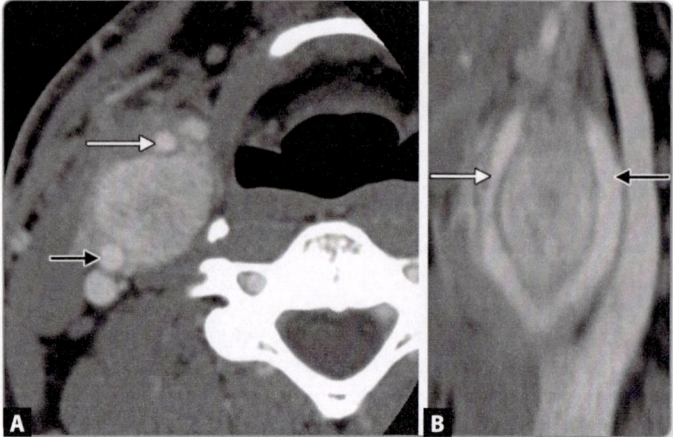

**Figures 13.7A and B** Carotid body tumor. Contrast-enhanced CT images [axial] (A); [sagittal] (B) demonstrate a strongly enhancing mass at the right carotid bifurcation, splaying the internal (black arrows) and external (white arrows) carotid arteries

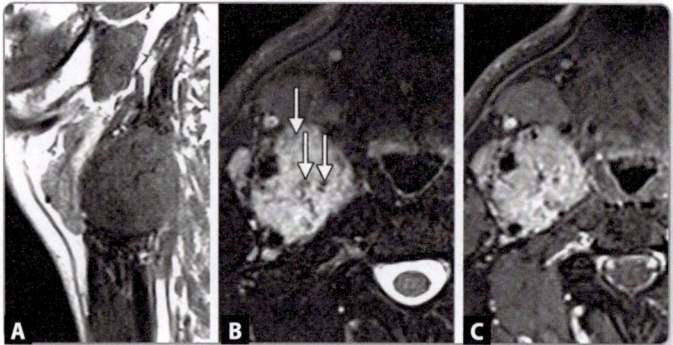

**Figures 13.8A to C** Carotid body tumor. Sagittal T1-weighted (A), axial T2-weighted (B), and postgadolinium axial T1-weighted images. There is a mass at the right carotid bifurcation, with multiple small flow voids (arrows) and strong enhancement postgadolinium

adventitia of the artery. Arterial supply is predominantly via branches of the external carotid artery. A carotid body tumor characteristically splays the bifurcation, filling the crotch between the ICA and ECA. A carotid body tumor may encase the carotid artery, but does not narrow it. Differential considerations include hypervascular nodal metastases (such as thyroid carcinoma, renal cell carcinoma, and melanoma), schwannoma, ICA aneurysm or pseudoaneurysm, and type 3 branchial cleft cyst.

## Glomus vagale tumor (Figures 13.9 and 13.10)

Glomus vagale tumor is a neoplasm of the paraganglia around the vagus nerve. These paraganglia are not a compact mass like the carotid body, but dispersed within the nerve. The vagus nerve resides posterior to the ICA, so glomus vagale tumors displace the ICA anteriorly. They typically arise just below the skull base. A large

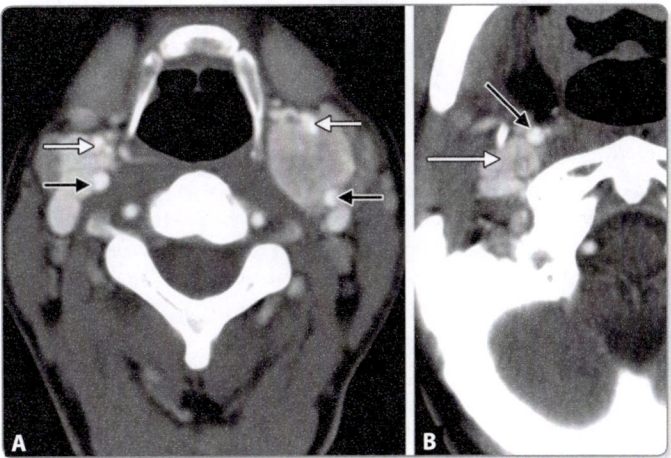

**Figures 13.9A and B** Carotid body tumors and glomus vagale tumor. Contrast-enhanced axial CT images demonstrate a strongly enhancing mass splaying the right internal (black arrow) and external (white arrow) carotid arteries, and a similar larger mass on the left side, consistent with carotid body tumors. (B) Demonstrate an enhancing mass (white arrow) just posterior to the internal carotid artery (black arrow) just below the skull base, consistent with a glomus vagale tumor

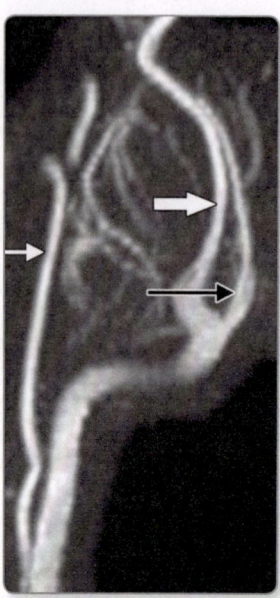

**Figure 13.10** Glomus vagale tumor. Maximum intensity projection from a MR angiogram demonstrates marked anterior bowing of both the internal (thick white arrow) and external (black arrow) carotid arteries and distal common carotid artery, consistent with a mass centered posteriorly in the carotid sheath (Small white arrow labels a vertebral artery)

glomus vagale tumor may extend far inferiorly and splay the ICA and ECA, but unlike a carotid body tumor, it will not usually fill the crotch between the ICA and ECA. Arterial supply of the tumor is typically via an enlarged ascending pharyngeal artery. Glomus vagale tumor grows within the nerve, so it is nearly impossible to remove the tumor without sacrificing the nerve, and patients usually have vocal cord paralysis after surgery.

## Glomus jugulare tumor (Figures 13.11A to D)

Glomus jugulare tumor is less common the carotid body and glomus vagale tumors. Glomus jugulare tumors arise from vagus nerve paraganglia in the jugular fossa. They typically spread both above and below skull base, classically eroding the jugular spine. If the tumor extends into the middle ear cavity, it can be called a "glomus jugulotympanicum tumor". Malignancy is less common than for carotid

Carotid, prevertebral, and perivertebral spaces

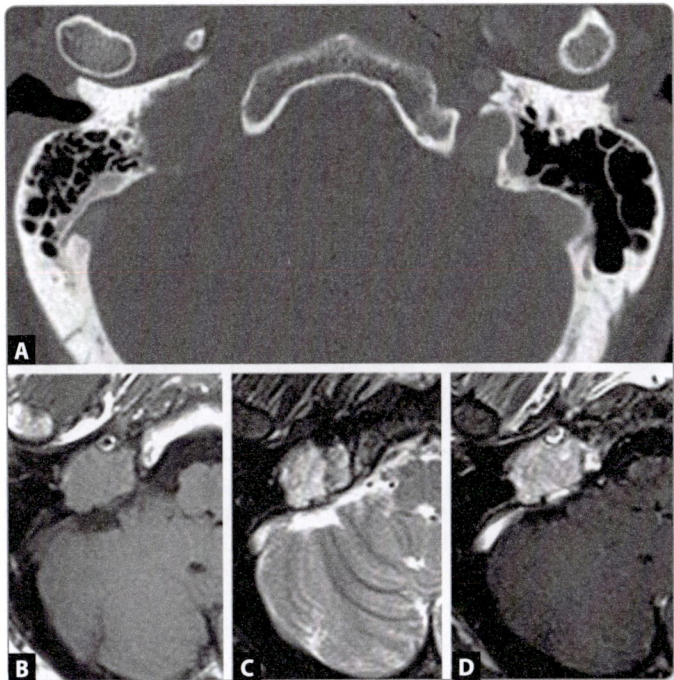

**Figures 13.11A to D** Glomus jugulare tumor. Axial CT image (A) demonstrates a mass centered in the right jugular fossa, with permeative destruction of the jugular fossa. Axial T1-weighted (B), T2-weighted (C), and postgadolinium T1-weighted (D) images showing a corresponding mass with a slightly speckled appearance on T2-weighted images and strong enhancement postgadolinium

body or glomus vagale tumors. Differential includes meningioma, metastasis, and schwannoma.

# Nerve sheath neoplasms

## Carotid space schwannoma

Schwannomas are benign encapsulated neoplasms arising from nerve sheath Schwann cells, and not infiltrating the nerve itself.

There is an association with neurofibromatosis type 2. Carotid space schwannomas most commonly present as an asymptomatic neck mass in a young or middle age adult. They usually undergo slow progressive growth. Treatment of choice is total resection with vagus nerve preservation.

Carotid space schwannomas most commonly arise from the vagus nerve. The vagus nerve resides posterior to the ICA, so like glomus vagale tumors, vagal schwannomas displace the ICA anteriorly. On imaging (**Figures 13.12 and 13.13**), carotid space schwannomas are fusiform (that is, spindle-shaped) with a smooth well-defined margin. Paragangliomas commonly have a speckled texture, but they are grossly relatively homogeneous, that is, one part of the tumor looks like the other parts. In contrast, schwannomas may be more grossly heterogeneous due to intramural hemorrhage or necrosis. They are typically hyperintense on T2-weighted images. A lack of flow voids differentiates them from paragangliomas. Schwannomas are hypovascular, but they accumulate extravascular space contrast over time, and several minutes following intravenous contrast injection, schwannomas will enhance even more than paragangliomas that wash-out quickly. A schwannoma extending to the skull base will result in smooth enlargement of the jugular foramen, in contrast with paragangliomas which cause aggressive-appearing permeation

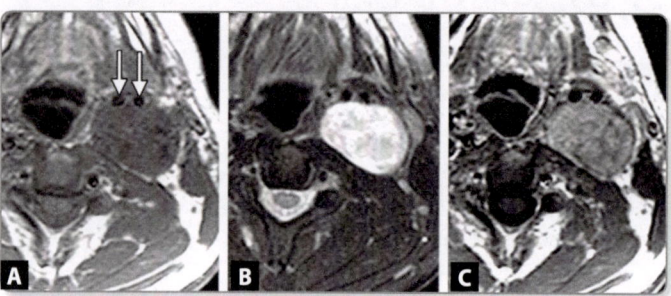

**Figures 13.12A to C** Vagus nerve schwannoma. Axial T1-weighted (A), T2-weighted (B), and postgadolinium T1-weighted (C) images demonstrate a mass which displaces both the internal and external carotid artery anteriorly. The mass is quite hyperintense on the T2-weighted images

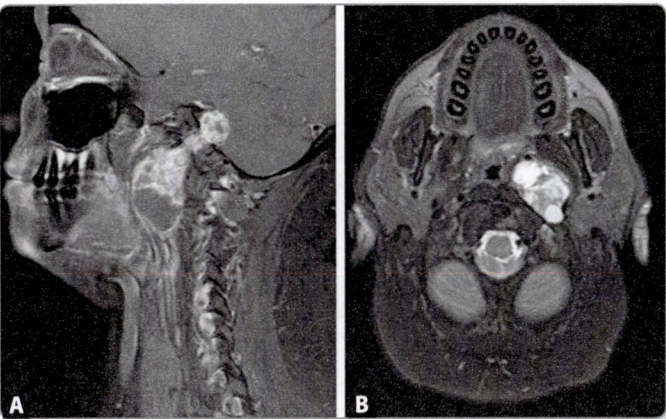

**Figures 13.13A and B** Another schwannoma of the carotid space. (A) a fat-saturated postgadolinium enhanced scan that shows the elongated nature of the schwannoma. Intracranial extension is present. (B) a fat saturated T2 image showing the presence of internal cystic change. The carotid is being displaced anteriorly

of the bone. Malignant peripheral nerve sheath tumors are rare. They usually have a similar imaging appearance to schwannomas, and the diagnosis of malignancy is usually made only after resection.

If there is uncertainty as to whether a tumor is a paraganglioma or schwannoma, one additional technique that can be employed is dynamic contrast-enhanced imaging. Paraganglioma enhancement peaks at 30 to 45 seconds, whereas as schwannomas show continuous accumulation of contrast over minutes. If there is still uncertainty, the lesions may be differenentiated by FNA or a conventional angiogram showing the hypervascularity of paraganglioma.

## Neurofibroma (Figure 13.14)

Neurofibromas are much less common than schwannomas. Whereas schwannomas are encapsulated tumors arising from nerve sheath Schwann cells, neurofibromas are nonencapsulated neoplasms containing all elements of the nerve of origin. They typically exist as

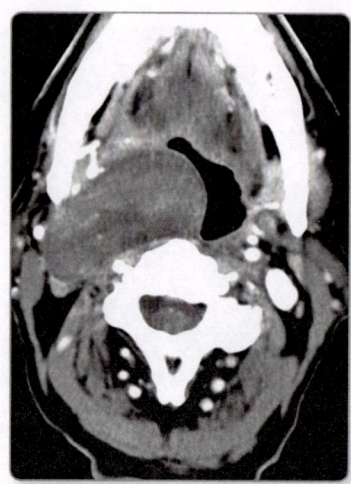

**Figure 13.14** Sympathetic chain neurofibroma. Contrast-enhanced axial CT image demonstrates a well-defined soft tissue mass centered in the right carotid space. The mass displaces the internal and external carotid arteries anterolaterally, and extends into the retropharyngeal region on the right side, with mass effect on the hypopharynx. The mass is quite low in attenuation

multiple neurofibromas. Only 10 percent of patients with neurofibromas have neurofibromatosis. Neurofibromas may undergo fatty degeneration and have lipid signal on MRI and hypoattenuation on CT.

## Lymphadenopathy (Figure 13.15)

The carotid space contains the internal jugular chain of lymph nodes (levels II, III, IV). The most cranial node in this chain, the "jugulodigastric" node, resides at the level where the digastric muscle passes the internal jugular vein. Above this level, a node in the region of the carotid space actually resides in the lateral aspect of the retropharyngeal space. Carotid space nodes are considered enlarged if they are greater than 10 mm in maximum transverse diameter, with the exception of the jugulodigastric nodes, for which the threshold is 15 mm. Carotid space nodes are a final common lymphatic drainage

Carotid, prevertebral, and perivertebral spaces 547

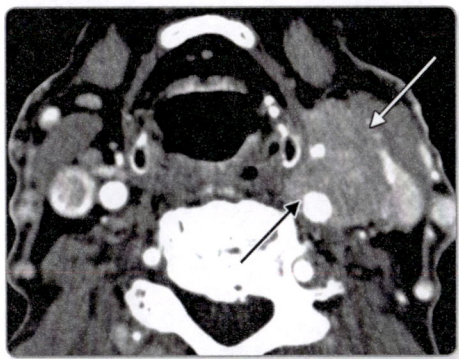

**Figure 13.15** Medullary thyroid carcinoma metastasis. Contrast-enhanced axial CT image demonstrates a soft tissue mass (arrows) in the left carotid space, encasing the left common carotid artery and left internal jugular vein

pathway for the head and neck, so most head and neck pathology can yield carotid space lymphadenopathy. The most common malignancy of the carotid space is squamous cell nodal metastases.

Nodes may be present in any part of the space relative to the vessels, and may displace the vessels in any direction. Lymphadenopathy tends to displace the carotid and jugular vessels together, and not to splay them. Extracapsular spread may result in encasement of the internal carotid artery. CT and MRI have limited ability to determine the degree of vascular invasion (that is, unresectability), but in general, greater circumferential contact between the tumor and artery suggests invasion is more likely, and 270 degrees is sometimes used as a threshold between likely resectable and likely not resectable. Carotid artery involvement is not only a problem for surgical resection. Radiation therapy also poses a major risk of hemorrhage if the carotid artery is invaded.

## Direct spread of malignancy to the carotid space

This is most commonly from nasopharyngeal carcinoma (**Figure 13.16**).

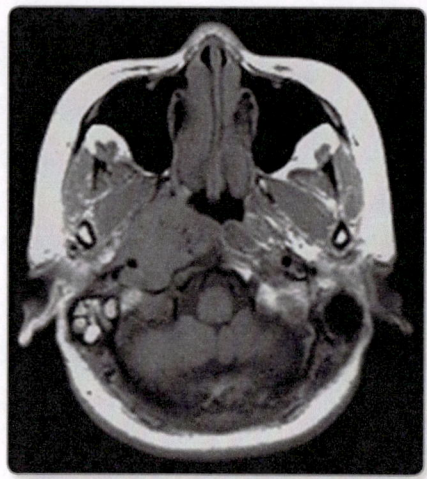

Figure 13.16 Axial T1-weighted image shows posterolateral extension of a large nasopharyngeal carcinoma to encase the right carotid artery

# Retropharyngeal space

## Anatomy

The retropharyngeal space is bounded posteriorly by the deep layer of deep cervical fascia (alar fascia) that is situated anterior to and parallel to the prevertebral fascia. Laterally (on each side), the retropharyngeal space is bounded by the carotid space. Anteriorly, the retropharyngeal space is bounded by the middle layer of deep cervical fascia that surrounds the aerodigestive tract (the buccopharyngeal fascia). The retropharyngeal space extends from the skull base into the mediastinum (to the T3 level). It is at this level that the alar fascia fuses with the anteriorly located visceral fascia/buccopharyngeal fascia. A space located posterior to the retropharyngeal space which is bound by the alar fascia and prevertebral fascia extends from the skull base down to a level just above the diaphragm. This is the "danger space" and can be a potential tract by which infection can spread from the neck into the mediastinum. On imaging is not possible to visually separate these two spaces. The suprahyoid retropharyngeal space contains fat and lymph nodes. Nodes are categorized into a medial group and a lateral group (nodes of Rouviere). The infrahyoid retropharyngeal space does not contain lymph nodes.

# Infectious or inflammatory

## Retropharyngeal abscess

Retropharyngeal abscess most commonly occurs in the context of oropharyngeal infection: infection spreads from the pharynx to retropharyngeal nodes, with intranodal abscess formation (suppurative adenitis), and node rupture yielding retropharyngeal abscess. The most common organism is group A beta-hemolytic *Streptococcus*, but a variety of other organisms may cause retropharyngeal abscess, and often the infection is polymicrobial. Other causes include foreign body penetration of the pharynx, and direct spread of infection from vertebral osteomyelitis or discitis, middle ear infection, or paranasal sinusitis. Clinically, retropharyngeal abscess typically presents with neck pain and stiffness, dysphagia, fever, posterior pharyngeal swelling on exam, and leukocytosis. This is a life-threatening disorder, requiring urgent ENT referral for airway management. Treatment is intravenous antibiotics with or without surgical drainage.

The initial imaging of a patient with suspected retropharyngeal space infection is usually a lateral radiograph of the neck. Findings may include prevertebral soft tissue swelling, air in the prevertebral soft tissues, and loss of the usual cervical lordosis. Attention to radiographic technique is important as neck flexion or incomplete inspiration may mimic prevertebral soft tissue thickening. Further evaluation with CT is preferable to MRI. As the retropharyngeal space extends into the mediastinum, it is essential to image these patients from the skull to the carina, to assess the full craniocaudal extent of disease. On CT, suppurative lymphadenopathy (**Figures 13.17A and B**) appears as central regions of hypoattenuation within lymph nodes, with peripheral enhancement. There may be surrounding inflammatory changes

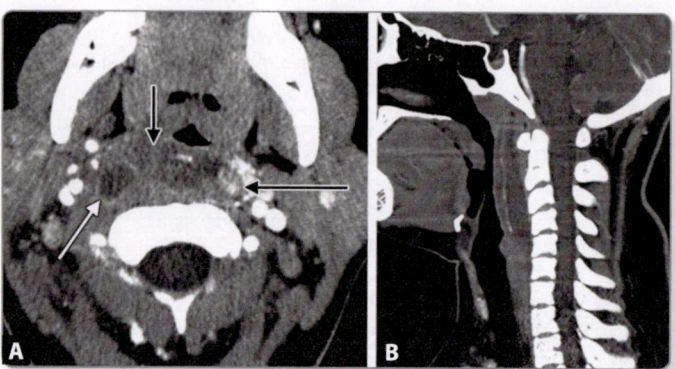

**Figures 13.17A and B** Retropharyngeal intranodal abscess. Contrast-enhanced axial CT image (A) demonstrates a smoothly-marginated rim-enhancing ovoid fluid collection in the right lateral aspect of the retropharyngeal space (white arrow) at the level of the oropharynx, consistent with intranodal abscess. There is associated fluid in the retropharyngeal space (black arrow). There is an enlarged lymph node, without abscess formation, in the left lateral retropharyngeal space (long black arrow). Sagittal image nicely shows the craniocaudal extent of the abscess collection

in the retropharyngeal fat. Untreated, these nodes may rupture into the retropharyngeal space, resulting in an abscess (**Figures 13.17A and B**). A retropharyngeal abscess appears as a fluid collection with enhancing rim. This collection distends the retropharyngeal space. There may be gas within the abscess cavity. Once a retropharyngeal abscess is diagnosed, look for evidence of the cause (such as vertebral endplate erosion from discitis), penetrating foreign body (**Figures 13.18A and B**), and look for complications: airway narrowing, carotid artery narrowing, thrombosis or microbial aneurysm, internal jugular vein thrombosis, extension of infection into mediastinum or epidural space of the spine.

One must differentiate between retropharyngeal abscess and retropharyngeal edema (**Figures 13.19 and 13.20**). Edema may represent an early retropharyngeal infection (which does not require surgical drainage), but also occurs secondary to calcific tendinitis, venous obstruction (from IJV thrombosis), or lymphatic obstruction (for example, from prior nodal dissection).

Carotid, prevertebral, and perivertebral spaces 551

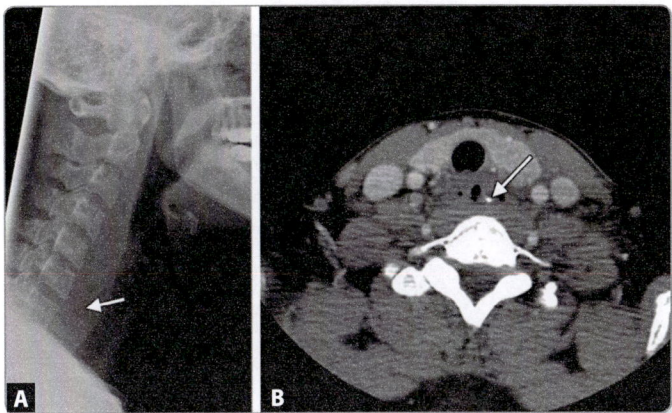

**Figures 13.18A and B** Lateral radiograph shows marked soft tissue swelling anterior to the vertebral column. There is a small focus of gas lucency visible (short arrow). CT of the same patient shows a small pocket of gas lucency as well a hypodense foreign body which was a fish bone (long arrow)

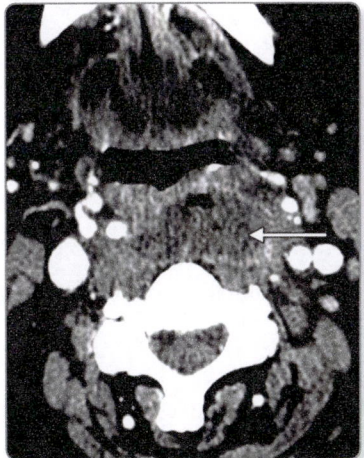

**Figure 13.19** Retropharyngeal abscess. Contrast-enhanced axial CT image demonstrates a large rim-enhancing fluid collection (arrow) in the retropharyngeal space. The collection contains locules of gas. There was a history of oropharyngeal infection

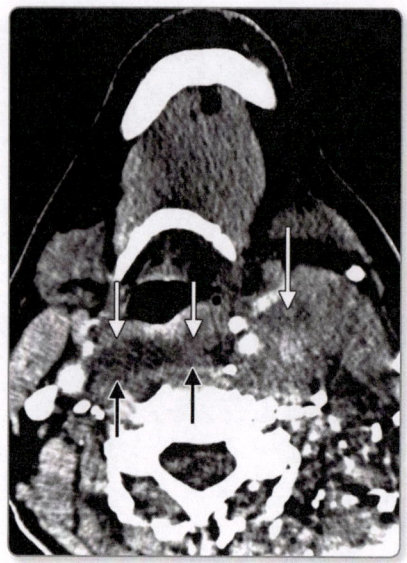

**Figure 13.20** Retropharyngeal edema. Contrast-enhanced axial CT image demonstrates a distended retropharyngeal space of fluid density (small white and black arrows). The left internal jugular vein is not opacified with contrast, and there is fat stranding throughout the left carotid space (large white arrow), consistent with internal jugular vein thrombosis

# Neoplastic

## Benign neoplasms

Lipomas, hemangiomas, and fibromyxomas are some of the benign tumors that arise in this space.

## Lymphadenopathy (Figures 13.21A and B)

The retropharyngeal lymph nodes primarily drain the nasal cavity, nasopharynx, oropharynx, hypopharynx, middle ear and Eustachian tube. The retropharyngeal nodes then drain into level II nodes. Retropharyngeal nodes are considered enlarged if they are greater than 8 mm in maximum diameter.

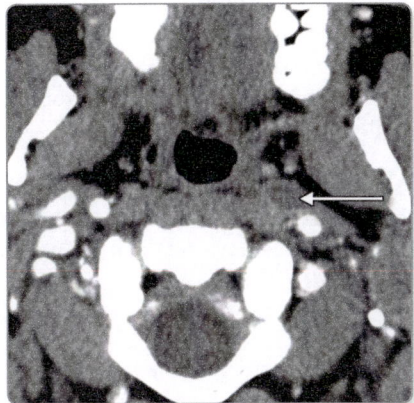

**Figure 13.21A** Retropharyngeal lymphadenopathy in a patient with adenoid cystic carcinoma. Contrast-enhanced axial CT image demonstrates an enlarged and centrally necrotic lymph node of Rouviere

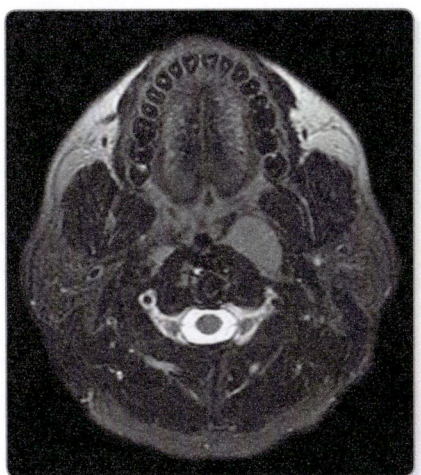

**Figure 13.21B** Large left retropharyngeal node in a patient with a nasopharyngeal carcinoma

## Direct spread of malignancy

Direct spread of nasopharyngeal carcinoma is an important cause of retropharyngeal space disease. More than one-third of patients with nasopharyngeal carcinoma patients have retropharyngeal space involvement at the time of diagnosis.

## Postradiation changes

Patients may develop edema in the retropharyngeal space following external beam radiation therapy, and this may persist for months or years.

## Multinodular goiter

Multinodular goiter may extend cranially into the retropharyngeal space (**Figures 13.22A and B**). On imaging, look for contiguity with an enlarged thyroid.

## Vascular

Retropharyngeal hematoma occurs mainly in the context of trauma or coagulopathy.

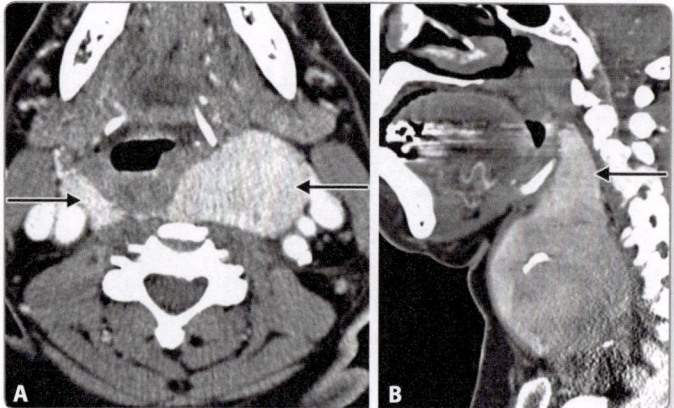

**Figures 13.22A and B** Multinodular goiter extending into the retropharyngeal space. Contrast-enhanced axial and sagittal CT images demonstrate extension of a large thyroid gland into the retropharyngeal space bilaterally (arrows)

# Perivertebral space

## Anatomy

The "perivertebral space" is bounded by the deep layer of deep cervical fascia that surrounds the vertebral column and associated musculature. Anterior to the vertebral column, the perivertebral space is more specifically called the "prevertebral space." The prevertebral space extends from the skull base to the coccyx. The deep layer of deep cervical fascia is attached to the cervical transverse processes, and then posterior to this, it envelops the paravertebral musculature, and attaches to the ligamentum nuchae. The portion of the perivertebral space posterior to the transverse processes is more specifically called the "paravertebral space". The prevertebral space contains the longus colli and longus capitis muscles, the scalene muscles, brachial plexus roots, the phrenic nerve, vertebral artery and vein, and vertebral bodies. The paravertebral space contains the posterior elements of the vertebrae, and the paravertebral muscles.

The prevertebral space is immediately posterior to the retropharyngeal space. These spaces have different differential diagnoses, so it is important to distinguish between them. On imaging, this is done by evaluating the relationship of a lesion to the prevertebral muscles. If the lesion displaces the longus colli/longus capitis muscles posteriorly, then it resides within the retropharyngeal space. If the lesion is within the prevertebral muscles or displaces the muscles anteriorly, then it is in the prevertebral space.

## Infectious or inflammatory

### Acute calcific tendinitis of longus colli

This disorder is characterized by acute inflammation of the longus colli tendon into the anterior arch of the C1 vertebra. The inflammation, similar to calcific tendonitis elsewhere in the body, is caused by deposition of hydroxyapatite crystals in the tendon. Patients are typically middle age adults or elderly. The clinical presentation is acute neck pain and stiffness, sometimes with odynophagia,

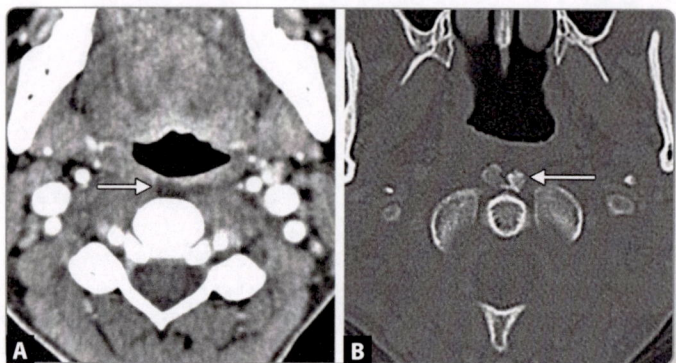

Figures 13.23A and B Acute calcific tendonitis of longus colli. Contrast-enhanced axial CT images with soft tissue (A) and bone (at a slightly higher level, right) algorithm demonstrate a small volume of fluid in the retropharyngeal space (arrow, left) and amorphous calcification just superior the fluid, anterior to the odontoid process (arrow right)

sometimes with fever. This is self-limiting, with symptoms typically resolving spontaneously in 1 to 2 weeks. Treatment is nonsteroidal anti-inflammatory drugs.

On imaging, (**Figures 13.23A and B**) acute calcific tendinitis manifests as amorphous calcifications in the prevertebral space of the upper cervical spine, with associated prevertebral space edema or fluid collection. The effusion originates in the prevertebral space but may extend into the retropharyngeal space. The most important point about this disorder is to avoid mistaking it for a retropharyngeal abscess. CT is helpful at differentiating between calcific tendinitis and abscess, with the former demonstrating fluid that lacks rim enhancement and tapers inferiorly, and the latter demonstrating a collection with rim enhancement and rounded margins.

## Perivertebral abscess

The two greatest risk factors for perivertebral abscess are intravenous drug abuse and surgery. The most common organism is *Staphylococcus aureus*. On imaging (**Figure 13.24**), evaluate for an

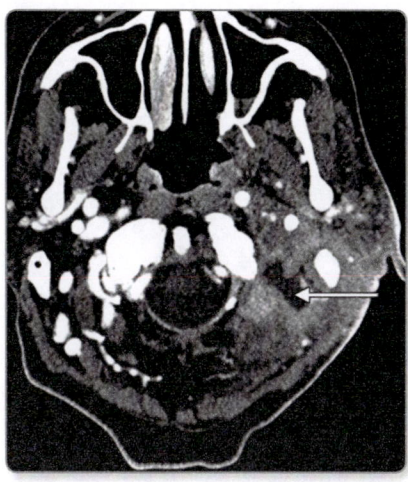

**Figure 13.24** Paravertebral abscess secondary to malignant otitis externa. Contrast-enhanced axial CT image demonstrates a rim enhancing fluid collection (arrow) in the left paravertebral space with surrounding inflammatory changes

underlying source of infection (such as discitis) and for complications (such as epidural extension with spinal cord compression). The important MR sequences are T2-weighted imaging with fat suppression, and T1-weighted imaging postgadolinium with fat suppression.

## Neoplastic

A variety of benign and malignant tumors may involve the perivertebral space. Benign lesions include schwannomas and neurofibromas arising from the brachial plexus, other soft tissue lesions such as lipomas, and benign lesions arising from the vertebra such as osteoblastoma. Malignant lesions include direct spread of mucosal tumors (**Figures 13.25A and B**), primary vertebral lesions such as giant cell tumor or myeloma (**Figures 13.26A to D**), lymphoma/leukemia (**Figure 13.27**), and metastases.

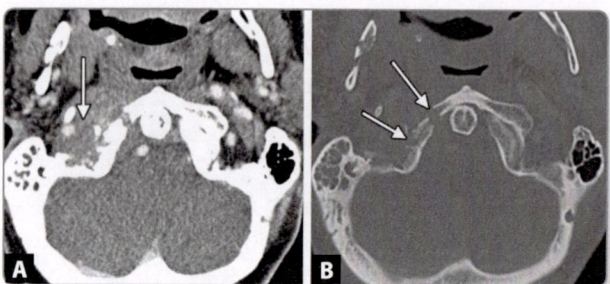

**Figures 13.25A and B** Carcinoma of retromolar trigone with direct spread to prevertebral space. Contrast-enhanced axial CT images with soft tissue (A) and bone (B) algorithm. A soft tissue mass (arrow, left) in the right prevertebral space extends into the right carotid space and encases the right internal carotid artery and internal jugular vein. There is pathological fracture of the arch of C1 and the right occipital condyle (arrows, right). Tumor extends into the epidural space of the upper spinal canal. There is fluid in the right mastoid air cells

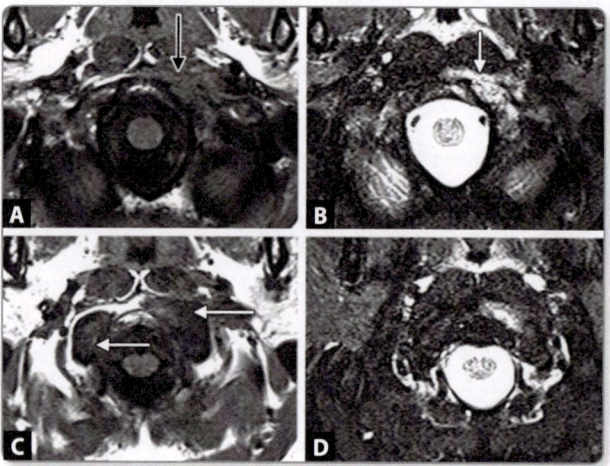

**Figures 13.26A to D** Myeloma involving the prevertebral space. T1 (left) and T2 (right) weighted fat suppressed axial MR images at (bottom) and just above (top) the level of the C1 vertebra anterior arch. There is loss of the normal marrow hyperintensity on T1-weighted images (arrows, bottom left image). Tumor in the prevertebral space elevates the left prevertebral musculature (arrows, upper images).

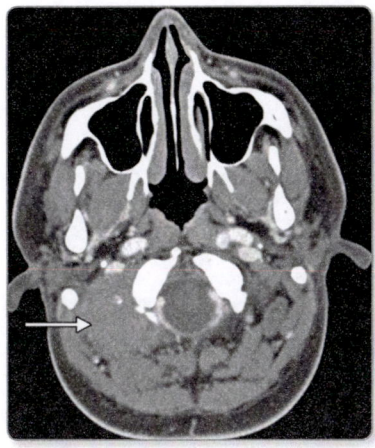

**Figure 13.27** Acute myelogenous leukemia with paravertebral leukemic mass. Contrast-enhanced axial CT image demonstrates a soft tissue mass in the right paravertebral space, obliterating the normal fat planes

# Bibliography

1. Chong VF, Fan YF. Pictorial review: Radiology of the carotid space. Clinical Radiology. 1996;51(11):762-8.
2. Davis WL, Harnsberger HR. CT and MRI of the normal and diseased perivertebral space. Neuroradiology. 1995;37(5):388-94.
3. Davis WL, Harnsberger HR, Smoker WR, Watanabe AS. Retropharyngeal space: Evaluation of normal anatomy and diseases with CT and MR imaging. Radiology. 1990;174(1):59-64.
4. Fruin ME, Smoker WR, Harnsberger HR. The carotid space in the suprahyoid neck. Seminars in Ultrasound, CT and MR. 1990;11(6):504-19.
5. Fruin ME, Smoker WR, Harnsberger HR. The carotid space of the infrahyoid neck. Seminars in Ultrasound, CT and MR. 1991;12(3):224-40.
6. Kurihara N, Takahashi S, Higano S, Nakamura M, Tsuda M, Saito H. Edema in the retropharyngeal space associated with head and neck tumors: CT imaging characteristics. Neuroradiology. 2005;47(8):609-15.
7. Tardy J, Pariente J, Nasr N, Peiffer S, Dumas H, Cognard C, Larrue V, Chollet F, Albucher JF. Carotidynia: A new case for an old controversy. European Journal of Neurology. 2007;14(6):704-5.

# Vascular lesions of the head and neck

chapter **14**

Juan Pablo Cruz, Timo Krings, Tom Marotta

### Abstract

This chapter covers the imaging features of the various types of vascular malformations that affect the head and neck. Traumatic vascular lesions such as AV fistula and vessel dissection are also covered. The chapter ends with a discussion on vascular neoplasms and hypervascular lymphadenopathies.

### Keywords

Vascular malformations, high flow, low flow, AVM, venous vascular malformations.

Vascular lesions of the head and neck are a heterogeneous group of diseases that range from congenital disorders (i.e. vascular malformations) to acquired conditions. These include traumatic, autoimmune, neoplastic or as a manifestation of a syndrome. Lesions will be more frequently located in the anterior parapharyngeal space (carotid space), but can be found anywhere in the neck, cervical spine or skull base. They can be asymptomatic and come to attention as an incidental finding, or present with a wide variety of symptoms according to their nature and location. We will try to group these lesions according to etiology rather than location, so as to create a more systematic and comprehensible approach for an otherwise complex subject.

## Vascular malformations

Vascular malformations of the head and neck region are a vast topic, with many different manifestations, locations and treatment strategies. In an attempt to simplify the discussion of these lesions we will present a conceptual approach to vascular malformations in general. Vascular malformations are non-neoplastic mass lesions that are present at birth, but may become clinically apparent later in life, grow in relation to the body volume and do not spontaneously involute. They are subdivided into high-flow and low-flow groups. High-flow vascular malformations have an arterial component and include both arteriovenous malformations and arteriovenous fistulas. Low–flow vascular malformations include lymphangiomas and venous malformations. Goals of imaging of vascular malformations are: (1) lesion characterization and (2) anatomic location/extent.

## Low flow vascular malformations

### Lymphatic or venolymphatic malformations

Lymphatic malformations, also called lymphangioma or cystic hygroma are lesions of unknown etiology. They usually include both lymphatic and venous components (mixed venolymphatic vascular malformations). Possible etiologies include failure of the lymphatic system to connect with or separate from the venous system, abnormal budding of lymphatic structures from the cardinal vein, or sequestration of lymphatic tissue in early embryogenesis. Acquired processes that may be involved in the formation of these lesions include trauma, infection, chronic inflammation, or lymphatic obstruction. From a practical point of view they should be separated into macrocystic, microcystic, or mixed types. However, this gross morphology does not necessarily correlate with histologic subtypes.

Head and neck lymphangiomas are uncommon, representing less than 6 percent of benign tumors of childhood. Their incidence is estimated at 2.8 per 1000 population or less and there is no gender predilection. The majority (90%) will be diagnosed by 2 years of age. In the suprahyoid neck, the masticator and submandibular spaces are most commonly involved, whereas in the infrahyoid neck, the posterior cervical space is the most commonly affected. Orbital lesions are often multicompartmental involving pre- and postseptal regions as well as intra- and extraconal portions of the orbit.

Symptoms depend on size and location. The majority will present as a slow-growing cystic mass. The most significant symptom is respiratory compromise, especially with suprahyoid involvement. Sudden enlargement after intracystic hemorrhage or after an upper airway infection may result in airway obstruction or sudden painful proptosis depending on location. Puberty and pregnancy have been associated to lesion enlargement. Skeletal distortion, dental malocclusion, mandibular overgrowth, anterior open bite, and lateral cross-bite will be seen as consequences in larger lesions.

MR is the preferred imaging modality for this type of lesions given its superior soft tissue contrast. It will better differentiate the different vascular components and the anatomic extent of the lesion. In addition, the brain can be evaluated for associated vascular anomalies. In general terms, these lesions will show a low to intermediate signal intensity on T1WI and a marked hyperintensity in T2WI, though this may vary depending on the presence and state of degradation of blood products. No enlarged feeding vessels or flow voids are seen; this helps to differentiate them from capillary hemangiomas or arteriovenous shunting malformations. Lymphangiomas can involve multiple compartments, a feature that is characteristic of this lesion. Enhancement is heterogeneous and quite variable depending on the amount of venous component and presence of hemorrhage/infection. The cystic areas will show no internal enhancement (**Figures 14.1 and 14.2**). CT may show phleboliths associated to the venous component of the lesion and will better characterize the associated bone abnormalities. Differential diagnoses depend on the location and include branchial cleft cysts, thyroglossal duct cysts, venous malformations, hemangioma and abscess.

Treatment options include complete surgical excision versus percutaneous sclerotherapy for macrocystic lesions. In spite of gross

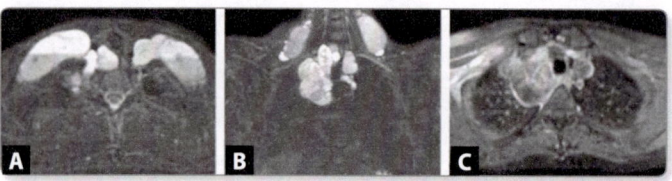

**Figures 14.1A to C** Cervical venolymphatic vascular malformation. (A and B) Axial and coronal fat saturated T2WI and (C) gadolinium enhanced fat saturated T1WI. Large multicompartmental cystic mass involving the base of the neck and the medium mediastinum with fluid-fluid levels, showing patchy delayed enhancement of the venous component, but no internal enhancement of the cystic regions

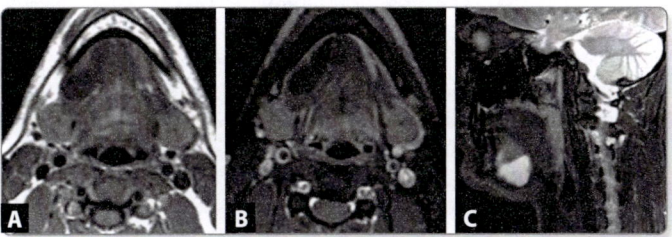

**Figures 14.2A to C** Venolymphatic vascular malformation. (A) Axial T1WI, (B) Axial gadolinium enhanced fat saturated T1WI and (C) Sagittal fat saturated T2WI. Cystic lesion in the sublingual space, without any internal enhancement

resection, these lesions may continue to enlarge and recur in up to 30 percent. The rate of complications is directly correlated with the size and extent of the lesion and the degree of involvement of the adjacent structures ranging from 17 percent in smaller circumscribed lesions to as high as 100 percent in complex bilateral multicompartmental lesions. Complications after surgery include facial nerve injury, infection, and airway compromise requiring tracheostomy, dental caries, episodic bleeding, hypoglossal nerve injury, and significant functional and cosmetic deformity. Common side effects after sclerotherapy include fever lasting between 2 to 4 days and local inflammatory reaction with tenderness and erythema, which may last for up to 3 weeks. Massive swelling is the most dangerous complication because of potential airway involvement.

## Venous vascular malformations

Venous vascular malformation (VVM) is the second most common vascular lesion of the head and neck after hemangiomas and is the most common vascular malformation in this region. VVMs have an equal sex distribution and do not regress spontaneously. They consist of dysplastic venous channels with minimal connection to adjacent veins and no arteriovenous shunting. Histologically they are composed of thin-walled, dilated, sponge-like abnormal channels of variable size and thickness.

Venous malformations are considered congenital lesions, but they may remain clinically silent for years. Superficial lesions will clinically present as soft, compressible, nonpulsatile lesions that gradually refill when pressure is released, and a bluish skin discoloration. Position related swelling is seen as patient head is placed below the heart level. Deeper lesions may not be visible on clinical exam. VVMs have a slow growth rate, but rapid exacerbated growth has been reported after trauma, sepsis, or hormonal changes (puberty, pregnancy). Patients have often, episodic painful swelling, likely secondary to spontaneous thrombosis of venous sacs. Repeated thrombosis and recanalization leads to formation of phleboliths.

Soft tissue lesions are located most frequently on the face followed by the suprahyoid neck spaces (mandibular, sublingual, tongue) and orbit (also called orbital varix). Although they are predominantly soft tissue masses, they may infiltrate deeply along facial planes. Deep or intramuscular lesions may present with pain most severe in the morning. The adjacent bone may become thinned or eroded. Intraosseous lesions involve the calvarium and the mandible.

Lesions that are superficial in the facial and orbital region can show distensibility on clinical (and imaging) evaluation when the patient is asked to perform a Valsalva maneuver.

Venous malformations are often asymptomatic. There is however a wide range of associated symptoms and potential complications. These include disfiguration, venous stasis, ischemia, skeletal abnormalities and consumptive coagulopathy. Local mass effect with airway involvement or optic neuropathy may be seen when they reach a massive size.

On MRI they will show a lobulated, well-defined lesion, markedly hyperintense on T2WI and intermediate T1 signal with variable degrees of enhancement (**Figures 14.3A to D**). Phleboliths, which are a pathognomonic feature, will appear as low T1WI and T2WI small rounded foci within the lesion (**Figure 14.4B**). When complicated with hemorrhage or after treatment, the T1 and T2 signal will be heterogeneous related to the various states of blood product degradation. Flow voids are not a common feature given the low flow nature of the lesion; however, occasional dysplastic draining veins may be visualized.

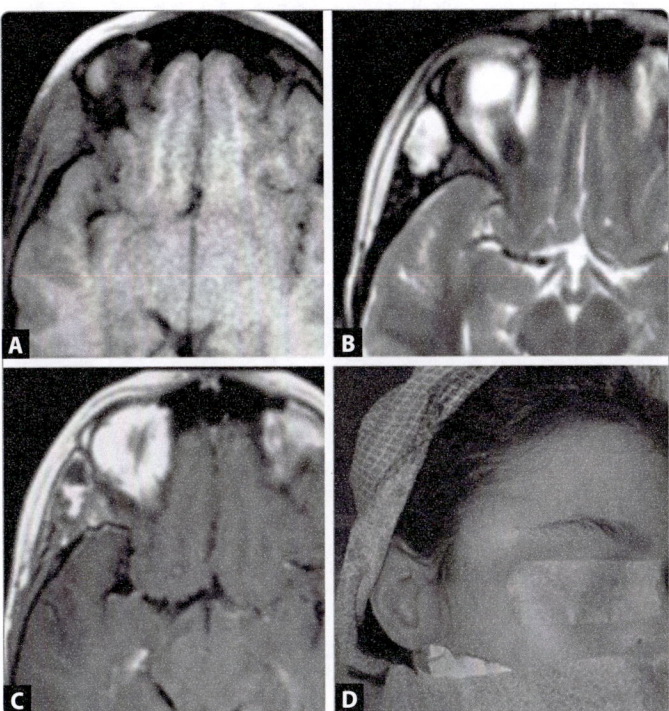

**Figures 14.3A to D** VVM. (A) Axial T1WI, (B) Axial T2WI, (C) Gadolinium enhanced T1WI and (D) Intraoperative picture. Superficial intramuscular VVM located in the temporalis muscle, with intermediate T1 signal, markedly hyperintense T2 signal and internal delayed enhancement after gadolinium administration. Intraoperative picture shows the corresponding local volume increase (*for color version of Figure 14.3D see Plate 17*)

On CT these lesions are isodense, lobulated, heterogeneously enhancing, well circumscribed solid mass, occasionally with associated dysplastic veins and phleboliths (**Figure 14.4A**). Delayed images show a more homogeneous pattern of enhancement. Intraosseous lesions may be seen as focal areas of cortical thinning with increased trabeculae, non-sclerotic margins and a radial sunburst pattern.

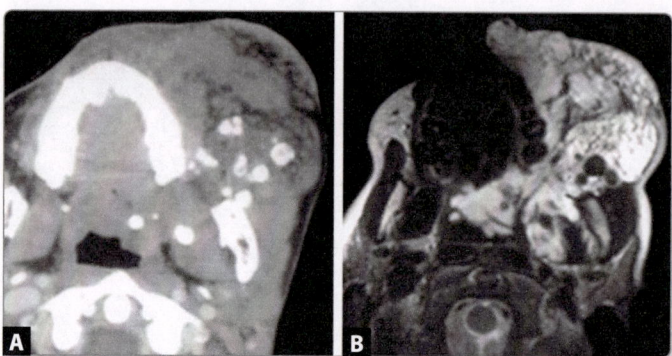

**Figures 14.4A and B** Venous vascular malformations. (A) Non-enhanced CT, (B) Axial T2WI. Complex deep and superficial VVM centered in the parotid space, extending to the parapharyngeal and parapharyngeal mucosal space. Note the pronounced hyperintensity in the T2WI and the presence of phleboliths in the NECT

Diagnostic angiography is rarely necessary unless strong pulsation or bruits are present, suggesting a large vascular connection.

In symptomatic venous malformations, percutaneous sclerotherapy is the mainstay treatment. Direct phlebography must be performed to delineate multiple compartments of the malformation and the venous drainage for adequate treatment planning. Multiple punctures and injections are usually required to evaluate different components. Treatment response should be assessed after months, allowing time for the transient inflammatory reaction to resolve (**Figures 14.5A to D**). Complications of sclerotherapy are rare and include skin necrosis, neuropathy, pain and swelling, muscle atrophy, deep vein thrombosis, pulmonary embolism, pulmonary vasospasm, disseminated intravascular coagulation, and cardiac arrest (as a result of direct cardiotoxicity).

## High flow vascular malformations

### Arteriovenous malformations

Arteriovenous malformations (AVM's) are congenital vascular lesions constituted by abnormal vascular channels connecting the arterial

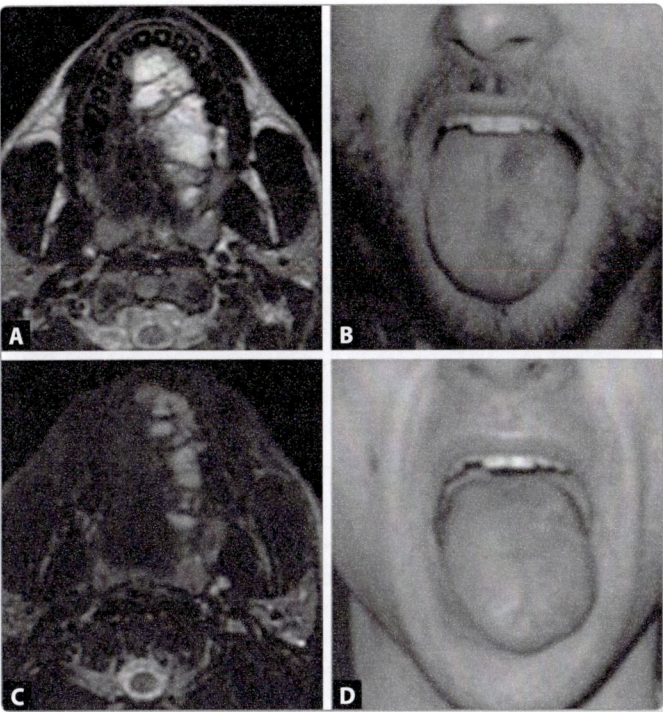

**Figures 14.5A to D** VVM (A, B) Pre- and (C, D) Postembolization axial T2WI and picture of a lingual VVM. High T2 signal multicystic lesion involving the left side of the tongue and sublingual space. Note the interval decrease in size after the embolization procedure and the almost complete resolution of the clinical mass effect and bluish discoloration of the tongue (*for color version of Figure 14.5B and D see Plate 18*)

and venous system, without an intervening normal capillary bed, and a variable degree of arteriovenous shunting. They are considered the most aggressive of all the vascular malformations leading to dramatic deformity, functional impairment, and possible mortality. The head and neck is the most common location for extra-CNS AVM's. Seventy percent will involve the midface, 14 percent will affect the upper third of the face and 17 the lower third. This is proportional to the volume of tissue seen during the embryonic stage. Invasion of the underlying bone is often seen and complicates therapy.

Symptoms vary depending on location, the degree of arteriovenous shunting, and venous hypertension. They usually manifest as a warm palpable pulsatile mass, with a bruit and engorged venous structures. In cases when the shunt is less significant, symptoms will be less pronounced and the objective bruit may be the only manifestation. The fast-flow character of AVMs usually becomes evident in childhood or during puberty. Rapid expansion has been reported following pregnancy, trauma, or inadequate surgical intervention. Schobinger described 4 clinical stages: (1) quiescence, (2) expansion, (3) destruction, including pain, bleeding, or ulceration, and (4) decompensation, (e.g. cardiac failure). Pain associated with an AVM is a worrisome sign for progression on to the next stage.

CTA and MRA will show the prominent tortuous vascular structures without a discrete enhancing soft-tissue mass and flow voids on spin-echo imaging. The absence of a discrete soft tissue mass differentiates the AVM from the infantile hemangioma. As previously stated, cross-sectional imaging will show better the anatomic relation with the adjacent structures and the extent of the lesion. Conventional catheter angiography is mandatory for a more detailed characterization of flow dynamics within the lesion, the arterial supply, the venous drainage pathways and potential dangerous anastomoses between the extracranial and intracranial arteries. This information is fundamental for treatment planning. Classic angiographic features are multiple hypertrophied feeding arteries rapidly shunting into enlarged draining veins across a nidus (**Figures 14.6A to D**).

In small, asymptomatic lesions, observation is often a good initial approach. Pain, expansion, ulceration, bleeding, and cardiac decompensation can occur after a quiescent period given the dynamic ever-changing nature of these lesions. In this clinical setting, intra-arterial embolization with or without complete surgical resection is the treatment of choice. In some cases excision may be impossible because of the location and extent of the malformation so embolization alone may be used as a palliative therapy to control symptoms. In contrast to intracranial AVMs, occlusion of the venous side is a

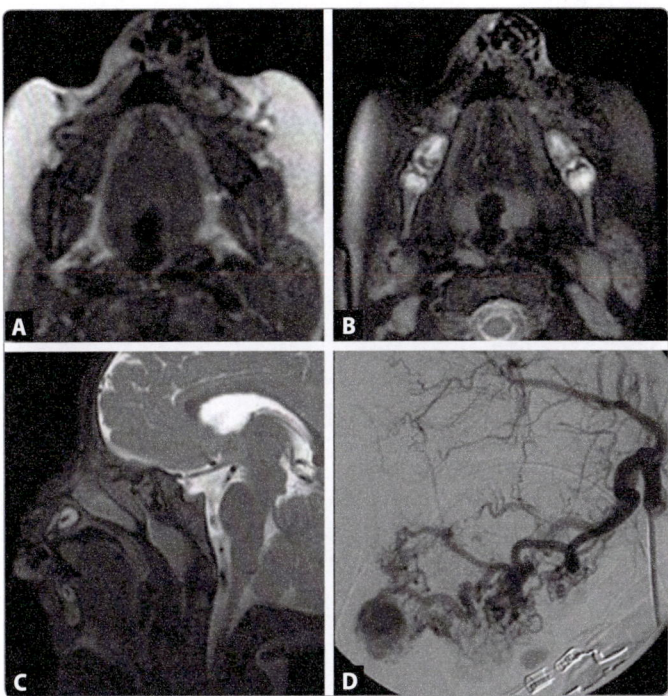

**Figures 14.6A to D** AVM. (A) Axial T1WI, (B and C) axial and sagittal fat saturated T2WI, (D) Lateral angiogram after distal ECA injection. Inferior labial AVM with local mass effect and multiple flow voids seen on MR imaging. Catheter angiogram shows and AVM supplied mainly by the facial artery with a venous pouch in the inferior lip. Note the early opacification of the venous structures seen in the arterial phase of the angiogram

potential treatment option. Ligation embolizations, proximal occlusions and particle embolization should be avoided at all costs since these will trigger lesion growth and indirect recruitment, which will be difficult to reach with an endovascular approach. Extracranial arteriovenous malformations are difficult to cure, but all efforts should be made in curing the lesion early in the development of the disease ("all or nothing" approach). Each treatment session will trigger the release of different angiogenic factors that will promote recurrence and growth, so every failed attempt will make cure or control of the AVM progressively more difficult. For the aforementioned reasons, partial treatment should never be the aim of any surgical or interventional procedure.

A multidisciplinary approach is best to determine appropriate management strategy and must evaluate each patient individually. Long-term complications include cardiac hypertrophy, cardiac failure, hemorrhage and stroke.

## False maxillofacial vascular malformations

### Sinus pericranii

Since it was first described by Stromeyer in 1850, there have been multiple definitions of a sinus pericranii (SP). Gandolfo et al recently defined it as a "an emissary vein (in terms of its transosseous disposition and associated diploic drainage) with an increased subgaleal drainage (instead of an interperiostodural, i.e. sinus, drainage)." It represents an extreme form of brain venous drainage outside the cranial cavity through a network of thin-walled veins that form a varix on the external table of the skull.

Sinus pericranii is a relatively rare entity of unknown etiology, but it may be related to abnormal cellular signaling during embryonic development, which eventually may lead to overtriggering of the diploic veins that converge in a SP.

Clinically, it will present most usually as a midline lesion, commonly located in the frontal region, with swelling after Valsalva maneuvers, and no bruit or plasticity. It behaves as a venous lesion. They are usually asymptomatic and patients will come seeking for medical attention due to cosmetic issues.

The venous anatomy inside the cranial cavity is generally missbuilt and there is a large bony channel in the skull, which allows extracranial drainage of intracranial blood. SP may be associated to other venous abnormalities as developmental venous anomalies, hemangiomas, VVMs and vein of Galein aneurysmal malformation.

Surgical or endovascular treatment of SP is usually indicated for cosmetic reasons. For treatment planning DSA is mandatory so to assess whether the lesion is "dominant" (constitutes a main venous drainage pathway for the brain) or "accessory" (small part of the venous outflow is seen through the lesion). This is extremely important because if a dominant lesion is "treated", it would lead to venous congestion and hemorrhagic venous infarction.

## Facial venous dilations associated to intracranial vascular lesions

The facial veins may provide an alternative draining route for the brain parenchyma in intracranial disorders with a hemodynamic through flow rerouting to the cavernous sinus and via ophthalmic veins and subsequently to the facial veins. Two different situations are associated with transorbital drainage: (1) the brain drains through the orbit, while the intracranial AVS drains separately into the posterior sinuses or (2) the jugular foramen is occluded and both the brain and the lesion drain through the orbit.

These lesions should be suspected when there are added symptoms from the shunt itself or derived from venous congestion. In this cases catheter angiogram is mandatory even if CT or MR studies are negative. Treatment should aim to exclude the underlying AV shunt and as a consequence the facial venous dilatation may resolve. Resolution is less common in AV shunts with associated venous outlet obstruction.

## Idiopathic facial vascular dilations

In the setting of an asymptomatic patient with a dilated facial vein (usually naso-orbital region) with an associated bruit, and MR study should be performed to rule out an intracranial AV shunt or a sinus occlusion. If there are no symptoms and no associated imaging abnormality, this can be regarded as an idiopathic facial venous dilatation. This entity is seen in infants and young children, extremely rare in neonates and nonexistent in the adult population. It is considered a benign entity and shows spontaneous resolution usually before the age of 7 years. Clinical follow-up is mandatory to document resolution.

In theory, these venous dilatations represent an early opening of the brain venous outlets into the cavernous sinus in a still under developed skull base.

## Traumatic vascular lesions

Traumatic vascular lesions of the head and neck are associated with a high morbidity and mortality. Two major mechanisms are involved, penetrating and blunt trauma with the latter being the most common one. The carotid arteries are two times more often injured than the vertebral arteries. Carotid injury should be suspected in patients with fractures of the sella turcica-sphenoid sinus complex or air within the carotid canal. Indicators for vertebral artery injury are spinal cervical injuries with dislocation/rotation mechanisms or fractures involving the foramen transversarium. The incidence ranges from 0.18 to 1.55 percent of all trauma patients. Motor vehicle accidents are the main cause with young males (below 30 years old) being the most commonly affected. There are 3 major types of injuries: arterial dissection, pseudoaneurysms and traumatic AV fistulas.

### Traumatic dissections

An arterial dissection is a hematoma within the blood vessel wall that might produce a stenosis, luminal irregularity and/or aneurysmal dilatation. This intramural hematoma may evolve with an intraluminal rerupture, creating a double lumen or through the adventitia leading to vessel rupture. It usually occurs in association with cervical hyperextension/rotation injuries. The most common location is the cervical and petrous internal carotid artery, sparing the carotid bulb, secondary to stretching of the artery across the transverse processes of the cervical vertebrae. Vertebral artery dissections are usually located between the skull base and C2, and may happen due to arterial stretching or fractures extending through the foramen transversarium.

Dissections account for the majority of cerebrovascular trauma sequels. Delayed onset of ischemic brain infarcts is the most common manifestation. Patients may be asymptomatic in 20 to 33 percent of the cases. Other clinical manifestations include neck pain along the course of artery and Horner's syndrome (**Figure 14.7**).

Imaging findings in CTA and MRI/MRA can show luminal narrowing with an intramural hematoma (best seen on nonenhanced T1 fat-saturated sequences) (**Figures 14.8A to F**) or an intimal flap

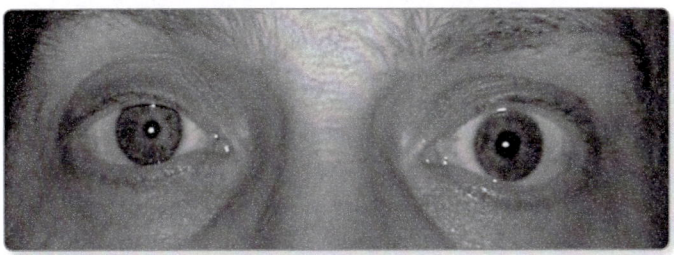

**Figure 14.7** Horner's syndrome. Patient with a right ICA dissection and Horner's syndrome characterized by right ptosis, miosis and anhydrosis (*for color version see Plate 18*)

(**Figures 14.9A to C**). On angiography findings may vary between circumferential long segment narrowing to smooth tapered occlusions (string sign) (**Figures 14.10A to C**).

Medical management with anticoagulation therapy is the treatment of choice for preventing thromboembolic complications. This has been subjected to controversy with several publications showing no difference between anticoagulation versus antiplatelet therapy. Endovascular treatment (stents or vessel occlusion) or surgical treatment are reserved for patients with contraindications for anticoagulation or medical therapy failure and only exceedingly rarely indicated.

The prognosis depends on the associated injuries. Compared to spontaneous dissections where 85 percent improve, traumatic dissection improve in only 55 and 25 percent progress to complete occlusion.

## Traumatic aneurysms

Traumatic aneurysms are not true aneurysms, i.e. their "wall" consists of coagulated hematoma surrounding the vessel disruption. They may result as a consequence of a dissection (dissecting aneurysm) or an organized hematoma (pseudoaneurysms). Extracranial traumatic aneurysms are more commonly seen in penetrating trauma, while skull base aneurysms are seen in blunt head injury with skull base fractures. Iatrogenic aneurysms following neck surgery, tracheostomy,

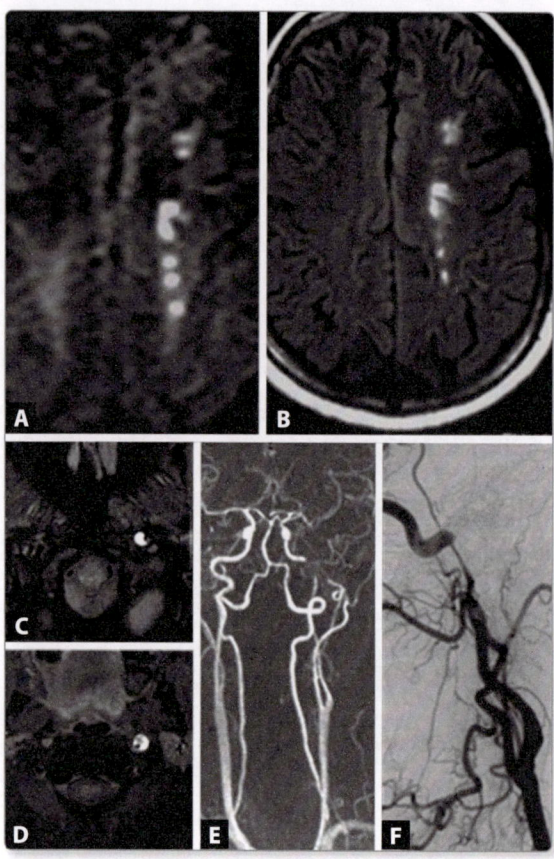

**Figures 14.8A to F** Arterial dissection. (A) DWI, (B) Axial FLAIR, (C) Axial fat saturated T1WI, (D) Contrast enhanced MRA and (E, F) Lateral angiogram after common carotid artery injection. Multiple recent infarcts in a watershed distribution seen in the left supratentorial deep white matter. The far saturated images show a hyperintense crescentic shaped intramural hematoma in the cervical left ICA secondary to the presence of meta hemoglobin. Angiographic pictures reveal a smooth, tapered severe narrowing of the ICA with decreased flow distally, in keeping with an arterial dissection

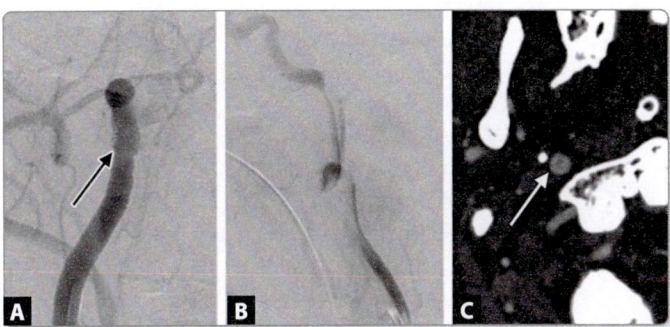

**Figures 14.9A to C** Iatrogenic arterial dissection. (A, B) AP and lateral angiograms, (C) CTA source images. Patient undergoing endovascular treatment for a ruptured intracranial aneurysm who had a catheter related ICA dissection. Note the linear filling defect (black arrow on (A) corresponding to the dissection flap, and the contrast stagnation with decreased distal flow on (B). Follow-up CTA shows the dissection flap (white arrow) with a patent right ICA

or intraoral procedures are far less common. Distal cortical and subcortical traumatic intracranial aneurysms will not be discussed in this chapter. Other locations less commonly seen are the distal superficial temporal artery and occipital artery.

There are a wide variety of clinical manifestations, including asymptomatic, pulsatile cervical or superficial scalp mass, local mass effect, rupture with massive bleeding and death. Delayed onset of symptoms is common.

Angiographic findings on extracranial traumatic aneurysms include small saccular lesions, fusiform dilatations and large cavitated hematomas. Skull base aneurysms will usually have more irregular contours. Clinical history is fundamental (**Figures 14.11A and B**).

Treatment strategy should consider that these types of aneurysms do not have a true wall so the use of coils or liquid embolic materials should be avoided. The main objective in an acute setting is to stop the hemorrhage. Vessel occlusion, either surgical or endovascular, surgical reconstitution of the vessel or the use of stent grafts are the main treatment options.

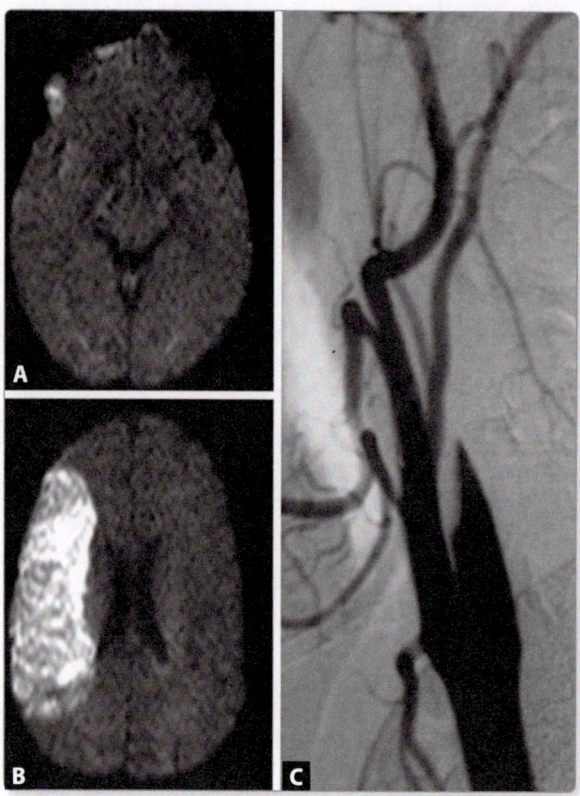

**Figures 14.10A to C** Arterial dissection. (A) DWI and (B and C) Lateral angiogram. Large right MCA infarct seen in DWI. Angiogram revealed a tapered caliber reduction of the proximal cervical ICA with distal occlusion (flame shaped occlusion), classical for ICA dissection

## Traumatic AV fistula

Traumatic AVFs can occur anywhere in the head and neck region where there is a close spatial relationship between an artery and a vein. In clinical practice, the two most common locations for traumatic AVFs are the carotid-cavernous fistula (CCF) and the vertebrovenous

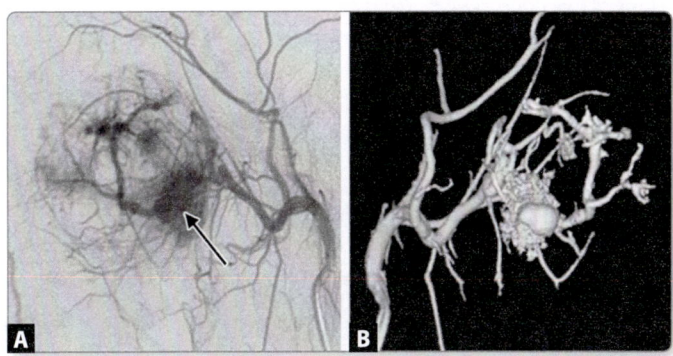

**Figures 14.11A and B** Iatrogenic pseudoaneurysm. (A) Lateral distal ECA angiogram and (B) VR images from the 3D rotational angiogram. Patient with massive epistaxis after biopsy of a vascular nasal polypoid tumor. Angiogram revealed a saccular dilatation within the vascular tumor, at the biopsy site, in keeping with an iatrogenic pseudoaneurysm

fistulae (VVFs). In CCFs the mechanism of fistulization is a direct high flow arteriovenous shunt due to tearing of the ICA or avulsion of one of the small meningeal arteries. Each of these "connects" with the multiseptated venous spaces of the cavernous sinus to produce an A-V shunt. The most common etiology is a skull base fracture. Less frequently this can be seen in the setting of a ruptured traumatic skull base aneurysm.

Clinical manifestations of a traumatic CCF may appear days to weeks after trauma. Signs and symptoms include pulsatile exophthalmos, chemosis, bruit, ophthalmoplegia and glaucoma due to venous congestion, leading to transient or permanent visual loss. When there is deep venous drainage, subarachnoid hemorrhage or parenchymal hematomas can be seen. In more severe trauma, a CCF can be associated with massive, life-threatening epistaxis.

CT and MR images may show an enlarged cavernous sinus and, depending on the drainage pattern a dilated vein, with the superior ophthalmic vein being most commonly involved. Cross-sectional imaging may in these instances also show proptosis. Time resolved MRA or CTA will demonstrate early opacification of the cavernous sinus. Associated skull base fractures and aneurysms are best seen in CT. Catheter angiography is the exam of choice, given the superior spatial and temporal resolution (**Figures 14.12A to D**). The main goal of angiography is to assess the draining pattern of the fistula and collateral circulation for treatment planning. Draining routes include: (1) ophthalmic vein into the angular vein and subsequently the facial vein (most common pathway), (2) inferior petrosal sinus into the sigmoid sinus, (3) superior petrosal sinus, which usually

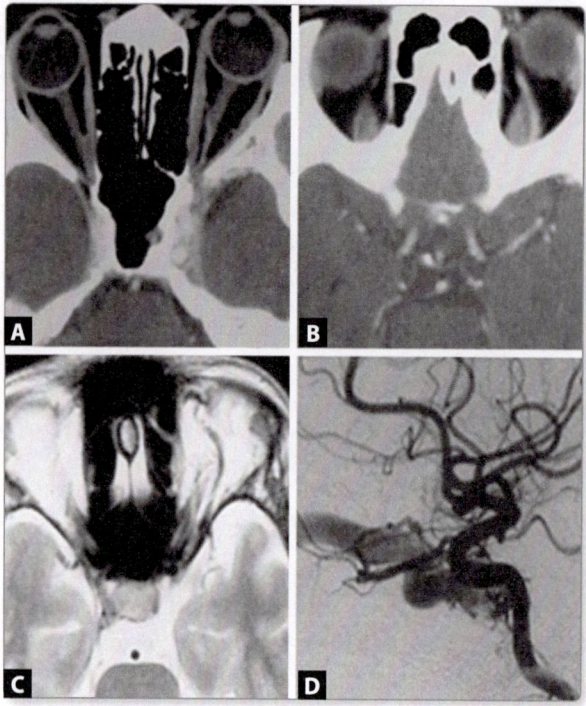

**Figures 14.12A to D** Carotid-cavernous fistula (CCF). (A, B) CTA, (C) Axial T2WI and (D) Lateral ICA angiogram. Mild left proptosis with enlargement and early opacification of the left superior ophthalmic vein (SOV). The patient worsened and follow-up angiogram showed a type I CCF with interval progression of the SOV dilatation

connects to the transverse-sigmoid sinus, but may have connections with the posterior fossa veins, (4) sphenoparietal sinus into cortical veins further draining into the superior sagittal sinus, or (5) basal vein of Rosenthal into the vein of Galen and the straight sinus. Prognosis depends on the venous drainage routes with the latter ones resulting in more venous congestion and subsequent potential hemorrhagic infarction.

External carotids AVFs represent 11 percent of all carotid artery fistulae. They are classified according to their location and draining pattern (extracranial, intracranial [i.e. middle meningeal artery] with or without cortical drainage). They can present with a pulsatile mass, bruit and brain parenchymal hemorrhage in those with cortical drainage.

Vertebral artery AVFs are ten times less common than CCFs. They are secondary to an abnormal communication between the vertebral artery or its muscular branches and the surrounding venous plexuses (**Figures 14.13A to C**). The most common clinical manifestations are pulsatile tinnitus or a cervical bruit. Other symptoms include neck pain, steal phenomenon with posterior fossa TIAs, and spinal cord or nerve root compression from enlarged venous pouches.

Treatment options include endovascular occlusion of the parent artery, transarterial endovascular occlusion of the fistula using balloons or coils, transvenous occlusion from the venous side (**Figures 14.14A to F**). The use of covered stent grafts has also been reported for cervical and carotid cavernous AVFs.

# Other vascular diseases

## Fibromuscular dysplasia

Cervicocephalic FMD is an uncommon segmental, nonatheromatous, noninflammatory arterial disease of unknown origin that affects small to medium-sized vessels. Three main pathologic subtypes exist: intimal, medial and adventitial (or periarterial). The medial type is the most common (90–95%), followed by the intimal type (5%), with the adventitial type being the least common.

# 580 Introductory head and neck imaging

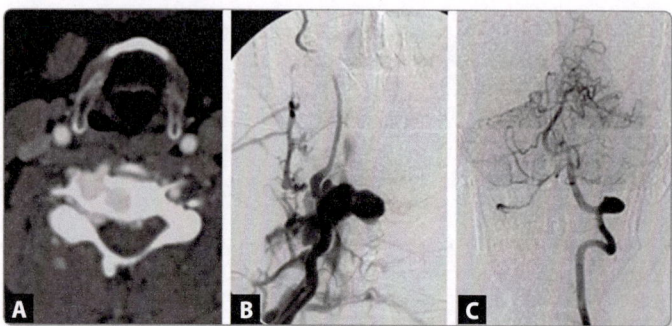

**Figures 14.13A to C** Vertebrovenous AVF. (A) CTA source images, (B) Right and (C) Left vertebral AP angiograms. Patient with pulsatile tinnitus following remote trauma, evolved with right C6 nerve root compression. CTA images show enlarged venous structures remodeling the adjacent C6 vertebral body and displacing the right foraminal fat tissue, in keeping with a vertebrovenous AVF. Findings were corroborated in the diagnostic catheter angiogram

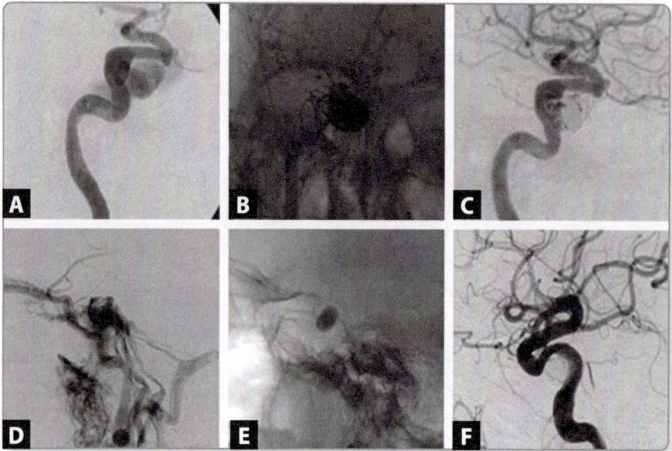

**Figures 14.14A to F** CCF. (A, D) Pre- and (B, C, E, F) post-treatment ICA angiograms. Examples of type I direct CCF treated with coils and detachable balloon respectively. The pretreatment angiograms show a direct CCF in both cases with impaired distal flow due to the amount of AV shunting. Post-treatment angiograms show no AV shunt and marked improvement of the opacification of the intracranial circulation

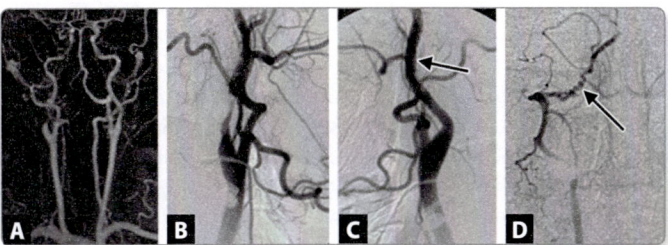

**Figures 14.15A to D** FMD. (A) Contrast enhanced MRA, (B) Right, (C) Left lateral ICA angiograms (D) AP right vertebral angiogram. Patient with a right ICA dissection (note the smooth tapered severe narrowing of the right ICA in A and B). Angiogram showed the classic "beaded appearance" of the contralateral ICA and right vertebral seen in patients with medial FMD (black arrows)

This is a rare disorder in the head and neck, with a prevalence of 1/100.000, more common in females in the fifth decade. It involves the extracranial ICA in nearly 75 percent and is classically bilateral. The extracranial vertebral artery is involved in 15 to 25 percent of patients.

It is usually asymptomatic, but it can present with TIA or stroke. Patients are more prone to arterial dissection and have a higher prevalence of intracranial aneurysms. The mid and distal cervical segment of the ICA is the most commonly affected, with sparing of the carotid bulb. The most common imaging finding on CTA, MRA or DSA is a multifocal concentric luminal narrowing alternating with areas of mural dilatation (string-of-beads appearance), seen in 80 to 90 percent (**Figures 14.15A to D**). Less common findings are tubular stenosis (6–12%), a septum, or a diverticulum.

If there is dissection associated with FMD, management includes anticoagulation or antiplatelet therapy. In cases with an expanding or symptomatic pseudoaneurysm, endovascular or surgical therapy may be considered.

## Large and medium vessel arteritis

Giant cell arteritis is a large and medium vessel granulomatous inflammatory vasculitis that especially involves the superficial temporal arteries, cervical and vertebral arteries, the aorta and its branches, and coronary arteries. It is the most common vasculitis in the elderly in North America and Europe.

Takayasu arteritis is an acute and chronic granulomatous inflammatory of medium and large vessels vasculitis, with stenotic and occasionally dilated lesions in the aorta, its main branches, pulmonary artery, and coronary arteries. It affects mainly young and middle aged Asian women. Patients with chronic vasculitis progress to atherosclerosis.

Etiology for both entities remains unknown, but is presumed to be secondary to cell mediated autoimmunity. Even though these are two distinct entities, seen in different population groups, both have similar clinical features, such as size of affected vessels, ischemic symptoms due to stenosis, and good response to steroid therapy.

MR is the most useful technique for assessment of large and medium vessel arteritis. It will show circumferential, homogenous arterial wall thickening, with adjacent mild edema on T2WI and delayed wall enhancement after contrast administration. The degree of enhancement usually correlates with the degree of disease activity. These findings may be associated with multiple areas of smooth long segment luminal narrowing or segmental occlusions. The most commonly affected vessels are the aortic arch, right subclavian, left common carotid and left subclavian, but any large or medium vessel may be involved (**Figures 14.16A and B**). Giant-cell arteritis also shows a preferential involvement of the superficial temporal arteries, where high resolution MR imaging may play an important role. In Takayasu arteritis, CT may show dystrophic arterial wall calcifications.

FDG PET may reveal the distribution and degree of inflammatory activity in larger vessels in giant cell arteritis and Takayasu arteritis, with increase glucose uptake by the wall of the artery. 18F-FDG PET may be more sensitive than MR on early stages of the disease.

Corticosteroid therapy is the first line of treatment in patients with giant cell arteritis or Takayasu arteritis. Immunosuppressants can be used as a second line treatment in addition to corticosteroids. Tapering of corticosteroids may cause relapses.

Giant cell arteritis has a favorable prognosis given its late onset and reduced incidence of long-term complications. Early treatment is

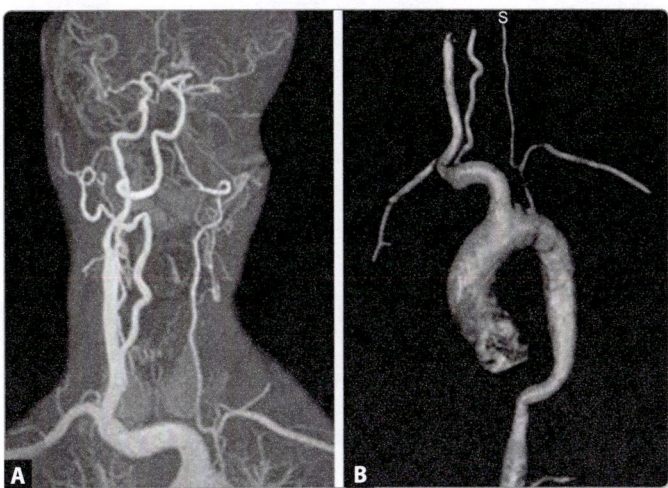

**Figures 14.16A and B** Takayasu's arteritis. (A) Contrast enhanced MRA and (B) VR images from an aortic CTA. There is occlusion of the left common carotid artery and severe diffuse circumferential narrowing of the left subclavian artery secondary to long standing arteritis. The distribution of the disease is more in keeping with a Takayasu's arteritis (*for color version of Figure 14.16B see Plate 19*)

important for more favorable outcomes. Residual arterial stenosis may persist despite resolution of inflammation. Morbidity and mortality in Takayasu arteritis is due to hypertension and stroke, and congestive heart failure is the primary cause of death. Even so, 15 year survival is high (90–95%).

## Cervical septic thrombophlebitis (Lemierre's syndrome)

Lemierre's syndrome, also called postanginal sepsis or necrobacillosis, was described in 1936 by the French microbiologist, Andre Lemierre. It is defined by the triad of internal jugular vein thrombophlebitis, systemic sepsis, and disseminated abscesses following oropharyngeal infection. It is considered a rare disease in the antibiotic era, with an incidence between 0.6 and 2.3 per million. It is more common in males, with a male-to-female ratio of approximately 2:1. The most common agent is *Fusobacterium necrophorum*, a commensal bacillus of the oral

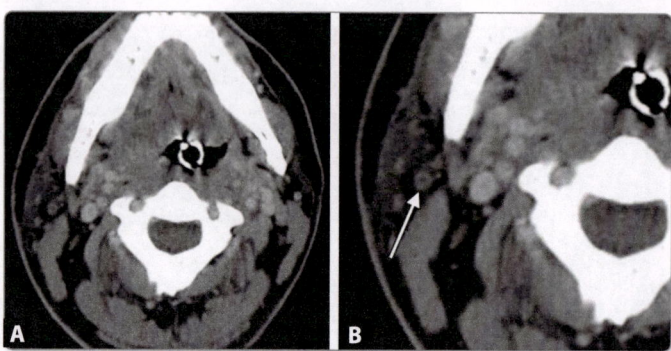

**Figures 14.17A and B** Septic cervical thrombophlebitis. (A, B) Axial neck CECT. Patient with peritonsilar abscess drained 48 hrs ago, evolved with fever, neck pain and multiple cranial nerve palsies. CT shows a soft tissue mass in the tonsilar fossa with inflammatory changes of the parapharyngeal fat. The retromandibular vein has a central filling defect consistent with a thrombus. *Fusobacterium necrophorum* was cultured from the abscess sample. Although the classic Lemierre's syndrome is referred to the jugular vein, it may be seen in any of the main cervical venous structures

cavity, but several other microorganisms have been implicated alone or in combination with *Fusobacterium necrophorum*.

CT images will show internal jugular vein thrombus with adjacent inflammatory changes in the parapharyngeal space fat tissue, with or without an oropharyngeal or parapharyngeal space abscess. Other cervical veins may be involved (**Figures 14.17A and B**). Chest CT may show septic emboli to the lungs, a finding described in 79 to 100 percent of the patients. Joints are the second most common site of involvement, with the hip, shoulders, and knee joints most frequently affected.

# Vascular tumors

## Infantile hemangiomas

In comparison to the vascular malformations described above, hemangiomas are true neoplasms. Hemangiomas are a distinct type of tumor from endothelial origin. In the early proliferative phase, the lesion is composed of densely packed, hyperplastic endothelial cells, which may show numerous mitotic figures. If there is development of an involutional phase, endothelial cells become flatter and more mature, the vascular lumen becomes more conspicuous and there is progressive replacement with fibrous and fatty tissue leading finally to fibrosis and eventual regression of the lesion.

The term hemangioma has been used to describe both a vascular tumor and a venous vascular malformation. Especially, the term "cavernous hemangioma" has been used with confusion in the literature. To attempt to simplify this we will use the classification scheme proposed by Waner and Suen, who separate hemangiomas into superficial, deep, and combined and these correspond respectively to the capillary, cavernous, and mixed capillary-cavernous types proposed by Mulliken and Glowacki. The differentiation between a deep hemangioma and a venous vascular malformation (VVM) may be difficult even with histology.

Hemangiomas are the most common tumor in the pediatric population, occurring in 8 to 12 percent of infants. They have a clear female preponderance ranging from 3:1 to 5:1. Most of these lesions are small and solitary but 60 percent arise on the facial region, giving rise to significant cosmetic issues. They also may occur in association with other manifestations in various syndromes.

A hemangioma usually appears few weeks after birth and grows more rapidly than the infant does. Natural history consists of a proliferative phase (3–9 months) followed by a slow regression phase, with a resolution rate of 10 percent per year. After complete regression, normal skin is restored in 50 percent of patients, but 10 to 38 percent will develop scarring, ulceration, skin atrophy or fibrofatty residuum, and 80 percent of them will have significant residual cosmetic deformity. On the other hand, vascular malformations are structural anomalies present at birth but may be clinically silent; they have a normal growth rate and normal rates of endothelial turnover, and grow in relation to body volume is classically seen.

Clinically, orbital hemangiomas may cause proptosis, globe displacement, and, occasionally, amblyopia. They may expand slightly during crying or straining. Laryngeal hemangiomas or congenital subglottic hemangiomas present usually with sudden biphasic stridor during the first few months in an otherwise healthy infant. The location in the subglottis makes it potentially fatal during the proliferative phase, requiring a rapid and effective intervention. If untreated, these tumors may have a mortality rate as high as 70 percent.

On imaging these lesions are seen as a retroseptal extraconal mass. Laryngeal hemangiomas are submucosal masses usually located in the posterolateral subglottic region. All hemangiomas share the same imaging characteristics and appear as a lobulated, irregularly marginated, and heterogeneous mass with intense delayed homogeneous enhancement after contrast administration. On MR they are usually hypointense on T1WI, and hyperintense on T2WI, with lobules with thin septa, combined with intralesional and perilesional flow voids (**Figures 14.18 and 14.19**). CT will show better the adjacent bone remodeling, especially seen in orbital lesions.

Complications occur in 20 percent of all hemangiomas, with ulceration being the most common (10% of patients), which is seen most often during the rapid proliferation phase. Complications will depend on the location and include permanent scarring or disfigurement for facial hemangiomas; ocular axis occlusion, astigmatism, amblyopia and tear-duct occlusion in orbital hemangiomas; airway hemangioma ulceration, disfigurement, feeding difficulties for perioral hemangiomas; airway obstruction in laryngeal hemangiomas.

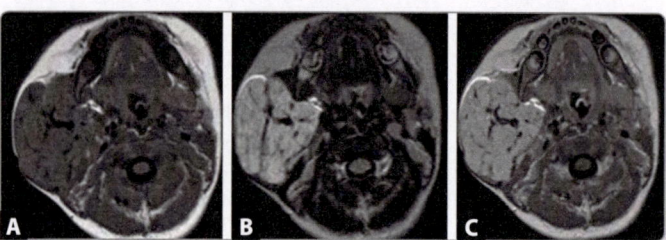

**Figures 14.18A to C** Parotid hemangioma. (A) Axial T1WI, (B) T2WI and (C) contrast enhanced T1WI. Infant with left parotid region mass. The MR shows a multilobulated low T1, high T2 well-circumscribed enhancing mass in the parotid region, with some prominent venous structures (flow voids). Location and imaging characteristics are typical for a parotid hemangioma

Vascular lesions of the head and neck 587

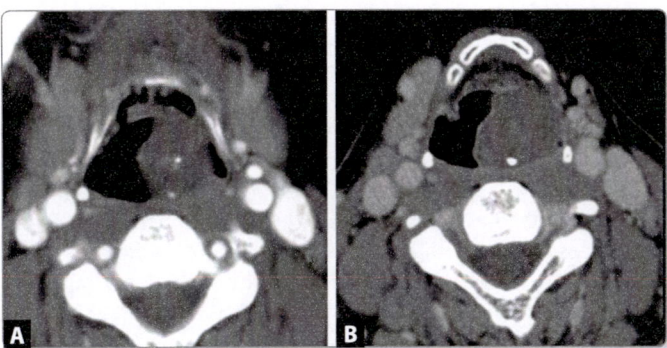

**Figures 14.19A and B** Laryngeal hemangioma. Axial neck CT images in (A) Arterial and (B) Venous phase. Submucosal hypodense, lobulated mass in the left larynx, in a child with biphasic stridor. The mass shows well-defined borders, delayed enhancement and no abnormal vascular structures. Location and imaging characteristics are typical for a laryngeal hemangioma

Indications for treatment are tissue destruction or disfigurement, severe bleeding, obstruction of vital functions (subglottic locations), functional impairment (eyelid lesions may lead to amblyopia), high-output cardiac failure, necrosis of cartilage (tip of the nose, ear) or platelet trapping with coagulopathy. Maxillofacial lesions may lead to dysmorphisms because they interfere with the bilabial, alveolar, and tongue to palate contact, which are fundamental "oral references" for the correct development of the maxilla. For these reason the skeletal malformations may persist even if the hemangioma involutes and may require further surgical correction.

Treatment options include systemic or local steroids, which produce a growth arrest so there is a far better response during the rapid proliferative phase. Results are variable, with a dramatic response in 30 percent, equivocal response in 40 percent, and no response in 30 percent. Side effects include cushinoid effects, adrenal suppression, infections, and growth suppression. Intralesional steroid therapy has been used predominately in cases of periorbital hemangiomas. The main complication is eyelid necrosis.

Surgical therapy is used as a last resort for complicated lesions. Arterial embolization may be used for inoperable lesions, hemorrhaging lesions, or failed response to other therapies, but results are usually temporary.

## Kasabach-Merritt syndrome

Kasabach-Merritt syndrome (KMS) was originally described in 1940 and was defined as a consumptive thrombocytopenia and coagulopathy associated with a hemangioma. Recent evidence however has shown that KMS is not related to a true hemangioma, but rather to a kaposiform hemangioendothelioma (KHE) and tufted angioma (TA). KHE is a locally aggressive tumor, with borderline malignant potential, composed by round and spindle-shaped endothelial cells infiltrating the dermis and subcutaneous tissue with microthrombi and hemosiderin deposits. TA is characterized by large dermal capillary tufts, much larger than those seen in infantile hemangiomas (IH). Both types may be found in a KMS lesion. Other vascular lesions that may present in association with KMS are angiosarcomas and AVMs.

Onset of symptoms occurs in early infancy, with a median age of 5 weeks. Unlike classic infantile hemangiomas (IH), KMS lesions are solitary, do not have a clear female predominance (male to female ratio 1:1–1.6), and more than 50 percent of lesions associated to KMS will be present at birth. They appear as brownish, infiltrative and painful (rather than red and nontender like most IH) showing a rapid growth, with common associated signs as purpura, edema, induration, and an echymotic margin. They may be subcutaneous or deep dermal and may extend deeper into the surrounding fat tissue and adjacent anatomic structures. The most common locations are the upper extremities, trunk and retroperitoneum, but up to 25 percent may appear in the head and neck region.

Chronic or intermittent consumptive coagulopathy can be seen in other conditions as in blue rubber bleb nevus syndrome or Klippel-Trenaunay-Weber syndrome, but this does not correspond to a KMS, where a single lesion (KHE or TA) is the underlying cause.

MR is the imaging technique of choice and will show a usually large vascular tumor involving multiple tissue planes with edema and thickening of the overlying dermoepidermic plane. Tortuous, dilated feeding arteries and draining veins around the mass are common, with flow voids on T2WI. Intratumoral foci of signal dephasing may be noted secondary to hemosiderin deposits.

First line of treatment still relies in the use of systemic steroids and/or interferon. In nonresponders, chemotherapy (vincristine) has shown a dramatic response and almost complete resolution of symptoms and of the KMS lesion. Cases of "chemotherapy dependence" have been reported with rebound after treatment withdrawal. Transarterial embolization is reserved for failure of medical treatment or as a coadjuvant treatment for palliation. Radiotherapy increases risk of sarcomatous degeneration, so it should be avoided. Curative surgical excision may be considered in clinical stable patients and depending on the location and size of the KMS lesion, as well as the degree of involvement of the adjacent anatomical structures. However, it must take in consideration that, even though they may be large lesions, spontaneous involution is still expected.

## Adult orbital hemangiomas

Adult orbital hemangiomas (AOH), also referred as cavernous hemangiomas of the orbit, are considered by many authors in the category of nondistensible VVMs. Even though, as stated before, the term cavernous hemangioma may be confusing, these lesions represent a distinct clinical and imaging entity, so for practical purposes they will be described as a separate type of vascular mass lesion.

AOHs are non-neoplastic masses composed of dilated vascular channels lined with flattened endothelial cells, separated by fibrous septae, surrounded by few layers of smooth muscle, and will have no signs of cellular proliferation. They are the most common intraorbital mass in adults and represent 4.3 percent of all the orbital mass lesions. They usually manifest in 30- to 50-year-old patients, with a slight female predilection.

These lesions may grow slowly and will present usually as painless, progressive unilateral proptosis. Less commonly diplopia, decreased visual acuity, ophthalmoplegia, compressive optic neuropathy, or encroachment of adjacent structures may be seen.

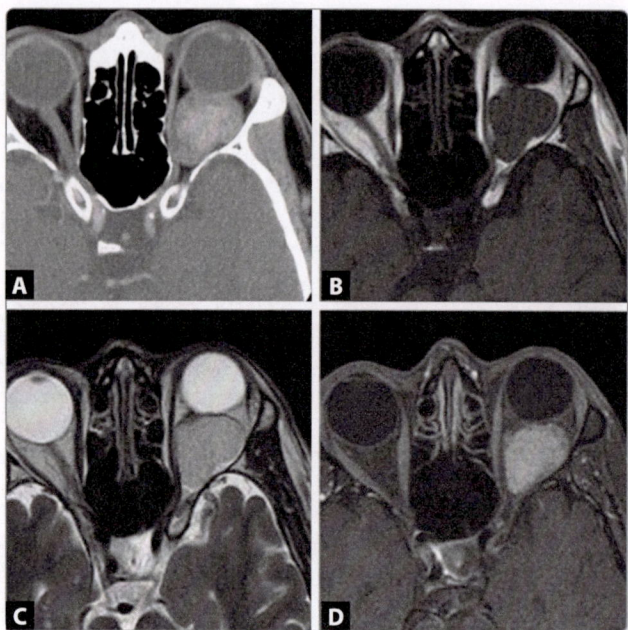

**Figures 14.20A to D** Adult orbital hemangioma. (A) CECT, (B) Axial T1WI, (C) T2WI and (D) Contrast enhanced fat saturated T1WI. Lobulated intraconal mass in an adult with proptosis. The mass is well-defined, with low T1 signal, high T2 signal and diffuse delayed internal enhancement after gadolinium administration

Cross-sectional imaging studies will show a retroseptal, intraconal, well-defined rounded mass. MRI is the preferred imaging technique. This lesion will typically have a markedly high signal on T2WI and may show internal septations. A low T1 and T2 fibrous pseudocapsule is also one of the characteristic features. On dynamic contrast enhanced CT or MRI they will show a characteristic pattern of enhancement with patchy irregular enhancement on early arterial phase and a complete, progressive, intense homogenous enhancement on delayed images (**Figures 14.20A to D**).

Surgical excision is the treatment of choice in cases where there is significant mass effect or cosmetic issues. Prognosis is invariably good, with extremely low recurrence and complication rates.

## Nasopharyngeal angiofibroma (juvenile nasal angiofibroma)

Nasopharyngeal angiofibroma is a benign encapsulated neoplasm derived from cartilage precursor cells that arises in the pterygopalatine fossa, and that is composed of a collagen matrix with a network of vascular channels and fibrous stroma (fibroblasts/myofibroblasts). These lesions demonstrate aggressive local growth and a tendency for skull base and intracranial invasion. Malignant conversion can occur, but is rare in tumors not previously irradiated. It is the most common benign tumor of the nasopharynx, but represent only 0.5 percent of all head and neck tumors. It occurs almost exclusively in adolescent males with a peak incidence between 14 to 17 years, being exceedingly rare over 25 years. Its occurrence in female patients should raise the suspicion of mosaicism and chromosomal analysis must be conducted.

These tumors are initially asymptomatic but once they have grown enough they exert local mass effect and produce nasal obstruction and recurrent epistaxis. If drainage is impeded by the tumor, sinusitis or otitis may develop. Anosmia, proptosis, facial or temporal swelling, and extraocular muscle palsies have been reported depending in the direction of the tumor spread. Staging is according to the tumoral spread with 4 different stages: (1) tumor located in the nasopharynx only; (2) extension into nasal cavity and/or sphenoid sinus; (3) involvement of the antrum, ethmoid sinus, infratemporal fossa, orbit, or cheek; (4) intracranial extension.

CT and MR imaging are fundamental tools in the diagnosis, staging and treatment planning of these tumors. CT images with bone window show bone remodeling and destruction, extending to the medial pterygoid plate with anterior bowing of the posterior wall of the maxillary sinus. MRI demonstrates a heterogeneous T1W and T2W signal mass with internal flow voids. Pre and postcontrast CT and MR imaging demonstrates the soft-tissue extent of the tumor with an intense early enhancement, allowing differentiation between obstructed sinus secretions versus soft tissue mass as well as intracranial extension. Large tumors are dumbbell-shaped or bilobed, with one portion of the tumor filling the nasopharynx and the other portion extending into the pterygopalatine fossa (**Figures 14.21 and 14.22**). These tumors can spread extensively along natural tissue planes; anteriorly into the nasal cavity or medially toward the opposite nasal cavity; superiorly into the sphenoid sinus, cavernous sinus, sella, and middle cranial fossa; laterally into the pterygomaxillary and sphenopalatine fossa and invading the infratemporal region. On occasion, the greater wing of the sphenoid bone may be eroded, exposing the dura of the middle cranial fossa. Given the better soft tissue contrast, MR is better characterizes these findings.

Angiographic features include minimally dilated supplying arteries from the ECA and ICA, and an early-appearing, intense, inhomogeneous vascular blush that persists until late in the venous phase (**Figures 14.21C and 1422C, D**). Arteriovenous shunting can be seen. Arterial supply is mainly derived from branches of the IMA (the sphenopalatine and descending palatine branches), the anterior division of the ascending pharyngeal and the accessory meningeal artery. In larger lesions there can be recruitment of branches from the facial artery (ascending palatine artery), ophthalmic artery (ethmoidal branches), and ICA (mandibulovidian branch and other arteries arising from the petrous portion, meningohypophyseal trunk and

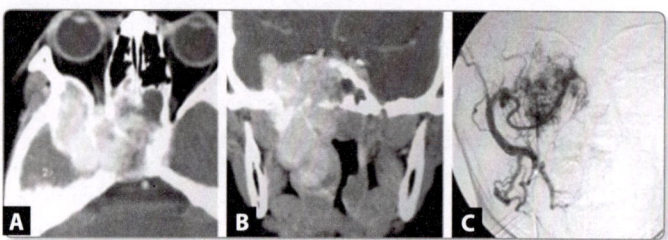

**Figures 14.21A to C** JNA. (A) Axial and (B) Coronal CECT. (C) Distal right ECA AP angiogram. Large hypervascular mass centered in the right pterygopalatine fossa extending to the infratemporal fossa and nasal cavity. The angiogram shows the hypervascular nature of the mass supplied mainly by the internal maxillary artery

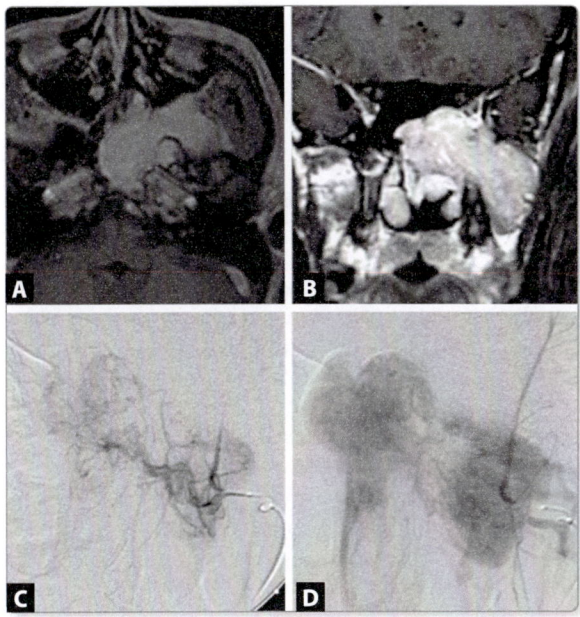

**Figures 14.22A to D** JNA. (A) Axial and (B) Coronal CE fat saturated T1WI, and (C and D) Distal left ECA AP and lateral angiogram. Another example of a left JNA showing the marked hypervascularity of the lesion

inferolateral trunk). In cases in which the tumor crosses the midline angiography should include bilateral internal and external carotid arteries.

Preoperative endovascular embolization followed by surgical removal of the tumor is the treatment modality of choice for extracranial disease, to decrease the intraoperative blood loss, with less benefit for smaller tumors. Preoperative biopsy should not be performed given the high vascularity of the lesion and risk of massive bleeding. The goal of surgery is to achieve a complete en bloc resection and it should be performed from 24 to 72 hours after embolization to prevent recanalization of the occluded arteries or formation of collateral channels. The recurrence rate after surgical treatment varies from 20 percent up to 40, typically due to incomplete resection.

Radiotherapy is reserved on poor surgical candidates, inoperable recurrent or residual disease or large invasive tumors in which surgical removal may threaten vision or require carotid artery resection. Embolization with radiotherapy has been used with good results in cases of residual disease.

## Paragangliomas

Paragangliomas are a locally invasive, benign, highly vascular type of tumors that arise from neural crest cells of the autonomic nervous system, composed of nests of neoplastic chief cells surrounded by reticulin fibers and numerous blood vessels (zellballen). Malignant paragangliomas are described in 3 percent of the cases and are considered a clinical diagnosis, made when local invasion or metastases are present with no histological features distinguishing both groups. This type of tumor represents 0.6 percent of the head and neck neoplasms and is seen more frequently in women (4 – 6 times more often than in men) with a peak incidence between 40 and 60 years of age. A higher prevalence of carotid body tumors has been reported in patients who live under chronic hypoxic conditions (chronic obstructive pulmonary disease and populations living at high altitudes). Seven to 9 percent correspond to familial paragangliomas, with 90 percent of them arising from the carotid body at a younger age (average age 38.8 years). Inheritance mode is autosomal dominant with variable penetrance. Multiplicity is seen in 10 percent of nonfamilial and 25 to 50 percent of familial cases.

There are typically 5 types of paragangliomas described in the head and neck region, named after their site of origin. They are the carotid body, jugular bulb, vagus nerve (nodose ganglion), Jacobson's nerve within the middle ear mucosa (tympanicum), and laryngeal nerve. The clinical symptoms vary according to the size and location of the paraganglioma. Approximately 1 to 3 percent of patients will suffer symptoms from tumor secretion of catecholamines and vasoactivity (palpitations, hypertension, and flushing).

Carotid paragangliomas (CP) are the most common paragangliomas of the head and neck representing a 60 percent of the total. They usually present as a nontender slowly growing painless mass along the anterior border of the sternocleidomastoid muscle and in larger lesions vocal cord paralysis, hoarseness, stridor, tongue paresis, vertigo or mild dysphagia can be seen.

Jugular paragangliomas (JP) are the second most common head and neck paragangliomas, accounting for 20 to 25 percent of the total. They are centered in the jugular foramen and, when symptomatic, present as objective pulsatile tinnitus with Horner syndrome and/or cranial nerve palsies occurring late (Vernet syndrome: motor paralysis of cranial nerves IX, X, and XI. Collect-Sicard syndrome: Vernet syndrome with additional involvement of cranial nerve XII). When there is extension to the middle ear they are referred as jugulotympanic paragangliomas, appearing as a vascular retrotympanic mass on otoscopic exam.

Vagal paragangliomas (VP) represent only the 2.5 percent of the major paragangliomas. They most commonly arise at the nodose ganglion but may occur anywhere along the course of the vagus nerve. They manifest as a slowly growing, painless mass most frequently located behind the angle of the mandible. Multiplicity is seen in 5 percent of sporadic cases and in up to 90 percent of familial cases. Cranial nerve deficits appear late in the clinical course and they include vagal, hypoglossal, accessory or glossopharyngeal nerve deficits. Infiltration of the cervical sympathetic chain with Horner's syndrome occurs in 25 percent of patients.

Tympanic paragangliomas (TP) arise from Jacobson's or tympanic nerve (branch of the IX cranial nerve on the cochlear promontory. They are the most common tumor of middle ear, being nonsecretory in this location and rarely associated with multicentric paragangliomas.

Laryngeal paragangliomas (LP) are rare, with only 76 acceptable cases reported. They usually arise from the superior laryngeal paraganglia (82% of the cases) above the anterior part of the vocal folds near the aryepiglottic fold. They have a female preponderance (3:1 ratio), and are usually benign. Most common symptoms include hoarseness and dysphagia.

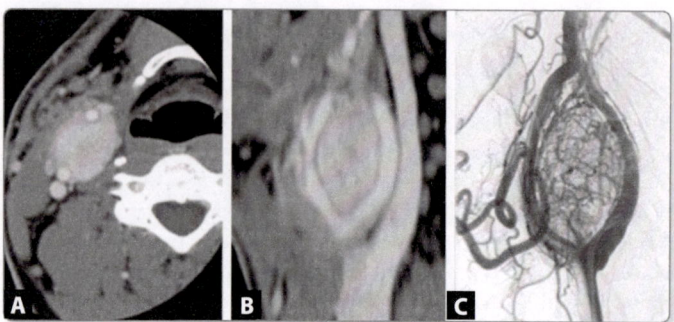

**Figures 14.23A to C** Carotid body paraganglioma. (A) Axial and (B) Coronal CECT, and (C) Right CCA lateral angiogram. Well circumscribed hypervascular mass in the carotid space, splicing the carotid bifurcation (lire sign), typical of a CP. The angiogram shows the hypervascular nature of the tumor and the multiple prominent peritumoral and intratumoral vessels

Imaging features include in both CT and MRI a well-circumscribed hypervascular mass, which, depending on its size, will have prominent vessels seen as flow voids in the MR and cystic hemorrhagic areas (salt and pepper appearance). CPs cause splaying of the carotid with posterolateral displacement of the ICA, and anterolateral or anteromedial displacement of the ECA, splicing the carotid bifurcation (lire sign) (**Figures 14.23 and 14.24**). Also, encasement of the ICA and ECA may be seen. JPs show bony erosions along the margin of the jugular foramen, differentiating it from other jugular foramen masses (i.e. vagal schwannoma, meningioma) and can encase the intrapetrous segment of the ICA or the internal jugular vein. They can also encase the facial nerve canal (**Figures 14.25A to D**). VPs are located in the carotid space, centered higher than the CPs and displacing the ECA and ICAs anteromedially, without splaying the carotid bifurcation (**Figures 14.26A to D**). TPs are flat-based soft tissue masses in the cochlear promontory, with pronounced enhancement in MRI. They usually do not destroy the surrounding bony structures, except for larger lesions, which can erode the ossicles. If bony erosions of the inferior wall of the middle ear are seen, the diagnosis of a jugulotympanic paraganglioma should be made.

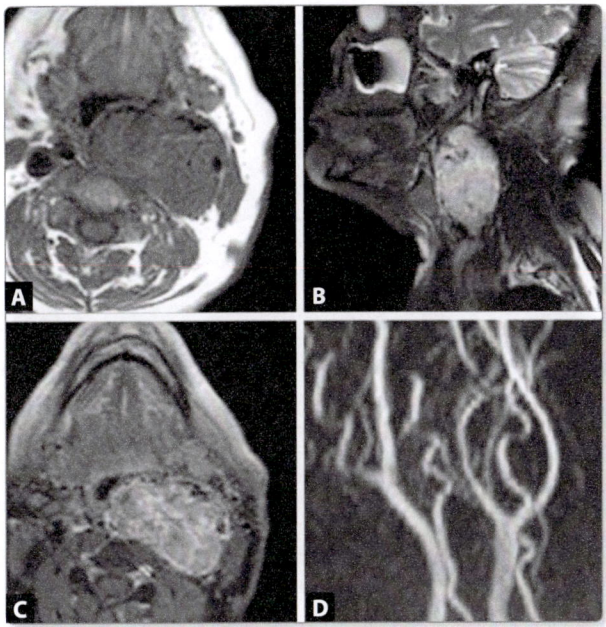

**Figures 14.24A to D** Carotid body paraganglioma. (A) Axial T1WI, (B) Sagittal T2WI, (C) Axial contrast enhanced fat saturated T1WI and (D) CE MRA. Another example of a carotid body paraganglioma with pronounced high T2 signal and avid contrast enhancement. There are subtle areas of low signal within the tumor corresponding flow voids. No intratumoral hemorrhage was seen in this case. Note the lire sign on the CE MRA

On angiography all paragangliomas subtypes will demonstrate an intense tumor blush, and may show enlarged feeding arteries and variables amounts of A-V shunting. The main vascular supply for these tumors will almost invariably come from the ipsilateral ascending pharyngeal artery.

Treatment options include surgery, embolization, radiation therapy, or any combination of these modalities, depending on the size, extension, location, and multicentricity, along with the patient's age, general health, and symptoms. Complete surgical resection is

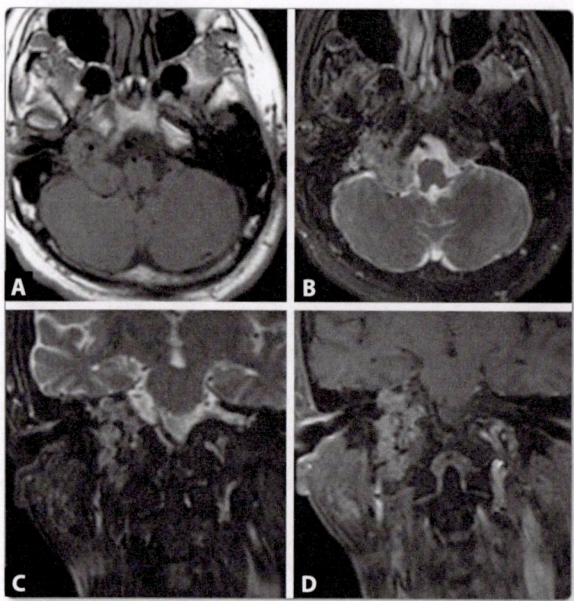

**Figures 14.25A to D** Jugulotympanic paraganglioma. (A) Axial T1WI, (B) Axial and (C) Coronal fat saturated T2WI, and (D) Coronal fat saturated contrast enhanced T1WI. Well-circumscribed hypervascular mass in the right jugular foramen region, with bone erosion and extending to the middle ear cavity, typical for a jugulotympanic paraganglioma

possible in younger patients with small tumors. Alternatives should be considered in patients in which radical surgical resection carries a high-risk of iatrogenic cranial nerve deficit. Surgical resection carries a mortality rate of 3 to 15 percent. Cranial nerve deficits can be expected in 18 to 50 percent, after surgical excision, especially in JTP and large VP, leading to permanent neurological damage in 32 to 44 percent of all patients. Vascular complications occur in 9 to 28 percent of cases, with an estimated risk of stroke up to 11 percent. Tumors larger than 5 cm have greater rates of complications. Transarterial embolization with particles or liquid embolic material, though still controversial, has been used to minimize blood loss during surgery,

Vascular lesions of the head and neck **599**

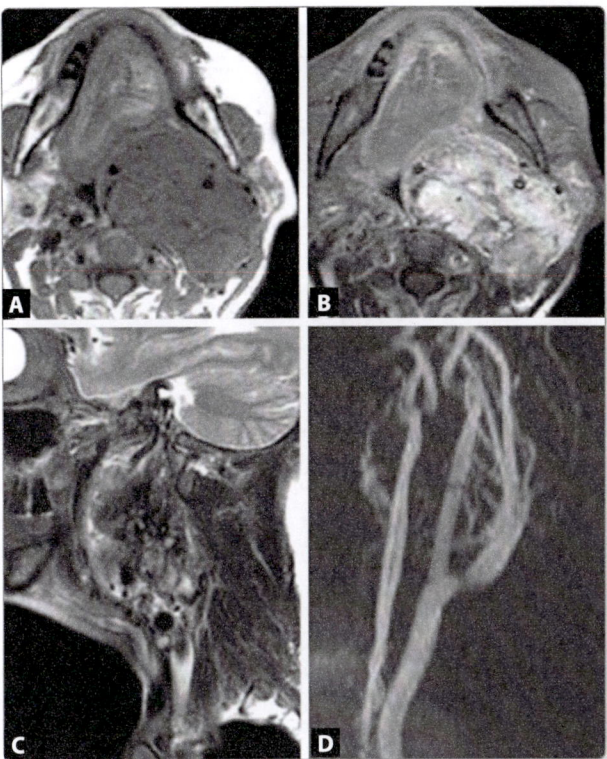

**Figures 14.26A to D** Vagal paraganglioma. (A) Axial T1WI and (B) Contrast enhanced fat saturated T1WI, (C) Sagittal T2WI and (D) CE MRA. Well-circumscribed hypervascular tumor in the left carotid space with the classic "salt and pepper" appearance on T2WI, displacing the ICA and ECA anteriorly, without splicing the bifurcation (no lire sign), which is a classic feature that distinguishes this tumor form the CP

with best results in larger than 3.0 cm. In cases were transarterial embolization is considered unsafe, direct tumor puncture with liquid embolic materials has also been reported. Radiation can be used for local control but total resolution of the mass is seen infrequently.

## Angiosarcoma

Angiosarcoma is a term used for all sarcomas with endothelial differentiation (vascular or lymphatic endothelium). These are rare tumors and represent 2 percent of all sarcomas, with almost half of the cases involving the head and neck region. The most common locations are in the scalp and facial skin, neck, oropharynx, and sinonasal tract in decreasing order. Still, they only represent 1 percent of the head and neck malignancies.

Head and neck angiosarcomas occur more often in the elderly and have no gender predilection, and rarely affect African-American patients. Chronic lymphedema and radiation have been described as the most important etiological factors in the pathogenesis of angiosarcomas. Other predisposing factors include exposure to Thorotrast, vinyl chloride, arsenic, and radiation. Also there is a predilection for this tumor in patients with Wilms' tumor, retinoblastoma and von Recklinghausen disease. The three clinical patterns described are superficial spreading, nodular, and ulcerating. The clinical differential diagnosis includes pyogenic granuloma, hemangioma, hemangioendothelioma, Kaposi's sarcoma, and ulcerative squamous cell carcinoma.

CT and MRI are nonspecific, but will show the hypervascular nature of the lesions, with T1, high T2 and marked enhancement after contrast administration. Given the superior soft tissue contrast of MRI, this exam is the image modality of choice to evaluate the extension of the tumor and the presence of metastasis. Diagnosis has to be made with histology and immunohistochemistry.

Surgery is the mainstay of treatment for angiosarcomas. Very wide margins are required, because these lesions are often multifocal and extend well beyond visible margins. Half of the patients present with metastatic disease, both through vascular and lymphatic channels, most commonly to cervical lymph nodes, lungs, and liver. Postoperative radiation and chemotherapy are used to increase the local control and the metastasis free survival rate.

Angiosarcomas of the head and neck have a poor prognosis with a 5-year survival rate of 10 to 35 percent. Prognostic factors include age, tumor size larger than 5 cm, high grade, positive margin, lymphedema and location, with grade being the most important factor. Females have worse prognosis than men. It is unknown whether estrogen or testosterone plays any role in this difference.

## Hemangiopericytoma

The hemangiopericytoma is a very rare tumor in the head and neck region. It arises from the pericapillary pericytic cells. On histologic examination the tumor shows a proliferation of oval and spindle-shaped pericytic cells. Signs for a malignant transformation are an increased mitotic activity, a higher cell density, an appearance of undifferentiated cells, as well as necrotic and hemorrhagic zones in the tumor tissue. Clinically, malignant hemangiopericytoma is characterized by hematogenic metastases.

Of all hemangiopericytomas, between 16 and 33 percent are located in the head and neck region. The most frequent locations are the lower and the upper limbs as well as the brain. They occur more frequently in middle age adults, with no clear sex predominance. Symptoms will depend on the location, with nose congestion, facial swelling, and proptosis being the most frequent.

Hemangiopericytomas enhance intensely and may be confused with adult orbital hemangiomas (AOHs) when located in the orbit. Dynamic contrast-enhanced CT may help as hemangiopericytomas have an early arterial phase and early venous phase enhancement followed by rapid washout. At MR imaging, the signal intensity of hemangiopericytomas is similar to that of gray matter on T1- and T2-weighted image that helps to differentiate them from AOHs. Digital subtraction angiography demonstrates prominent arterial supply with early florid blush and persistent tumor staining, unlike schwannomas, which typically show no tumor blush (**Figures 14.27A to D**).

Surgical radical resection is the main treatment option for hemangiopericytomas. The utility of postoperative radiotherapy is not well-established, but is frequently used in incompletely excised lesions. Local recurrence is seen in approximately 30 percent and lesions may recur up to 30 years after treatment. Although metastases are uncommon, they have been reported in up to 15 percent of patients, with the lung being the most common site.

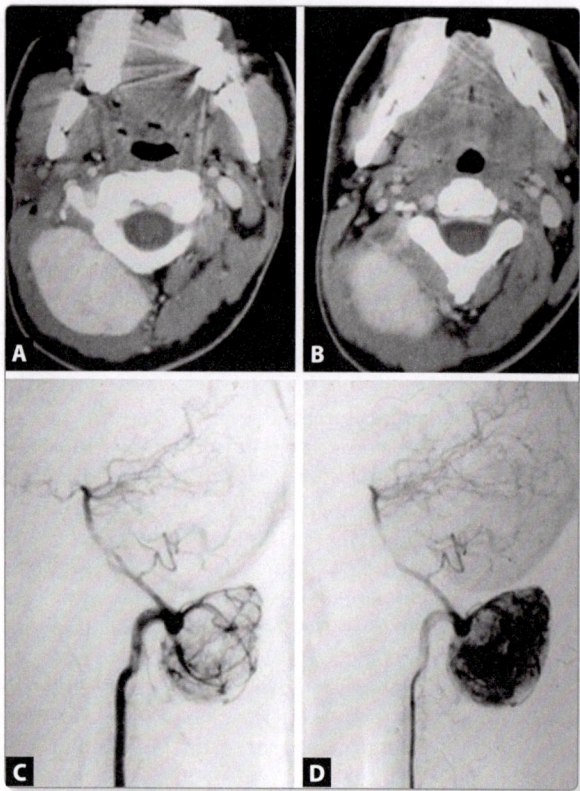

**Figures 14.27A to D** Neck hemangiopericytoma. (A, B) Axial CECT and (C, D) Right VA lateral angiograms. Large well-circumscribed hypervascular right paraspinal tumor, recruiting arterial supply from the V3 segment of the right VA. This tumor turned out to be a neck hemangiopericytoma

## Kaposi's sarcoma

Kaposi's sarcoma (KS) is an angioproliferative disorder characterized by proliferation of spindle-shaped cells, neoangiogenesis, inflammation, and edema. It is an intermediate neoplasm due to the absence of conventional features of malignancy.

It is a rare lesion, with a decreased incidence in Europe and USA, but in Africa, a dramatic increase in KS has been noticed, being the most common cancer in males (40%) in some countries.

Four major forms have been identified: classic, African endemic, immunosuppression-associated or transplant-associated, and AIDS-associated. Kaposi's sarcoma involves skin, oral cavity, sinonasal, gastrointestinal tract, lung, and lymph nodes. In the head and neck area, cutaneous lesions predominate (66%), followed by mucosal (56%) and deep structures lesions (13%). Oral lesions represent the first KS sign in 22 percent of HIV-positive individuals and eventually, 71 percent of them will show KS.

Imaging manifestations are nonspecific and include thickening of the mucosa or the dermoepidermic tissue plane and enlarged lymph nodes with marked hypervascularity and a hypodense/hypointense center.

Therapeutic options depend mainly on the KS type and the disease stage. For early stage classic KS, options include follow-up, surgical excision, or radiotherapy. For patients in a later stage or with rapid evolution, chemotherapy is recommended. For AIDS related KS highly active antiretroviral therapy (HAART) is the treatment of choice, particularly in early stages. Poor prognostic factors are visceral and pulmonary involvement, tumor size, associated edema or ulceration, a CDU count less than 200 cells/mm$^3$, and history of opportunistic infections.

# Hypervascular lymphadenopathies

## Castleman's disease

Castleman's disease was described by Castleman et al in 1956. It is characterized by massive lymph node enlargement, with mediastinum being the most common site, but it may involve any part of the lymphatic system. Other terms that have been used for Castleman's disease are giant lymph node hyperplasia, angiomatous lymphoid hamartoma, follicular lymphoreticuloma, and angiofollicular lymph node hyperplasia.

The etiology remains unknown, but theories include a form of lymphoid hypertrophy because of sustained antigenic stimuli, or a hamartomatous overgrowth of lymphoid tissue.

There are two basic subtypes, the hyaline vascular and plasma cell types with the former being the most common, representing more than 90 percent of the cases. Plasma cell type may present with systemic symptoms such as fever, fatigue, perspiration, anemia, high sedimentation rate, hypergammaglobulinemia and hypoalbuminemia.

The imaging findings of Castleman's disease are not specific. The MRI signal may be iso-, hypo-, or hyperintense in on T1WI, hyperintense on T2WI and postcontrast images will usually show it hypervascular nature. Complete surgical resection provides definitive diagnosis and treatment.

## Angioimmunoblastic T-cell lymphoma

Angioimmunoblastic T-cell lymphoma is a subtype of T-cell lymphoma. The majority of the patients are over 60 years old, and there is no gender predilection. They present with acute onset of generalized peripheral lymphadenopathy, hepatosplenomegaly, and systemic symptoms including fever, chills, night sweats, malaise, anorexia, weight loss, or a combination of these. Most have a normochromic, normocytic anemia, leukocytosis, with neutrophilia or eosinophilia, and lymphopenia.

The hystologic differential diagnosis is broad, and includes atypical reactive processes, Hodgkin's disease (HD), B-cell lymphomas, and other peripheral T-cell lymphomas.

The prognosis is poor, with a median survival of less than 3 years. Factors associated with poor prognosis include patient age over 60 years, advanced stage disease, B symptoms, rash or pruritus, edema, and ascites.

## Hypervascular metastasis

The most common hypervascular nodal metastasis in the head and neck region are metastatic papillary thyroid carcinoma, renal cell carcinoma, and melanoma (**Table 14.1**). Imaging characteristics are nonspecific and vary according to the tumor type. Papillary thyroid carcinoma metastasis may show microcalcifications, which are best seen on ultrasound. Melanoma metastasis may have spontaneous high T1 signal on MR depending on its melanin content. Renal cell metastasis will be located most commonly in the lower cervical nodes (group IV and V) and supraclavicular nodes.

| | |
|---|---|
| • | Skull base |
| | – Esthesioneuroblastoma |
| | – Inverting papilloma |
| | – Malignant meningioma |
| | – Chordoma |
| | – Osteogenic sarcoma |
| | – Chondrosarcoma |
| | – Peripheral nerve sheath tumors |
| • | Nasopharynx **(Figures 14.28A to D)** |
| | – Salivary tumors |
| | – Inverting papilloma |
| | – Lymphoma |
| | – Rhabdomyosarcoma |
| • | Thyrolarynx |
| | – Primary spine bone tumors |

Note: Any nonvascular tumor of head and neck is likely SCC

**Table 14.1** Other vascularized malignant tumors

## 606  Introductory head and neck imaging

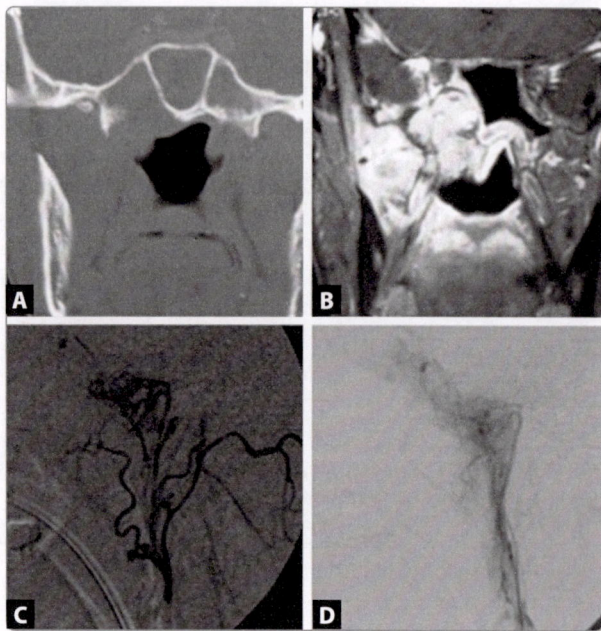

**Figures 14.28A to D** Hypervascular tumor. (A) Coronal NECT, (B) Coronal CE T1WI (C, D) Lateral right ECA angiograms. Large hypervascular nasopharyngeal tumor, with adjacent bone erosion/invasion and extension to the right infratemporal fossa. Angiogram shows a large tumor blush, with the mass supplied mainly by the right ascending pharyngeal artery. This tumor turned out to be a large SCC, which is the most likely histology for a hypervascular mucosal or submucosal H and N tumor in the adult population

# Bibliography

1. Adams DM, Lucky AW, Cervicofacial vascular anomalies. I. Hemangiomas and other benign vascular tumors. Semin Pediatr Surg. 2006;15(2):124-32.
2. Ansari SA, et al. Cervical dissections: Diagnosis, management, and endovascular treatment. Neuroimaging Clin N Am. 2009;19(2):257-70.
3. Antonitsis P, et al. Management of cervical paragangliomas: Review of a 15-year experience. Langenbecks Arch Surg. 2006;391(4):396-402.

4. Beletsky V, et al, Cervical arterial dissection: Time for a therapeutic trial? Stroke. 2003;34(12):2856-60.
5. Bloom DC, Perkins JA, Manning SC. Management of lymphatic malformations. Curr Opin Otolaryngol Head Neck Surg. 2004;12(6):500-4.
6. Choi DJ, et al. Neurointerventional management of low-flow vascular malformations of the head and neck. Neuroimaging Clin N Am. 2009;19(2):199-218.
7. Chung EM, et al. From the archives of the AFIP: Pediatric orbit tumors and tumor like lesions: Nonosseous lesions of the extraocular orbit. Radiographics: A review publication of the Radiological Society of North America, Inc. 2007;27(6):1777-99.
8. Chung EM, Specht CS, Schroeder JW. From the archives of the AFIP: Pediatric orbit tumors and tumor like lesions: Neuroepithelial lesions of the ocular globe and optic nerve. Radiographics: A review publication of the Radiological Society of North America, Inc. 2007;27(4):1159-86.
9. Connor SEJ, Flis C, Langdon JD. Vascular masses of the head and neck. Clin Radiol. 2005;60(8):856-68.
10. Cox MW, et al. Traumatic pseudoaneurysms of the head and neck: Early endovascular intervention. J Vasc Surg. 2007;46(6):1227-33.
11. De Monyé C, et al. MDCT detection of fibromuscular dysplasia of the internal carotid artery. AJR Am J Roentgenol. 2007;188(4): W367-9.
12. Diaz-Daza O, et al. Endovascular therapy of traumatic vascular lesions of the head and neck. Cardiovasc Intervent Radiol. 2003;26(3):213-21.
13. Elluru RG, Azizkhan RG. Cervicofacial vascular anomalies. II. Vascular malformations. Semin Pediatr Surg. 2006;15(2):133-9.
14. Elsayes KM, et al. Vascular malformation and hemangiomatosis syndromes: Spectrum of imaging manifestations. AJR Am J Roentgenol. 2008;190(5):1291-9.
15. Engelter ST, et al. Antiplatelets versus anticoagulation in cervical artery dissection. Stroke. 2007;38(9):2605-11.
16. Enjolras O, et al. Residual lesions after Kasabach-Merritt phenomenon in 41 patients. J Am Acad Dermatol. 2000;42(2 Pt 1):225-35.
17. Ferry JA. Angioimmunoblastic T-cell lymphoma. Adv Anat Pathol. 2002; 9(5):273-9.
18. Flis CM, Connor SE. Imaging of head and neck venous malformations. Eur Radiol. 2005;15(10):2185-93.
19. Flis CM, Jäger HR, Sidhu PS. Carotid and vertebral artery dissections: Clinical aspects, imaging features and endovascular treatment. Eur Radiol. 2007;17(3):820-34.
20. Furie DM, Tien RD. Fibromuscular dysplasia of arteries of the head and neck: Imaging findings. AJR Am J Roentgenol. 1994;162(5):1205-9.
21. Gandolfo C. et al. Sinus pericranii: Diagnostic and therapeutic considerations in 15 patients. Neuroradiology. 2007;49(6):505-14.
22. Geibprasert S, et al. Dangerous extracranial-intracranial anastomoses and supply to the cranial nerves: Vessels the neurointerventionalist needs to know. AJNR Am J Neuroradiol. 2009;30(8):1459-68.
23. Gemmete JJ, Ansari SA, Gandhi D. Endovascular treatment of carotid cavernous fistulas. Neuroimaging Clin N Am. 2009;19(2):241-55.

24. Gemmete JJ, et al. Embolization of vascular tumors of the head and neck. Neuroimaging Clin N Am. 2009;19(2):181-98.
25. Georgiadis D, et al. Aspirin vs. anticoagulation in carotid artery dissection: A study of 298 patients. Neurology. 2009;72(21):1810-5.
26. Hall GW, Kasabach-Merritt syndrome: Pathogenesis and management. Br J Haematol. 2001;112(4): 851-62.
27. Hetts SW, English JD. Acute Neurointerventional Therapies. Neuroimaging Clinics of NA. 2010;20(4):493-510.
28. Hoang JK, Eastwood JD, Glastonbury CM. What's in a name? Eponyms in head and neck imaging. Clinical Radiology. 2010;65(3):237-45.
29. Jayarajan J, Azad A. A rare cause of bilateral parotid enlargement: Angioimmunoblastic T-cell lymphoma. ANZ J Surg. 2009;79(10):769.
30. Koscielny S, Bräuer B, Förster G. Hemangiopericytoma: A rare head and neck tumor. Eur Arch Otorhinolaryngol. 2003;260(8):450-3.
31. Krings T, Geibprasert S, Lasjaunias PL. Cerebrovascular trauma. Eur Radiol. 2008; 18(8):1531-45.
32. Lacey B, Rootman J, Marotta TR. Distensible venous malformations of the orbit: Clinical and hemodynamic features and a new technique of management. Ophthalmology. 1999;106(6):1197-209.
33. Lambert M, et al. Large vessel vasculitis without temporal artery involvement: Isolated form of giant cell arteritis? Clin Rheumatol. 1996;15(2):174-80.
34. Lasjaunias P, Berenstein A, Brugge KG. Cervicofacial Vascular Malformations, in Surgical Neuroangiography Clinical and Interventional Aspects in Children. Lasjaunias P (Ed). Springer-Verlag: Berlin, Heidelberg 2006.
35. Maguiness S, Guenther L. Kasabach-Merritt syndrome. J Cutan Med Surg. 2002;6(4): 335-9.
36. Marsot-Dupuch K, Quillard J, Meyohas MC, Head and neck lesions in the immunocompromised host. Eur Radiol. 2004;14: E155-67.
37. Mazumdar A, et al. Update on endovascular management of the carotid blowout syndrome. Neuroimaging Clin N Am. 2009;19(2):271-81.
38. McIntosh BC, Narayan D. Head and neck angiosarcomas. J Craniofac Surg. 2005;16(4):699-703.
39. Menon R, et al. Treatment of cervical artery dissection: A systematic review and meta-analysis. J Neurol Neurosurg Psychiatr. 2008;79(10):1122-7.
40. Myssiorek D, et al. Laryngeal paraganglioma: An updated critical review. Acta Otolaryngol. 2004;124(9):995-9.
41. Olsen WL, et al. Lesions of the head and neck in patients with AIDS: CT and MR findings. AJR Am J Roentgenol. 1988;151(4):785-90.
42. Osborn AG. Nonatheromatous Vasculopathy, in Diagnostic cerebral angiography, Osborn AG, Jacobs JM (Eds). 1999, Lippincott-Raven: Philadelphia. p. xi, 462 p.
43. Persky MS, et al. Combined endovascular and surgical treatment of head and neck paragangliomas—a team approach. Head Neck. 2002;24(5):423-31.
44. Pipitone N, Versari A, Salvarani C. Role of imaging studies in the diagnosis and follow-up of large-vessel vasculitis: An update. Rheumatology (Oxford). 2008;47(4):403-8.

45. Plouin PF, et al. Fibromuscular dysplasia. Orphanet J Rare Dis. 2007;2:28.
46. Poyanli A, et al. Cervical Castleman's disease: imaging findings. Eur Radiol. 2000;10(7):1190-2.
47. Ramírez-Amador V, Anaya-Saavedra G, Martínez-Mata G. Kaposi's sarcoma of the head and neck: A review. Oral Oncology. 2010;46(3):135-45.
48. Redekop G, Marotta T, Weill A. Treatment of traumatic aneurysms and arteriovenous fistulas of the skull base by using endovascular stents. J Neurosurg. 2001;95(3):412-9.
49. Rootman J, Marotta T, Graeb D. Vascular lesions in diseases of the orbit: A multidisciplinary approach. Rootman J, (Ed). 2003, Lippincott Williams & Wilkins: Philadelphia, Pa. p. xx, 628 p.
50. Scheschonka A, et al. Pre- and post-treatment MR imaging in AIDS-related Kaposi sarcoma of the conjunctiva and lacrimal gland. AJNR Am J Neuroradiol. 2003;24(7):1327-9.
51. Schroeder JW, Baskaran V, Aygun N. Imaging of traumatic arterial injuries in the neck with an emphasis on CTA. Emerg Radiol. 2010;17(2):109-22.
52. Seko Y. Giant cell and Takayasu arteritis. Curr Opin Rheumatol. 2007;19(1):39-43.
53. Siu WW, et al. Arteriovenous malformation of the mandible: Embolization and direct injection therapy. J Vasc Interv Radiol. 2001;12(9):1095-8.
54. Smoker WRK, et al. Vascular lesions of the orbit: More than meets the eye. Radiographics: A review publication of the Radiological Society of North America, Inc. 2008;28(1):185-204; quiz 325.
55. Tsai YH, et al. Stent-graft treatment of traumatic carotid artery dissecting pseudoaneurysm. Neuroradiology. 2010;52(11):1011-6.
56. Tucci FM, et al. Head and neck vascular anomalies in children. International Journal of Pediatric Otorhinolaryngology. 2009;73:S71-6.
57. Turowski B, Zanella FE. Interventional neuroradiology of the head and neck. Neuroimaging Clin N Am. 2003;13(3):619-45.
58. Vargiami EG, Zafeiriou DI. Eponym: The Lemierre syndrome. Eur J Pediatr. 2010;169(4):411-4.
59. Werner JA, et al. Current concepts in the classification, diagnosis and treatment of hemangiomas and vascular malformations of the head and neck. Eur Arch Otorhinolaryngol. 2001;258(3):141-9.
60. Willems PWA, Farb RI, Agid R. Endovascular treatment of epistaxis. AJNR Am J Neuroradiol. 2009;30(9):1637-45.
61. Woo EK, Connor SEJ. Computed tomography and magnetic resonance imaging appearances of cystic lesions in the suprahyoid neck: A pictorial review. Dentomaxillofac Radiol. 2007;36(8):451-8.
62. Wu IC, Orbach DB. Neurointerventional management of high-flow vascular malformations of the head and neck. Neuroimaging Clin N Am. 2009;19(2):219-40.
63. Yang XJ, et al. Angiosarcomas of the head and neck: A clinico-immunohistochemical study of 8 consecutive patients. Int J Oral Maxillofac Surg. 2010;39(6):568-72.

# Diseases of the thyroid gland

chapter 15

Andrew Law, Andrew Thompson

### Abstract
Developmental, inflammatory diseases including autoimmune thyroiditis are covered. Imaging features of thyroid neoplasm is also included.

### Keywords
Thyroid, papillary, medullary, anaplastic carcinoma, thyroiditis, Grave's disease, goiter.

## Embryology

Development of the thyroid gland commences around the 5th week of gestation. The thyroid gland is derived from invagination of endoderm at the foramen cecum, which is located at the base of the developing tongue. It migrates ventrocaudally through the thyroglossal duct, which eventually atrophies and degenerates. The thyroid reaches its final location at the 7th gestational week and is endocrinologically functional by the end of the 1st trimester.

## Anatomy

The thyroid gland is an encapsulated bilobed gland united by a central isthmus. Each lobe is located on either side of the trachea and is approximately 5 cm long with a narrow upper pole and a broad lower pole (**Figure 15.1**). The upper margin is located near the oblique line of the thyroid cartilage and the lower margin at the level of the fourth or fifth tracheal cartilage rings. Occasionally there is an accessory lobe called the pyramidal lobe that projects superiorly from the thyroid isthmus (**Figures 15.2A and B**). The thyroid gland moves with swallowing as it is attached to the larynx and trachea by an envelope of pretracheal fascia, and attached to the cricoid by the suspensory ligament of Berry.

Diseases of the thyroid gland  611

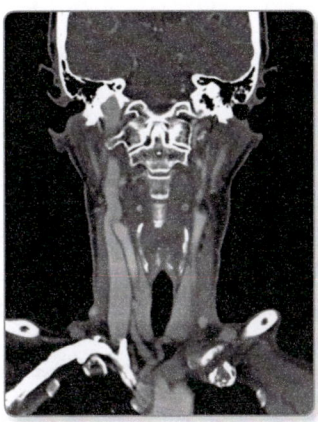

**Figure 15.1** Coronal contrast-enhanced CT showing the normal thyroid gland

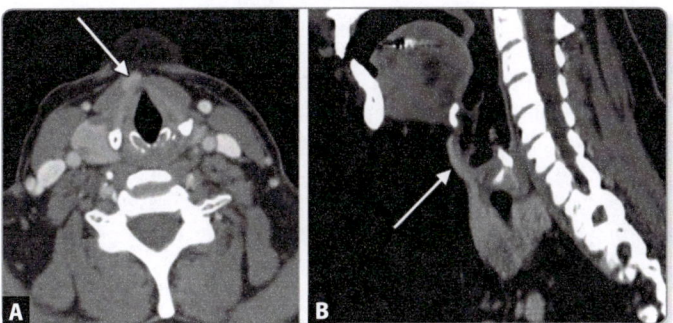

**Figures 15.2A and B** Axial and sagittal enhanced CT. Prominent pyramidal lobe in a 45-year-old female with a mildly enlarged and multinodular gland

Arterial supply to the thyroid is from the superior and inferior thyroid arteries, which are branches of the external carotid artery and subclavian artery respectively. The thyroidea ima artery is a normal variant in 3 percent of the population and commonly arises from the aortic arch, right common carotid artery, or brachiocephalic artery. Venous drainage is to the internal jugular vein and into a pretracheal venous plexus. Thyroid lymphatics drain into the deep cervical nodal chain.

## Imaging overview

### Ultrasound

Ultrasound of the thyroid gland is performed using a high-frequency (>10 MHz) linear-array transducer. The normal thyroid gland is uniformly hyperechoic and has a higher echogenicity compared to surrounding muscle (**Figure 15.3A**). Ultrasound is able to accurately differentiate between cystic (**Figure 15.3B**) and solid lesions and detect microcalcifications. Fine-needle aspiration performed under real-time ultrasound guidance is the preferred method for obtaining cytology from suspicious thyroid lesions or lymphadenopathy.

Whilst there are no definite sonographic features to differentiate between malignant and benign thyroid nodules, some signs are suspicious for malignancy and warrant fine needle aspiration (FNA). Microcalcifications are 10 to 100 μm deposits of crystalline calcium that appear as punctate echogenic foci without posterior acoustic shadowing. They are found in up to 60 percent of all primary thyroid carcinoma and have a specificity of 85 to 95 percent and a positive predictive value of 42 to 94 percent for malignancy. Dystrophic calcifications are most commonly found in multinodular goiters secondary to necrosis and are usually benign in this setting. If present in a solitary nodule, the rate of malignancy is around 75 percent.

A solid, hypoechoic nodule has a low specificity but high sensitivity for either carcinoma or lymphoma. An ill-defined or irregular margin, direct invasion of adjacent structures, and the presence of nodal disease are also highly specific for malignancy. A nodule that is taller than it is wide (anteroposterior to transverse ratio of greater than or equal to 1) has a specificity of 91.4 percent for being malignant.

Conversely, a cystic nodule with a complete smooth surrounding hypoechoic rim, or a nodule that is entirely avascular is very unlikely to be malignant. Nodules with multiple microcystic components forming more than 50 percent of nodule volume are termed spongiform, an imaging feature highly specific for a benign lesion.

Diseases of the thyroid gland 613

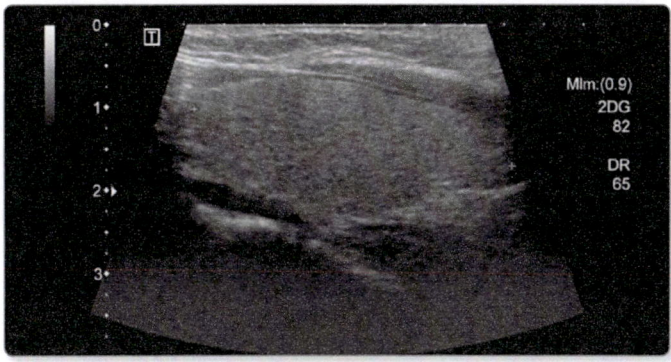

**Figure 15.3A** Normal sagittal sonographic view of the thyroid demonstrating normal uniform echogenicity

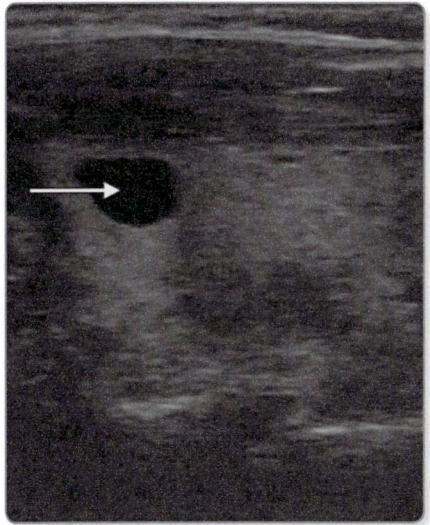

**Figure 15.3B** Sagittal sonographic view of the thyroid cyst which is seen as an anechoic clear mass with acoustic enhancement (white arrow)

Patients who are considered at high-risk for thyroid malignancy include those with a family history of thyroid cancer in one or more first degree relatives, family history of a thyroid cancer syndrome, history of the head and neck or whole body irradiation during childhood, prior hemithyroidectomy with history of thyroid cancer, and FDG-avid nodules on PET imaging.

The revised American Thyroid Association 2009 guidelines recommend thyroid FNA in the following scenarios based on good or fair evidence:
- Nodules >5 mm in size in patients with a high-risk history, with or without suspicious sonographic features.
- Nodules of any size in the presence of abnormal cervical lymphadenopathy.
- Nodules ≥ 10 mm with microcalcifications.
- Solid and hypoechoic nodules > 10 mm
- Mixed solid and cystic nodules ≥ 15 to 20 mm with suspicious sonographic features.

The revised American Thyroid Association recommendations suggest thyroid FNA in the following scenarios based on expert opinion:
- Solid and iso- or hyperechoic nodules ≥ 10 to 15 mm.
- Mixed solid and cystic nodules >20 mm without suspicious sonographic features.
- Spongiform nodule > 20 mm (or sonographic monitoring without biopsy).

## Nuclear medicine

Iodine 131 (radioiodine, I-131); Iodine 123 (I-123); and sodium (Tc-99m) pertechnetate are used to assess the morphology of the thyroid gland. As radioiodine emits both beta and gamma radiation, it can be used in treatment of thyroid carcinomas that concentrate iodine. To reduce the radiation dose to the thyroid, sodium pertechnetate or I-123 is preferred over I-131 for morphological assessment. These radionuclides are taken up by the thyroid gland as part of the normal process of thyroid hormone synthesis, which can be affected by excess exogenous iodine intake. Certain medications such as amiodarone and interferon, and iodinated contrast media will cause spurious results on radionuclide-uptake studies for up to 6 weeks after administration. Nuclear scintigraphy should ideally be performed prior to a contrast-enhanced CT.

Up to 85 percent of all thyroid nodules are cold and the rate of malignancy in this subset is around 10 percent. This compares with a malignancy rate in hot nodules of less than 1 percent. All cold nodules require further investigation (**Figures 15.4A and B**). Due to a low specificity, radionuclide imaging does not have a role in the initial investigation of a thyroid nodule except to confirm a hyperfunctioning nodule in the setting of thyrotoxicosis and exclude the patient from fine needle aspiration. In the follow-up of thyroid carcinoma in the setting of an elevated thyroglobulin with no sonographic evidence of recurrence, iodine nuclear scintigraphy can be performed. For non-I-131 avid tumors, a thallium or FDG PET scan can be performed instead.

Increased and uncontrolled cellular proliferation seen in all malignancies is reflected by an increase in the rate of glucose metabolism. Fluorodeoxyglucose positron emission tomography (FDG-PET) utilizes this principle but in the thyroid is unable to differentiate between benign and malignant nodules. Its current role is primarily in the assessment of recurrent or metastatic disease in noniodine avid thyroid malignancies. Incidental FDG-avid thyroid nodules occur in 1 to 2 percent of all PET studies and require further evaluation as the risk of malignancy in these nodules is approximately 33 percent.

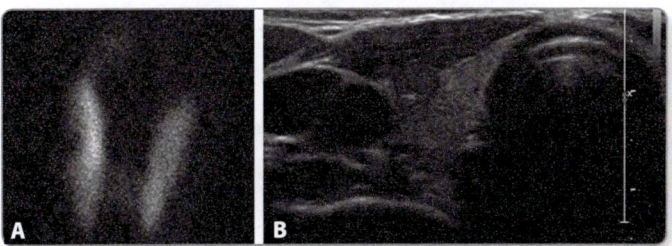

**Figures 15.4A and B** A cold nodule is noted in the right upper thyroid on a pertechnetate thyroid scan (B) and corresponds to a nodule on sonography (A)

## Computed tomography and magnetic resonance imaging

Cross-sectional imaging is usually performed in the setting of thyroid malignancy for accurate local and distant staging of disease. Invasion of locoregional and deep structures necessitates different management strategies with the aim of preserving respiration, speech, and alimentation. The normal thyroid is hyperattenuating (80–100 HU) on noncontrast CT due to its iodine concentration and demonstrates homogenous enhancement following administration of iodinated contrast media (**Figure 15.5**). A poorly functioning thyroid gland has reduced iodine uptake and therefore gross assessment of function can be made on a noncontrast CT, where the thyroid gland will have lower-than-normal attenuation and may be difficult to visualize. The normal thyroid gland has slightly hyperintense compared to muscle on T1-weighted imaging and is hyperintense on T2-weighted imaging.

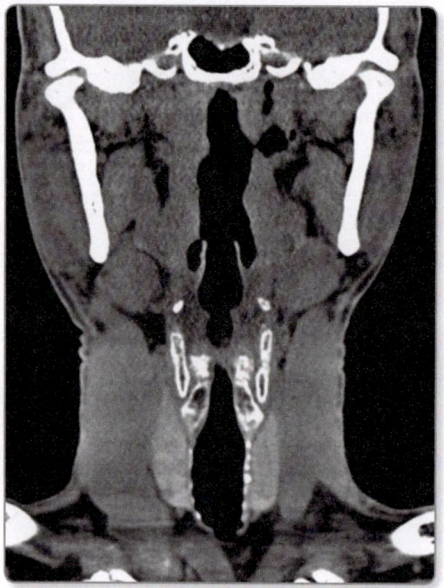

**Figure 15.5** Coronal unenhanced CT shows mild hyperattenuation of the thyroid lobes

Diseases of the thyroid gland 617

## Pathology

### Developmental

#### Thyroglossal duct anomalies

Thyroglossal duct abnormalities are the most common congenital lesion of the head and neck, with formation of a thyroglossal duct cyst or a persistent fistulous tract. Fifty percent are located at the level of the hyoid bone and 25 percent are infrahyoid and between the strap muscles. The majority of these lesions are located in the midline, but up to 25 percent can be parasagittal in location. The most common presentation is in childhood as a palpable, painless midline neck lump.

Simple cysts have a thin, smooth rim lined by squamous epithelium containing homogenous fluid attenuation or signal. With secondary infection, there is stranding of the surrounding fat, with thickening and enhancement of the cyst wall. The cyst contents may become proteinaceous, reflected by an increase in CT attenuation and altered MR signal characteristics, these changes can persist after resolution of infection (**Figures 15.6A and B**).

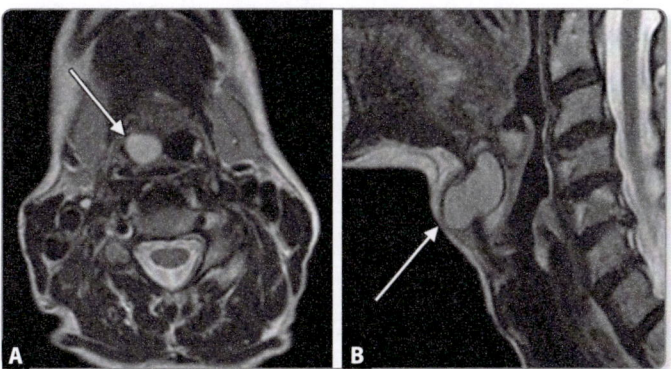

**Figures 15.6A and B** Sixty-six-year-old female, anterior neck lump. Axial and sagittal T2 weighted MRI: Bilobular hyperintense thyroglossal duct remnant, suprahyoid component (A) fills the right vallecula, infrahyoid midline component between strap muscles (B)

Thyroglossal duct cysts can contain functioning thyroid tissue and if cyst resection is considered and the thyroid gland is unable to be palpated, thyroid scintigraphy is necessary to avoid inadvertently rendering the patient acutely hypothyroid. Malignant transformation of ectopic thyroid tissue is more common than in normally located tissue, and the incidence within a thyroglossal duct cyst is around 1 percent. This should be suspected if soft tissue nodularity and calcification is present, with the overwhelming majority of such malignancies being of the papillary type on histopathology.

## Lingual thyroid

Failure of thyroid gland descent is rare and is much more common in females compared to males. Arrest of migration can occur at any point but most commonly occurs at the foramen cecum causing a palpable mass at the base of tongue. In 75 percent, there is an absence of any other functional thyroid tissue within the neck and failure to recognize this may result in removal of the only functioning thyroid tissue present in the patient.

Ectopic thyroid tissue may result in dysphagia, a globus sensation, and rarely, airway obstruction. Sudden enlargement secondary to hemorrhage may precipitate acute symptoms. As with all thyroid tissue, a lingual thyroid has high attenuation on noncontrast CT and high signal on T1- and T2-weighted imaging compared to muscle (**Figures 15.7A and B**).

# Inflammatory

## Branchial apparatus anomalies

These are most frequently classified as 4th branchial apparatus lesions, although some authors believe that they may arise from the third arch. A congenital cystic lesion, most often involving the left superolateral thyroid lobe, may be associated with a fistula that arises from the lateral neck and parallels the course of the recurrent laryngeal nerve terminating in the apex of the pyriform fossa. These cysts are predisposed to bacterial infection and subsequent acute suppurative thyroiditis and abscess formation.

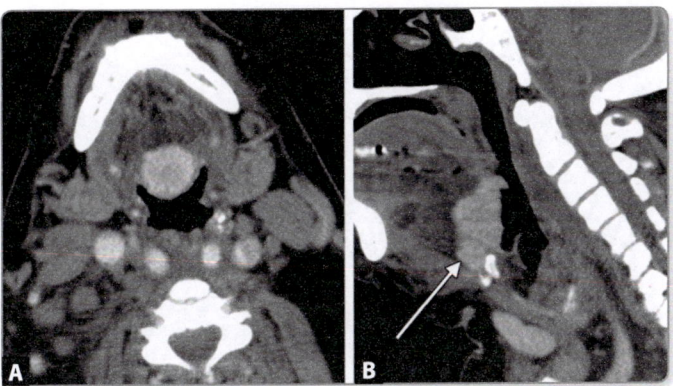

**Figures 15.7A and B** Axial, sagittal enhanced CT, 49-year-old woman. Incidental lingual thyroid tissue, no thyroid gland was visualized in the neck

## Autoimmune disease and thyroiditis

Thyroiditis is caused by a number of clinically and pathologically varied conditions and is characterized by infiltrates of inflammatory cells.

## Graves' disease

Graves' disease is a common cause of hyperthyroidism and is around 7 times more common in females compared to males. Autoantibodies are directed against thyrotropin receptors on follicular cells mimicking the action of thyroid stimulating hormone (TSH) and resulting in unchecked thyroid hormone production. Thyroid ophthalmopathy is present in up to 30 percent of patients with Graves' disease, characterized by exophthalmos, periorbital edema, ophthalmoplegia, and extraocular muscle swelling that classically spares the muscle tendon. On ultrasound there is glandular enlargement with a diffuse increase in echogenicity and hypervascularity on color Doppler imaging. Radionuclide studies using Tc-99m pertechnetate or I-131 or I-123 typically demonstrate uniformly increased uptake, the degree of which is proportional to the severity of thyrotoxicosis (**Figure 15.8**). Focal nodules are seen in up to 10 percent of patients. Cross-sectional

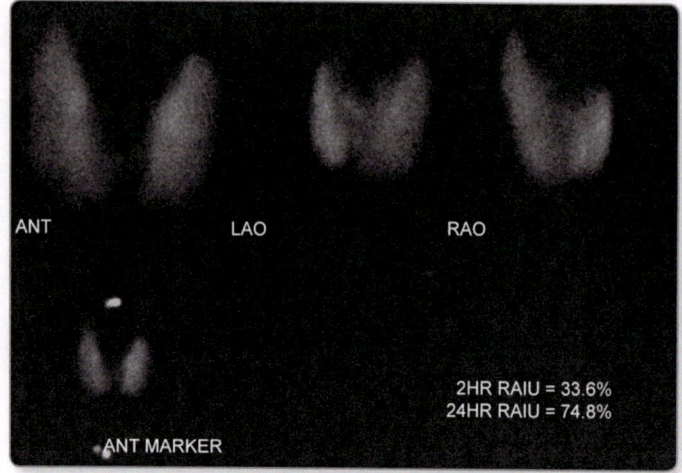

**Figure 15.8** Graves' disease. Pertechnetate scan shows elevated 24 hour uptake

imaging may show mild gland enlargement, enlargement of the pyramidal lobe and edema (**Figure 15.9**).

## Hashimoto thyroiditis

Hashimoto thyroiditis (chronic autoimmune lymphocytic thyroiditis) is the second most common cause of goitrous hypothyroidism behind iodine deficiency. It is 10 to 20 times more common in females, with a higher incidence in people with down syndrome and turner syndrome. Autoantibodies are formed against thyroglobulin and thyroid peroxidase, and TSH-receptors.

Computed tomography (CT) imaging may show nonspecific gland enlargement. There may be areas of focal lower attenuation (**Figures 15.10A and B**).

Sonographically distinct forms of diffuse or nodular Hashimoto's thyroiditis have been described, with varying opinion as to whether differences are secondary to a spectrum of progression or if they are indeed separate clinical entities. In the diffuse form, the thyroid is

Diseases of the thyroid gland 621

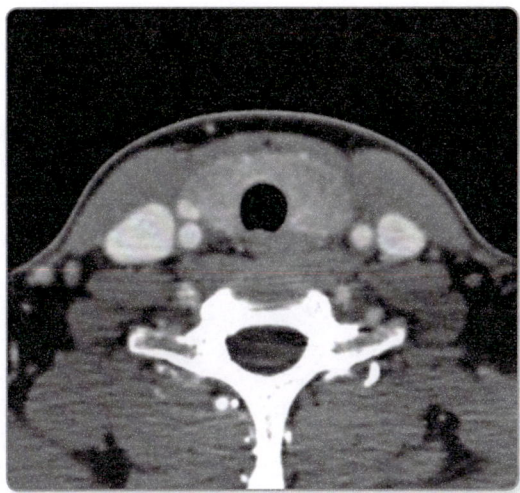

**Figure 15.9** Axial enhanced CT. Graves' disease: The gland, including the isthmus shows diffuse enlargement. The glandular parenchyma and is mildly heterogenous and of reduced attenuation due to diffuse edema

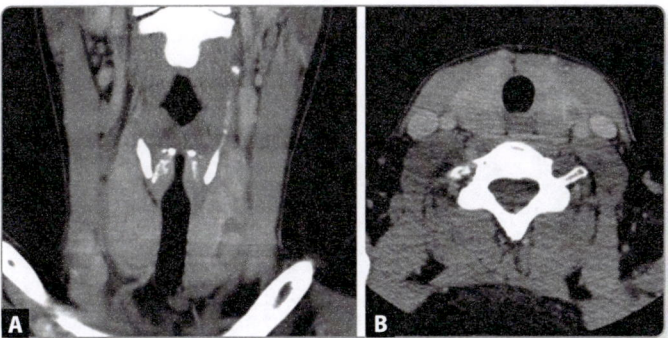

**Figures 15.10A and B** Coronal and axial contrast CT of Hashimoto's thyroiditis shows a generalized lower glandular attenuation with areas of internal heterogeneity

enlarged and hypervascular with a coarse and diffusely hypoechoic appearance. Hypoechoic micronodules (1–7 mm in size) may be seen in the diffuse form. The nodules in nodular disease are larger than micronodules and are variable in appearance but most commonly hyperechoic with irregular margins. They can occur with diffuse parenchymal changes or in an otherwise normal appearing thyroid (**Figures 15.11A and B**).

Hashimoto thyroiditis has a variable appearance on radionuclide studies. In the thyrotoxicosis phase, there is diffuse or nodular increased uptake of Tc-99m pertechnetate and I-123 or I-131. With tissue destruction and the development of hypothyroidism, there is reduced uptake of pertechnetate and iodine uptake may be borderline-low or reduced.

There are two forms of subacute thyroiditis. De Quervain's thyroiditis (subacute granulomatous thyroiditis) is a painful swelling of the thyroid that develops following a viral infection. It is 3 to 5 times more common in females and usually occurs between 10 and 40 years of age. Subacute lymphocytic thyroiditis is most common in middle-aged women, especially in the postpartum period. It is painless and silent form of thyroiditis that is autoimmune in nature. In both forms, there is transient hyperthyroidism for 2 to 6 weeks due to release of preformed thyroid hormone. This is followed by a period of hypothyroidism typically lasting between 2 to 4 months. The majority of patients return to a euthyroid state, however there is persisting hypothyroidism in up to 5 to 10 percent.

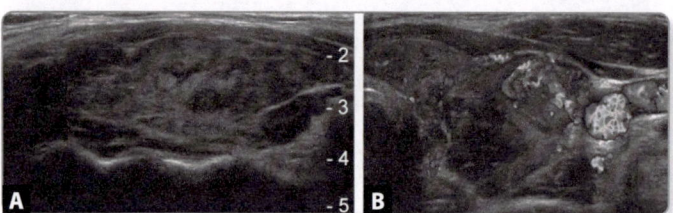

**Figures 15.11A and B** Sagittal sonographic image (A) through the right thyroid and axial Doppler image through the left thyroid and a patient with Hashimoto's thyroiditis (*for color version of Figure 15.11B see Plate 19*)

## Thyroid goiter

Thyroid goiters are common lesions arising from follicular hypertrophy secondary to reduced thyroid hormone production. Endemic goiters develop in children living in areas of iodine deficiency. Sporadic goiters have a strong female predominance with peak incidence during adolescence. Computed tomography is the best imaging modality for assessing retrosternal extension, which occurs in around 33 percent, and tracheal compression. Multiple nodules are often formed within the enlarged thyroid gland over time, referred to as a multinodular goiter. Clinically a hypothyroid or hyperthyroid state may exist and the nodules can eventually become autonomous with production of hormone independent of normal regulatory-feedback pathways.

The imaging of multinodular goiter reveals a heterogenous gland with areas of nodularity (**Figures 15.12 and 15.13**). Calcifications, fibrosis, cystic degeneration, and hemorrhage can all be present. The overall risk of thyroid malignancy in multinodular goiter is 5 percent, the same as a person with a solitary nodule. Ultrasound is indicated to determine nodule morphology and identify the dominant nodule. All nodules with suspicious sonographic appearances as outlined by the American Thyroid Association should be aspirated. If none of the nodules appear suspicious, the dominant nodule should be aspirated.

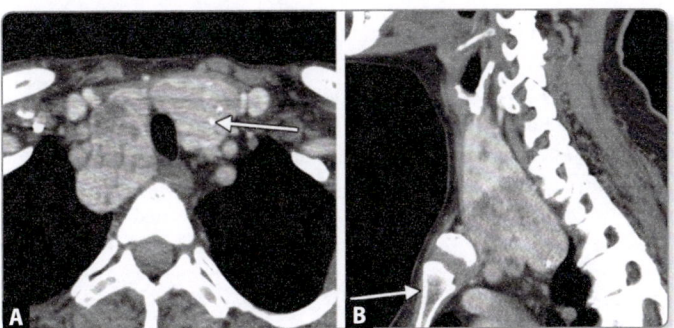

**Figures 15.12A and B** Axial, sagittal enhanced CT, 69-year-old woman. Multinodular goiter, the gland is enlarged by innumerable heterogeneous nodules, some with dystrophic calcification (arrow, left). Note mild compromise of the transverse luminal airway dimension and caudal extent to the level of the manubrium (arrow, right)

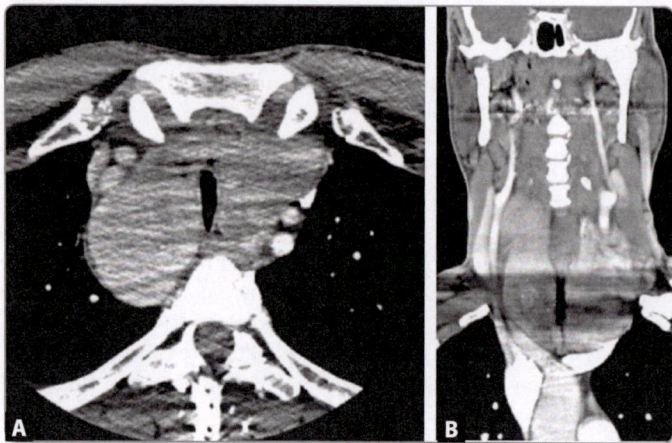

**Figures 15.13A and B** Axial, coronal enhanced CT in a patient with a large goiter. There is mediastinal extension with associated narrowing of the trachea

Nuclear scintigraphy can assist in nodule characterization and risk assessment, with cold nodules having a much higher malignant risk compared to hot nodules.

## Malignant neoplasms

In general terms, malignant thyroid lesions typically present as a palpable mass and initial imaging and cytological assessment is usually with ultrasound and fine needle aspiration. CT is often employed to facilitate accurate locoregional and cervical nodal staging. There is ongoing debate in the literature as to the use of contrast material in staging examinations. Uptake of iodinated contrast media does render thyroid tissue temporarily insensitive to subsequent treatment with radioactive iodine.

However, enhanced CT may improve identification of suspicious lymph nodes in papillary thyroid cancer. This may have implication for subsequent recurrent cervical disease and long-term morbidity.

The CT appearance of the primary cancer is often nonspecific and may reveal a thyroid mass of heterogeneous texture; there may

Diseases of the thyroid gland 625

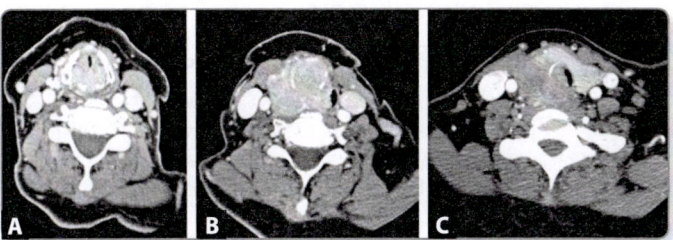

**Figures 15.14A to C** Axial CT of anaplastic carcinoma showing invasion into the hypopharynx, larynx and trachea

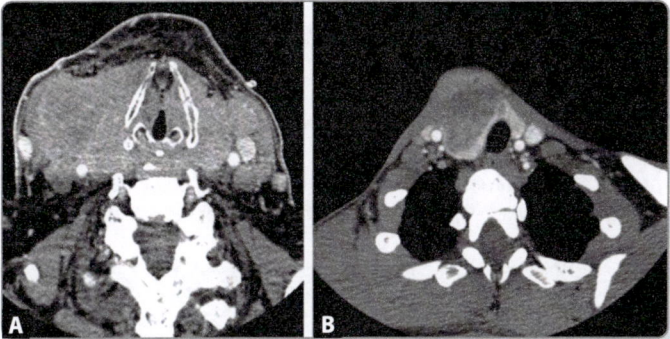

**Figures 15.15A and B** Axial CT images show thyroid carcinoma extending outside the gland capsule to elevate the sternocleidomastoid musculature (A) and the strap muscles (B)

be associated calcifications and necrosis. Anaplastic carcinomas tend to be larger at presentation often with aggressive extracapsular and locoregional soft tissue invasion. CT is also important in documenting retrosternal extension, vascular, tracheal and esophageal invasion (**Figures 15.14 and 15.15**).

## Differentiated thyroid carcinoma

Papillary carcinoma and follicular carcinoma account for the majority of all forms of thyroid malignancy, representing up to 80 and 10 percent respectively. Thyroid carcinoma is rare overall, and accounts for only 1 percent of all malignant tumors.

Peak incidence occurs between 20 and 40 years of age and is 3 times more common in females compared to males. Radiation-exposure is one of the main risk factors for developing differentiated thyroid carcinoma. The most common presentation for differentiated thyroid carcinoma is a painless, palpable, firm and solitary nodule. These malignancies are usually well-encapsulated and low grade and carry a generally excellent prognosis, especially in the absence of capsular invasion.

Papillary carcinoma spreads predominantly through the lymphatic system, with microscopic nodal involvement in up to 50 percent of all cases at presentation compared with 10 percent of all cases of follicular carcinoma. CT imaging may be variable and demonstrate features ranging from a normal appearing gland to the presence of a mass lesion with associated heterogeneity, cystic change and calcifications (**Figures 15.16A and B**). Lymphatic drainage is generally initially to the medial compartment (levels 6 and 7) and subsequently to the jugular chain and retropharyngeal nodes. Pathologically involved nodes have a variable appearance on CT and US, and apart from an enlarged size, other suspicious features include: cystic change,

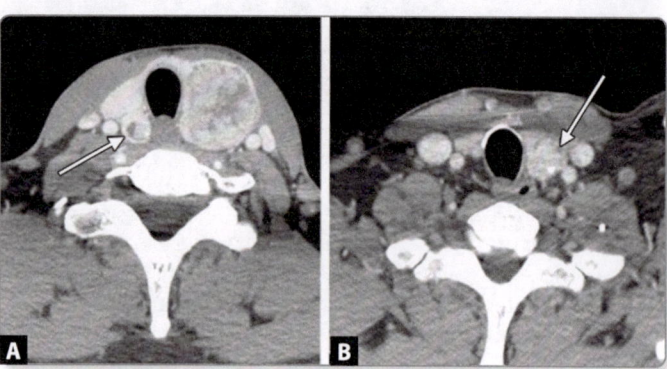

**Figures 15.16A and B** Axial enhanced CT, left lobe papillary thyroid carcinoma in two different patients. Note the heterogeneous and nonspecific CT appearance of the primary lesion. The case on the right shows calcification in the primary mass (arrow) and on the left, note a cystic and enhancing metastatic level 6 node (arrow)

calcifications, loss of the normal fatty hilum, a rounded or irregular shape, peripheral as opposed to central vascularity, and increased enhancement (**Figures 15.17 and 15.18**).

Follicular carcinoma favors hematogenous spread, with distant metastases to lung, bone, and central nervous system found in 20 percent at presentation, compared with 5 to 10 percent of patients with papillary carcinoma. CT imaging will be indistinguishable from other types of thyroid carcinoma (**Figures 15.19A and B**). Both papillary and follicular carcinomas have an excellent prognosis with 20-year survival rates of 90 to 95 percent and 85 percent respectively. Whilst differentiated thyroid carcinoma is an indolent disease, recurrence rates are high and range from 15 to 30 percent.

The mainstay of postoperative surveillance consists of serial serum thyroglobulin measurements and neck ultrasound. Radioiodine I-131 scanning can also be performed to identify residual and recurrent disease (**Figure 15.20**).

FDG-PET can be helpful for detecting recurrent disease in the setting of a raised thyroglobulin level and a normal ultrasound and radioiodine scan. It has a sensitivity of 50 to 83 percent, which is directly proportional to the thyroglobulin level.

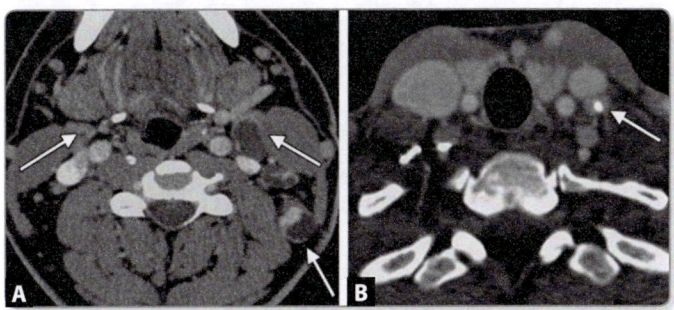

**Figures 15.17A and B** Metastatic jugular chain nodal disease in papillary carcinoma, two different patients. Note the multiple cystic nodes with rim enhancement (A), and focal metastatic nodal calcification (B)

## 628 Introductory head and neck imaging

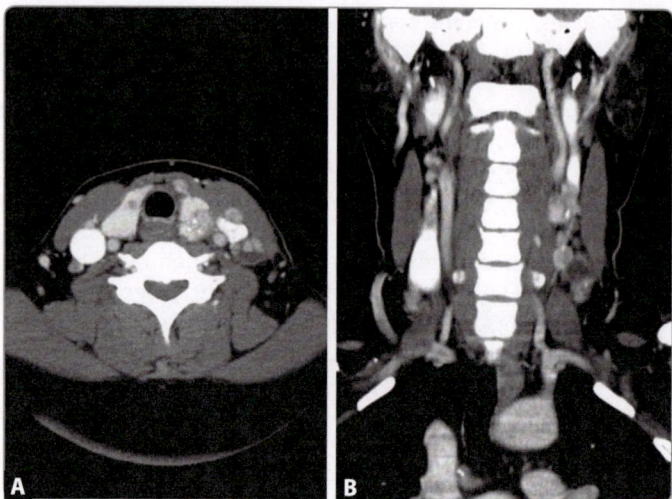

**Figures 15.18A and B** Contrast enhanced axial and coronal imaging of a papillary carcinoma in the left lobe. Note the presence of small punctate calcifications in the nodule. Neck adenopathy is also present showing suspicious features: cystic change, calcifications and marked enhancement

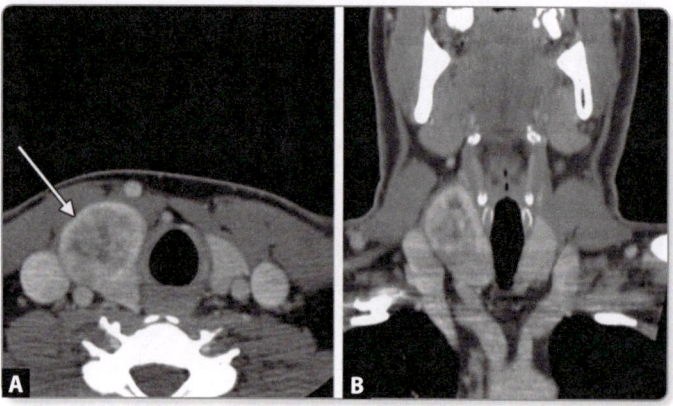

**Figures 15.19A and B** Axial and sagittal enhanced CT, solitary right thyroid mass with a nonspecific CT appearance, follicular carcinoma

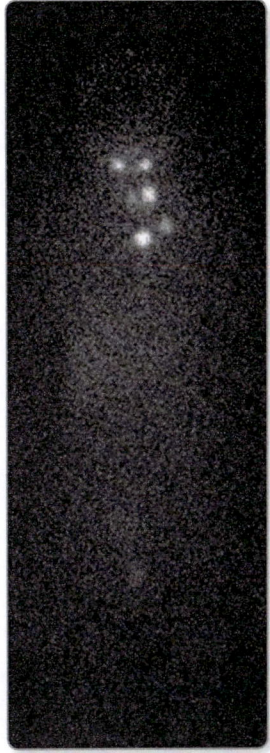

Figure 15.20 Iodine 131 scan shows areas of uptake in the neck and mediastinum corresponding to areas of residual thyroid carcinoma

## Medullary carcinoma

Medullary carcinomas are neuroendocrine tumors that arise from the parafollicular calcitonin secreting cells. The majority of cases are sporadic, most common above 60 years of age. Bilateral disease is present in two-thirds of sporadic malignancy. The familial form is associated with mutations of the RET proto-oncogene on chromosome 10. Adolescents are affected with multifocal and bilateral disease in almost all cases. Sixty-five percent of the familial form of medullary carcinoma is associated with multiple endocrine neoplasia (MEN) syndrome IIA and IIB, with disease in the latter tending to be a more aggressive variant with detectable metastases in 70 percent of patients at presentation.

Medullary carcinoma and differentiated thyroid carcinoma can have similar sonographic features, typically appearing as an irregular, ill-defined thyroid nodule with central necrosis and punctate or coarse calcification. Unlike differentiated thyroid carcinomas, medullary carcinoma does not usually take up iodine and is unable to be treated with radioiodine therapy (**Figures 15.21A and B**). Like other neuroendocrine tumors, there is uptake of I-131-MIBG and in-111-octreotide.

Up to 90 percent of medullary carcinomas secrete calcitonin, which can also be used to monitor disease activity and response to treatment. Medullary carcinoma has a poorer prognosis compared to differentiated thyroid carcinoma with overall 10-year survival rate of 60 to 90 percent for patients without metastatic or locally advanced disease. If metastases are present at presentation, 5-year survival rates are around 50 percent.

## Anaplastic carcinoma

Anaplastic carcinoma encompasses a group of high-grade and highly aggressive malignancies with a propensity for invasion of surrounding

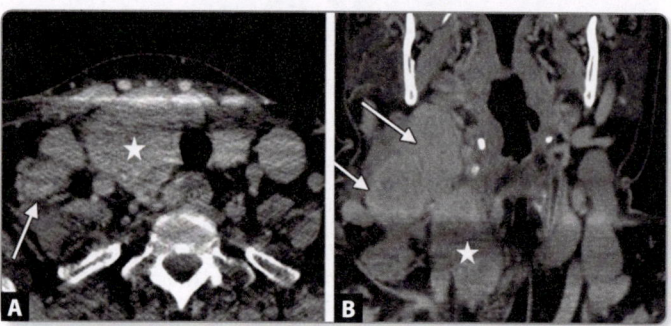

**Figures 15.21A and B** Axial, coronal enhanced CT, 34-year-old male: medullary carcinoma with extensive local nodal disease. Note the nonspecific right lobe primary mass (star) and bulky jugular chain metastatic adenopathy (arrows)

soft tissue and vascular structures (**Figures 15.14 and 15.22**). Most common in females over 60 years of age, they are usually hypoechoic on ultrasound with infiltrative margins, necrosis, and dystrophic calcification. Lymphadenopathy is present in the majority of patients at diagnosis. Anaplastic carcinomas do not usually concentrate radioiodine but may have increased uptake of thallium-201 radioisotope. Average survival ranges from 6 to 12 months from diagnosis with a 5-year survival rate of 5 percent.

## Lymphoma

Primary lymphoma is a rare disease, defined as an extranodal, extralymphatic lymphoma arising from the thyroid gland. It accounts for less than 5 percent of all thyroid malignancies with an estimated incidence of 2 cases per million. It is most common in females over 60 years of age, with a history of Hashimoto thyroiditis seen in 40 to 80 percent of cases. Treatment is dependant on the histopathological classification, as the more common diffuse large B-cell non-Hodgkin lymphoma carries a worse prognosis compared to the relatively indolent mucosa-associated lymphoid tissue (MALT) lymphoma.

The most common imaging appearance is that of a single, large (5–10 cm) homogeneous thyroid mass (**Figures 15.23A and B**) with

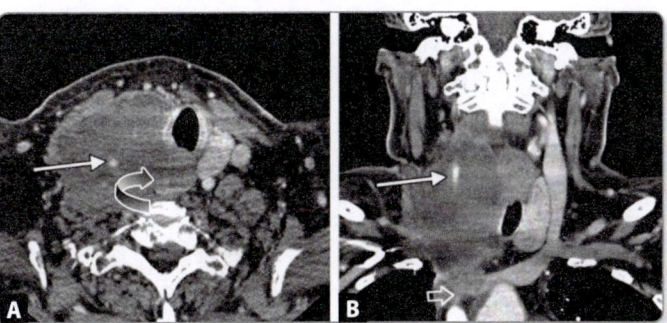

**Figures 15.22A and B** Axial, coronal enhanced CT, anaplastic thyroid carcinoma. Note the large mass with ill-defined margins and extensive locoregional soft tissue invasion, evidence by encasement and narrowing of the common carotid artery (arrows), invasion of the esophagus (curved arrow) and of mediastinal venous structures (open arrow)

## 632 Introductory head and neck imaging

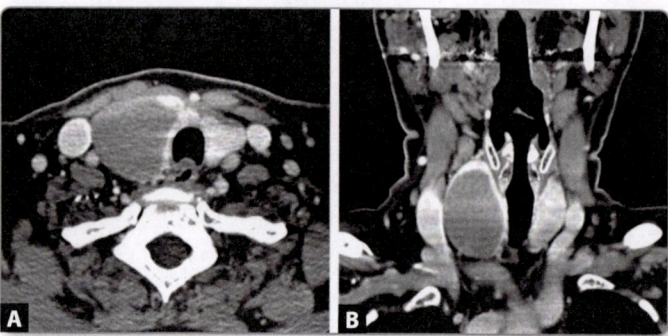

**Figures 15.23A and B** Axial, coronal enhanced CT, primary thyroid lymphoma. The large well-circumscribed right lobe mass shows typical CT imaging features, homogeneous and of low-attenuation compared with the remaining normal thyroid parenchyma

lymphadenopathy in a patient with a history of Hashimoto thyroiditis. The mass is hypoechoic on ultrasound and of low-attenuation on contrast-enhanced CT compared to background thyroid tissue. Less commonly, multiple masses or diffuse infiltration is present. Necrosis and calcification are uncommon findings. Lymphomas do not concentrate radioiodine and are cold on I-131 scintigraphy. Avid uptake of gallium-67 is not found in other thyroid malignancies and this can be used to monitor progress or assess for recurrence.

## Bibliography

1. Anderson L, Middleton WD, Teefey SA, et al. Hashimoto thyroiditis: Part 1, sonographic analysis of the nodular form of Hashimoto thyroiditis. AJR. 2010;195:208-15.
2. Anderson L, Middleton WD, Teefey SA, et al. Hashimoto thyroiditis: Part 2, sonographic analysis of benign and malignant nodule are patients with diffuse Hashimoto thyroiditis. AJR. 2010;195:216-22.
3. Baldini M, Orsatti A, Bonfanti MT, Castagnone D, Cantalamessa L. Relationship between the sonographic appearance of the thyroid and the clinical course and autoimmune activity of Graves' disease. J Clin Ultrasound. 2005;33:381-5.
4. Bomeli SR, LeBeau SO, Ferris RL. Evaluation of a thyroid nodule. Otolaryngol Clin N Am. 2010;43:229-38.

5. Clarke SEM, Rankin SC. The thyroid gland. Imaging. 2002;14:103-14.
6. Clayman GL, El-Baradie TS. Medullary thyroid cancer. Otolaryngol Clin North Am. 2003;36:91-105.
7. Cooper DS, Doherty GM, Haugen BR, et al. Revised American Thyroid Association Management Guidelines for patients with thyroid nodules and differentiated thyroid cancer. Thyroid. 2009;19:1167-1214.
8. Dackiw APB. The surgical management of medullary thyroid cancer. Otolaryngol Clin N Am. 2010;43:365-74.
9. Graff-Baker A, Roman SA, Thomas DC, Udelsman R, Sosa JA. Prognosis of primary thyroid lymphoma: Demographic, clinical, and pathologic predictors of survival in 1.408 cases. Surgery. 2009;146:1105-15.
10. Hoang JK, Lee WK, Lee M, Johnson D, Farrell S. US features of thyroid malignancy: Pearls and Pitfalls. Radiographics. 2007;27:847-65.
11. Hurley DL, Gharib H. Evaluation and management of multinodular goiter. Otolaryngol Clin North Am. 1996;29:527-40.
12. Ito Y, Amino N, Miyauchi A. Thyroid ultrasonography. World J Surg. 2010;34:1171-80.
13. Johnson NA, Tublin ME. Postoperative surveillance of differentiated thyroid carcinoma: Rationale, techniques and controversies. Radiology. 2008;249:429-44.
14. Jones R, Spendiff R, Fareedi S, Richards PS. The role of ultrasound in the management of nodular thyroid disease. Imaging. 2007;19:28-38.
15. Kim HC, et al. Primary thyroid lymphoma: CT findings. Eur J Radiol. 2003;46:233-9.
16. Knudsen N, Laurberg P, Perrild G, Bulow I, Ovesen L, Jorgensen T. Risk factors for goiter and thyroid nodules. Thyroid. 2002;12:879-88.
17. Lee S, Shin JH, Han BK, Ko EY. Medullary thyroid carcinoma: Comparison with papillary thyroid carcinoma and application of current sonographic criteria. AJR. 2010;194:1090-4.
18. Madana J, Yolmo D, Saxena SK, Gopalakrishnan S. True thyroglossal fistula. Laryngoscope. 2009;119:2345-7.
19. Marsh DJ, Learoyd DL, Robinson BG. Medullary thyroid carcinoma: Recent advances and management update. Thyroid. 1995;5:107-24.
20. McCoul ED, de Vries EJ. Concurrent lingual thyroid and undescended thyroglossal duct thyroid without orthotopic thyroid gland. Laryngoscope. 2009;119:1937-40.
21. Sheth S. Role of ultrasonography in thyroid disease. Otolaryngol Clin N Am. 2010;43:239-55.
22. Som PM, Curtin HD. Head and Neck Imaging. 4th edn. St Louis: Mosby; 2003.
23. STAT dx. Salt Lake City, Utah: Amirsys; c2005-2010 [cited 2010 October 18]. Available from: https://my.statdx.com/
24. Thomas B, Shroff M, Forte V, et al. Revisiting imaging features and the embryologic basis of third and fourth branchial anomalies. AJNR. 2010;31:755-60.
25. Urken ML. Prognosis and management of invasive well-differentiated thyroid cancer. Otolaryngol Clin N Am. 2010;43:301-28.
26. Wunderbaldinger P, Harisinghani MG, Hahn PF, et al. Cystic lymph node metastases in papillary thyroid carcinoma. AJR. 2002;178:693-7.

# Introduction to radiation oncology

chapter 16

Karen P Chu, Annie Hsu, Arjun Sahgal

### Abstract
The purpose of this chapter is to provide an overview of radiobiology, radiation physics and the principles of radiation oncology for the nonradiation oncologist. We then focus on radiation planning as it pertains to head and neck radiation therapy with detailed case examples. We explain the advent of modern radiation planning using intensity modulated radiotherapy and image-guided radiotherapy which have revolutionized radiation delivery for head and neck indications.

### Keywords
Radiation oncology, radiobiology, radiation physics, intensity modulated radiotherapy, image-guided radiotherapy.

## Introduction

Radiation oncology has been defined as the medical discipline "concerned with the generation, conservation, and dissemination of the knowledge of causes, prevention, and treatment of cancer and other special expertise in the therapeutic application of ionizing radiation". Since the first observation that X-rays can be used to treat cancers, we now have a much more advanced understanding of how radiation works to kill cancer cells and have evolved technologically to maximize our ability to target tumor and avoid surrounding critical normal tissues.

### Types of radiation
X-rays are part of a continuous spectrum of electromagnetic radiation that can be considered as moving packets, or quanta of energy referred to as photons. Photons with sufficient energy can interact with matter and cause displacement of an electron orbiting the

nucleus of an atom. If an electron has been displaced into a higher energy level orbital without actual ejection, the process is referred to as excitation. Ionization occurs when the electron receives sufficient energy from radiation causing it to be ejected from the molecule or atom. A key characteristic of ionizing radiation is the release of large amounts of energy locally.

Ionizing radiation is divided into two types: electromagnetic and particulate. Two common forms of electromagnetic radiation are X-rays and γ-rays. X-rays are produced when electrons are accelerated to a high energy and abruptly stopped by a target, commonly tungsten or gold. The kinetic energy released is converted into X-rays. Machines that deliver ionizing radiation based on generating X-rays are called linear accelerators, or better known as a linac. Conversely, γ-rays are produced intranuclearly. That is, they are emitted when excess energy is released from an unstable nucleus that breaks up and decays to reach a stable form. These photons carry varying amounts of energy that are absorbed in the body and deposited in various tissues and cells in discrete packets. For these photons to be referred to as ionizing radiation, it must have a minimum amount of energy per quanta – 124 electron volts (eV). The energy of these beams of radiation is sufficient to cause a break in a chemical bond and lead to biologic change. Machines that house a radiation source that emit γ-rays have largely been replaced by linacs, however, Gamma Knife technology is still based on the arrangement of multiple Co-60 sources and used for specific indications—particularly in brain tumors.

The other form of radiation is particulate. In radiation oncology, some forms of particulate radiation are commonly used clinically:

1. *Electrons*: These are small, negatively charged particles that are accelerated to very high energies (nearly the speed of light) by an electrical device such as a linear accelerator. Electrons are the most commonly used form of particulate radiation in radiation oncology and mainly for superficial diseases as they have a limited depth of penetration.
2. *Protons*: These are positively charged particles with a mass 2000 times greater than an electron. Because of the increased mass, they require more complex equipment such as a cyclotron to be

accelerated for use in cancer therapy. Proton beam therapy is an emerging area in clinical radiation oncology that has garnered increased interest due to its finite depth of dose deposition. This key feature could potentially increase the precision of radiotherapy dose deposition and potentially decrease the dose to surrounding normal structures. However, it remains to be seen if proton therapy has any clinical advantage over modern X-ray based radiotherapy.

## Biologic effects of radiation

The energies used in radiation oncology most commonly create absorption processes such as Compton and photoelectric absorption.

In the Compton process, the photon will interact with an orbital electron which has a small binding energy. The energy of the photon is divided into kinetic energy delivered to the electron to overcome the binding energy and cause its release from the atom and the remaining photon energy is released as another photon, or a scattered photon. This scattered photon can go on to cause other interactions (**Figure 16.1**).

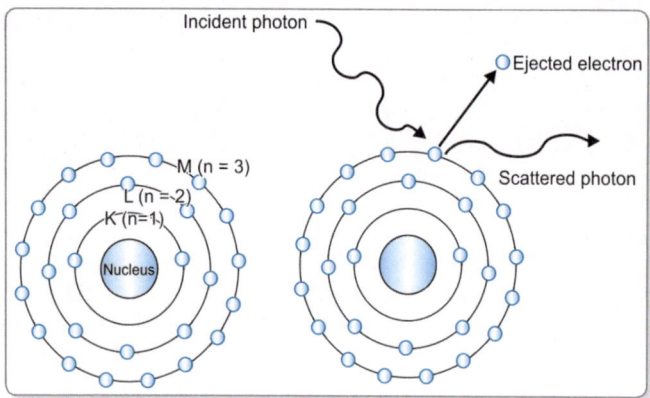

**Figure 16.1** The Compton process. An incident photon interacts with an orbital electron. If the photon has sufficient energy, it will overcome the binding forces of the orbital electron causing its release from the atom. The remaining energy of the incident photon is redirected and will continue on to create other interactions

In the photoelectric process, the photon interacts with an inner shell electron. All the energy of the photon is absorbed into the electron. Some of the energy will be used to overcome the binding energy of the electron, but the remainder will be given to the electron as kinetic energy thereby allowing it to create other interactions in matter. The vacancy in the atomic orbital is then filled by an outer electron falling into its place to stabilize the atom. When an outer orbital electron falls into the inner shell, the change in potential energy causes the release of another photon referred to as a characteristic X-ray. Characteristic radiation generally has very low energy in the range of 0.5 kV and therefore, has little biological impact (**Figure 16.2**).

While the photoelectric effect only requires ≤500 keV, the majority of the Compton process occurs in a higher energy range from approximately 500 keV to 5 MeV. Therefore, in radiation oncology, the Compton process dominates.

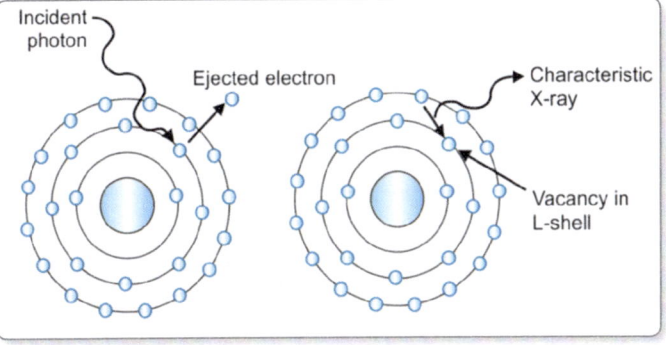

**Figure 16.2** Photoelectric effect. In contrast to the Compton process, in the photoelectric effect, the incident photon interacts with an inner shell electron. This electron absorbs all of the photon's energy. Part of this energy is used to overcome the binding forces. The rest is absorbed by the electron which can be subsequently used in further interactions in matter. The vacancy in the shell left by the ejected electron will be filled by an outer electron. When this outer electron falls to the inner shell, it releases energy in the form of a characteristic X-ray

## Mechanism of radiation damage

DNA damage by radiation is created by breaks in the chromosomes. Single strand breaks occur commonly from irradiation, but they can be repaired easily using the opposite strand sequence as a template. If there is an error in repair (misrepair), a mutation can occur. As long as this mutation does not impede replication, the mutation will be carried forth in subsequent replications of the cell. Double strand breaks occur when there are breaks in both strands opposite to one another or within a few base pairs. These breaks occur much less frequently than single strand breaks. If the breaks can be repaired in the same pattern, no damage will be noticed. But if the breaks do not rejoin in the proper configuration, this creates an aberration that may subsequently lead to cell death (**Figure 16.3**).

DNA damage created by radiation occurs either directly or indirectly (**Figure 16.4**). When particulate radiation directly releases sufficient kinetic energy that causes damage to tissues or cells leading to biologic changes, the process is referred to as directly ionizing. Electromagnetic radiation such as X-rays and γ-rays are indirectly ionizing because they do not cause any damage directly to tissues or cells. Instead, the energy is absorbed by molecules. When sufficient energy is absorbed, fast moving particles, such as electrons or free radicals are released from the atom and produce the biologic changes through damage to tissues or cells.

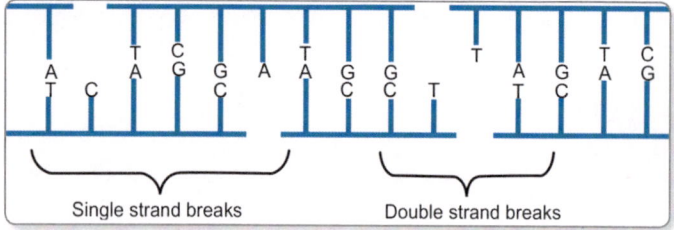

**Figure 16.3** DNA damage by radiation. Damage caused by radiation can lead to single strand breaks where the cell can use the other strand as a template for repair. Double strand breaks occur when there is damage to both strands of DNA that have a higher probability of causing a lethal chromosomal aberration that will inhibit cell replication. Ultimately, this will lead to cell death

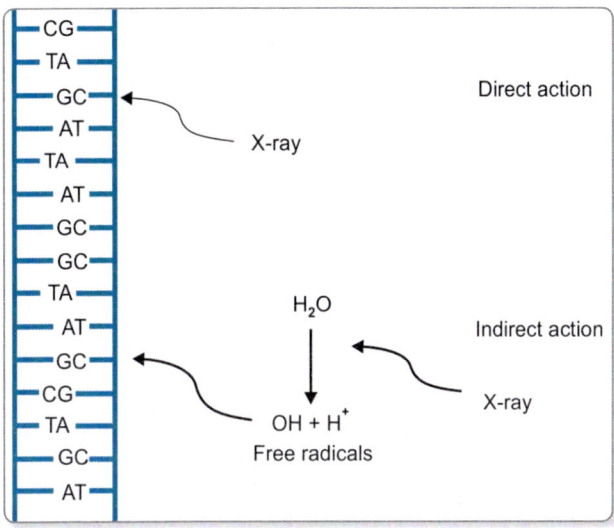

**Figure 16.4** Direct and indirect action of radiotherapy. Direct action by radiation occurs when the photon or radiation itself interacts with the DNA to cause damage. Conversely, indirect action occurs when the photon or radiation interacts with another molecule—most commonly water—which will create free radicals that subsequently interact and damage DNA. Indirect DNA damage can also occur from electrons that are released from an atom by radiation

To understand damage created by irradiation, a basic understanding of cell replication is required (but is beyond the scope of this chapter). Cell death from radiation occurs most commonly by a process called mitotic death. Mitotic death occurs when cells with damaged chromosomes attempt to divide. The other method of cell death is apoptosis, or programmed cell death. Apoptosis is a multistep process where the dying cell separates from its neighbors. Chromatin condenses and the nucleus fragments. The cell shrinks from cytoplasmic condensation until the cell completely separates into several membrane-bound fragments called apoptotic bodies.

## Radiation damage, repair, and dose rate effect

Radiation damage can be classified into three groups:
1. *Lethal damage*: Irreversible damage (due to large number of double strand breaks) that irrevocably leads to cell death.
2. *Sublethal damage*: While there is damage present, DNA is still repairable if sufficient time is provided. However, if additional sublethal damage is delivered, this may convert the sublethal to lethal damage.
3. *Potentially lethal damage*: This type of radiation damage can be modified by manipulation of the environment (e.g. altering the environment to slow down the cell cycle thereby allowing more time for cell repair). However, under normal circumstances, this type of damage leads to cell death.

The relationship between cell survival and chromosomal aberrations can be illustrated with the linear quadratic relationship (**Figure 16.5**). At low doses of radiation where there may only be a

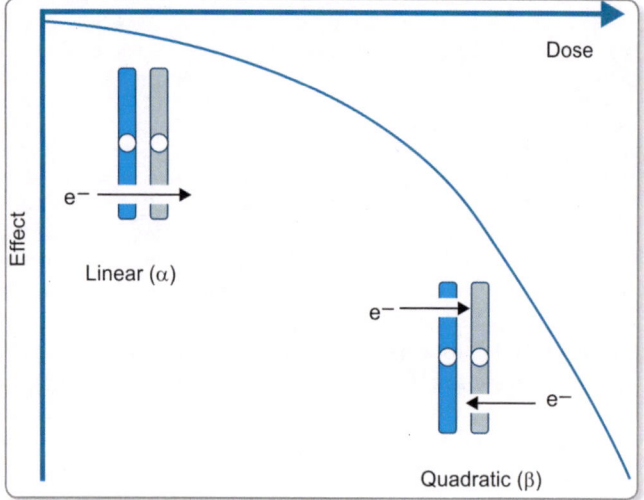

**Figure 16.5** Linear quadratic relationship. At lower doses of radiation, the probability of DNA damage is linear (α). But as dose increases, the probability of DNA damage becomes quadratic (β) due to increased frequency of cellular interactions

single electron creating an aberration, the probability of a chromosomal break is proportional to dose (linear). When the radiation dose increases, there are more cellular interactions. That is, chromosomal breaks may occur from separate electrons which increase the probability of creating an aberration proportional to the square of the dose (quadratic).

The α/β ratio is an important concept in radiation oncology where both α and β are proportionality constants that represent the damage created during the linear and quadratic portion of the cell survival curve respectively. Tumors in general have a high α/β ratio (~10) compared to normal tissues (α/β ≈ 2). Therefore, for optimal dose fractionation, smaller dose per fraction would allow for multiple repetitions of the shoulder of the survival curve = shallower curve. This is referred to as the dose-rate effect. As the dose rate is decreased and the exposure time is increased, the biologic effect of a given dose is reduced. Further, the survival curve becomes shallower and the shoulder disappears making the survival curve an exponential function of dose. The magnitude of the dose rate effect from the repair of sublethal damage varies among different cell types. For each cell type, any deviation from the dose rate range will result into little change in the survival curve relative to the dose rate. Sublethal damage that occurs during long radiation exposure would be repaired.

## Concept of fractionation

Based on the dose-rate effect, the total dose of radiation is divided into several fractions delivered over weeks to maximize the effect of repeating the shoulder portion of the survival curve. For example, head and neck cancers are generally treated at our institution with 70 Gy of radiation divided into daily fractions of 2 Gy — resulting in a total of 35 fractions. The high dose volume treated to 70 Gy includes visible tumor with an appropriate margin to account for set up errors and potential microscopic areas of spread (typically 1 cm). A lower dose of 56 to 60 Gy, delivered over the same 35 fractions (1.6 – 1.7 Gy per fraction), is also delivered to those areas at risk of tumor spread (for example the relevant lymph node levels where the cancer is likely to spread to). This will be explained in further detail below. Given the tolerance of the normal structures within this area, we are unable to deliver these doses (for example) over a single fraction without essentially destroying all the structures in the region. To provide some perspective:

- 5 to 12 Gy to the whole body in a single fraction will cause death within days due to extensive destruction of the mucosa of the gastrointestinal tract.
- The tolerance of the lens to cause cataracts in 5 percent of the population in 5 years is only 10 Gy in 5 fractions (2 Gy fractions).
- 45 Gy divided into 2 Gy fractions is sufficient to cause hypothyroidism in 5 percent of patients treated with radiotherapy 5 years later.

The benefits of fractionation are to maximize repair and repopulation of the normal tissue cells between fractions and to enhance tumor cell kill by allowing time for reoxygenation of the tumor and reassortment to more sensitive phases of the cell cycle prior to the next radiation exposure. The disadvantage to fractionation is the potential for the tumor to repopulate during the 7th week course of treatment. The "4 R's" of radiobiology are summarized as follows:

1. *Repair*: Sublethal damage requires time to be repaired. The balance in radiation oncology is to allow sufficient time for normal tissues to be repaired without allowing too much time for tumor cells to repair.
2. *Reassortment*: The timing of radiation is important to coincide with the cell cycle and each mitotic division. Therefore, both repair and radiation damage may not be evident until the cell completes another cycle. Cells are most sensitive to radiation in the G2 phase.
3. *Repopulation*: The delivery of radiation over weeks allows for cells to double between exposures to radiation. This allows for normal tissue repair during the course of radiation.
4. *Reoxygenation*: As tumors grow, they outstrip their blood supply making the core of the tumor hypoxic. As radiation kills the peripheral cells, they slough off and expose the inner layers of cells which can subsequently reach the blood supply and oxygenation. Oxygenation of these cells is thought to increase the

effect of radiation by the following mechanisms: production of free radicals that cause chromosomal damage; "fixation" of the damage produced by radiation; promoting the production of peroxides that can damage the cell membrane.

## Clinical radiation oncology

In radiation oncology, the SI unit for absorbed dose is the gray (Gy) which is defined as:

$$1\ Gy = 1\ J/kg$$

That is the absorption of one joule of ionizing radiation by a kilogram of matter or tissue. The most commonly used radiotherapy machines include the following:

1. *Orthovoltage therapy*: X-ray treatment with potentials between 150 to 500 kV. Given the low potential of these X-rays, they are limited for very superficial lesion ≤1 cm from the surface such as skin cancers.
2. *Linear accelerator*: This is the most common radiation generator. High frequency electromagnetic waves are used to accelerate electrons to high energy. Once these fast electrons hit their target, the energy released as photons are directed for use in radiotherapy. Alternatively, the accelerated electrons can also be used from a linear accelerator to treat patients. This type of radiation generator is discussed in more detail in the next section.
3. *Cyclotron*: This machine accelerates charged particles to produce high energy protons or neutrons. It can also be used to produce radionuclides.
4. *Cobalt-60 unit*: Here an embedded isotope constantly emits γ-rays which are shaped by a collimator and aimed at the target. 60Co is most commonly used. These units have largely been replaced by linac units but still used for Gamma Knife radiosurgery due to physical characteristics that provide some advantage in the treatment of small brain lesions.
5. *Brachytherapy*: Radionuclides are also used in brachytherapy where radioactive material is used to locally deliver radiation to the tumor by implanting them permanently or temporarily into

the tumor tissue. Common radioactive sources include 125I, 103Pd, and 192Ir.

## Linear accelerators

Similar to the production of X-rays with electrons hitting a target at the anode, a linear accelerator, or linac, also uses an accelerated electron to hit a target to produce photons. The basic schematic of a linac can be seen in **Figure 16.6**. A power supply provides the current that will be modulated into a pulse forming network. These pulses are directed to both the electron gun and the magnetron/klystron. The magnetron/klystron inject pulsed microwaves into the accelerator tube where the electrons will "surf" across to the treatment head. As the electrons travel along these waves in the accelerator tube, it gains more energy until it reaches the target, commonly tungsten. The resulting bremsstrahlung X-rays are directed by a bending magnet to be used therapeutically to treat a patient.

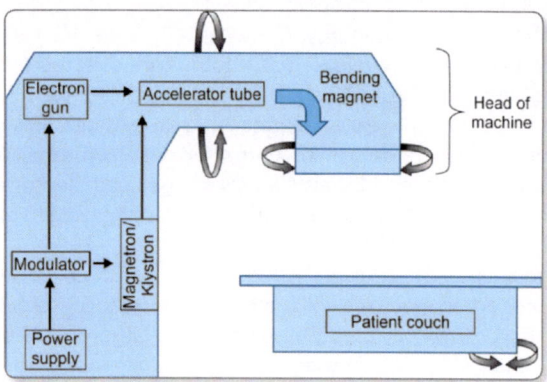

**Figure 16.6** Linear accelerator. Energy modulated from a power source is pulsed by a magnetron/klystron allowing electrons to "surf" through the accelerator tube. The resulting accelerated electrons are redirected by a bending magnet to the target within the head of the machine to produce photons. If electrons are to be used instead, the target is moved out of the pathway of the beam

Introduction to radiation oncology 645

The beam is modulated with two collimators into the desired shape (**Figure 16.7**). The first or primary collimator is fixed and is found just below the X-ray target that helps to decrease the leakage of radiation from the head of the machine. The secondary collimator is more dynamic and can be used to sculpt the radiation to an appropriate size and shape suitable for an individual tumor using multileaf collimators (MLC). MLCs are individual leaves that are composed of a high atomic number material (e.g. tungsten). As each of these leaves can independently move in and out of the radiation beam, they can modulate the dose delivered. This is the basis of intensity modulated radiotherapy (IMRT), which creates highly shaped dose distributions that effectively treat the head and neck cancer while sparing critical structures from a toxic dose.

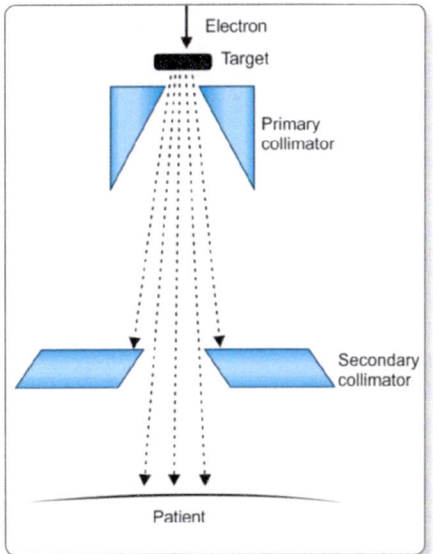

**Figure 16.7** Linear accelerator treatment head components. When the electrons strike the target, photons are released which are shaped using collimators prior to reaching the surface of the patient

## Clinical radiotherapy planning

When patients come for radiation, the first step is the initial consultation with the multidisciplinary team that includes the radiation oncologist. Cases are often discussed in a multidisciplinary setting where all members of the oncology team will help make a decision for the patient's treatment.

In radiation oncology, approximately 50 percent of patients are treated with a radical or curative intent. In these situations, the doses range from 50 to 70 Gy over 5 to 7 weeks depending on the clinical scenario. However, radiotherapy is also effective for symptom management in the metastatic or palliative setting. Common palliative roles for radiotherapy include the management of pain, prevention of pathologic fractures, and to stop bleeding that result from a metastases or incurable primary tumor. The dose-fractionation schemes range from a single treatment of 8 Gy, to approximately 30 Gy in 10 fractions. These low doses are sufficient to provide control of symptoms and the tumor in the short term, but not necessarily durable long-term local control.

> **Case example:** A 60-year-old male presented to his family physician with increasing headaches and cranial nerve palsies. The patient was referred to an ear, nose, and throat specialist who performed a debulking surgery which demonstrated an EBV positive nasopharyngeal carcinoma. A staging PET/CT scan was performed. The scan demonstrated a highly metabolic posterior left nasopharyngeal mass measuring 6 x 4 cm in size. The mass extended and eroded into the posterior left sphenoid, clivus, and petrous apex (**Figure 16.10**). The mass crossed the midline and caused a mass effect on the oropharynx. There was also a large 1.7 x 1.2 cm left level II lymph node with an SUV of 24.
>
> The patient was assessed in the oncology clinic by the surgeon, radiation oncologist, and medical oncologist. On flexible nasopharyngoscope, a left sided nasopharyngeal mass was noted that extended to the right. The tumor extended down the lateral wall of the oropharynx down to just superior to the pyriform sinus. The soft palate was partially involved.

Given the substantial tumor burden, the patient was staged as a T4N1, WHO 2 nasopharyngeal carcinoma. The consensus within the multidisciplinary group was for the patient to receive chemoradiation. With respect to the radiation, he was treated with a total dose of 70 Gy that was delivered over 33 fractions.

Once a decision is made to proceed with radiotherapy, the first step is a CT simulation where a patient is set up, or simulated, in the same position as they would be for their daily radiation treatments. Based on the location of the tumor, a variety of immobilization devices exist to help the patient maintain the same position during the course of treatment. Most commonly for head and neck cancer radiation, a thermoplastic mask that is moulded to the specific contour of the patient's head and shoulder region is used (**Figure 16.8**). For each radiation treatment, the patient is set-up in this mask, and once aligned in the proper position, treatment begins.

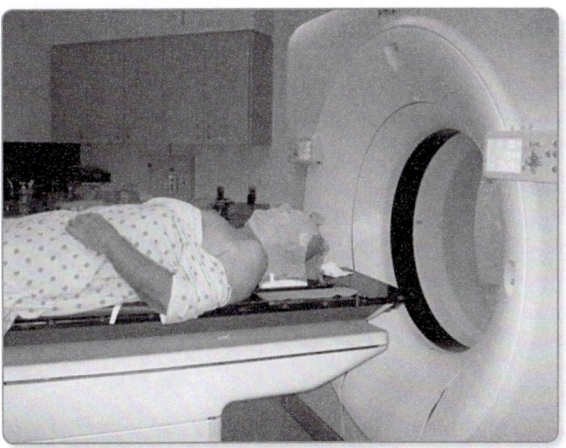

**Figure 16.8** CT simulation set-up. A mask is molded to the patient's facial anatomy (and often, for increased reproducibility, a longer mask is used to mold to the patient's facial and shoulder anatomy) such that it can be reproduced daily. The mask is anchored to the table top using pegs to fasten the mask to the table. A head rest is positioned to support the head and neck. Arms are kept at the side to ensure no radiation beams are passed through the arms to reach the target in the head and neck region

A CT with a field of view that included the entire circumference of the patient's body at the level of interest is obtained. For example, a nasopharyngeal tumor is scanned from the brain to below the clavicles as opposed to a smaller field of view centered on the area of disease alone. This creates complete electron density information required for the treatment planning system to model the effect of the beams entering and exiting the patient for dose calculation. Newer technology has also made it feasible to use MRI in the simulation process, however, treatment planning on MRI alone is not possible due to the lack of electron density information needed to calculate dose. Therefore, MRI images are fused onto the CT in order to delineate the anatomy. **Figures 16.9A and B** illustrate these points.

Planning of radiotherapy is a complex process involving a number of oncology staff including radiation dosimetrists and physicists that work alongside the radiation oncologist. Various programs are available for the radiation oncologist to outline or contour the tumor

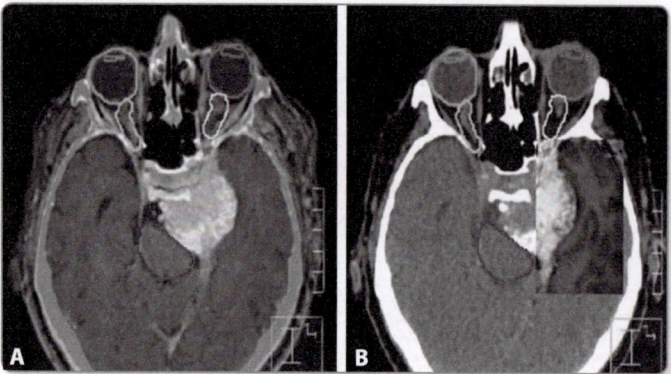

**Figures 16.9A and B** Fusion of MRI and CT data to plan radiotherapy for a cavernous sinus meningioma case. In this example, (A) demonstrates an MRI fused to the planning CT. (B) The CT simulation alone but with an overlying clipbox that allows visualization of the MRI data set for the purpose of illustrating the fusion. As can be seen on the (A), the advantage of CT to identify the bony anatomy is combined with the superior soft tissue delineation of MRI (*for color version see Plate 19*)

volume. Standard definitions of tumor volumes have been outlined by the International Commission on Radiation Units (ICRU):
1. *Gross tumor volume (GTV)*: It is defined as the tumor based on clinical assessment aided by pathology and imaging available.
2. *Clinical target volume (CTV)*: This is defined as the volume encompassing areas at risk of tumor progression or areas of microscopic spread of tumor.
3. *Planning target volume (PTV)*: During treatment, there are a number of potential errors that can occur from daily set-up and from normal organ motion. This volume accounts for these potential changes from day-to-day treatments.
4. *Organs at risk (OAR)*: In addition to the tumor and target volumes that define where the radiation should target, the organs at risk are those normal structures that the radiation oncologist would like to avoid receiving a substantial dose of radiation.

In some cases, especially in the postoperative setting where the tumor has been removed, it is imperative to have the preoperative imaging available to help delineate the previous location of the tumor. If possible, this preoperative imaging is "fused" or overlaid onto the CT simulation imaging to better define the tumor volumes.

**Case example: Figure 16.10**, the volume receiving 70 Gy was the primary tumor and the involved level II lymph node. The dose delivered to the subclinical disease—that is, the areas at risk of involvement—was 56 Gy delivered over the 33 fractions. In a locally advanced nasopharyngeal tumor such as the one the patient presented with, the areas at risk including the remaining nasopharynx, clivus, sphenoid and maxillary sinuses, posterior nasal cavity, parapharyngeal space, and pterygoid fossa.

The PTV generated from the areas at risk (CTV) was an additional 3 to 5 mm margin. The volumes created are based on both the imaging and clinical judgment. Therefore, in areas where the tumor is in very close proximity to normal structures such as the brainstem, the PTV is decreased to as little as 1 mm to prevent overdose of the brainstem. Further, even if not evident on imaging, such as on the PETCT scan in this patient's case, the tumor

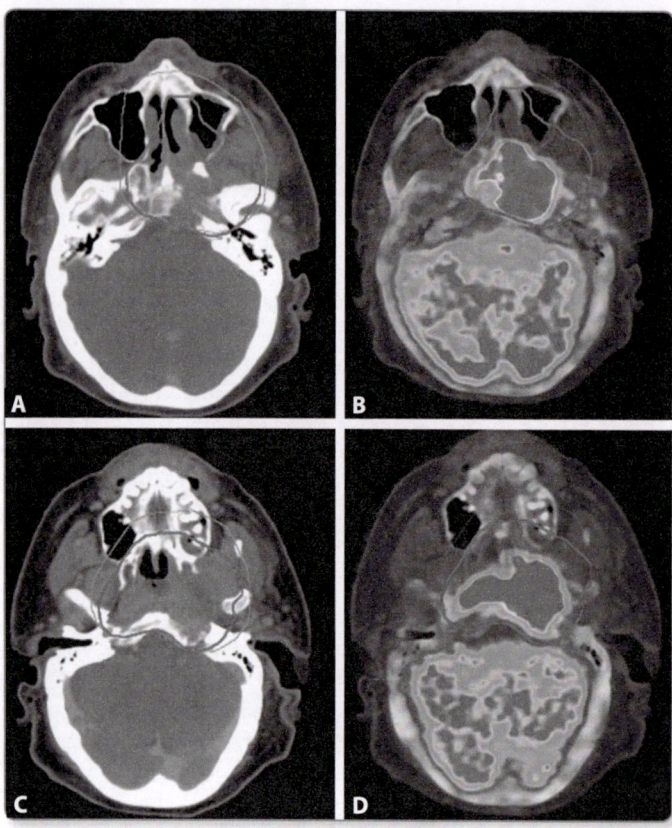

**Figures 16.10A to D** Tumor volumes. The patient had a PETCT simulation to design his therapy. The red outline illustrates the planning target volume (PTV) that encompasses the gross tumor volume (GTV) with a margin to include the areas of potential microscopic spread clinical target volume (CTV) and a margin to account for potential daily errors in set up or from patient motion. This volume was treated to 70 Gy. The orange line represents the PTV that included all potential areas of disease spread based on the known disease progression and potential pathways of spread in nasopharyngeal cancer. The volume was treated to 56 Gy (*for color version see Plate 20*)

volume is adjusted to account for all areas of disease that may have been more easily visualized clinically.

Treatment planning in radiation oncology has progressed over the past 50 years. Initially, plans were simplistic using, for example, fluoroscopy to aid in outlining the treatment field using a limited number of fields. X-rays were the dominant form of visualization to determine the tumor location based on bony anatomy.

With the advent of CT simulation, treatment planning progressed to the above tumor and target volumes to define the treatment fields. Using CT simulation in conjunction with delivery using MLCs, the radiation oncologist is now able to shape the beam to the profile of the tumor using multiple beams in a process referred to as 3D conformal radiotherapy (3DCRT) (**Figures 16.11 and 16.12**).

Most recently, radiation oncology has increasingly moved towards IMRT as a standard of care for complex curative radiation treatments.

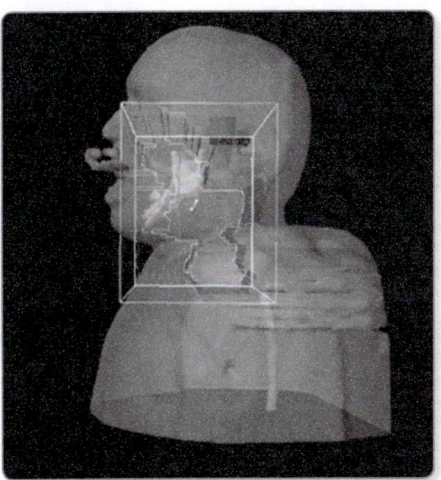

**Figure 16.11** Three-dimensional conformal radiotherapy (3DCRT). The tumor and target volumes are outlined along with the organs at risk. Using computer based programming, the structures can be reconstructed in three-dimensional imaging and overlaid on a surface rendering of the patient based on the CT simulation (*for color version see Plate 21*)

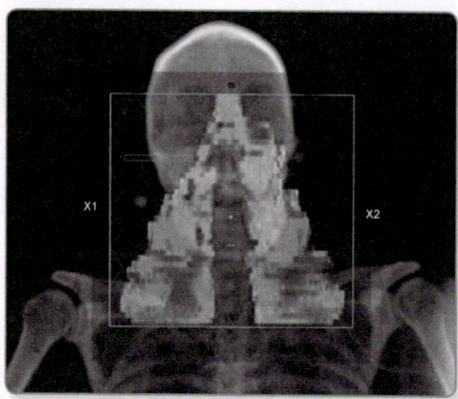

**Figure 16.12** Radiation dose distribution. Using computer software, the doses to the tumor and target volumes can be constructed and illustrated on the bony anatomy of the patient. The hotter (red/orange/yellow) colors indicate areas of higher dose while the cooler (green/blue) colors demonstrate areas receiving a lower dose. One can appreciate the large volumes of tissue that will be radiated in treating a head and neck cancer for cure as this is a typical volume treated in a nasopharyngeal cancer patient (*for color version see Plate 21*)

Intensity modulated radiotherapy (IMRT) improves the ability to shape the dose distribution around the target area while minimizing dose to surrounding normal tissues. Using MLCs, the intensity of the radiation is modulated by adjusting the MLC leaf position throughout the course of treatment (**Figure 16.13**). In simple terms, the intensity is greater in areas of target and less in areas of normal tissues that are to be spared. This is a very powerful development in the specialty and has allowed major clinical advances in reducing the toxicity of head and neck treatment. For example, parotid sparing radiation has reduced the incidence of long-term xerostomia (**Figures 16.14A and B**). Moreover, significant gains in tumor control have been specifically observed using conformal radiation among several cancer sites including nasopharyngeal cancer.

Intensity modulated radiotherapy (IMRT) is still based on the CT simulation. Computer algorithms determine the optimal means of delivering dose to the tumor. Dose is calculated throughout the body

Introduction to radiation oncology 653

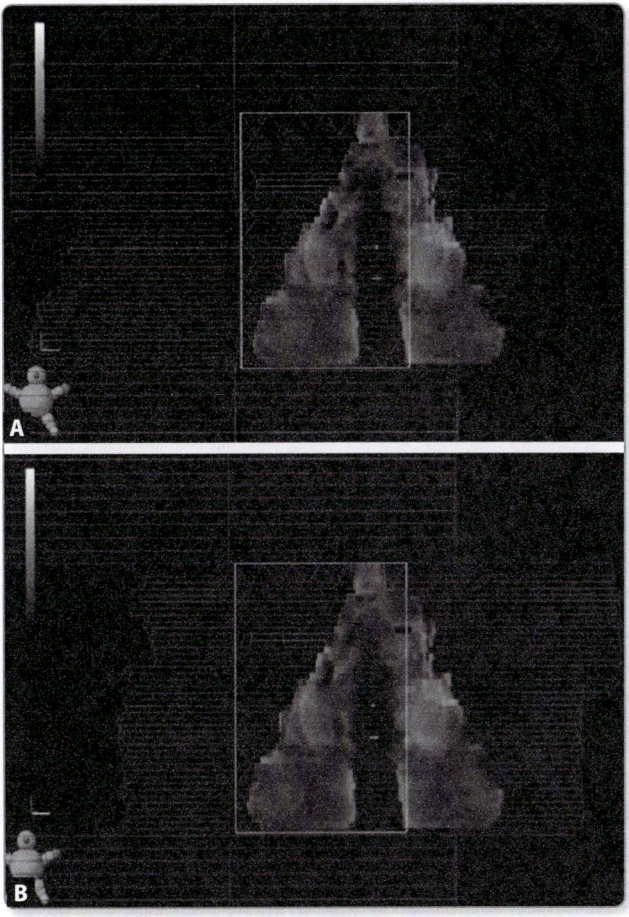

**Figures 16.13A and B** Sequencing of multileaf collimators (MLCs). In intensity modulated radiotherapy (IMRT), the dose is modulated by the MLCs within the head of the machine. The MLCs can vary their position and the time held in a single position. In this way, the beam is shaped to the tumor and target volumes. Using multiple beams with the MLCs allows for sculpting of the dose to match the tumor shape and minimize toxicities to normal structures (*for color version see Plate 22*)

## 654 Introductory head and neck imaging

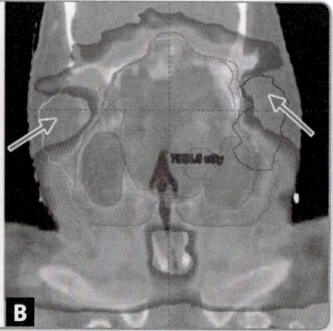

**Figures 16.14A and B** Dose sparing with intensity modulated radiotherapy. A common side effect of radiation therapy to the head and neck region is xerostomia due to the dose received by the parotids (arrows). IMRT allows the radiation oncologist to spare the parotid to a dose below the mean tolerance of 26 Gy. In the figure above, the dose distributed on the transverse and coronal slices represents a minimum of 26 Gy (dark blue) and progressively increases to 70 Gy that is focused on the actual tumor (red). The majority of the parotids is not within this dose distribution and therefore, receives less than 26 Gy (*for color version see Plate 23*)

based on densities of the tissues the photon beam will pass through. Once the optimal sequencing of the MLCs to modulate the beam is determined and the plan is deemed acceptable, then a complex process of quality assurance is undertaken and treatment can be delivered. The ultimate goal is for the target volumes to receive the full dose of radiation within +/– 5 to 10 percent of the prescription. The other goal is for the organs at risk to receive the minimal amount of radiation. Therefore, not only is a great deal of effort and time spent on defining tumor volumes and optimizing a treatment plan, a substantial amount of time is spent delineating and evaluating the dose to the normal tissues. A dose-volume histogram is generated for the targets and organs at risk and carefully scrutinized (**Figure 16.15**). The final acceptability of a treatment plan is based on achieving the required dose to the tumor while respecting known dose thresholds limits for toxicity.

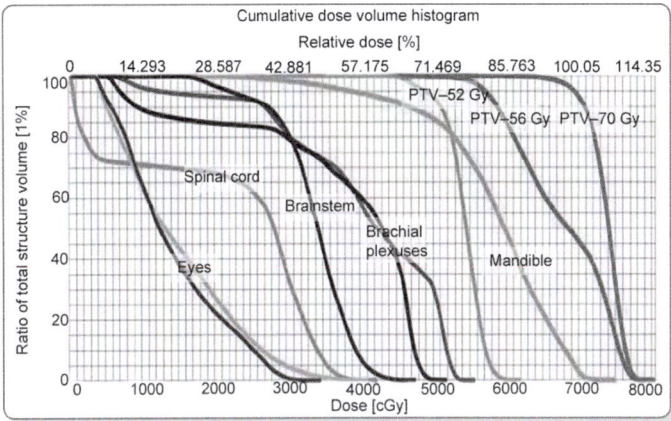

**Figure 16.15** Dose volume histogram (DVH). A DVH is a graphical representation of the dose received by all structures outlined by the radiation oncologist. The target volumes should receive the prescribed dose within approximately 5 to 10 percent. The tolerances of normal structures are known and therefore, can be used to help guide the evaluation of dose to these structures. The goal is to maximize the tumor coverage while minimizing the dose received by normal tissues. In this case the target volumes included the 70 Gy volume to cover the visible tumor, 56 Gy volume to cover high-risk areas, and a 52 Gy volume to much lower risk areas such as the low neck and supraclavicular region (*for color version see Plate 23*)

**Case example:** The volumes for the patient were designed by the radiation oncologist and were used to plan the radiation treatments.

During the daily radiation treatments, radiation therapists will set up the patient in the same positioning as when he was simulated for treatment planning. Throughout the course of radiotherapy, the patient is imaged using an electronic portal imaging device (EPID). This allows for the radiotherapy team to match the patient's bony anatomy with the bony anatomy reconstructed from the CT simulation. These images are reviewed by the radiation oncologist. If the patient's position differs significantly, the team will be alerted to change the positioning to ensure accurate treatment.

However, with increased precision of radiotherapy, there is also an increased risk of errors. The goals in radiation oncology are to maximize the dose to the tumor while minimizing the dose to the critical or normal structures. One method to do which decrease the uncertainty in daily treatments—that is, the PTV margin. To do this, there must be a way to ensure accuracy of the daily treatments which often involves frequent imaging during the course of radiotherapy. This concept is referred to as image-guided radiotherapy (IGRT). Simply defined, IGRT refers to the use of various types of imaging to help guide the radiotherapy planning and daily treatments such that the tumor region can be imaged just prior to treatment and any adjustments made to ensure that the position of the tumor is in the intended location. Forms of IGRT include kV imaging, ultrasound, and various techniques of using CT imaging (**Figure 16.16**). Two commonly used forms of CT based IGRT are cone-beam CT and megavoltage CT. In both cases, the linac is equipped with a mounted CT scanner that can be used to image the patient prior to each daily fraction of radiotherapy to ensure proper set-up (**Figure 16.17**). In contrast to megavoltage CT, cone-beam CT uses kV energies for imaging.

**Case example:** In our case example, the patient had weekly CBCT to ascertain the accuracy of the set-up prior to beginning the daily fraction of radiation (**Figure 16.16**).

## Follow-up

During the course of radiotherapy, patients are followed weekly by the radiation oncologists to monitor for acute toxicities. Side effects from radiotherapy are limited to the area being treated. In general, patients will feel fatigued from radiation and will have some degree of skin reaction or radiation dermatitis. Other side effects will be site specific. That is, the side effects patients experience from radiotherapy is localized to the area that receives radiotherapy. For example, while a head and neck cancer patient may receive mucositis, a rectal cancer patient will not. Instead, this patient is more likely to experience diarrhea from their radiotherapy.

Some side effects from radiotherapy are permanent such as lymphedema from breast and axillary radiotherapy or xerostomia from head and neck radiotherapy. Further, there are late toxicities

Introduction to radiation oncology 657

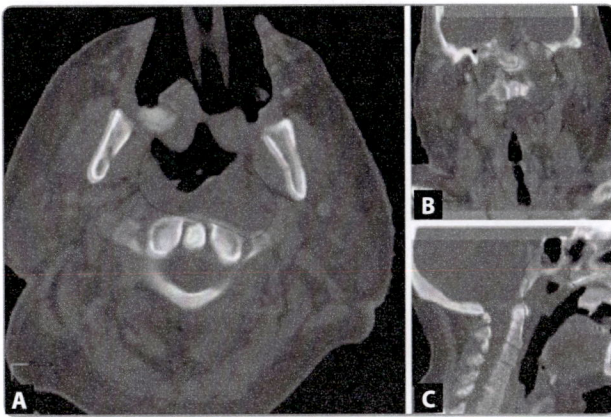

**Figures 16.16A to C** Cone-beam computed tomography (CBCT). With the proximity of critical structures such as the brainstem and the spinal cord, the room for error is minimal. Using a CBCT when the patient is set-up for daily radiation treatments allows the radiation oncologist to match the patient's soft tissue and bony anatomy with the CT simulation. The CBCT and the CT simulation images are superimposed. In addition to ensure proper patient set-up, the tumor response to radiotherapy can also be monitored (*for color version see Plate 24*)

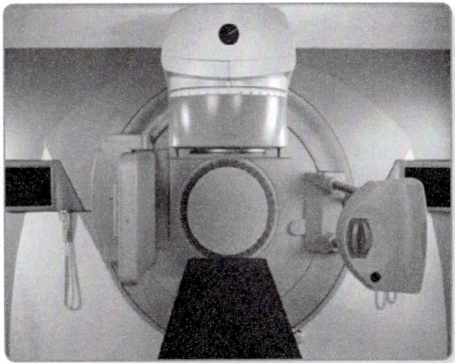

**Figure 16.17** Image guided radiotherapy (IGRT). This is one example of a linac equipped with a cone-beam CT (CBCT) image guidance system. The CBCT scanner is mounted onto the head of the linac and allows the target to be imaged prior to treatment to ensure set-up accuracy

that can occur years after radiation such as esophageal strictures from radiotherapy to the head and neck or chest region. One concern in radiotherapy is the risk of developing a malignancy due to the radiation. These cancers occur >20 years after receiving radiation.

## Conclusion

The basis of radiation oncology is the "therapeutic application of ionizing radiation". The field is based on a solid foundation of radiobiology and radiation physics principles and key points include:

- Ionizing radiation refers to electromagnetic (X-rays, γ-rays) and particulate (electrons, protons, neutrons, alpha particles, heavy charged particles) forms.
- The target of radiotherapy is DNA.
- Clinical radiation is most commonly generated and delivered by a linear accelerator.
- Patients undergo a CT simulation to plan the radiation treatments. Additional imaging can be superimposed onto the CT to assist the radiation team to design the tumor volumes.
- The goal in clinical radiation oncology is to maximize dose to the tumor while minimizing toxicities to normal structures.
- Intensity modulated radiotherapy (IMRT) allows for dose sculpting to create highly refined plans and has resulted in improved local control and less long-term permanent side effects.
- Image-guided radiotherapy (IGRT) refers to imaging the target just prior to radiation delivery such that any positional deviations can be corrected. This has allowed for improved the accuracy of our treatments.

## Bibliography

1. Emami B, Lyman J, Brown A, et al. Tolerance of normal tissue to therapeutic irradiation. Int J Radiat Oncol Biol Phys. 1991;21(1):109-22.
2. Hall, EJ. Radiobiology for the radiologist, 5th edn. Philadelphia, PA. Lippincott Williams & Wilkins; 2000.
3. Halperin EC, Perez CA, Brady LW. Principles and practice of radiation oncology, 5th edn. Philadelphia, PA. Lippincott Williams & Wilkins; 2008.

# Index

Page numbers followed by *f* refer to figure and *t* refer to table.

## A

Aberrant internal carotid artery 48
Abnormal course of facial nerve 64
Accessory parotid tissue 360
Acinic cell carcinoma 120, 386, 387*f*
Acoustic schwannoma 77*f*
Acquired
    cholesteatoma 56
    diseases 38, 52, 64, 73
Acute
    calcific tendinitis of longus colli 555
    fulminant invasive fungal sinusitis 192
    inflammation of lacrimal gland 122
    internal jugular vein thrombosis 538*f*
    labyrinthitis 73*f*
    lymphoblastic leukemia 114
    myelogenous leukemia 114, 559*f*
    otomastoiditis 52
    rhinosinusitis 171
    secretions 172*f*
    sinusitis 172*f*
    subperiosteal abscess 102*f*
Adenocarcinoma 212
    of lung 494*f*
Adenoid
    cystic carcinoma 120, 386, 415*f*
        of sinus 210*f*
    hypertrophy 473*f*
Adenolymphoma 371
Adult orbital hemangiomas 589, 590*f*, 601
AJCC general nodal staging system for
    head and neck cancers 495*t*
    nasopharyngeal carcinoma 496*t*
    thyroid carcinomas 496*t*
AJCC nodal staging system for
    cutaneous squamous cell carcinoma 497*t*
    melanoma 498*t*
    merkel cell carcinoma 497*t*
Allergic fungal sinusitis 183, 184*f*
Ameloblastoma 270*f*, 323*f*
American Joint Committee on Cancer 247, 324, 425
Amyloidosis 251
Anaplastic carcinoma 630
Angiofibroma 216, 218*f*
Angiofollicular lymph node hyperplasia 485, 486*f*, 487*f*
Angioimmunoblastic T-cell lymphoma 604
Angiosarcoma 600
Anophthalmia 92
Anterior
    cervical nodes 430
    cranial fossa 204*f*
    ethmoid arteries 154*f*, 169*f*
    scalene muscle 445*f*
    stapes anterior crura 19*f*
    tympanic segment of facial nerve 20*f*
Antineutrophil cytoplasmic antibodies 196
Antrochoanal polyps 186*f*
Apical turn of cochlea 31*f*

Appearance of
    nodal calcifications 465f
    sinonasal tumors 202f
    tumor 201
Arterial dissection 574f, 576f
Arteriovenous malformation 137, 566
Ascending palatine artery 592
Assessment of orbital invasion 210f
Asymmetric size of internal jugular veins 532
Atelectatic sinus syndrome 191f
Auriculotemporal nerve 406
Autoimmune disease and thyroiditis 619
Autosomal dominant polycystic kidney disease 534

# B

Bacillary angiomatosis 477
Bacterial lymphadenitides 475
Basal
    cell carcinoma 46f
    turn of cochlea 21f, 31f, 33f
Behçet's syndrome 327
Bell's palsy 64, 65, 65f, 397, 419
Benign
    lesions 215
    lymphoepithelial lesions 376
    mixed tumor 251, 370
    neoplasms 369, 552
    osteoma of ethmoid sinus 222f
    reactive lymphadenopathy 457t
Bilateral
    coloboma 97f
    disease 629
    haller air cells 166f
    internal auditory canal 45f
    lacrimal gland malt lymphoma 121f
    parotid calculi 363f
    phthisis bulbi 94f
    retinoblastoma 117f
    retropharyngeal adenopathy 242f
    temporal bones 57f, 58f
    Warthin's tumors 376f
Blowout fracture of medial orbital wall 130
Bony
    and choanal atresia 227f
    atresia 37f
    modiolus of cochlea 23f
Boundaries of oropharynx 334f
Brachytherapy 643
Branchial
    apparatus anomalies 618
    cleft cyst 462f
Breast metastasis 120f
Bulla ethmoidalis 144
Buphthalmos 95

# C

Calcified tornwaldt cyst 236f
Capillary hemangioma 111
Carcinoma
    ex-pleomorphic adenoma 386
    *in situ* 248
    of lung metastasis 265f
    of retromolar trigone 558f
Carotid
    artery 445f
        dissection 295f, 534
    body
        paraganglioma 596f
        tumor 539, 540f, 541f
    canal 33f
    cavernous fistula 576, 578f
    encasement 346
    paragangliomas 595
    space 531, 547
        schwannoma 543, 544
Castleman's disease 485, 586f, 587f, 603, 604

Catheter angiography of angiofibroma 221*f*
Cat-scratch disease 477
Causes of
    cervical lymphadenopathy 488
    neural-perineural enhancement 419*t*
    reactive lymphadenopathy 480
Cavernous
    hemangioma 109, 111*f*
    sinus 135, 398, 411*f*, 412*f*, 418*f*
        thrombosis 104, 105*f*
Cerebrospinal fluid 89
Cervical
    lymph node 421, 424
        classifications 424
        staging 489
    lymphadenopathy 470, 481
    nodal calcifications 464
    node 422
    septic thrombophlebitis 583
    venolymphatic vascular malformation 562*f*
Chiasm glioma 137
Choanal atresia 226
Cholesterol granuloma 59, 60*f*
Chondrosarcoma 605
    of larynx 526*f*, 528*f*
Chordoma 605
Chronic
    autoimmune lymphocytic thyroiditis 620
    denervation 278*f*
    invasive fungal sinusitis 194
    lymphocytic leukemia 114
    myelogenous leukemia 114
    odontogenic sinusitis 179*f*
    otomastoiditis 56
    rhinosinusitis 162, 171, 177, 178, 181
    sinus disease 8*f*
    sinusitis 204*f*

Classification of cervical lymph nodes 424, 442*t*
Cobalt-60 unit 643
Cochlea 20*f*, 21*f*, 35*f*
Cochlear
    aperture 23*f*, 32*f*
    division of vestibulocochlear nerve 27*f*
    modiolus 32*f*
    otosclerosis 71*f*
    promontory 20*f*
Collect-Sicard syndrome 595
Coloboma 95
Comet tail 11*f*
    appearance 11*f*
    ring 11
Common carotid artery 521*f*
Complex temporal bone fracture 79*f*
Conal tissues 135
Concha bullosa of left middle turbinate 164*f*
Cone-beam computed tomography 657*f*
Congenital
    absence 361
    anomalies 37, 48, 64, 68, 92
    cholesteatoma 50
    disorders 223
    epithelial inclusion 330
    frontonasal masses 223
Consequence of peritonsillar abscess 263*f*
Coxsackie viruses 363
Cranial
    nerves 86
    neuro-schistosomiasis 419
Cricoid cartilage 529*f*, 530*f*
Cricothyroids 513
Crista galli 147*f*
*Cryptococcus neoformans* 419
Cutaneous malignancy 397
Cytomegalovirus infection 104

## D

Dacryoadenitis 122
Dentigerous cyst 269f, 323f
Dermatopathic lymphadenopathy 484
Dermoid
    and epidermoid cysts 96
    cysts 330
Desmoplastic melanoma 397
Development of parotid glands 355
Diffuse interstitial skeletal hyperostosis 351
Digital
    subtracted angiogram 112f
    subtraction sialography 359, 362
Dilatation of vestibular aqueduct 72f
Direct spread of malignancy 547, 554
Diseases of
    nasopharynx 229, 231
    parotid gland 355
    thyroid gland 610
Dose volume histogram 655f
Drainage pathways of paranasal sinuses 144
Duct laceration 369

## E

Electronic portal imaging device 655
Embryology of auricle 16f
Endotracheal enchondroma 526f
Eosinophilic mucus 183
Epithelial tumors of lacrimal gland 121f
Epitympanum 20f
Epstein-Barr virus 363
*Escherichia coli* 364
Esophageal carcinoma 12f
Esophagus 13
Esthesioneuroblastoma 213, 214f, 605
Ethmoid air cells 145, 147f, 148f
Ethmoidal bone 87f

External
    auditory canal 16, 30f
    atresia 37
    ear 16, 37
Extraosseus chordoma 251
Extraocular muscles 90f

## F

Facial
    nerve 25, 26f, 27f, 35f, 63, 399f, 402, 415f
        hemangioma 67
    node 428
    recess 19f
    venous dilations 571
False maxillofacial vascular malformations 570
Fetal alcohol syndrome 379
Fibromuscular dysplasia 534, 536, 579
Fibro-osseous lesions 220
Fibrous dysplasia 222
Fine needle aspiration 370
First branchial cleft cyst 360
Floor of mouth 306
    abscess 311f
    carcinoma 315
Fluorodeoxyglucose positron emission tomography 615
Focus of nodular internal enhancement 491f
Foramen
    ovale 276f, 400f
    rotundum 400f, 409f
Foramina 88f
Foreign body lymphadenopathies 488
Frontal
    recess 160f
    sinuses 145, 147f
    sinusitis 172f
Frontoethmoidal encephaloceles 226
Functional endoscopic sinus surgery 161

Fungal
    and protozoan lymphadenitis 480
    balls 191
    sinusitis 191
*Fusobacterium necrophorum* 537, 583, 584

## G

Giant cell 533
Glandular parenchyma 621*f*
Glomus
    jugulare 296*f*
        tumor 542, 543*f*
    jugulotympanicum 61*f*, 62*f*
        tumor 542
    tumors 61, 295
    tympanicum 62*f*, 63*f*, 296
    vagale 297*f*, 298*f*
        tumor 297, 541, 541*f*, 542*f*
Granulomatosis 419
Granulomatous
    diseases 196*f*
    sinusitis 196
Graves'
    disease 619, 620*f*, 621*f*
    dysthyroid ophthalmopathy 126
Greater
    and lesser palatine foramina 409
    superficial petrosal nerve 318, 402, 405, 406, 414*f*
Gross tumor volume 649

## H

Hairpin turn of facial nerve 28*f*
Haller cells 166*f*
Hard palate 308, 318
Hashimoto's thyroiditis 620, 621*f*, 622*f*
Haversian bone 71
Healing stage of labyrinthitis 75*f*
Hemangioma 137, 251, 419
Hemangiopericytoma 112, 137, 601
Hematological malignancies 112
*Hemophilus influenzae* 364
Herpes zoster ophthalmicus 102
Hiatus semilunaris 165*f*
High flow vascular malformations 566
Highly active antiretroviral therapy 603
HIV related lymphadenopathy 473*f*
Hodgkin's
    disease 604
    lymphoma 501*f*
Honeycomb bony appearance 67
Horizontal semicircular canal 23*f*, 26*f*, 28*f*, 33*f*-35*f*
Horner's syndrome 295, 535, 572, 573*f*
Human
    immunodeficiency virus 376
        infection 471
    papilloma virus 526
Hyoid bone 444*f*, 530*f*
Hyperplastic adenoid 233
Hypervascular
    lymphadenopathies 603
    metastasis 605
    tumor 606*f*
Hypoglossal
    nerve 403
    palsy 295
Hypopharynx 13, 505, 516, 519
Hypoplasia 361
Hypotympanum 20*f*

## I

Iatrogenic
    arterial dissection 575*f*
    pseudoaneurysm 577*f*
Idiopathic
    carotiditis 533, 534*f*
    facial vascular dilations 571
    hypertrophic cranial pachymeningitis 419
    orbital inflammatory disease 113, 122, 123*f*

Incus
    body 19f-22f
    lenticular process 21f
    long process 19f
    short process 19f
Infantile hemangiomas 584
Infectious mononucleosis 473
Inferior
    alveolar nerve canal 413f
    oblique muscle 91f
    orbital
        canal 151f
        fissure 150, 409
Infiltrative squamous carcinoma 320f
Inflammatory
    diseases 171
        of orbit 122
    myositis 263f, 264f
    nodes 449
    pseudotumor 251
Infraorbital
    foramen 88f
    nerve 416f
Infratentorial subdural abscesses 178f
Infrazygomatic
    mastication 260f
    masticator space 259f
    temporalis muscles 260
Injection of internal maxillary artery 221f
Inner ear 25, 68
Innervation of larynx and hypopharynx 518
Intensity modulated radiotherapy 645, 652
Internal
    auditory canal 21f, 28f, 33f, 35f
    carotid artery 20f, 170f, 533f, 541f
    jugular vein 445f, 521f
        thrombosis 537, 552f
    nodal
        architecture and homogeneity 458
        heterogeneity 459f, 461f, 462f
Intracranial
    complications of sinusitis 177f
    extension of
        *Aspergillus* sinusitis 195f
        diseases 13
    vascular lesions 571
Intraocular
    detachments 133
    hemorrhage 134f
    tumors 117
Intrinsic laryngeal
    muscles 513t
    musculature 513
Invasive fungal sinusitis 192
Inverted papilloma 215, 217f

# J

Jacobson's nerve 296
Jugular
    bulb 20f
        dehiscence 49
    paragangliomas 595
    tubercle 404f
    vein 584f
Jugulo-omohyoid node, 436
Jugulotympanic paraganglioma 598f
Juvenile
    angiofibroma 234, 238f
    nasal angiofibroma 591

# K

Kaposi's sarcoma 251, 463, 472, 502, 602
Kaposiform hemangioendothelioma 588

Kasabach-Merritt syndrome 588
Kawasaki's syndrome 487
Keratosis obturans 38, 39*f*
Kikuchi
	disease 464, 483*f*
	Fujimoto disease 481, 482
Kimura's disease 464, 481
Kissing carotids 532
Klippel-Trenaunay-Weber syndrome 588
Koerner's septum 23*f*, 56

# L

Labyrinthine
	ossificans 74
	segment of facial nerve 28*f*
Labyrinthitis 73
Lacrimal
	apparatus 118
	bone 87*f*
	gland 135, 91*f*
Lamina papyracea 87*f*
Langerhan's cell 501
	histiocytosis 125, 126*f*
Large
	and medium vessel arteritis 581
	artery vasculitis 533
	vascular tumor blush 221*f*
	vestibular aqueduct syndrome 72
Laryngeal
	cartilages 509
	hemangioma 587*f*
	papillomatosis 526, 527*f*, 528*f*
	paragangliomas 595
Laryngocele 520
Larynx 13, 505, 509, 519
Lateral
	cervical nodes 431
	cricoarytenoid 513
	nasal wall 143*f*
	pterygoid muscle 265*f*
	wall of nasal cavity 142

Left
	internal carotid artery dissection 535*f*
	maxillary sinus mucocele 189*f*
Lemierre's syndrome 476, 538*f*, 583, 584*f*
Lenticular process of incus 19*f*
Leprosy 239
Lethal damage 640
Letterer-Siwe disease 502
Leukemia 114
Linear accelerator 643, 644*f*
Lingual thyroid 618
Lip carcinoma 313
Lipoma 251
Liposarcoma 251
Long process of incus 23*f*
Longitudinal intrinsic muscle of tongue 304*f*
Low flow vascular malformations 561
Lung metastasis 119*f*
Lyme disease 419
Lymph node 423
	classification 425, 436
	drainage 519
	inclusions 488
Lymphadenopathy 13, 546, 552
Lymphangioma 381*f*
Lymphatic malformations 379
Lymphoepithelial cysts 473*f*
Lymphoid hyperplasia 233
Lymphoma 112, 137, 247, 387, 605, 631
Lymphoproliferative disorders 498

# M

Macrophthalmia 94
Maffucci syndrome 526, 526*f*, 527*f*
Maintenance of airway 505
Major salivary gland tumor 397
Malignant
	lesions 212
	melanoma 134

meningioma 605
neoplasms 115, 382, 624
otitis externa 44f, 557f
peripheral nerve sheath tumors 106
tumors 301
Malleolar head 19f, 22f, 32f
Malleus
anterior process 19f
lateral process 19f
Mandibular schwannoma 275f
Mantle cell lymphoma 347f
Manubrium of malleus 19f, 20f, 22f
Marfan syndrome 534
Masseter muscles 260f
Massive lymphadenopathy 482
Masticator space 257, 259–261
muscle denervation 277f
Mastoid
nodes 427
segment of facial nerve 29f, 30f, 31, 31f
Maxillary sinus 145, 158f
Maximal longitudinal diameter 453
Meckel's cave 275f, 276f, 398, 412f
Medial pterygoid 260f
Medialization thyroplasty 523
Medullary
carcinoma 629
thyroid
cancer 493f
carcinoma metastasis 547f
Melanoma 212
Menigoencephalocele 251
Meningioma 78, 107, 419
Merkel cell
carcinoma 492
skin carcinoma 491f
Metastasis of orbit 118
Metastatic
disease 388
jugular chain nodal disease 627f

lymph nodes 489
nodal disease 2f
thyroid carcinoma 493
Microphthalmia 93
Middle ear 18, 48
ossicles 19f
Mild hyperattenuation of thyroid lobes 616f
Minimum axial diameter 453
Minor salivary gland tumor 251
Mondini's malformation 68
Motor paralysis of cranial nerves 595
Mucoepidermoid carcinoma 120, 382, 385f
Mucosa-associated lymphoid tissue 112, 423, 631
Mucosal
malignancy 397
primary neoplasm 397
surfaces of endolarynx 513
Mucous retention cyst 187, 188f
Multileaf collimators 645
Multinodular goiter 554
Multiple
enchondromas 527f
endocrine neoplasia 630
lytic foci 527f
necrotic lymph nodes 2f
parotid lymphoepithelial cysts 473f
Muscles
of mastication 262
regulating tension in vocal ligaments 513
varying rima glottidis 513
Mycobacterial lymphadenitis 478
*Mycobacterium*
*avium*-intracellulare 479
*kansasii* 479
*scrofulaceum* 479
*tuberculosis* 480

## N

Nasal
    dermal sinus 224
    gliomas 226
    polyposis 183
Nasoethmoidal patterns of spread 199*f*
Nasolacrimal
    drainage system 135
    duct 150*f*
Naso-orbital fractures 130
Nasopharyngeal
    angiofibroma 591
    carcinoma 6*f*, 235*f*, 240, 243*f*, 293*f*, 300*f*, 466*f*, 553*f*
        staging 247, 248*t*
    cysts 231
    disorders 251
    encephalocele 251
    lymphoma 249*f*
    tuberculosis 237
Nasopharyngitis 231
Nasopharynx 13, 229, 230, 346, 605
Neck hemangiopericytoma 602*f*
Neoplastic
    causes of cervical lymphadenopathy 489
    nodal pathology 454
Nerve 406
    sheath
        neoplasms 543
        tumors 380, 419
Neural tumors of orbit 105
Neurofibroma 545
Neurogenic lesions 273
Neurovascular bundle 346
Nodal
    calcification 464
        in tuberculosis 464*f*
    chain classification 440
    enhancement 463
    neoplasms 502
Node size 454
Nodes 427-434
    of Rouviere 549
Non-Hodgkin's lymphoma 247, 347*f*, 500*f*, 501*f*
Noninvasive fungal sinusitis 191
Nonmelanoma skin cancers 497*f*
Nonoptic pathway neoplastic lymphoma/leukemia, metastases 137
Nonspecific
    inflammation 137
    inflammatory sialadenitis 367*f*
Noonan's syndrome 379
Normal
    appearance of anterior commissure 525*f*
    lymph node 10*f*
    nodes 449
    thyroid gland 611*f*
Nuclear medicine 359, 614

## O

Occipital nodes 427
Ocular
    infections 104
    melanoma 117
Odontogenic tumor 269
Olfactory
    fossa 167*f*
    neuroblastoma 213
Oncocytic neoplasms 377
Onodi air cell 159*f*, 169*f*
Ophthalmic
    artery 592
    vein 176*f*
Ophthalmoplegic migraine 419
Optic
    canal 88*f*, 89*f*
    glioma 106*f*
    nerve 137, 148*f*, 159*f*
        canal 148*f*, 156*f*

glioma 105
insertion 135f
sheath complex 135, 137
sheath meningioma 107, 137
neuritis 126, 127f, 137
pathway 89f
Oral
cavity 302
tongue 306, 316
Orbit 13, 86
apex and foramina 135
walls 135
Orbital
abscesses 101
cellulitis 174f
complications 173
infections 98, 102
invasion 208
neoplasms 105
pseudotumor 122
walls 87f
Organization of compartmentalizing orbit 134
Oropharynx 13, 333
Orthovoltage therapy 643
Osteogenesis imperfecta 534
Osteogenic sarcoma 605
Osteoma 41, 221f
Osteonecrosis of jaw 270, 272
Osteosarcoma 205f, 270
of mandible 271f
Otitis externa 41
Otosclerosis 69, 70f
Ox eye 95

## P

Panophthalmitis 103f
Papillary thyroid
cancer 491f, 492f
carcinoma 11f
Paradoxical middle turbinates 165f
Paragangliomas 539, 594

Paranasal sinuses 135, 142
Parapharyngeal space 257, 279-282
schwannoma 291f
Paravertebral
abscess 557f
leukemic mass 559f
space 555
Parotid
acinic cell carcinoma 291f
duct 306, 356
gland 388
hemangioma 586f
laceration 369
masses 473f
nodes 427
pleomorphic adenoma 290f
tumor 66f
Patterns of
parapharyngeal fat displacement 284
tumor spread 199
Periapical cyst 268f
Perineural
disease 275f
in head and neck 394
extension of disease 411f
spread 394, 410t
of diseases 13
of tumor 65
tumor spread 211
Perioptic tissues 135
Peripheral nerve sheath tumors 106, 605
Perivertebral
abscess 556
space 555
Persistent
generalized adenopathy 472
hyaloid artery 94f
hyperplastic primary vitreous 93
Petrous apex 33f
Peyer's patches 424

Pharyngeal canal 409
Planning target volume 649
Planum sphenoidale 155*f*
Plasma cell tumors 114
Plasmacytoma 115*f*, 272*f*
Pleomorphic adenoma 121*f*, 289*f*, 370
Posterior
    cricoarytenoid 513
    semicircular canal 23*f*, 32*f*
    stapes crura 19*f*
Postinfectious and demyelination disorders 419
Postradiation
    mucositis 251
    neuritis 419
Postseptal cellulitis 98, 100*f*
Post-transplantation lymphoproliferative disorders 499
Potentially lethal damage 640
Potts puffy tumor 173*f*
Preseptal
    cellulitis 98, 99*f*, 136
    tissues and orbital septum 134
Prestyloid parapharyngeal space 283
Prevertebral
    muscles 346
    space 555
Primary
    imaging modality 13
    lymphoma 631
    Sjögren's syndrome 364
    spine bone tumors 605
    tumor 324, 383
Proliferative histiocytic disorders 501
Prominent tonsillar crypts 339*f*
Protection against aspiration 505
Prussak's space 56, 21*f*
*Pseudomonas aeruginosa* 46
Pterygoid plates 151*f*, 152*f*
Pterygomaxillary fissure 158*f*, 409
Pterygopalatine fossa 150*f*, 151, 159*f*, 218*f*, 405, 407, 407*f*, 411*f*, 413*f*, 414*f*, 416*f*
Puffed cheek technique 3*f*
Pyogenic sialadenitis 363
Pyramidal eminence 19*f*
Pyriform sinus
    contours 529*f*
    perforation 529, 529*f*

## R

Radiation
    dose distribution 652*f*
    induced sialadenitis 368
    osteitis 46
Radicular cyst 268*f*
Radiographic anatomy and pathology of oral cavity 302
Radionecrosis of mandible 273*f*
Ranula of left sublingual space 329*f*
Reactive or inflammatory nodes 449
Recurrent
    adenoid cystic carcinoma 412*f*
    papillary thyroid cancer 465*f*
Regional lymph node 248, 325, 338, 383
    metastasis 496
Reichert's cartilage 16
Renal cell carcinoma 493*f*
Residual thyroid carcinoma 629*f*
Retention cysts 231
Retinal detachment 135
Retinoblastoma 116
Retrobulbar
    intraconal tissues 135
    orbit 134, 137
    space 118*f*
Retromolar trigone 318
Retropharyngeal
    abscess 549, 551*f*
    carotid arteries 532, 533*f*
    edema 552*f*
    intranodal abscess 550*f*
    lymphadenopathy 553*f*
    nodes 428
    space 548

Retrostyloid parapharyngeal space 294
Rhabdomyosarcoma 115, 116f, 251, 605
Rhinocerebral
   mucormycosis 419
Right
   hypoglossal canal and nerve 404f
   inferior orbital foramen 88f
   internal carotid artery dissection 536f
   superior orbital foramen 88f
Rosai-Dorfman disease 484f, 501
Round window niche 31f
Routes of
   drainage of nodes 427-434
   perineural spread 397t
Routine suppurative lymphadenitis 475
Rouvière classification of cervical nodes 434t

## S

Salivary gland
   and ducts 13
      epithelial malignancies 382
   tumors 605
Sarcoidosis 124, 367, 484
Schwann cells 543
Schwannoma 137
   of carotid space 545f
Schwartze's sign 71
Scrofula 464f, 479f
Scutum 20f, 21f
Secondary
   Sjögren's syndrome 365
   tumor 265f
Septic cervical thrombophlebitis 584f
Sequencing of multileaf collimators 653f
Severe pharyngitis 452f
Sialocele 369
Sialolithiasis 361
Sialosis 368
Silent sinus syndrome 190
Simplified nodal classification 519t
Sinochoanal polyp 185
Sinonasal
   cavities 13
   tumors 198
   undifferentiated carcinoma 214
Sinus
   histiocytosis 482
   pericranii 570
   tympani 19f, 31f
Sjögren's
   disease 377
   syndrome 125, 364, 365, 366f, 387
Skull base 346
Soap-bubble cystic lesion 269
Sphenoethmoid recess 155f, 156f, 160f, 187f
Sphenoid
   body 227f
   meningocele 227f
   ostium 160f, 187f
   sinus 146, 148f, 157f, 159f, 161f, 169f, 230f
      secretions 180f
Sphenopalatine foramen 156f, 218f, 409
Spinal nerves 405
Squamous cell carcinoma 5f, 48, 212, 312, 340f, 343f, 469f, 507, 519, 521f
   of oral
      cavity 7f
      tongue 9f
   of posterior oropharyngeal wall 345f
   of sinonasal cavity 8f
   of tongue 460f

Stapes
    anterior
        crura 21*f*
        crus 23*f*
    capitellum 19*f*
    footplate 19*f*
    posterior crus 23*f*
*Staphylococcus aureus* 364, 476, 556
Staphyloma 95
Stensen's duct 306, 356, 360
Sternocleidomastoid muscle 445*f*, 451*f*, 452, 467*f*
*Streptococcus*
    *pneumoniae* 364
    *pyogenes* 364, 476
    *viridans* 364
Subglottic
    larynx 516*f*
    stenosis 524
Sublethal damage 640
Sublingual nodes 429
Submandibular
    gland 444, 444*f*, 445*f*, 451*f*, 452*f*
    nodes 429
Submental nodes 429
Superficial layer of deep cervical fascia 259*f*, 260*f*, 261*f*
Superior
    oblique muscle 91*f*
    ophthalmic vein 93*f*, 176*f*
    orbital fissure 88*f*
    semicircular canal 34*f*
    sphenoid sinus 187*f*
Supraglottic larynx 515*f*
Supra-zygomatic temporalis muscles 260
Sympathetic chain neurofibroma 546*f*
Syphilis 239

## T

Takayasu's arteritis 533, 583*f*
Tegmen tympani 21*f*, 76*f*
Temporal
    arteritis 533, 581
    bone 13, 15, 16
        pathology 37
Temporomandibular joint 80*t*, 406
Tenon's capsule 90
Tensor vascular styloid fascia 280*f*
Teratoma 251
Thyroglossal duct anomalies 617
Thyroid
    associated orbitopathy 126
    carcinoma 625
    cartilage 529*f*, 530*f*
    goiter 623
    nodules 13
    orbitopathy 126
Tolosa-Hunt syndrome 123, 123*f*, 419
Tongue
    carcinoma 299*f*
    denervation 299*f*, 328*f*
    musculature 304*f*
    squamous cell carcinoma 459*f*
Tonsillar carcinoma 293*f*
Tornwaldt cysts 233, 253
Tracheal enchondroma 526, 526*f*
Transverse
    arytenoid 513
    intrinsic muscle of tongue 304*f*
    thyroid ultrasound 11*f*
Trauma 13, 79, 369
    of orbit 129
Traumatic
    aneurysms 573
    AV fistula 576
    dissections 572
Traumatic vascular lesions 572
Trigeminal nerve 399*f*, 405
Tripod fracture 131*f*
Tuberculous
    cervical lymphadenitis 479*f*
    lymphadenopathy 464*f*

Tumor 287, 295, 337
    of external auditory canal 47
    reactive lymphadenopathy 488
Turner's syndrome 379
Tympanic
    paragangliomas 595
    segment of facial nerve 21*f*, 29*f*
Types of
    radiation 634
    tumors 395
Typical
    appearances of nasopharyngeal carcinoma 243*f*
    molar tooth appearance of incus and malleus 31*f*
    of nasopharyngeal carcinoma 242*f*

## U

Ultra small iron oxide particles 470
Upper parapharyngeal space 346

## V

Vagal
    paraganglioma 595, 599*f*
    schwannomas 297
Vagus nerve schwannoma 544*f*
Valsalva maneuver 564
Vascular
    diseases 533, 579
    lesions of head and neck 560
    malformations 310, 378, 560
    tumor 584
        of orbit 109
Vascularized malignant tumors 605*t*
Vein of Galen 579
Venolymphatic
    malformations 561
    vascular malformation 563*f*
Venous
    thrombosis 137
    vascular malformation 310*f*, 563, 566*f*, 585
Vernet syndrome 595
Vertebral erosions 346
Vertebrovenous AVF 580*f*
Vestibular
    aqueduct 35*f*
    division of vestibulocochlear nerve 27*f*
    schwannoma 76
Vestibulocochlear nerve 26*f*, 35*f*
Vidian
    canal 409
    nerve 405, 406
Viral
    infections 475
    lymphadenitis 471
    sialadenitis 363
Vocal cord paralysis 520, 523*f*

## W

Waldeyer's ring 247, 262, 345, 473*f*
    structures 422, 500
Warthin's tumors 359, 371, 375
Wegener's granulomatosis 124, 124*f*, 137, 196, 196*f*, 239, 479, 524, 525*f*

## X

X-ray esophagram 12

## Z

Zygomatic arch 130, 258
Zygomaticomaxillary
    complex 130
    fractures 129